Physiotherapy in Paediatrics

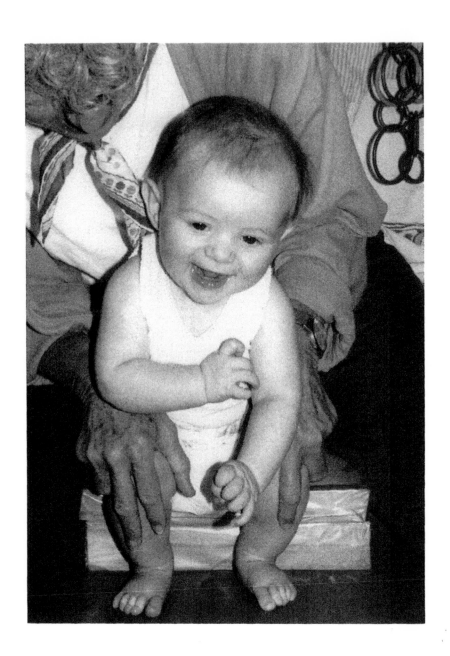

Physiotherapy in Paediatrics

Third edition

Roberta B. Shepherd, Ed. D., M.A. (Columbia), Dip. Phty.

Fellow of the Australian College of Physiotherapists
Foundation Professor of Physiotherapy,
Faculty of Health Science, The University of Sydney, Australia

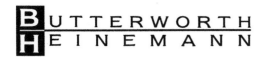

Butterworth-Heinemann
An imprint of Elsevier Science Limited

First published 1974
Second edition 1980
Third edition 1995
Reprinted 1997, 1998, 1999, 2000, 2002
Transferred to digital printing 2005

British Library Cataloguing in Publication Data
Shepherd, Roberta B.
  Physiotherapy in Paediatrics. – 3Rev.ed
  I. Title
  618.920062

ISBN 0 7506 0620 7

Library of Congress Cataloging in Publication Data
Shepherd, Roberta B.
  Physiotherapy in paediatrics/Roberta B. Shepherd. – 3rd ed.
  p. cm.
  Includes bibliographical references and index.
  ISBN 0 7506 0620 7
  1. Physical therapy for children. I. Title.
  [DNLM: 1. Physical Therapy – in infancy & childhood. WB 460 S548p]
  RJ53.P5S48
  615.82–dc20

94–3907
CIP

Printed and bound by Antony Rowe Ltd, Eastbourne

To my parents
for their encouragement and generosity

Just a little more
And we shall see the almond trees in blossom
The marbles shining in the sun
The sea, the curling waves.

Just a little more
Let us rise just a little higher

George Seferis (transl. Rex Warner)*

*Quoted from George Seferis, *Poems*, by kind permission of The Bodley Head

Contents

Preface   ix

Preface to the first edition   xi

Acknowledgements   xii

Section I: Introduction to paediatrics
1   The child, the parents and the
    physiotherapist   3
2   The development of movement
    and skill   9
3   Training motor control and optimizing
    motor learning   43

Section II: Neurological disorders
4   Maturational, pathophysiological and
    recovery processes in the CNS   91
5   Cerebral palsy   110
6   Acute brain injury   145
7   Minimal brain dysfunction: learning
    disability, attention deficit disorder,
    clumsiness   154
8   Mental retardation: cognitive
    impairment and developmental delay   165
9   Infections of the nervous system   185
10 Brachial plexus lesions in infancy   196

Section III: Congenital abnormalities
11 Talipes equinovarus   207
12 Talipes calcaneovalgus   224
13 Congenital dislocation of the hip   228
14 Arthrogryposis multiplex congenita   235
15 Spina bifida   238
16 Congenital limb deficiencies   261

**Section IV: Disorders of bones, joints, muscles
and skin**
17 Introduction   275
18 Muscle disorders (myopathies)   280
19 Torticollis   293
20 Structural scoliosis   303
21 Inflammatory disorders of soft
    tissues and joints   311
22 Burns in childhood   322

Section V: Disorders of the respiratory system
23 Introduction   335
24 The development and mechanics of
    respiration   338
25 Respiratory disorders in the neonatal
    period and infancy   344
26 Respiratory disorders in childhood   350
27 Physical evaluation and treatment   363

Appendices
1   Tests for reflexive and prefunctional
    activity   387
2   Guide to developmental assessment
    of the infant   393
3   The blind infant   397

Index   399

Preface

Physiotherapy as a clinical science is in a process of continual evolution, new clinical practices being developed out of relevant findings from scientific and clinical investigations. New theoretical perspectives and data-based findings are providing considerable challenge to paediatric physiotherapy, requiring a rethinking of traditional methods of practice and the ability to function with the flexibility needed to keep abreast of new developments. If physiotherapists are to take up the exciting challenges ahead, it will be mandatory for physiotherapy education to be updated to include a rigorous and relevant scientific preparation for clinical practice.

The impact of new scientific developments is particularly obvious in the area of human movement, its development and control. The last two decades have seen a substantial increase in the number of investigations into normal movement, motor development, muscle adaptability, how humans acquire skill in movement and the effects of environmental factors on movement control. In addition, there is now a greater understanding of the pathological mechanisms underlying motor dyscontrol and about the motor performance deficits associated with different lesions.

In the face of these new research findings, physiotherapy for movement-disabled individuals is in the process of changing from therapeutic approaches developed 30–40 years ago to a science-based approach. The importation into physiotherapy of knowledge gained in sciences outside physiotherapy now enables clinical practice to be built on a framework of scientific theories and data from studies of both able-bodied and disabled subjects.

In preparing this new edition, the author has set out to illustrate the clinical relevance of some recent scientific developments and, by including expanded reference and reading lists, provide some guidance to additional reading for the student of paediatric physiotherapy. New chapters have been written on motor development and the acquisition of skill, and on the maturational, dyscontrol and recovery processes associated with neural lesions. Based on the work done for many years by the author in collaboration with J.H. Carr, a new chapter on training motor control and optimizing motor learning in infants and children with movement disability has also been written for this edition (Chapter 3). The objective of this chapter is to illustrate how the physiotherapist can derive clinical implications from scientific research into human movement and generate methods of training movement control in infants and children. The reader will need to refer to this chapter when reading the chapters related to movement disability resulting from lesions of the neuromusculoskeletal system.

A greater understanding of the need to measure outcome, together with recent developments in technology, are stimulating research into the effects of physiotherapy. Recent advances in knowledge and technology also mean that the scientifically educated physiotherapist is in an excellent position to contribute to the investigation of movement control and dyscontrol. The systematic measurement of motor performance in disabled infants and children and the generating and testing of hypotheses related to clinical practice are critical endeavours both to increase the knowledge base on human movement and to optimize the functional abilities of disabled children.

Preface to the first edition

This book has been written for undergraduates as a guide to physical treatment in the field of paediatrics. I hope they will study in greater detail the subjects which interest them, and that they will have as teachers people who will demonstrate the use of practical techniques in the actual treatment of patients, something which a textbook can never do.

I have concentrated on relating pathology, anatomy and physiology to the problems found in sick and disabled children, suggesting the rationale for physical treatment. Actual techniques for treatment are outlined only briefly, in the belief that the acquisition of wisdom is not the collection of recipes for all occasions but the development of an understanding which makes possible an intelligent and imaginative planning of treatment for each particular patient. I hope the book will stimulate students to question many established practices in physiotherapy, and to seek out new and more effective methods of treatment.

I gratefully acknowledge the advice and encouragement given to me by friends and teachers, especially by Professor James McLeod, Drs Janet McCredie, Corrie Reye and Edward Bates, and Mrs Berta Bobath, Miss Nancie Finnie, Miss Janet Clarke, Miss Jennifer Harrison and Miss Janet Carr. To the latter I owe particular thanks for the patience with which she read and re-read the manuscript in its various forms, and for the kindness with which she gave praise and criticism where they were most needed. The Council of the New South Wales branch of the Australian Physiotherapy Association and the Director of the School of Physiotherapy, Miss Jeanette Salmon, were generous in giving me study leave.

I would also like to thank Mrs Penny Eamer, medical artist, for the drawings and diagrams, and the Departments of Photography of the Royal Alexandra Hospital for Children and the Royal Prince Alfred Hospital for their help. Finally, I must thank the parents of the children whose photographs appear on these pages.

Acknowledgements

The author wishes to acknowledge the assistance given by many colleagues, and to thank in particular Dr Janet Carr for her collaborative work over many years, and Dr Elizabeth Ellis, Jenny Alison, Louise Ada, Dr Nick O'Dwyer and Dr Mary Westbrook for valuable comments and suggestions on particular chapters. Many other colleagues and students also generously gave their time in stimulating discussions during the writing of the book. Thanks are due to David Robinson who so skilfully and patiently took many of the new photographs for this new edition, and to the children and parents who agreed to participate in this intellectual adventure.

Section I

Introduction to paediatrics

1   The child, the parents and the physiotherapist
2   The development of movement and skill
3   Training motor control and optimizing motor learning

1

The child, the parents and the physiotherapist

The child is not a miniature adult. The period of development into a fully integrated human being which begins with the embryo does not cease until growth is complete. Development itself continues throughout life as we learn and adapt. In the physical sense, development does not merely mean that the child grows larger but also that components change and adapt according to genetically determined maturational processes as well as to the infant's experiences and the demands of the environment.

The infant's central nervous system is not fully developed at birth, and the acquisition of motor control and skill follows upon a progressive change in the nervous system. Nerve fibres grow, new connections between nerve cells are made and neurotransmitters become operative. Brain growth is characterized by changes in synaptic connections, with functional connections apparently depending upon stimulation and use. Although the child cannot be expected to achieve skills in advance of neural development, practice and opportunity to interact effectively with the environment may be critical influences on neuromuscular development.

Similarly, the infant's respiratory system is not fully developed at birth. Further structural development, including an increase in the number of terminal airways as well as an increase in their relative size, must occur before optimal adult respiratory function is acquired. These considerable changes which occur with growth and development must be taken into account in

order that respiratory physiotherapy can be appropriate to infant and child and not merely reflect treatment principles and practices developed for the adult.

The effect of the environment on the child appears to be critical. It is generally considered that a child's emotional development may be impeded by a lack of parental warmth and affection, but the child's physical development may also be retarded or deformed by many factors during growth and development. Retention of secretions within the lungs of an infant may have a more disabling effect upon ventilatory function than in an adult because damage to immature structures may prevent their normal development or differentiation. Abnormal posturing resulting from muscle imbalance and length-associated changes in soft tissues may cause maldevelopment of bone in growing children which could result in more severe and disabling deformity than a similar muscle imbalance in adult life. Bones develop and are shaped and influenced to some extent by the stresses put upon them. If these stresses are abnormal, skeletal development may also be abnormal.

Since interactions with the environment and functional interactions between body segments must affect growth and development, early physiotherapy intervention in infants with neuromuscular dysfunction is probably critical. Bony deformity due to abnormal stresses put on growing bones by inextensible soft tissues may be avoided by intervention designed to maintain muscle length. An inability to take weight through the feet in order to stand up or to take steps may be avoided if calf muscle length is maintained and these actions are practised from early infancy. The ability to make functional neuronal connections may be optimized by practice (i.e. experience) of functionally relevant actions.

Knowledge of the nature of development will help the adult to understand and accept the child; to understand that the child's behaviour is to some extent the result of physical, cognitive, emotional and social immaturity. A small child may not be able to sit still when asked to do so. The child cannot always conform to social and environmental pressures as can an adult.

A child's potential for growth and development appears to depend upon the presence of caring adults and a challenging environment. A child who must stay in a hospital or other institution for a long period may be deprived of both close human warmth and challenge, and may as a result demonstrate developmental retardation. The effects of separation of a child from the mother have been documented by many authors (e.g. Bowlby 1953; Winnicott 1964). The age at which a child is most likely to suffer from separation is said to be between 6 and 9 months and the effects are particularly evident if the infant has had a close and loving relationship with the mother (Bowlby 1953). An infant may demonstrate the effect of deprivation by becoming quiet, by moving and vocalizing less, by failing to respond to the overtures of an adult and by seeming withdrawn. Motor development may also be affected and the infant may develop more slowly compared to peers. A substitute parent who is personally responsible for the child while in the institution may modify some of these effects in an infant under 1 year of age, but a 2- or 3-year-old may reject the substitute, refuse to be comforted, refuse to eat, cry inconsolably, and eventually become apathetic and start bed-wetting and thumb-sucking. Bowlby (1953) suggested that at this age a violent reaction to another adult is a healthy reaction, and a quiet resigned attitude a sign of unhealthy emotional development. Between 3 and 5 years the child is beginning to grasp the idea that parents will return in the future, and this probably helps the child cope emotionally with the separation. An older child may still suffer considerable anxiety, worrying that the stay in hospital may be a form of punishment.

In an attempt to overcome these problems which it is thought may result in serious emotional difficulties in both childhood and adult life, paediatric hospitals allow free visiting for parents and many have facilities for a parent to stay with the child. In addition, hospital stays are limited to day stays where possible and other treatment may be carried out at home. The child in hospital is kept as much as possible in touch with home if the therapist talks about the family and pets and encourages parents to bring in a favourite toy. The child treated in the therapist's rooms may need to be given time to adjust to the new surroundings. Furniture can be suited to the child's needs and painted in bright colours. Where possible, visits to the physiotherapist are kept to a minimum with parents supervising a programme at home, returning to the physiotherapist for further advice. In some cases, a period of intensive treatment may be required with the child attending daily.

A child may also suffer deprivation at home, and may lack 'mothering', that is, a stable figure with whom a bond can be formed (Rendle-Short 1971). A child may suffer physical or emotional abuse, and the health professional should be aware of this possibility if a child presents with multiple bruising or burns, and report it to the child's physician. The abuse of young children by their parents is not uncommon and is more often a manifestation of neurosis or drug-related factors in the parents than of calculated cruelty. The situation can become very serious and the child may die as a result of physical ill-treatment (Rendle-Short 1971; Green 1975).

The disabled child may also experience rejection within the family, and, although rejection may not be overt, the child may suffer emotionally as a result and become attention-seeking, manipulative or destructive. The situation may become serious enough to require psychiatric help. However, most parents of disabled children come to terms with their child's disability and develop a positive approach which communicates itself to the child, giving considerable encouragement and motivation.

A child's development cannot be considered in isolation from the family unit. As a result, the physiotherapist encourages a close involvement of parents and other family members in the child's treatment or motor training. The physiotherapist develops a concern for the family's welfare as it relates to the child's disability and this may consist of advice about caring for a severely disabled infant, or a suitable chair for a child who needs to practise standing up and sitting down at home, methods of bathing or feeding a brain-injured or mentally retarded infant, or providing an understanding ear for a depressed or anxious parent.

Parents should not be bombarded with suggestions for treatment or advice. Therapy or exercise programmes should reflect the family's needs and level of competency. Most parents are able to carry out short periods of treatment, the relevance of which they understand, rather than more lengthy periods or treatment techniques which have little apparent meaning to them. Parents may prefer to write down the home programme themselves as the therapist explains it to them, finding their own notes a better reminder than a printed sheet supplied by the therapist. However, videotapes of normal motor performance or sketches of particular aspects of an action to be practised are usually helpful. Where family and therapist do not speak the same language, an interpreter is necessary to gain information and to describe details of treatment and of the home programme.

The therapist's approach to a child depends to some extent on the child's age. An infant responds to someone who smiles and makes encouraging noises provided the person is close enough to be seen. A small child may prefer to be undressed by a parent than by a stranger. A child may need to be assessed initially on a parent's lap and need not be undressed until more familiar with the new surroundings. In children with movement disabilities, it is preferable to carry out an assessment at home in order to evaluate how the child uses and explores the environment and interacts with the family. Observations can be both structured and unstructured, involving a variety of situations and tasks. The family's strengths and difficulties need to be assessed by observation and interview, and from time to time the therapist should monitor the family's ability to cope and their changing needs as the child grows and develops. It is useful to consider that the major goal of physiotherapy for the movement-disabled child is to train effective motor performance on a number of critical everyday actions.

It is wiser not to talk to a child as though an inferior. Explanations and requests may have to be simplified but conversations can centre on the child's particular interests or on the task of the moment in much the same way as in conversation with an adult. A child may not be able to use language clearly but understanding is probably in advance of speech. Since speech develops by listening, baby-talk is both unnecessary and regressive. Similarly, questions such as 'Would you like to do ...?' are best avoided with very young children since such questions are likely at certain stages to elicit a negative response.

Many adults find it difficult to play with children, and a physiotherapist needs to use skill and imagination to prevent a child from becoming bored with exercises and distracted. To play successfully requires a knowledge of development as well as an understanding of play as a means of learning. Toys should be appropriate to the infant's level of skill and, in infants with movement dysfunction, toys can be selected for their capacity to facilitate the motor performance to be learned.

Knowledge of the development, biomechanics and control of movement assists the therapist in finding ways to elicit the desired motor performance from an infant. For example, extension of the head and trunk may be obtained by moving the infant in the erect or prone position. The scheme of infant gymnastics designed by Neumann-Neurode (1967) and the methods of facilitation evolved by Bobath and Bobath (1964) demonstrate the ease with which specific motor behaviour may be elicited where active cooperation cannot be obtained. For skill to be acquired by the infant and child, however, the motor performance should be linked to some feedback about the success or otherwise of the action, and where possible it is preferable for even small infants to be helped to perform self-initiated and goal-directed actions.

It is the treatment of a child aged 2–4 years which is most likely to strain the tolerance and patience of an adult. Remaining still may be intolerable to a mobile child and attention may flit from one task to another. The therapist can, however, make use of natural curiosity and love of imitation to enable the child to accomplish the necessary objectives.

At 7–8 years most children are more interested in what is happening and become more conscious of themselves in relation to others.

At this stage, the therapist can begin explaining to the child the reasons for treatment or exercise. The older child can begin to take responsibility for part of the exercise programme under parental supervision.

It is usually possible to avoid upsetting or frightening a child if the therapist takes time to allow some adjustment. The therapist can usually anticipate imminent tears and by changing the emphasis of treatment avoid them. If the child does cry it may be better for the therapist to provide consolation in order to avoid a cycle in which every time the child cries he or she is handed back to the parent.

Some situations do constitute a perceived threat to the small child and care should be taken to avoid unnecessary fear. A child who must, for example, have a plaster cast removed may be under considerable strain until the situation has become familiar. A demonstration on an adult's limb that the plaster saw does not cut skin may help. Certainly another adult, and preferably a parent, should be there to provide reassurance. During treatment of a disabled child it is important that therapy is organized to allow the child to achieve some success at the activities being practised. Tools or the environment may be modified to allow a goal to be attained through the child's own efforts. The child's opinion can be sought as to the best way of achieving particular goals and the child should be encouraged to be an active problem-solver. Physiotherapy should be enjoyable and the child should look forward to sessions with the physiotherapist as times of achievement of desirable goals.

Disciplining the child is the responsibility of parents and not the health professional. However, if faced with a 'naughty' child, the therapist could consider the reason behind the behaviour. The child may be uninterested in what is happening and may fidget or run away. A child may misbehave through being too hot, too cold, hungry, thirsty, bored or in pain. The child could be pitting his or her wits against those of the adult or experimenting with a new form of behaviour. It is better to avoid threatening the child or bargaining and instead try to provide a distraction with a change to an activity or environment which is more absorbing. Parents may need to be dissuaded from threatening the child who does not meet their expectations of good behaviour while with the therapist.

When a child is born with severe musculo-skeletal deformities or neurological abnormalities such as arthrogryposis multiplex congenita, limb deficiency or spina bifida, it is a catastrophic event for the parents. As a result, parents may initially experience strong feelings of denial, disappointment, anger, guilt and depression. They move on then to a process of mourning the expected normal infant and this period can last a long time. Not all parents can express these feelings but staff who work with them to assist their infants to develop their optimum abilities should be aware that these feelings exist and if necessary refer parents for psychological help.

The effect of the environment on the development and behaviour of the child is now generally recognized (Sameroff and Chandler 1975; Sameroff 1986; see also Chapter 2). The family forms a critical part of the child's environment and interactions between family members and the child's influence within the family are recognized as important features in a child's overall development.

Involvement of the family as active participants is considered critical to the success of an intervention programme (Bronfenbrenner 1979). Kolobe (1991) reviews the history of parental involvement in intervention directed at children with disabilities. As Kolobe points out, family-focused intervention arises out of a systems and ecological view of family functioning and the child's needs. There are said to be various levels of family involvement in intervention (Simeonsson and Bailey 1990).

Parental involvement is critical to improvement in motor performance, since, for effective motor performance in various tasks to be learned, these actions must be practised. Parents' focus and expectations may need to be changed from one of dependence on the health professional for all active intervention to one in which the emphasis is on the need for the child to be assisted to practise whenever possible with the therapist acting as coach.

Parents of sick or disabled children may face considerable difficulty in coming to terms with the child's illness and require support from all those with whom they come into contact. Families of disabled children have been shown to experience more stress than other families (Kazak 1987; McKinney and Peterson 1987). Coping parents seem to use strategies which include maintaining social support networks and gaining an understanding of the nature of the child's disability and functional capacity (Bernheimer *et al.* 1983; Kolobe 1991). Factors that may contribute to a family's development of the ability to cope have been suggested to include the values and feelings of the family and the relative power of the disabled child within the family (Beavers *et al.* 1986). Parents may be helped by focusing on small gains (Abbot and Meredith 1986). Summers and colleagues (1989) discuss teaching coping skills to parents.

Where the child needs long-term treatment it may be the physiotherapist to whom the child becomes close and who is often the person best placed to understand some of the stresses experienced by child and family. However, the health professionals involved with the family should not add to the parents' stress by giving them conflicting advice and this requires a high level of communication and a consistency of goals among the various members of the health team.

Summary

Growth and development are the key concepts for understanding the behaviour and needs of a child. Since the child is part of a family unit, physiotherapy should be carried out with consideration of the child as part of that unit. In addition, other members of the family may need guidance and support. Growth and development are dependent not only upon genetically determined maturational processes but also on the infant's experiences and possibilities for interaction with the environment. The child's environment is also important for happiness and cooperation. Both infant and child will respond well to calmness and a lack of fuss. Treatment and play are inseparable in the young child, and physiotherapy should enable disabled children to learn about the world and to participate actively in it.

References

Abbot, D.A. and Meredith, W.H. (1986) Strengths of parents with retarded children. *Fam. Rel.*, **35**, 4, 371.

Beavers, J., Hampson, R.B., Hulgus, V.F. and Beavers, R.W. (1986) Coping in families with a retarded child. *Fam. Process*, **25**, 365.

Bernheimer, L.P., Young, M.S. and Winton, P.J. (1983) Stress over time: parents with young handicapped children. *Dev. Behav. Pediatr.* **4**, 3, 177.

Bobath, K. and Bobath, B. (1964) The facilitation of normal postural reactions and movements in the treatment of cerebral palsy. *Physiotherapy*, **50**, 8, 246.

Bowlby, J. (1953) *Child Care and the Growth of Love.* London: Pergamon.

Bronfenbrenner, U. (1979) *The Ecology of Human Development: Experiments by Nature and Design.* Cambridge, MA: Harvard University Press.

Green, F.C. (1975) Child abuse and neglect. A priority problem for the private physician. *Pediatr. Clin. North Am.*, **22**, 2, 329–339.

Kazak, A.E. (1987) Families with disabled children: stress and social networks in 2–3 samples. *J. Abnorm. Child Psychol.*, **15**, 137.

Kolobe, T.H.A. (1991) Family-focused early education. In: *Pediatric Neurologic Physical Therapy*, edited by S.K. Campbell. New York: Churchill Livingstone, pp. 397–432.

McKinney, B. and Peterson, R.A. (1987) Predictors of stress in parents of developmentally disabled children. *J. Pediatr. Psychol.*, **12**, 1, 133.

Neumann-Neurode, D. (1967) *Baby Gymnastics.* London: Pergamon.

Rendle-Short, J. (1971) *The Child.* Bristol: Wright.

Sameroff, A.J. (1986) Environmental context of child development, *J. Pediatr.*, **109**, 192.

Sameroff, A.J. and Chandler, M.J. (1975) Reproductive risk and the continuum of caretaking casualty. In: *Review of Child Development Research*, 4, edited by F. Horowitz, M. Hetherington, S. Scarr-Salapatek *et al.* Chicago: University of Chicago Press, p. 187.

Simeonsson, R.J. and Bailey, D.B. (1990) Family dimensions in early intervention. In: *Handbook of Early Childhood Intervention*, edited by S.J. Meisels and J.P. Schonkoff. New York: Cambridge University Press, p. 428.

Summers, J.A., Behr, S.K. and Turnbull, A.P. (1989) Positive adaptation and coping strengths of families who have children with disabilities. In: *Support for Caregiving Families: Enabling Positive Adaptation to Disability*, edited by S.H. Singer and L.K. Irvin. Baltimore, MD: Paul H. Brookes, p. 27.

Winnicott, D.W. (1964) *The Child, the Family and the Outside World.* London: Penguin.

Further reading

Axline, V. (1966) *Dibs: In Search of Self.* London: Gollancz.

Barker, R.G. and Wright, H.F. (1971) *Midwest and its Children.* Hamden: Archon Books.

Bowlby, J. (1969) *Attachment and Loss.* New York: Basic Books.

Bowley, A. and Gardner, L. (1969) *The Young Handicapped Child.* London: Livingstone.

Brazelton, T.B. (1969) *Infants and Mothers.* New York: Delacorte Press.

Brazelton, T.B. (1970) *Doctor and Child.* New York: Delacorte Press.

Brazelton, T.B. (1974) *Toddlers and Parents* New York: Delacorte Press.

Brazelton, T.B. (1976) Early parent–infant reciprocity. In: *The Family – Can it be Saved?* edited by V.C. Vaughan and T.B. Brazelton. New York: Year Book.

Campbell, D. and Draper, R. (1985) *Applications of Systemic Family Therapy.* London: Grune & Stratton.

Cherry, D.B. (1989) Stress and coping in families with ill or disabled children: application of the model to pediatric therapy. *Phys. Occup. Ther. Pediatr.*, **9**, 2, 11.

Dweck, C.S. and Reppucci, N.D. (1973) Learned helplessness and reinforcement responsibility in children. *J. Personality Soc. Psychol.*, **25**, 1, 109–115.

Featherstone, H. (1980) *A Difference in the Family: Life with a Disabled Child.* New York: Basic Books.

Illingworth, R.S. and Holt, K.S. (1955) Children in hospital; some observations on their reactions with special reference to daily visiting. *Lancet*, **2**, 1257.

Kagan, J. (1975) *The Nature of the Child.* New York: Basic Books.

Minuchin, P. (1988) Relationships within the family: a systems perspective on development. In: *Relationships Within Families: Mutual Infleunces*, edited by R.A. Hinde and J. Stevenson-Hinde. New York: Oxford University Press, p. 7.

Murphy, M.A. (1982) The family with a handicapped child: a review of the literature. *J. Dev. Behav. Pediatr.*, **3**, 73.

Ounsted, C., Oppenheimer, R. and Lindsay, J. (1974) Aspects of bonding failure. *Dev. Med. Child Neurol.*, **16**, 447.

Parette, H.P. and Hourcade, J.J. (1985) Parental participation in early therapeutic intervention programs for young children with cerebral palsy: an unresolved dilemma. *Rehab. Lit.*, **46**, 1, 2–7.

Richardson, S.A., Hastorf, A.H. and Dornbusch, S.M. (1964) Effects of physical disability on a child's description of himself. *Child Dev.*, **35**.

Robertson, J. (1958) *Young Children in Hospital.* London: Tavistock.

Schmitt, B.D. and Kempe, C.H. (1975) *Child Abuse.* Basle: Ciba-Geigy.

Sheridan, M.D. (1965) *The Handicapped Child and his Home.* London: National Children's Home.

Singer, S.H. and Irvin, S.L. (1989). Family caregiving, stress and support. In: *Support for Caregiving Families: Enabling Positive Adaptation to Disability*, edited by S.H. Singer and S.L. Irvin. Baltimore, MD: Paul H. Brookes, p. 3.

Thomas, A., Chess, S. and Birch, H.G. (1970) The origin of personality. *Scient. Am.*, **223**, 2, 102.

Turnbull, A.P. and Turnbull, H. (1985) *Parents Speak Out*, 2nd edn. Columbus, OH: Merrill.

Walsh, F. (1982). Conceptualizations of normal family functioning. In: *Normal Family Processes*, edited by F. Walsh. New York: Guildford Press, p. 3.

...re 4 months old (Bayley 1969). Perhaps, ...urprisingly, babies placed habitually in ... by their parents appear to develop more ...ly in this position than infants placed ...ually in supine (Holt 1977).

...s usually not recognized in the clinic that, ...fants as in adults, muscles will function ...effectively when conditions such as the ...ment of segments are optimal. For exam-...an infant who is slow to lift the head in the ...e position may be able to lift the head when ...against a parent's shoulder. In physiother-...when an objective is to assist a motor-...aired infant to achieve active head move-...t, the optimal position in which active con-...tion of the neck muscles can be gained ...uld be emphasized. The optimal position ...urs when the baby is held erect – a position ...which vision provides inputs facilitatory to ...d control, and not necessarily the prone ...ition.

...erarchical organization of CNS

...major obstacle to the use of a scientifically ...sed framework for the training of effective ...tor performance in infants is the view that ... nervous system is hierarchically organized, ...th motor development reflecting an invariant ...ogression from reflexive to voluntary beha-...our, reflexes becoming inhibited as higher ...ntres mature. In this view, motor develop-...ent is linked to a hierarchical progression or ...e maturation of the CNS. These views are still ...ominant in paediatric clinical practice.

...Recent studies raise questions regarding ...hether this hierarchical model accounts for ...he complexities of human motor develop-...ent. Although maturation must be regarded ...s a critical factor, perception, cognition, ...xperience and the environment are additional ...determinants. Development appears to be non-...inear, consisting of spurts, plateaus and regres-...sions that produce quantitative and qualitative ...changes in motor performance. Ages for emer-...gence of new behaviours are probably fixed to ...some extent by maturation and set a lower limit ...on independence, hence independent sitting is ...in general not seen before 5–6 months of age, ...and independent walking seldom before 9 ...months.

...Maturation may be to some extent reflected ...in a sequence of motor behaviours chronologi-...cally yoked to age but it is certainly dynamic

and complex, early stereotypical movements being modified to produce mature, skilled motor function. Forssberg (1985) and others (Zelazo 1983; Clark and Phillips 1987; Thelen and Cooke 1987) have shown the transition from neonatal to mature stepping, with step-ping being transformed from reflexive to volun-tary through the modification of innate conditions rather than the creation of a new form.

Milani-Comparetti (1980) has recorded the development of prenatal motor patterns and demonstrated fetal–infant continuity. He noted, for example, that the fetus practised pushing against the wall of the uterus in pre-paration, he suggested, for parturition. This innate pattern, when modified according to task and context, appears also to be utilized in those actions which involve extending the lower limbs on fixed feet, such as standing up and jumping.

Rather than conceptualizing CNS organiza-tion as a strict hierarchy, modern neuroscience holds that the CNS is organized in a distributed manner. A major recent development in our understanding of motor control, which stems from early work by Bernstein (1967), the Russian physiologist, is the view of motor beha-viour as emergent, developing out of the inter-action between the individual and the environment. Movement is viewed, therefore, as controlled not only from CNS internally generated sources (motor nerve impulses) but also by external sources (by visual, tactile impulses) and by sources originating in the movement of linked segments themselves (gravitational, interactional, inertial forces). This modern view sees movement as produced not only by muscle innervation through the nervous system but also by forces generated by segmental movement itself. That is, the CNS appears to take advantage of and utilize the dynamics inherent in the musculoskeletal system and the attributes of the muscles them-selves. These attributes include the potential for storing and releasing elastic energy in a stretch-shortening cycle (e.g. Cavagna 1977) and the power-transferring capacity of biarticular mus-cles (e.g. Gregoire *et al.* 1984). The newborn infant's task becomes, in effect, one of learning how to match the biodynamical potential of linked body segments to the task to be accom-plished and the environment in which it is being performed.

2

The development of movement and skill

Introduction

An understanding of motor development is cri-tical for paediatric clinical practice. This is par-ticularly so where the infant has, or is at risk of having, motor dysfunction as a result of neural lesion or musculoskeletal abnormality, asso-ciated with, for example, cerebral palsy, spina bifida, brachial plexus paralysis or talipes equi-novarus.

Traditionally, most of our understanding of motor development has been shaped by obser-vational studies performed in the first half of the century (e.g. Shirley 1931; McGraw 1945) and from a view of the central nervous system (CNS) as a reflex-hierarchical system. Recently there has been a renewed research interest in early motor development and new theoretical perspectives and experimental findings in the broad area of the movement sciences, particu-larly in neurobiology (motor control), biome-chanics and psychology (motor learning, cognitive psychology). These developments have resulted in challenges to more traditional views and expanded insights into motor perfor-mance and motor control. As a result, motor development is viewed as dependent on biol-ogy, behaviour and the environment rather than being solely reliant on neurological maturation.

In considering the development of motor activity in childhood, it is useful to consider the issue of the acquisition of skill in perform-ing motor actions. The phrase 'development of

movement' is usually taken to describe the effects of maturation of the nervous system in the early years of life. However, it is also of interest to the physiotherapist to study how the child acquires the skills needed for recrea-tion, sport, work and adult life. There are a number of interesting texts on this topic (e.g. Kelso and Clark 1982; Wade and Whiting 1986; Whiting and Wade 1986; Gentile 1987) and some details of the methods by which skill is acquired in movement are outlined in Chapter 3.

The early observers of infant movement kept detailed records of the developmental progress of infants and children in terms of activity descriptions and the age of onset of certain behaviours. Virtually all these studies were of children of European origin. Normative data which form the basis of our understanding of motor development and of our developmental scales are, therefore, data concerning princi-pally this cultural group. Although these obser-vational studies contain descriptive information about what can be observed of motor perfor-mance, with a few exceptions, details of motor performance in specific motor actions were not, until recently, examined or measured.

The development of new methods of investi-gating motor performance by motion analysis and the increased interest in child-rearing as practised in other cultures have been joined in the last 10 years or so by changing views of motor control in which the task itself and the environment in which it is performed are seen to be powerful factors in the production of controlled movement. These views have become dominant in neuroscience and are variously referred to as the ecological approach (e.g. Reed 1982) and the dynamic systems perspective (e.g. Kelso and Tuller 1984).

The result of this research and theoretical development has been an explosion of investigations into human movement, including motor development, which provide information critical to the physiotherapist involved in evaluating performance and in intervening to improve the effectiveness of motor performance in disabled infants, children and adults. The information currently available provides us with methods of measuring motor performance and details of the dynamics of actions such as walking, reaching and manipulation, together with the anticipatory and ongoing postural adjustments (see, for example, Thelen and Lockman 1993). This should enable us to develop more scientifically based and effective clinical programmes.

As a result of this research endeavour, it is now possible to build a scientific framework for physiotherapy for the movement-disabled out of research findings that provide more relevant detail about the motor performance of humans at different ages than has been available previously.

A new look at some traditional views

In the field of motor development, interest has principally been focused on descriptive studies of the development of motor milestones. In terms of assessing an infant's neural maturation, of major interest has been the reflexive behaviours of the neonate (e.g. stepping, tonic reaction of the finger flexors, asymmetrical and symmetrical tonic neck reflexes) and the infant's responses to movement initiated from externally evoked postural reactions (righting and equilibrium reactions). The so-called 'primitive reflexes' of the neonate have been held to be inhibited as the CNS matures; the responses to externally imposed movement have been considered evidence of the development of balance. Descriptions of reflexes and responses are included in Appendix 1.

Renewed interest in motor development is currently focused on biomechanical studies of performance at different ages under different conditions (e.g. Zernicke and Schneider 1993). In addition, the nature and purpose of reflexes have been the focus of much recent research and theorizing. While it has generally been considered that neonatal reflexes need to be inhibited before mature behaviour can develop, the current view is that many of these early behaviours are prefunctional, an immature form of motor behaviour illustrating an innate motor pattern which, as the infant learns to move about and interact with the environment, is fine-tuned into task- and context-relevant action.

Surprisingly, the postural righting and equilibrium reactions, despite their dominant position in the clinical literature, have been subjected to very little research effort, with one or two exceptions. Clinicians have developed a rather stereotyped view of postural reactions, which are facilitated in response to predictable and stereotyped perturbations applied by the therapist. Postural reactions are, however, more flexible. That a certain behaviour in response to externally imposed movement (such as being picked up and moved about) strengthens as the infant gets older is undoubtedly so. It is also obvious that with developing maturity and experience, responses to externally imposed perturbations become flexible, and can be adapted according to task and context (e.g. standing on a moving footpath, sitting in a car). It is very likely that these postural responses represent the infant's developing ability to activate muscles with sufficient force to ensure the body and head remain upright, eyes positioned horizontally, together with a growing awareness by the infant of the relevance of the erect position, head aligned for optimal vestibular and visual input. In addition, balance during self-initiated movements is now extensively studied, indicating that we balance ourselves during such actions as reaching out to an object by making postural adjustments that are both preparatory and ongoing.

Maturation

Traditional theories of motor development suggested that development occurs in an invariant, hierarchically ordered sequence, principally dependent on cortical maturation (Halverson 1931, 1933; Shirley 1931; McGraw 1935, 1945). Motor milestones were thought, there-

fore, to mirror CNS maturation. Cardinal rules based on Gesell's work have remained prominent, with little role for learning or experience (Leonard 1990). Maturation has been conceptualized as uniform, invariant and marked by the passage of time.

Motor milestones have been considered by clinicians and others to occur in an invariant neurodevelopmental sequence (e.g. Shirley 1931), with earlier activities providing the necessary conditions for the ones that follow, that is, as prerequisites for subsequent actions. It is perhaps not surprising that this viewpoint arose when so little was known of the details of human motor performance. In the first year of life in particular there is an obvious progression in terms of the acquisition of skill. The infant increases his or her repertoire of actions; movement becomes more effective and matches more efficiently the infant's intentions. However, although the ability to perform certain movements emerges as the system matures, it is not necessarily so that, because a particular action occurs before another, the earlier movement must occur first or that its earlier occurrence facilitates in any way the acquisition of the later action (Roberton 1978).

Motor development has also been described as progressing in a cephalocaudal direction, for example, head control before trunk control. However, this appears an illusion (Green and Nelham 1991), as close scrutiny of some motion analysis studies shows that control apparently develops simultaneously in different parts of the body or a limb.

Although many western-reared children crawl before they walk, crawling is not a necessary condition for walking; variations in the path to bipedalism include scooting and hitching. Crawling is an action which is biomechanically, and in terms of muscle function, quite different to walking, particularly in terms of postural adjustments, since the base of support is composed of different body segments (Abitbol 1993). Quadrupedalism is also more inefficient in terms of energy consumption than bipedalism (Sparrow *et al.* 1987) and the child walks upright as soon as postural adjustments can be controlled in standing.

In childhood and in adult life it is not usual for previously acquired activities to be considered critical to the acquisition of a new skill. It is known, for example, that in order to develop the action of surfboard riding or archery, it is

necessary to practise these
opportunity to experience
under which these actic
Nevertheless, arbitrary co
placed in the clinic on, for
development, by such assu
for a disabled infant to pa
progression sequence, with a
proximodistal progression t
the standing position. Som
gest such an invariant seque
condition for developing hig
tions such as reading (Del
view that the sequence is itsel
to disabled babies being denie
to experience erect sitting and

The view that, for example,
extension in prone lying mus
standing, or crawling before
sitting on the floor before sit
has been in the physiotherapy
erature for some time. Neverthe
logical foundation, together wit
ity between the biomechanical e
such actions as lifting the head i
standing, for example, should e
siotherapists to move on from
In real life, control of the head
control of vision probably de
infant is carried about, held in
ported in standing and walked a
ents.

Indeed, several studies have sho
ent effect of child-rearing and pare
on the developmental sequenc
humans and animals, motor b
highly context-dependent, with th
initiating a complex movement n
than typically observed if certain
are met (Bradley 1990). For examp
tion in postural control requiremen
shown to allow earlier acquisition
nated limb movements (Fentre
Infants from certain African cult
been shown to be advanced com
American babies in independent sitti
parents facilitate sitting behaviour b
a hole in the sand and sitting the inf
It has been shown that infants wi
attempts to catch a target moving a
field of vision in the first month if
supported in a semireclined positic
Hofsten 1982). It has been typical, how
assume that babies cannot reach for a ri

they
not
pron
quick
habi

It
in in
mos
align
ple,
prop
held
apy
imp
mer
trad
sho
occ
in
hea
po

Hi

A
ba
m
th
w
p
vi
ce
m
th
d

This dynamical perspective is an attractive theory for physiotherapists, in that, instead of focusing analysis and intervention solely on the neural system, a framework is provided for clinical practice in which movement is seen as emerging from external as well as internal constraints which are acting on the dynamic system of the developing infant. According to this view, the task and environmental demands dictate the pattern of coordination. To base movement analysis and training on this theory is to shift from eliciting responses to conditions imposed by the therapist to providing an environment and goals which will enable the individual to learn to perform self-initiated active body movements within naturally occurring restraints (Shepherd and Carr 1991).

This dynamic systems perspective emphasizes the self-organizing properties of the sensorimotor system and their role in the development of movement (Thelen *et al.* 1987). It views motor development as dependent on task and environmental demands. For example, the desire to look around or to respond to an auditory or visual input in prone lying causes the infant to raise the head. To describe this action as a righting reaction is to miss the point of intention or the driving nature of an environmental stimulus. After all, an intellectually impaired infant may not lift the head even when sufficient muscle strength is present. Since motor behaviour emerges as a result of the infant's interaction with the environment, it is closely linked to visual, speech and cognitive development. Accordingly, the infant's behaviour changes and becomes more flexible and more related to intention as the CNS matures. Performance will also change as the infant's morphology changes, for example, as the relationship between head size and body size changes. In the course of their development, infants have to learn to manage both system and environmental constraints.

Neonatal reflex activity

Recent studies have raised questions about the traditional view of neonatal reflexes. A traditional view of motor development is that neonatal reflexive or primitive motor activity should disappear before reappearing again in a more mature form (e.g. McGraw 1945). This is said to be due to the takeover of behaviour from lower brain centres through a process of inhibition by cortical centres. For example, stepping at birth is typically regarded as reflexive; it is considered to disappear at the end of 2–3 months due to inhibition by maturing higher cortical centres. This view is questioned as a result of investigations which have shown, for example, that the neonatal stepping reflex does not disappear in infants whose parents train them to maintain their stepping (Zelazo *et al.* 1972). Stepping appears to be an example of an innate motor pattern which becomes modified by practice as the infant matures. To call these neonatal movements reflexes may in this case be erroneous. Instead Katona (1989) has referred to these early movements as 'elementary neuromotor patterns' and Zelazo (1983) as 'prefunctional movements'. Milani-Comparetti (1980) called them 'primary motor patterns' and pointed out that, although they are evoked by stimuli, this does not necessarily make them reflexes.

Movement patterns similar to those seen in the neonate have been described in the fetus from ultrasound studies (Milani-Comparetti 1980; De Vries *et al.* 1982). By 18 weeks of gestation, the fetus thrusts the feet against the uterine wall. This propulsion, sometimes called jumping, enables a change of position and during parturition will enable the fetus to assist the birth process. Around the seventh gestational month, reciprocal limb movements have been observed which are termed 'locomotor' because of their similarity to walking. A grasping pattern has been observed in a fetus of 10 gestational weeks. From 13 weeks the hand was observed to be open with increasing frequency and the fetus explored the surroundings with open hands. These findings support the view that the neural substrate to generate several motor behaviours is available very early in development, is present at birth and that the early movements are prefunctional in the sense that they become modified into mature motor actions. Rather than being reflexes which are inhibited as the brain matures, they are evidence of the early self-organizing capacity of the infant's system, the potential of which is realized through the emergence of motor actions suited to the infant's intentions and the affordances (Gibson 1979) or possibilities offered by the environment.

Considerable emphasis has been placed on the importance of reflexes in the clinical motor assessment of infants despite there being no agreement as to their significance. When the stepping reflex, for example, fails to disappear at the end of 3 months, this persistence is said to be the result of cortical disinhibition due to brain injury. Assumptions about neonatal reflexes include that they are suppressed by encephalization; that neonatal stepping and independent walking are unrelated; that failure of primitive reflexes to disappear indicates neuromotor pathology. The evidence is that these assumptions may be incorrect.

Associated movements

One aspect of the development of motor control which has undergone little investigation so far is the excessive and apparently unnecessary muscle activations accompanying immature motor performance. This spread of muscle activation has traditionally been termed 'associated movements' (Fog and Fog 1963), 'associated reactions' (Walsh 1923) and 'mirror movements' and appears to have been studied so far only in relation to manipulation.

The spread of muscle activation beyond those muscles principally involved in an action is generally regarded by clinicians as evidence of developmental delay or CNS dysfunction (Touwen and Prechtl 1970; Bobath 1971). Clinically, a relationship between associated movements and spasticity seems to be assumed, with associated reactions being described as an increased tone in certain parts of the body caused by movement in other body parts (Wilson 1991). Some clinicians make a distinction between associated reactions as increased tone in other body parts seen in brain-damaged infants and children and associative movements as mirror movements seen in normally developing children as well as disabled children (e.g. Wilson 1991).

Associated movements are particularly obvious in manipulation, although they would also occur during other movements as part of the gradual acquisition of motor control. As part of the development of independent finger control, the infant makes frustrating errors. For example, a toddler who holds a chocolate between thumb and index finger with the unwanted wrapping held in the palm by the remaining fingers may drop the chocolate when trying to get rid of the wrapping. Maintaining a grip with the fourth and fifth

fingers when releasing a grip between thumb and index finger is only possible when the child can control the individual parts of the hand separately (fractionate movement). The infant and young child may be unable to inhibit muscles which are unnecessary for a particular motor action. For example, in squeezing an object with one hand, involuntary squeezing occurs with the other hand. This unnecessary muscle activation is reported to decrease with increasing age (Fog and Fog 1963; Connolly and Stratton 1968; Todor and Lazarus 1986). Although, in an experimental clip-gripping task, older children were better able to control any tendency to activate gripping muscles in the opposite hand than younger children, the inhibition of involuntary muscle contractions became progressively harder to invoke at higher exertion levels (Todor and Lazarus 1986). At a high level of exertion, when an individual is attempting to generate maximum levels of force, the associated muscle activity apparently unrelated to the task may actually provide some reinforcement.

The presence of muscle activity in parts of the body not apparently required for the movement has been said to be typical of unskilled motor performance (Bruner 1973). The development of motor control in a particular task has been considered by some to depend more on the progressive inhibition of unwanted muscle activity than on the activation of additional motor units (O'Connell 1972; Basmajian 1977).

Mirror facilitation of bimanual hand or arm movements is frequently observed in actions which require both hands to move simultaneously in a coordinated manner. When people move both arms in a circle, they tend to synchronize the movements in space, moving their hands in either an inward or an outward direction so that one hand mirrors the other. The two movements tend to be synchronized in time also. This symmetry constraint has been suggested to have a strong effect on movement (Kelso *et al.* 1983). Symmetry constraints are also seen in young children and unintended mirror movements are often associated with unimanual activities, decreasing in the first decade of life (Wolff *et al.* 1983).

Clinically, it is important to understand that a spread of muscle activation which is not critical to the action being performed apparently occurs normally in development and occurs also in adult life, probably as a reflection of lack of skill as well as being associated with higher exertion levels. Since this phenomenon is as yet so little understood, physiotherapists should be cautious in interpreting this finding in the clinic. Physiotherapists are in a unique position to make comparative studies of this phenomenon in both disabled and normal infants and children.

A descriptive overview

Observations of the development of movement in a baby and young child have been described in detail by many authors. In this section, only a brief overview of the major events is given. The times at which infants can perform the different actions mentioned probably depend to some extent on the opportunity to practise and will vary according to child-rearing practices and the environment.

It is useful to keep in mind while reading of the gradual development of motor patterns that the newborn infant's overall goal is the accomplishment of adult (mature) motor performance. Specifically, the upper limbs have to be coordinated for reach and manipulation; the lower limbs for support, balance and propulsion over fixed distal segments in standing and sitting (the feet and/or thighs) in a gravitational environment. These are the main motor challenges in terms of motor development in the first year of life. They involve the infant gradually learning to use the morphological attributes of the linked-segment structure, such as the inertial and geometrical properties of the linked system, muscle characteristics, including viscoelastic properties and the properties of monoarticular and bi- or multiarticular muscles, all in relation to different environmental contexts and the infant's own intentions.

What seems critical to the development of movement is the opportunity to generate self-initiated movements and to be in a position to see the interaction between the environment and the limbs during active movement. The importance of active body movements to the development of motor control and of visual monitoring of the moving limbs to the development of eye–hand coordination and guided reaching behaviours have been shown in studies of kittens (Hein 1974; Held and Hein 1976). These studies of imposed passive versus active walking and of early visual deprivation

show how critical being able to initiate and carry out movement actively and see the body parts moving is for the development of kittens.

Mature human movement is very flexible in that movements are constantly adapting to different or changing situations (Higgins and Spaeth 1972; Gentile 1987). Although there appear to be certain components of an action which are invariant and are, therefore, considered essential to that action (Carr and Shepherd 1987a), provided these essential components or biomechanical necessities are present, the neuromusculoskeletal system seems to be able to adapt freely within these constraints as the need arises. To illustrate this point, there are certain critical features of standing up which are involved in moving the body's centre of mass forwards over the new base of support (the feet) in order that lower limb extension lifts the thighs from the seat. However, within these constraints, an individual can adapt the pattern of standing up according to seat height, seat characteristics, the intention of the action and the need to balance a hot cup of tea or hold a baby.

Although it has been assumed in the developmental literature that the result of practice and increased skill in an action is increased consistency in its performance (Connolly 1973; Glencross 1977), it appears that, just as in adults, this is not necessarily so. One study of children (Moss and Hogg 1983) has shown that consistency in grip patterns during manipulation (in a rod placement task) decreased as proficiency increased, suggesting that a greater repertoire of solutions became available to the child.

There is considerable evidence that the mechanics of human movement (kinematic, kinetic and muscle activation patterns) are task- and context-specific. Although early limb movements in infancy appear to occur without specific task demands or intentions, the infant's system seems to have an inbuilt task-specific organization (Jensen *et al.* 1989).

The neonate demonstrates what Milani-Comparetti (1980) calls 'competencies for survival', which are the Moro reaction (to facilitate the first inspiration), rooting, suckling and swallowing (to facilitate nutrition). The latter three have been observed from as early as 15 weeks of gestational age. Evidence even at this early age suggests that the infant is capable of a considerable degree of organization of body parts in order to produce movement. For example, phase plane plots (angular displacement graphed against angular velocity) of early kicking movements show that even 2-week-old infants display a similar pattern to adults, with peak velocities occurring in mid-range, indicating that the joint is decelerating considerably in advance of a change in direction (Jensen *et al.* 1989).

Behaviour in prone The young infant when placed in prone begins to lift the head soon after birth, as part of the protective turning of the head to keep the mouth and nose free. The infant will, however, show much better ability to lift the head when held against a parent's shoulder than when lying in prone, which reflects, even at this young age, that movement is most easily elicited when the mechanical conditions are optimal. Babies who spend some time exercising in prone develop extensor muscle strength and the ability to extend the head and trunk develops quickly. Within a few weeks the infant can activate the neck and upper trunk extensors strongly enough to raise the head and look around. After a few more weeks, the infant can raise the head and shoulders and take weight through the forearms (Fig. 2.1) and the hands. By 5 months the infant will be able to lift head, shoulders and lower legs from the support surface simultaneously, rocking back and forth in this position. At this stage, the infant will reach out for objects in prone and begin to develop the ability to shift the body mass laterally (Figs 2.2 and 2.3).

Changes in postural control in prone are illustrated by the infant shifting laterally on to a forearm (Fig. 2.3), before being able to use one hand for support (Fig. 2.2). One means of progression from one place to another develops around this time, as the infant pulls along on the floor using the arms.

Crawling Not all infants crawl, but for those who do, crawling is usually the next means of progression attempted, requiring first that postural adjustments can be made in four-point kneeling (Fig. 2.4).

These adjustments and the other aspects of motor control which are required in order to achieve skill in a quadripedal gait are acquired through much trial and error. The first movements practised are simple horizontal shifts of body mass backwards and forwards on to both hands. Both looking around and reaching out for objects probably help the infant develop the ability to shift laterally on to ipsilateral hand and leg. However, the crawling pattern is no doubt fine-tuned through practice of the action itself. Crawling is probably not a simple action to learn, requiring as it does that postural adjustments are appropriate as force is applied through diagonal limbs alternately.

Infants who crawl often go on to develop other quadripedal patterns, such as bear-walking (Fig. 2.5a) and other variations (Fig. 2.5b). Infants who do not crawl may shuffle, creep or roll from one place to another; others just get to their feet and walk (Robson 1984).

Behaviour in supine A normal newborn infant may show an initial head lag when pulled from

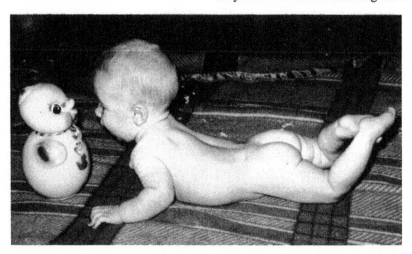

Figure 2.1   Aged 4 months, bearing weight through the forearms, with head and trunk well-extended.

they are 4 months old (Bayley 1969). Perhaps, not surprisingly, babies placed habitually in prone by their parents appear to develop more quickly in this position than infants placed habitually in supine (Holt 1977).

It is usually not recognized in the clinic that, in infants as in adults, muscles will function most effectively when conditions such as the alignment of segments are optimal. For example, an infant who is slow to lift the head in the prone position may be able to lift the head when held against a parent's shoulder. In physiotherapy, when an objective is to assist a motor-impaired infant to achieve active head movement, the optimal position in which active contraction of the neck muscles can be gained should be emphasized. The optimal position occurs when the baby is held erect – a position in which vision provides inputs facilitatory to head control, and not necessarily the prone position.

Hierarchical organization of CNS

A major obstacle to the use of a scientifically based framework for the training of effective motor performance in infants is the view that the nervous system is hierarchically organized, with motor development reflecting an invariant progression from reflexive to voluntary behaviour, reflexes becoming inhibited as higher centres mature. In this view, motor development is linked to a hierarchical progression or the maturation of the CNS. These views are still dominant in paediatric clinical practice.

Recent studies raise questions regarding whether this hierarchical model accounts for the complexities of human motor development. Although maturation must be regarded as a critical factor, perception, cognition, experience and the environment are additional determinants. Development appears to be non-linear, consisting of spurts, plateaus and regressions that produce quantitative and qualitative changes in motor performance. Ages for emergence of new behaviours are probably fixed to some extent by maturation and set a lower limit on independence, hence independent sitting is in general not seen before 5–6 months of age, and independent walking seldom before 9 months.

Maturation may be to some extent reflected in a sequence of motor behaviours chronologically yoked to age but it is certainly dynamic

and complex, early stereotypical movements being modified to produce mature, skilled motor function. Forssberg (1985) and others (Zelazo 1983; Clark and Phillips 1987; Thelen and Cooke 1987) have shown the transition from neonatal to mature stepping, with stepping being transformed from reflexive to voluntary through the modification of innate conditions rather than the creation of a new form.

Milani-Comparetti (1980) has recorded the development of prenatal motor patterns and demonstrated fetal–infant continuity. He noted, for example, that the fetus practised pushing against the wall of the uterus in preparation, he suggested, for parturition. This innate pattern, when modified according to task and context, appears also to be utilized in those actions which involve extending the lower limbs on fixed feet, such as standing up and jumping.

Rather than conceptualizing CNS organization as a strict hierarchy, modern neuroscience holds that the CNS is organized in a distributed manner. A major recent development in our understanding of motor control, which stems from early work by Bernstein (1967), the Russian physiologist, is the view of motor behaviour as emergent, developing out of the interaction between the individual and the environment. Movement is viewed, therefore, as controlled not only from CNS internally generated sources (motor nerve impulses) but also by external sources (by visual, tactile impulses) and by sources originating in the movement of linked segments themselves (gravitational, interactional, inertial forces). This modern view sees movement as produced not only by muscle innervation through the nervous system but also by forces generated by segmental movement itself. That is, the CNS appears to take advantage of and utilize the dynamics inherent in the musculoskeletal system and the attributes of the muscles themselves. These attributes include the potential for storing and releasing elastic energy in a stretch-shortening cycle (e.g. Cavagna 1977) and the power-transferring capacity of biarticular muscles (e.g. Gregoire *et al.* 1984). The newborn infant's task becomes, in effect, one of learning how to match the biodynamical potential of linked body segments to the task to be accomplished and the environment in which it is being performed.

fore, to mirror CNS maturation. Cardinal rules based on Gesell's work have remained prominent, with little role for learning or experience (Leonard 1990). Maturation has been conceptualized as uniform, invariant and marked by the passage of time.

Motor milestones have been considered by clinicians and others to occur in an invariant neurodevelopmental sequence (e.g. Shirley 1931), with earlier activities providing the necessary conditions for the ones that follow, that is, as prerequisites for subsequent actions. It is perhaps not surprising that this viewpoint arose when so little was known of the details of human motor performance. In the first year of life in particular there is an obvious progression in terms of the acquisition of skill. The infant increases his or her repertoire of actions; movement becomes more effective and matches more efficiently the infant's intentions. However, although the ability to perform certain movements emerges as the system matures, it is not necessarily so that, because a particular action occurs before another, the earlier movement must occur first or that its earlier occurrence facilitates in any way the acquisition of the later action (Roberton 1978).

Motor development has also been described as progressing in a cephalocaudal direction, for example, head control before trunk control. However, this appears an illusion (Green and Nelham 1991), as close scrutiny of some motion analysis studies shows that control apparently develops simultaneously in different parts of the body or a limb.

Although many western-reared children crawl before they walk, crawling is not a necessary condition for walking; variations in the path to bipedalism include scooting and hitching. Crawling is an action which is biomechanically, and in terms of muscle function, quite different to walking, particularly in terms of postural adjustments, since the base of support is composed of different body segments (Abitbol 1993). Quadrupedalism is also more inefficient in terms of energy consumption than bipedalism (Sparrow *et al.* 1987) and the child walks upright as soon as postural adjustments can be controlled in standing.

In childhood and in adult life it is not usual for previously acquired activities to be considered critical to the acquisition of a new skill. It is known, for example, that in order to develop the action of surfboard riding or archery, it is

necessary to practise these actions and have the opportunity to experience the varied conditions under which these actions are performed. Nevertheless, arbitrary constraints have been placed in the clinic on, for example, locomotor development, by such assumptions as the need for a disabled infant to pass through a prone progression sequence, with a cephalocaudal and proximodistal progression before experiencing the standing position. Some would even suggest such an invariant sequence is a necessary condition for developing higher cortical functions such as reading (Delacato 1966). The view that the sequence is itself critical can lead to disabled babies being denied the opportunity to experience erect sitting and standing.

The view that, for example, head and trunk extension in prone lying must develop before standing, or crawling before walking, or long sitting on the floor before sitting on a chair, has been in the physiotherapy (and other) literature for some time. Nevertheless, its lack of a logical foundation, together with the dissimilarity between the biomechanical elements of two such actions as lifting the head in prone and in standing, for example, should encourage physiotherapists to move on from this viewpoint. In real life, control of the head together with control of vision probably develops as the infant is carried about, held in sitting, supported in standing and walked about by parents.

Indeed, several studies have shown the apparent effect of child-rearing and parental handling on the developmental sequence. In both humans and animals, motor behaviour is highly context-dependent, with the individual initiating a complex movement much earlier than typically observed if certain conditions are met (Bradley 1990). For example, a reduction in postural control requirements has been shown to allow earlier acquisition of coordinated limb movements (Fentress 1981). Infants from certain African cultures have been shown to be advanced compared to American babies in independent sitting. Their parents facilitate sitting behaviour by digging a hole in the sand and sitting the infant in it. It has been shown that infants will initiate attempts to catch a target moving across the field of vision in the first month if they are supported in a semireclined position (von Hofsten 1982). It has been typical, however, to assume that babies cannot reach for a ring until be powerful factors in the production of con-trolled movement. These views have become dominant in neuroscience and are variously referred to as the ecological approach (e.g. Reed 1982) and the dynamic systems perspec-tive (e.g. Kelso and Tuller 1984).

The result of this research and theoretical development has been an explosion of investi-gations into human movement, including motor development, which provide information criti-cal to the physiotherapist involved in evaluating performance and in intervening to improve the effectiveness of motor performance in dis-abled infants, children and adults. The infor-mation currently available provides us with methods of measuring motor performance and details of the dynamics of actions such as walk-ing, reaching and manipulation, together with the anticipatory and ongoing postural adjust-ments (see, for example, Thelen and Lockman 1993). This should enable us to develop more scientifically based and effective clinical pro-grammes.

As a result of this research endeavour, it is now possible to build a scientific framework for physiotherapy for the movement-disabled out of research findings that provide more relevant detail about the motor performance of humans at different ages than has been available pre-viously.

A new look at some traditional views

In the field of motor development, interest has principally been focused on descriptive studies of the development of motor milestones. In terms of assessing an infant's neural matura-tion, of major interest has been the reflexive behaviours of the neonate (e.g. stepping, tonic reaction of the finger flexors, asymmetrical and symmetrical tonic neck reflexes) and the infant's responses to movement initiated from exter-nally evoked postural reactions (righting and equilibrium reactions). The so-called 'primitive reflexes' of the neonate have been held to be inhibited as the CNS matures; the responses to externally imposed movement have been con-sidered evidence of the development of balance. Descriptions of reflexes and responses are included in Appendix 1.

Renewed interest in motor development is currently focused on biomechanical studies of performance at different ages under different

conditions (e.g. Zernicke and Schneider 1993). In addition, the nature and purpose of reflexes have been the focus of much recent research and theorizing. While it has generally been con-sidered that neonatal reflexes need to be inhib-ited before mature behaviour can develop, the current view is that many of these early beha-viours are prefunctional, an immature form of motor behaviour illustrating an innate motor pattern which, as the infant learns to move about and interact with the environment, is fine-tuned into task- and context-relevant action.

Surprisingly, the postural righting and equili-brium reactions, despite their dominant posi-tion in the clinical literature, have been subjected to very little research effort, with one or two exceptions. Clinicians have devel-oped a rather stereotyped view of postural reac-tions, which are facilitated in response to predictable and stereotyped perturbations applied by the therapist. Postural reactions are, however, more flexible. That a certain behaviour in response to externally imposed movement (such as being picked up and moved about) strengthens as the infant gets older is undoubtedly so. It is also obvious that with developing maturity and experience, responses to externally imposed perturbations become flexible, and can be adapted according to task and context (e.g. standing on a moving footpath, sitting in a car). It is very likely that these postural responses represent the infant's developing ability to activate muscles with suf-ficient force to ensure the body and head remain upright, eyes positioned horizontally, together with a growing awareness by the infant of the relevance of the erect position, head aligned for optimal vestibular and visual input. In addition, balance during self-initiated movements is now extensively studied, indicat-ing that we balance ourselves during such actions as reaching out to an object by making postural adjustments that are both preparatory and ongoing.

Maturation

Traditional theories of motor development sug-gested that development occurs in an invariant, hierarchically ordered sequence, principally dependent on cortical maturation (Halverson 1931, 1933; Shirley 1931; McGraw 1935, 1945). Motor milestones were thought, there-

2

The development of movement and skill

Introduction

An understanding of motor development is critical for paediatric clinical practice. This is particularly so where the infant has, or is at risk of having, motor dysfunction as a result of neural lesion or musculoskeletal abnormality, associated with, for example, cerebral palsy, spina bifida, brachial plexus paralysis or talipes equinovarus.

Traditionally, most of our understanding of motor development has been shaped by observational studies performed in the first half of the century (e.g. Shirley 1931; McGraw 1945) and from a view of the central nervous system (CNS) as a reflex-hierarchical system. Recently there has been a renewed research interest in early motor development and new theoretical perspectives and experimental findings in the broad area of the movement sciences, particularly in neurobiology (motor control), biomechanics and psychology (motor learning, cognitive psychology). These developments have resulted in challenges to more traditional views and expanded insights into motor performance and motor control. As a result, motor development is viewed as dependent on biology, behaviour and the environment rather than being solely reliant on neurological maturation.

In considering the development of motor activity in childhood, it is useful to consider the issue of the acquisition of skill in performing motor actions. The phrase 'development of movement' is usually taken to describe the effects of maturation of the nervous system in the early years of life. However, it is also of interest to the physiotherapist to study how the child acquires the skills needed for recreation, sport, work and adult life. There are a number of interesting texts on this topic (e.g. Kelso and Clark 1982; Wade and Whiting 1986; Whiting and Wade 1986; Gentile 1987) and some details of the methods by which skill is acquired in movement are outlined in Chapter 3.

The early observers of infant movement kept detailed records of the developmental progress of infants and children in terms of activity descriptions and the age of onset of certain behaviours. Virtually all these studies were of children of European origin. Normative data which form the basis of our understanding of motor development and of our developmental scales are, therefore, data concerning principally this cultural group. Although these observational studies contain descriptive information about what can be observed of motor performance, with a few exceptions, details of motor performance in specific motor actions were not, until recently, examined or measured.

The development of new methods of investigating motor performance by motion analysis and the increased interest in child-rearing as practised in other cultures have been joined in the last 10 years or so by changing views of motor control in which the task itself and the environment in which it is performed are seen to parts in order to produce movement. For example, phase plane plots (angular displacement graphed against angular velocity) of early kicking movements show that even 2-week-old infants display a similar pattern to adults, with peak velocities occurring in mid-range, indicating that the joint is decelerating considerably in advance of a change in direction (Jensen *et al.* 1989).

Behaviour in prone The young infant when placed in prone begins to lift the head soon after birth, as part of the protective turning of the head to keep the mouth and nose free. The infant will, however, show much better ability to lift the head when held against a parent's shoulder than when lying in prone, which reflects, even at this young age, that movement is most easily elicited when the mechanical conditions are optimal. Babies who spend some time exercising in prone develop extensor muscle strength and the ability to extend the head and trunk develops quickly. Within a few weeks the infant can activate the neck and upper trunk extensors strongly enough to raise the head and look around. After a few more weeks, the infant can raise the head and shoulders and take weight through the forearms (Fig. 2.1) and the hands. By 5 months the infant will be able to lift head, shoulders and lower legs from the support surface simultaneously, rocking back and forth in this position. At this stage, the infant will reach out for objects in prone and begin to develop the ability to shift the body mass laterally (Figs 2.2 and 2.3).

Changes in postural control in prone are illustrated by the infant shifting laterally on to a forearm (Fig. 2.3), before being able to use one hand for support (Fig. 2.2). One means of progression from one place to another develops around this time, as the infant pulls along on the floor using the arms.

Crawling Not all infants crawl, but for those who do, crawling is usually the next means of progression attempted, requiring first that postural adjustments can be made in four-point kneeling (Fig. 2.4).

These adjustments and the other aspects of motor control which are required in order to achieve skill in a quadripedal gait are acquired through much trial and error. The first movements practised are simple horizontal shifts of body mass backwards and forwards on to both hands. Both looking around and reaching out for objects probably help the infant develop the ability to shift laterally on to ipsilateral hand and leg. However, the crawling pattern is no doubt fine-tuned through practice of the action itself. Crawling is probably not a simple action to learn, requiring as it does that postural adjustments are appropriate as force is applied through diagonal limbs alternately.

Infants who crawl often go on to develop other quadripedal patterns, such as bear-walking (Fig. 2.5a) and other variations (Fig. 2.5b). Infants who do not crawl may shuffle, creep or roll from one place to another; others just get to their feet and walk (Robson 1984).

Behaviour in supine A normal newborn infant may show an initial head lag when pulled from

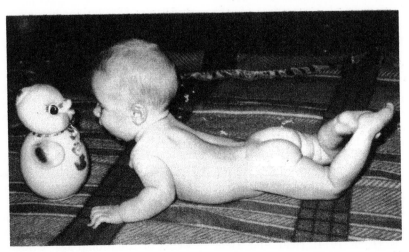

Figure 2.1 Aged 4 months, bearing weight through the forearms, with head and trunk well-extended.

skill as well as being associated with higher exertion levels. Since this phenomenon is as yet so little understood, physiotherapists should be cautious in interpreting this finding in the clinic. Physiotherapists are in a unique position to make comparative studies of this phenomenon in both disabled and normal infants and children.

A descriptive overview

Observations of the development of movement in a baby and young child have been described in detail by many authors. In this section, only a brief overview of the major events is given. The times at which infants can perform the different actions mentioned probably depend to some extent on the opportunity to practise and will vary according to child-rearing practices and the environment.

It is useful to keep in mind while reading of the gradual development of motor patterns that the newborn infant's overall goal is the accomplishment of adult (mature) motor performance. Specifically, the upper limbs have to be coordinated for reach and manipulation; the lower limbs for support, balance and propulsion over fixed distal segments in standing and sitting (the feet and/or thighs) in a gravitational environment. These are the main motor challenges in terms of motor development in the first year of life. They involve the infant gradually learning to use the morphological attributes of the linked-segment structure, such as the inertial and geometrical properties of the linked system, muscle characteristics, including viscoelastic properties and the properties of monoarticular and bi- or multiarticular muscles, all in relation to different environmental contexts and the infant's own intentions.

What seems critical to the development of movement is the opportunity to generate self-initiated movements and to be in a position to see the interaction between the environment and the limbs during active movement. The importance of active body movements to the development of motor control and of visual monitoring of the moving limbs to the development of eye–hand coordination and guided reaching behaviours have been shown in studies of kittens (Hein 1974; Held and Hein 1976). These studies of imposed passive versus active walking and of early visual deprivation

show how critical being able to initiate and carry out movement actively and see the body parts moving is for the development of kittens.

Mature human movement is very flexible in that movements are constantly adapting to different or changing situations (Higgins and Spaeth 1972; Gentile 1987). Although there appear to be certain components of an action which are invariant and are, therefore, considered essential to that action (Carr and Shepherd 1987a), provided these essential components or biomechanical necessities are present, the neuromusculoskeletal system seems to be able to adapt freely within these constraints as the need arises. To illustrate this point, there are certain critical features of standing up which are involved in moving the body's centre of mass forwards over the new base of support (the feet) in order that lower limb extension lifts the thighs from the seat. However, within these constraints, an individual can adapt the pattern of standing up according to seat height, seat characteristics, the intention of the action and the need to balance a hot cup of tea or hold a baby.

Although it has been assumed in the developmental literature that the result of practice and increased skill in an action is increased consistency in its performance (Connolly 1973; Glencross 1977), it appears that, just as in adults, this is not necessarily so. One study of children (Moss and Hogg 1983) has shown that consistency in grip patterns during manipulation (in a rod placement task) decreased as proficiency increased, suggesting that a greater repertoire of solutions became available to the child.

There is considerable evidence that the mechanics of human movement (kinematic, kinetic and muscle activation patterns) are task- and context-specific. Although early limb movements in infancy appear to occur without specific task demands or intentions, the infant's system seems to have an inbuilt task-specific organization (Jensen *et al.* 1989).

The neonate demonstrates what Milani-Comparetti (1980) calls 'competencies for survival', which are the Moro reaction (to facilitate the first inspiration), rooting, suckling and swallowing (to facilitate nutrition). The latter three have been observed from as early as 15 weeks of gestational age. Evidence even at this early age suggests that the infant is capable of a considerable degree of organization of body motor assessment of infants despite there being no agreement as to their significance. When the stepping reflex, for example, fails to disappear at the end of 3 months, this persistence is said to be the result of cortical disinhibition due to brain injury. Assumptions about neonatal reflexes include that they are suppressed by encephalization; that neonatal stepping and independent walking are unrelated; that failure of primitive reflexes to disappear indicates neuromotor pathology. The evidence is that these assumptions may be incorrect.

Associated movements

One aspect of the development of motor control which has undergone little investigation so far is the excessive and apparently unnecessary muscle activations accompanying immature motor performance. This spread of muscle activation has traditionally been termed 'associated movements' (Fog and Fog 1963), 'associated reactions' (Walsh 1923) and 'mirror movements' and appears to have been studied so far only in relation to manipulation.

The spread of muscle activation beyond those muscles principally involved in an action is generally regarded by clinicians as evidence of developmental delay or CNS dysfunction (Touwen and Prechtl 1970; Bobath 1971). Clinically, a relationship between associated movements and spasticity seems to be assumed, with associated reactions being described as an increased tone in certain parts of the body caused by movement in other body parts (Wilson 1991). Some clinicians make a distinction between associated reactions as increased tone in other body parts seen in brain-damaged infants and children and associative movements as mirror movements seen in normally developing children as well as disabled children (e.g. Wilson 1991).

Associated movements are particularly obvious in manipulation, although they would also occur during other movements as part of the gradual acquisition of motor control. As part of the development of independent finger control, the infant makes frustrating errors. For example, a toddler who holds a chocolate between thumb and index finger with the unwanted wrapping held in the palm by the remaining fingers may drop the chocolate when trying to get rid of the wrapping. Maintaining a grip with the fourth and fifth fingers when releasing a grip between thumb and index finger is only possible when the child can control the individual parts of the hand separately (fractionate movement). The infant and young child may be unable to inhibit muscles which are unnecessary for a particular motor action. For example, in squeezing an object with one hand, involuntary squeezing occurs with the other hand. This unnecessary muscle activation is reported to decrease with increasing age (Fog and Fog 1963; Connolly and Stratton 1968; Todor and Lazarus 1986). Although, in an experimental clip-gripping task, older children were better able to control any tendency to activate gripping muscles in the opposite hand than younger children, the inhibition of involuntary muscle contractions became progressively harder to invoke at higher exertion levels (Todor and Lazarus 1986). At a high level of exertion, when an individual is attempting to generate maximum levels of force, the associated muscle activity apparently unrelated to the task may actually provide some reinforcement.

The presence of muscle activity in parts of the body not apparently required for the movement has been said to be typical of unskilled motor performance (Bruner 1973). The development of motor control in a particular task has been considered by some to depend more on the progressive inhibition of unwanted muscle activity than on the activation of additional motor units (O'Connell 1972; Basmajian 1977).

Mirror facilitation of bimanual hand or arm movements is frequently observed in actions which require both hands to move simultaneously in a coordinated manner. When people move both arms in a circle, they tend to synchronize the movements in space, moving their hands in either an inward or an outward direction so that one hand mirrors the other. The two movements tend to be synchronized in time also. This symmetry constraint has been suggested to have a strong effect on movement (Kelso *et al.* 1983). Symmetry constraints are also seen in young children and unintended mirror movements are often associated with unimanual activities, decreasing in the first decade of life (Wolff *et al.* 1983).

Clinically, it is important to understand that a spread of muscle activation which is not critical to the action being performed apparently occurs normally in development and occurs also in adult life, probably as a reflection of lack of

This dynamical perspective is an attractive theory for physiotherapists, in that, instead of focusing analysis and intervention solely on the neural system, a framework is provided for clinical practice in which movement is seen as emerging from external as well as internal constraints which are acting on the dynamic system of the developing infant. According to this view, the task and environmental demands dictate the pattern of coordination. To base movement analysis and training on this theory is to shift from eliciting responses to conditions imposed by the therapist to providing an environment and goals which will enable the individual to learn to perform self-initiated active body movements within naturally occurring restraints (Shepherd and Carr 1991).

This dynamic systems perspective emphasizes the self-organizing properties of the sensorimotor system and their role in the development of movement (Thelen *et al.* 1987). It views motor development as dependent on task and environmental demands. For example, the desire to look around or to respond to an auditory or visual input in prone lying causes the infant to raise the head. To describe this action as a righting reaction is to miss the point of intention or the driving nature of an environmental stimulus. After all, an intellectually impaired infant may not lift the head even when sufficient muscle strength is present. Since motor behaviour emerges as a result of the infant's interaction with the environment, it is closely linked to visual, speech and cognitive development. Accordingly, the infant's behaviour changes and becomes more flexible and more related to intention as the CNS matures. Performance will also change as the infant's morphology changes, for example, as the relationship between head size and body size changes. In the course of their development, infants have to learn to manage both system and environmental constraints.

Neonatal reflex activity

Recent studies have raised questions about the traditional view of neonatal reflexes. A traditional view of motor development is that neonatal reflexive or primitive motor activity should disappear before reappearing again in a more mature form (e.g. McGraw 1945). This is said to be due to the takeover of behaviour from lower brain centres through a process of inhibition by cortical centres. For example, stepping at birth is typically regarded as reflexive; it is considered to disappear at the end of 2–3 months due to inhibition by maturing higher cortical centres. This view is questioned as a result of investigations which have shown, for example, that the neonatal stepping reflex does not disappear in infants whose parents train them to maintain their stepping (Zelazo *et al.* 1972). Stepping appears to be an example of an innate motor pattern which becomes modified by practice as the infant matures. To call these neonatal movements reflexes may in this case be erroneous. Instead Katona (1989) has referred to these early movements as 'elementary neuromotor patterns' and Zelazo (1983) as 'prefunctional movements'. Milani-Comparetti (1980) called them 'primary motor patterns' and pointed out that, although they are evoked by stimuli, this does not necessarily make them reflexes.

Movement patterns similar to those seen in the neonate have been described in the fetus from ultrasound studies (Milani-Comparetti 1980; De Vries *et al.* 1982). By 18 weeks of gestation, the fetus thrusts the feet against the uterine wall. This propulsion, sometimes called jumping, enables a change of position and during parturition will enable the fetus to assist the birth process. Around the seventh gestational month, reciprocal limb movements have been observed which are termed 'locomotor' because of their similarity to walking. A grasping pattern has been observed in a fetus of 10 gestational weeks. From 13 weeks the hand was observed to be open with increasing frequency and the fetus explored the surroundings with open hands. These findings support the view that the neural substrate to generate several motor behaviours is available very early in development, is present at birth and that the early movements are prefunctional in the sense that they become modified into mature motor actions. Rather than being reflexes which are inhibited as the brain matures, they are evidence of the early self-organizing capacity of the infant's system, the potential of which is realized through the emergence of motor actions suited to the infant's intentions and the affordances (Gibson 1979) or possibilities offered by the environment.

Considerable emphasis has been placed on the importance of reflexes in the clinical

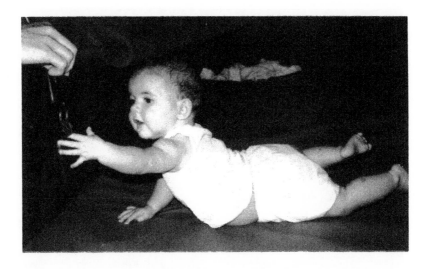

Figure 2.2 Aged 6 months, supported on one hand in order to reach forwards.

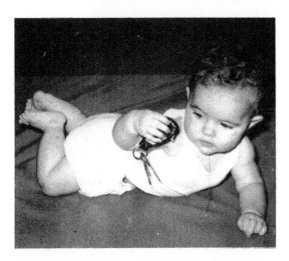

Figure 2.3 Aged 6 months, supported through forearm.

supine to sitting. However, when lowered from sitting to supine, the neck flexors may be able to contract and sustain the contraction for a large part of the movement. Some infants have a pronounced lag in this situation (see Fig. 5.1). This may be associated with CNS dysfunction but may also be the consequence of a prolonged delivery during which drugs with a depressing effect on the infant's CNS are ingested by the mother. In the first 4 months, the baby develops stronger neck and abdominal muscles and controlling the head in the midline is probably progressively facilitated by vision (Fig. 2.6). From the age of 5 months, when an adult puts out the hands to help the infant sit up,

neck and trunk flexor activity will be initiated in anticipation and, by 6 months, the infant will lift the head up spontaneously (Fig. 2.7). It is probable that infants given a great deal of experience in erect positions will acquire stronger and more controlled neck muscles than infants who spend their time horizontal.

Development of lower limb activity for support, balance and propulsion

Standing At birth, when held with the feet in contact with a support surface, the infant will extend the lower limbs and stand (Fig. 2.8) and when tilted forwards will take a few steps. Within a few weeks, this rather stereotyped walking cannot be elicited in many infants. At this time, when the infant is held in standing, the legs may collapse into flexion. A few weeks later, the infant is able to extend the legs and stand again when supported. Whether or not the infant goes through this stage of not supporting body weight through the legs seems to depend on the infant's cultural heritage and parental child-rearing practices. At approximately 8–10 months, the infant pulls to standing if there is something to hold on to. During these early standing sessions, the infant may stand on the toes. Having got into standing, it is usually difficult to sit down again, except by letting go the support and falling down. It is very likely that controlling eccentric muscle activity against the load of the body mass is

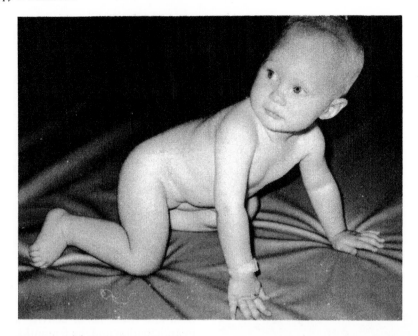

Figure 2.4   Aged 10 months, remaining balanced while shifting body mass laterally.

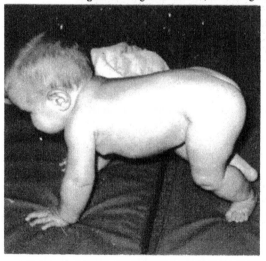

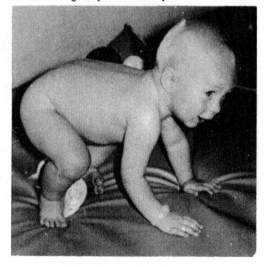

a   b

Figure 2.5   (a) Aged 8 months, supported through hands and feet but easily overbalances. (b) Aged 11 months, can move in and out of quadripedal position.

more difficult than concentric activity, making strength and control demands that the infant is not immediately able to produce. Nevertheless, it does not take much practice for the infant to master the action in both directions.

Sitting The acquisition of independent sitting increases the infant's scope for varied behaviour. Before this time, the infant is dependent upon being put into supported sitting by a par-

ent, and the amount of early sitting practice and hence the rate at which independent sitting is attained seem to depend on child-rearing practices. As in standing, the development of postural adjustments in sitting is dependent upon the opportunity to practise in sitting. In the early stages of developing independent sitting, the infant uses the hands for support, using them to compensate for immature postural

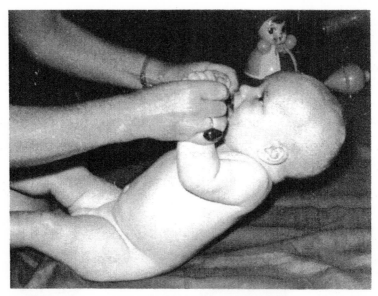

Figure 2.6 Aged 3 months, holds head steady and looks at parent when pulled to sitting.

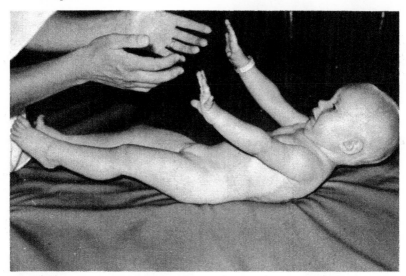

Figure 2.7 Aged 9 months, lifts head and shoulders in anticipation of being helped to sitting.

adjustments in this position. At first, the infant ensures maximum stability on a wide base of support by leaning forward on the hands (Fig. 2.9). Later, the hands can be used laterally as a means of saving balance when trunk and leg muscle activations are inadequate to prevent falling sideways (Fig. 2.10). By about 7–8 months, the infant has developed sufficient postural control to be able to move about in sitting without using the hands for support (Figs 2.11–2.13).

Postural adjustments in sitting require co-ordination between muscles which link the fixed distal body part (the lower limb) to the body part above (the trunk). Just as in standing, activation of these muscles needs to occur before the infant raises the arm to reach for an object; that is, they must be anticipatory, setting up the conditions for ensuring that when the perturbation (caused by the arm movement) occurs, it does not cause the infant to fall or to make post-arm movement reactive adjustments.

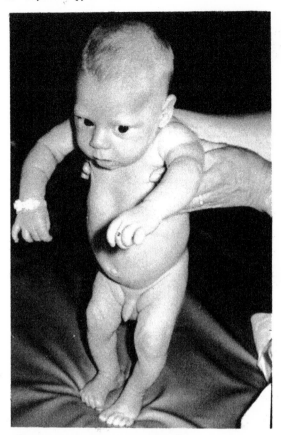

Figure 2.8   Neonatal standing.

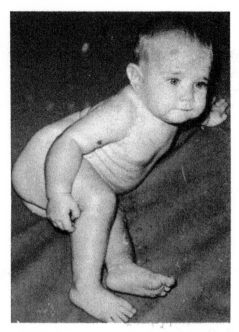

Figure 2.10   Aged 7 months, supporting on one hand laterally.

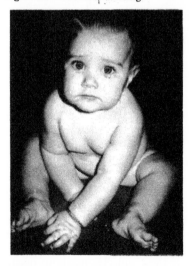

Figure 2.9   Aged 6 months, hands needed for support in independent sitting.

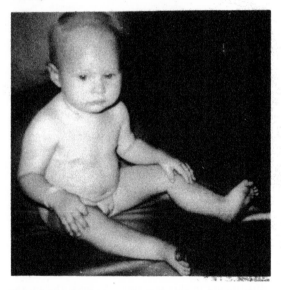

Figure 2.11   Aged 11 months, independent sitting without hands for support.

Development of sitting includes acquiring the skill of sitting on a stool, which requires specific postural adjustments which are differ-ent from the adjustments made when sitting on the floor. In sitting on a seat, the fixed base of support comprises the thighs and the feet, with muscle activity occurring in lower limbs both before and during arm movement when the movement is fast (Shepherd *et al.* 1994), but probably also during slower movements. There

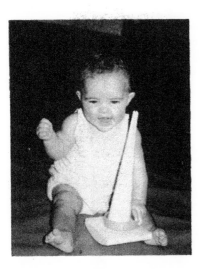

Figure 2.12 Aged 7 months, can move about in the sagittal plane without using the hands for support.

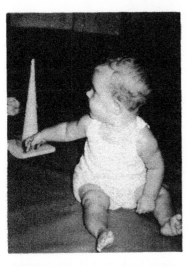

Figure 2.13 Aged 7 months, sitting balance sufficiently established to turn the head and upper body to look behind.

has been little interest in studying the development of independent sitting on a stool, perhaps because western-reared babies spend most of their sitting time on the floor. The development of the critical everyday actions of standing up from a stool and sitting down has similarly not been subject to much investigation, but, on observation, the infant can be pulled to standing if given assistance with the hands. The major component of the action of standing up to be acquired as the child devel-

ops may well be the ability to control forwards momentum of the body as the body mass is moved forwards from over the thighs to the feet, since this action poses a considerable threat to balance when uncontrolled, together with the ability to coordinate the horizontal and vertical phases of the action. Infants also develop the ability to stand up from the crouch or squat position, from kneeling and from half-kneeling.

Walking Some time before being able to walk alone, the infant 'cruises' the furniture or a parent's legs, walking sideways rather than forwards, occasionally letting go and sitting down. This sideways walking may assist the baby to learn one of the critical features of the initiation of walking – the ability to shift the body mass laterally and balance on one foot. Movement of the body mass laterally from one foot to another is probably easier to control than moving forwards as in walking, since the narrow base of support makes considerable demands on postural adjustments. It is notable that when the infant does eventually start walking independently, forwards progression is accomplished by small steps with feet turned out and legs abducted, giving a relatively wide base.

In standing, the infant practises controlling postural adjustments, in particular the muscle activations linking the fixed feet to the shank and other body segments, while looking around and reaching out for objects. Independent standing is assisted initially by support through both hands but the infant experiments, reaching out with one hand and sometimes with both hands. Initial walking is accomplished with arms abducted and postural adjustments are visible as they consist of excessive adjustment at the ankles and hips, followed by readjustment and frequent falling. As balance improves, the infant is able to carry objects without falling and walk on different surfaces (Figs 2.14 and 2.15). The infant is not able to jump on both feet until about 2–3 years of age, stand on one leg until 4 years, or hop until 5 years. Skill on the feet further develops into and through adult life, depending on interests, to comprise such activities as walking tightropes or traversing snow-covered alpine ridges.

From the start of independent walking and often earlier, the infant will utilize the environment to develop a wide repertoire of actions involving movement of the body mass over one or two fixed feet, moving between crouch

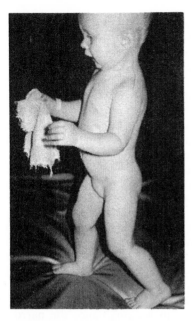

Figure 2.14 Aged 13 months, independent walking. The infant has developed sufficient balance to carry an object and walk on an unstable surface.

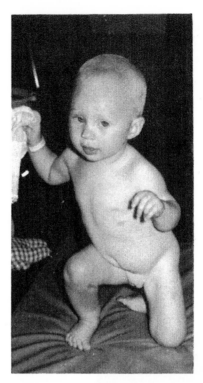

Figure 2.16 Aged 13 months, attempting to stand up through half-kneeling. Note that the infant needs some support as the surface is not firm.

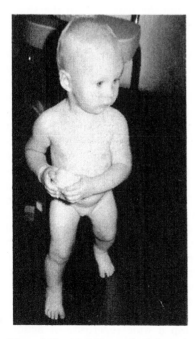

Figure 2.15 Aged 13 months, independent walking. Note the wide base of support in double-stance phase.

and standing, kneeling and standing (Fig. 2.16), standing up from a small seat and sitting down, walking up and down stairs (accomplished first on all fours), scrambling over and around large objects. The infant's explorations seem focused on gaining insights about the affordances of objects, their uses, their potential for use and the activities that objects will allow.

Development of upper limb activity for reaching and manipulation

A newborn infant holds the hands either fisted or loosely flexed. A grasp can be elicited by placing a finger across the infant's palm and giving gentle traction. When the arm is extended the hand tends to open. However, a few weeks later, when the infant extends the arm to reach out, the hand may be held tightly fisted. Although it used to be considered that arm movement in neonates and young infants is merely 'an excited thrashing of the arms' (White *et al.* 1964), recent evidence indicates that neonates held firmly supported in sitting will reach out towards objects if they are close enough and if they move across the infant's visual field (von Hofsten 1982).

The neonate will follow an object briefly with the eyes and follow a face from one side to another if it is close enough. It is probable that the conjunction of eye and hand control, that is, the ability to do simple grasping and to watch the hand, marks the start of functional use of the hand. By 3 months, the infant gets the two hands together in the midline and will clasp and unclasp them. By 4 months, reaching is more controlled but the infant will bat at objects rather than grasp them. At 5 months, voluntary grasping is seen more often, and the infant may grasp the toes when in supine (Fig. 2.17). In this early period of manipulation development, the strength of the grasp is not refined, and the infant tends to grasp too strongly and to have difficulty releasing. Release does not appear to become voluntary until the third trimester. When handed a biscuit, the infant will eat it but it may be crumbled before it reaches the mouth. Around 9 months, the infant will not hand back an object when given it, but by 12 months, the object will be handed back when the infant is asked. Some babies will feed themselves with a spoon by 9 months, most by 15 months. Until 12 months, most objects given to the baby are mouthed.

Early voluntary grasping is with the whole hand (Halverson 1931), tending towards the ulnar side. During the second half of the first year, the focus moves towards the radial side, and by 8 months, most objects will be held towards this side. An immature pincer grasp has usually developed by 9 months (Figs 2.18 and 2.19) and by 12 months the infant will hold small objects between the tip of the thumb and index finger (Gesell 1928). By the third year, most infants have developed what is often called a 'dynamic tripod grasp' (Wynn-Parry 1966), which involves thumb, index and middle finger being used together to make small highly cooordinated movements, such as are involved in writing. This grasp is said to be mature by the age of 6 years (Rosenbloom and Horton 1971).

Part of the development of control over the hand for function is the acquisition of skill in using fingers independently as well as together. Infants practise many diverse finger actions which are probably exploratory. Around 8 months, as part of the infant's increasing interest in faces, the index finger will be used to explore a parent's face, poking the finger into an ear or mouth. Rubbing, squeezing and banging are systematically used by infants soon after they have become effective at reaching and grasping. Patting, plucking and raking movements are practised as the infant discovers the potential of five fingers (Fig. 2.20). The principal feature of the motor system which enables independent finger movements and dexterity appears to be the corticomotoneuronal synapse (Kuypers 1982). In infant monkeys, these connections are manifested at the time when the animals first start to use their hands for precise

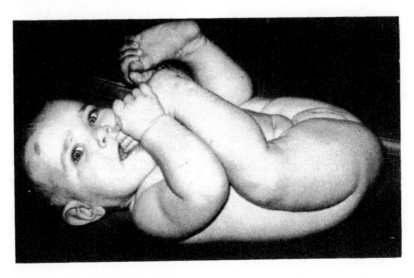

Figure 2.17 Aged 5 months, grasping toes.

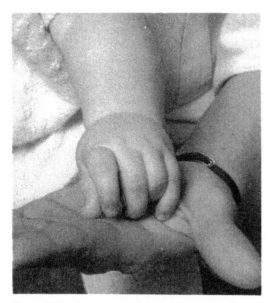

Figure 2.18 Grasp is radially oriented and the object is picked up between thumb, index and middle fingers.

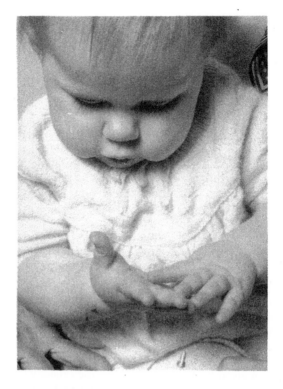

Figure 2.20 Although she has dropped the object (see bottom of picture), the infant is more intent on examining her hand.

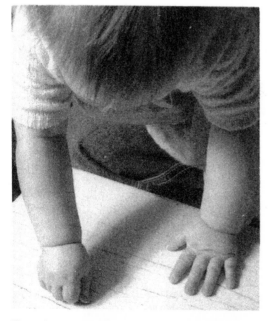

Figure 2.19 Immature pincer grasp. Small object is picked up between thumb and side of index finger.

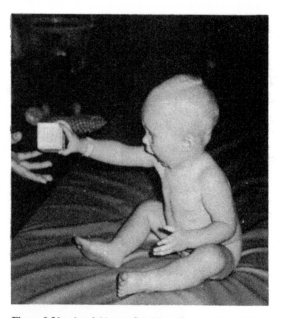

Figure 2.21 Aged 11 months. Note the opening of the mouth and increase in the left hand aperture accompanying grasping with the right hand.

manipulation, between 4 and 6 months of age (Flament *et al.* 1990).

When a task is difficult for a child, the action is usually accompanied, as it is in any unskilled person, by activity in muscles not normally involved in the action. For example, when grasping a large object, the 11-month-old baby in Figure 2.21 opens her mouth and the opposite hand. Acquiring skill in movement is known to be accompanied by a decrease in unnecessary muscle activity (Basmajian 1977).

Handedness varies in its time of establishment but many children show a hand preference by 15 months. Once grasp has been established, the development of manipulation probably depends upon experience and the possibilities offered by the environment. Skill in manipulating objects becomes increasingly object- and task-specific. Children who have blocks to play with can stack one on top of another at 12 months if the task is demonstrated, and by the age of 3 years the child will build a tower of 10 blocks. Voluntary undressing and dressing begin between 18 and 24 months. By 5 years, many western-reared children will be independent in most aspects of personal care. Children can throw a ball overarm in the standing position between 2 and 3 years and underarm by 3 years. Five-year-olds can catch a small ball.

Research findings related to the development of specific motor actions

Since much present-day physiotherapy practice is based on the traditional views of both motor development and the organization of the CNS (e.g. Perin 1989; Wilson 1991; Eckersley and King 1993), there is a need to examine recent research in order to update clinical practice. The following pages contain a brief review of some research findings on motor development which should form the basis of physiotherapy interventions. The reader who is working in paediatric practice should use the reference and additional reading lists provided at the end of the chapter to develop an understanding of the development of movement and the biomechanical details of motor performance necessary for a clinical movement scientist.

The development of postural control

Historically, descriptions of the development of postural control (or balance) have been confined to the first year of life and have been associated with such actions as controlling the head, independent sitting and standing. As Woollacott (1986) points out, the role of postural control in the execution of voluntary tasks has largely been ignored. In the health science literature on balance, the emphasis in treatment has traditionally been on the infant's response to being moved by the therapist (Perin 1989; Eckersley and King 1993). Indeed, it has been the reflexive or response aspects of postural adjustment which have been used for evaluating infant development and as the sole basis for intervention to improve balance (Bobath and Bobath 1964). Hence it is the tonic labyrinthine reflex, the tonic neck reflexes, the Landau reaction, righting and equilibrium reactions which have been the focus of attention in the assessment and treatment of motor-disabled infants. These responses have not, however, been the focus of much research since the early work which first described them, with one or two exceptions (Capute *et al.* 1985), so, although they are commonly part of the test procedure, their role in motor development is still not understood.

No doubt as a result of the historical neurophysiological view of balance as responsive and separate from action itself and the traditional emphasis placed on the reflexive nature of postural movement in the paediatric literature, physiotherapy for infants and children has dealt almost entirely with methods of facilitating automatic responses to perturbations caused by the therapist. Studies on the control of voluntary movement in animals, however, have shown that areas of the brain which control voluntary movement also activate postural adjustments (Gahery and Massion 1981). If, as seems likely, the voluntary and postural systems develop together, the emphasis in paediatric physiotherapy should be on training infants in a way that encourages the development of postural control associated with voluntary self-initiated actions. That is, it is probable that the emphasis should be on self-initiated movements made by the infant and not primarily on postural adjustments in response to movements imposed on the infant by another person.

The investigation of postural control in very young infants is still in its early stages. For example, a response to looming objects has been noted in newborns, causing a backwards movement of the head and arm raising (Bower *et al.* 1970). There has, however, been a considerable amount of research recently into postural control in adults and some studies of older infants and children (Shumway-Cook and Woollacott 1985; Forssberg 1985; Hirschfeld 1992). Much of this research has produced findings which are of direct relevance to physiotherapy and which should form part of the movement science framework of motor training in infants and children, as has been proposed by Carr and Shepherd for adults (1987b, 1990).

It seems very likely that both biomechanical and neuromotor processes are responsible for body stability and much of the recent research has been focused on questions related to these processes. Some investigations have been of relatively natural self-initiated movements, in which the postural muscle activity and various biomechanical parameters are studied as standing subjects raise an arm (Lee 1980), reach out or bend forwards (Oddsson and Thorstensson 1986). Most, however, have focused on the subject's response to external perturbation, invariably support surface perturbation in standing (e.g. Nashner 1982) and in sitting (Hirschfeld 1992).

It is important to consider the complexity of human movement, of which postural adjustments are a critical part. Postural adjustments vary according to the task being performed, the intention of the individual, the environmental context in which the task is performed, and to some extent the morphology of the individual. That is, research findings about muscle activation patterns and biomechanical parameters from a study in which the surface beneath the feet was unexpectedly moved may have relevance for real-life activities such as standing in a bus or sitting in a car but is probably irrelevant in terms of an action such as reaching out to take a glass from a table. In the former, the system is largely functioning in response mode; in the latter, postural adjustments would work in anticipatory mode as well as being ongoing throughout the action.

It is useful, therefore, to categorize balance in order to see the different types of context in which it plays a part. It could be said that balance is needed in everyday life under three types of conditions:

1   when segmental alignment has to be set or adjusted before a limb is moved voluntarily (e.g. in reaching for a glass) in order to allow for the reactive forces from the upcoming movement and, when the movement starts, to make ongoing adjustments;
2   when it is necessary to respond to movement of the surface on which we sit or stand (e.g. on a boat);
3   when it is necessary to brace the body to withstand displacement by some outside force (e.g. standing in a crowd).

Body equilibrium can therefore be distributed by two means: by an *internal* force generated by self-initiated body movement; and by an *external* force applied to the body, either by a direct perturbation such as a push or by movement of the support surface.

There are three major findings from recent postural control research on children and adults which are relevant to paediatric clinical practice since they provide information about the postural control which infants and children are striving to attain.

1   *Postural adjustments are anticipatory and preparatory*. Recent research into arm-raising and reaching in standing and sitting in adults has shown that lower-limb postural muscles are activated before prime mover arm muscle activation in order to minimize the subsequent perturbation caused by the self-initiated arm movement (e.g. Belenkii *et al.* 1967; Lee 1980; Cordo and Nashner 1982; Shepherd *et al.* 1994). Furthermore, it has been shown that these preparatory muscle activations are associated with joint rotations in the lower limbs and changes in the centre of pressure (Bouisset and Zattara 1981). These adjustments take place before the arm starts to move.
2   *Postural adjustments are task- and context-specific*. Many investigations reveal the dependence of postural adjustment on the task, the environment in which it is performed and the intention of the performer (e.g. Lee 1980; Zattara and Bouisset 1986). There are two of particular interest. In a study by Cordo and Nashner (1982), when standing subjects pulled on a handle, electromyogram (EMG) activity occurred in a calf muscle

(gastrocnemius) before EMG onset in the arm muscle (biceps brachii). However, when the subjects stood on a movable platform holding on to the stabilized handle and the platform was unexpectedly perturbed, the biceps brachii onset was evident before the gastrocnemius. This study showed that the temporal relationship between muscle onsets varied with the conditions of support. It also showed that the postural muscle is not necessarily a lower limb muscle, suggesting that muscles have a stabilizing function according to the needs of the moment. It is important to consider this when training postural adjustments in standing in disabled infants and children, since the use of aids such as parallel bars will encourage arm muscles to be used as postural muscles, and this may not always be desirable.

In another study on a movable platform, adults were shown to compensate for sway caused by the platform by using a stereotyped muscle activation pattern in which EMG onsets were seen first in distal muscles, that is, those muscles closest to the base of support (Nashner and Woollacott 1979). It is interesting that this distal-to-proximal activation of muscles has been found in infants aged from $1\frac{1}{2}$ to 3 years, although the activations were rather unrefined, being longer in duration and larger in amplitude than in the adult (Forssberg and Nasher 1982; Shumway-Cook and Woollacott 1985). Physiotherapists have to reconsider the prevalent view of the primacy of proximal stability or proximal control (e.g. Perin 1989; Kidd *et al.* 1992) which has led to insufficient consideration being given to muscle activity linking fixed distal segments to the segment(s) above.

Of course, many of these studies were carried out on individuals standing on a movable platform, and undoubtedly such studies have increased our understanding of the neural control mechanisms which occur in response to support surface perturbations. However, only studies in which freely moving subjects initiate movement themselves can give us information about such movements.

3 *Vision has a proprioceptive role in postural control.* In several studies of toddlers and adults (Lee and Aronson 1974; Lee and Lishman 1975; Lestienne *et al.* 1977; Butterworth 1986) it has been shown that vision plays an important exproprioceptive (Gibson 1979) role in postural control/stabilization in adults as well as in developing children.

The term exproprioceptive is used to indicate that visual inputs can be used to give information about the position of the body in relation to the surrounding environment.

In one experiment, toddlers aged 13–16 months were stood in a room in which the walls and ceiling could be moved backwards and forwards as a single unit (Lee and Aronson 1974). When the walls moved forwards, the optic flow pattern received by the infants would have been similar to that received if they were swaying backwards. When the walls moved backwards, the opposite illusion would also have occurred. When the infants responded to the non-existent sway, they swayed, staggered or fell in the direction of the optical movement. Since the infants would have also been receiving information from their ankle proprioceptors and vestibular systems, the authors proposed that these infants, who were learning to stand, were primarily using visual cues for postural control. Butterworth and Hicks (1977) performed a similar experiment on younger infants who were capable of sitting but not standing. These infants showed a similar response to the older infants, swaying forwards or backwards at the hips according to the optical movement. Interestingly, an apparent dominance of visual information under certain conditions has also been found in adults, who, in one study (De Wit 1972), swayed laterally in phase with an oscillating luminous rod when standing in a dark room.

It is apparent, therefore, that in acquiring balance control, individuals may use vision to fine-tune muscle activations by linking vestibular and proprioceptive inputs to pertinent information in the surrounding environment (Forssberg and Nashner 1982; Lee and Lishman 1975). In addition, vision acts as a means by which the individual can judge aspects of the environment such as the vertical and horizontal, thereby maintaining appropriate body position.

Integration of visual and kinaesthetic information is reported to undergo important changes between the ages of 6 and 8 (Birch and Lefford 1963). Butterworth (1986) suggested that there is a gradual shift towards a more dominant role for the vestibular-proprioceptive system in balance control as the nervous system matures. Experience of the upright position may be important in the development of the interaction between sensory inputs for the control of motor behaviour. This point will be considered later in discussing the means by which infants with severe disability (including lesions of the CNS) can be assisted to develop control over critical functional activities, all of which take place in the erect position.

The development of gait

In order to walk independently, the human infant must coordinate its multisegmental system to achieve both forwards mobility and postural control. Mature walking has been described as having a remarkably stable, typical structure which incorporates many characteristics for each individual (Bernstein 1967). Walking manages to be stable while also being flexible and adaptive.

Historically, the focus in gait development has been on antecedent motor behaviour – those actions which are seen before independent walking, such as sitting and crawling – rather than details of the walking action itself (McGraw 1945; Shirley 1931). This focus has also been obvious in the health sciences, where it has been assumed that there is some critical causal relationship between the development of these antecedent actions and walking.

More recently, however, there have been investigations of the biomechanical pattern of walking, giving details about the changes that take place as the neonatal stepping action is transformed into a mature walking pattern. Many of these studies give quantitative data on joint rotations, step length, support base, step frequency and EMG patterns (e.g. Wickstrom, 1983; Breniere *et al.* 1989). What is becoming increasingly evident is that by the time independent walking commences, the infant already demonstrates the basic locomotor pattern which is derived from simple patterning available from birth (e.g. Thelen 1986). After the onset of independent walking the infant's walking pattern gradually matures, the details emerging as the infant practises the action in different environments.

The neonate can stand if supported with the feet in contact with the floor and will take steps if tilted slightly forwards (Fig. 2.8). This *neonatal stepping* has traditionally been considered as reflexive or primitive; it certainly appears to be elicited automatically by the way in which the

infant is held. This neonatal activity is characterized by marked hip and knee flexion with phase coupling of joint motions, a digitigrade foot strike pattern, coactivation of agonist and antagonist muscles and the need for external support to maintain postural control and initiate the gait cycle (Forssberg 1985).

It has been shown by Thelen's studies of newborn infants that there are many similarities between the movement patterns of kicking in supine and of stepping, and it has been proposed that the two actions might be the same underlying movement, but with different biomechanical demands (Thelen and Fisher 1982).

Neonatal stepping decays by the third month and until the fifth month many infants go through a period of *locomotor inactivity* when no stepping can be elicited. However, it is now known that not all infants go through this stage and there is evidence from cross-cultural and training studies that infants from certain cultures and those who are given specific practice of stepping maintain their stepping ability. In other words, child-rearing practices in which parents handle their infants and provide an environment conducive to erect posture and walking specifically with a view to assisting motor development are associated with a different sequence of development. Furthermore, in infants from a cultural group which usually displays a period of locomotor inactivity, a similar result has been found when infants are specifically trained. For example, Zelazo and his colleagues (1972) showed that practice facilitates walking.

The disappearance by the third month of the stepping reflex in certain cultural groups has been thought to result from neural maturation factors, the reflexive behaviour being inhibited by maturation of higher cortical centres (McGraw 1945). The disappearance of the so-called stepping reflex has traditionally been taken to indicate healthy maturation and, conversely, its failure to disappear taken to indicate CNS dysfunction (e.g. Peiper 1963).

Alternative explanations are now being proposed. Zelazo (1983) has proposed that so-called primitive and reflexive stepping is an innate motor pattern which becomes modified by learning. The reflex is transformed from an automatically elicited to a volitionally controlled motor behaviour through practice and experience. Thelen offers a different explanation for the apparent loss of stepping. Thelen and Cooke (1987) suggested that Zelazo's findings were the result of a general increase in the infant's leg muscle strength due to the exercise, and that the period of locomotor inactivity in many infants could be due in part to a dramatic increase in the infant's leg mass (Thelen *et al.* 1982). This view is supported by a study which showed that infants who did not step when held in standing did so when held in water when their body mass was decreased (Thelen 1983).

The transformation from a reflexive to a mature form of walking is supported by EMG and kinematic studies which show the transitions which take place (e.g. Forssberg 1985). In one study (Thelen and Cooke 1987), the relationship between newborn stepping and later walking was investigated in 18 infants who were compared at 1 and 2 months of age, at 1 and 2 months before the first independent steps, and during the month when these first steps occurred. The tight synchronization between hip, knee and ankle movements present in the first month had changed by 2 months, when the ankle joint had begun to move out of phase with the other joints. A more adult-like pattern was evident before independent walking. In the early stages of independent walking, however, some of the characteristics of newborn stepping were evident. These organizational changes, from the basic stereotyped neonatal movement pattern evident in both stepping and kicking, to independent walking, may emerge from the dynamic functional demands on the lower limbs together with increased muscle strength and postural control in standing.

EMG studies of stepping in children have shown the development from coactivation of all antagonistic leg muscles in newborns (Forssberg and Wallberg 1980) to reciprocal leg muscle activation accompanying the appearance of mature action around 5–6 years of age (Berger *et al.* 1985).

Supported locomotion develops between 6 and 9 months and at this time the infant will initiate walking when supported. Support is provided by a parent and, just before the first independent steps are taken, by the furniture, along and around which the infant cruises. There have been no studies of the dynamics of sideways walking, but it may function as a means of developing postural control while moving from one foot laterally on to the other. This would be relevant training for walking forwards, in which one of the functions bringing about gait initiation involves a shift of body weight to the stance foot. Certainly the dynamics occurring prior to the first step in walking have been shown in adults to be critical to walking by setting up the postural and dynamic conditions necessary for progression forwards (Breniere *et al.* 1987).

Independent ambulation starts from 9 months onward (Forssberg 1985). It is characterized in the early stages by a more vertical posture than in the younger infant, with decreased hip and knee flexion and a desynchronization of hip, knee and ankle joints, and increased step length with full sole contact. By approximately 5 years of age, walking has been transformed to the adult pattern (Bernstein 1967; Sutherland *et al.* 1980).

There have been several recent studies which have examined infants in the first few months after they started to walk independently. Clark and Phillips (1987) showed that infants who have been walking for 3 months exhibit a step cycle organization very similar to mature walkers, with all four Phillipson phases present. These infants also adjust to differences in walking speed in the same manner as adults. After 3–6 months of unaided walking, the infant's system seems to be tuned to gravitational demands and reactive forces (Whitall *et al.* 1985). In other words, by this stage the child has apparently discovered the essential pattern of coordination for walking, having, for example, developed the ability to apply force from mid-stance to toe-off and the ability to make use of the dynamics of the swinging limb. Taking a dynamical perspective, the infant is able to utilize energy from the late stance phase and dissipate it through the remaining phases (Kugler *et al.* 1980).

Details of the mature walking pattern in terms of the integrative action of joints and forces emerge as dynamic phenomena resulting primarily from increasing postural control and strength in the stance phase. For example, new walkers may put the foot down flat instead of heel first because they need to contact the floor fast in order not to fall over (Thelen *et al.* 1987). However, by 18 months of age, heel strike is part of their walking pattern.

New walkers lack the strength and balance to sustain the full extension at the hip which is an essential feature of the stance phase of mature walking. Hip extension is considered to be essential in setting up the conditions for the upcoming swing phase. Firstly, it provides a stretch to the hip flexor muscles just before they are activated (Inman *et al.* 1981). Secondly, hip extension sets up the segmental alignment which enables power to be generated in the plantarflexors during push-off and utilized as a major energy source for accelerating the swing leg forward (Winter 1983). New walkers cannot apparently use the viscoelastic and inertial properties of the stretched leg to initiate swing but are more likely to use excessive muscle activity. However, within 2 months of walking independently, infants show the mature pattern of knee flexion preceding hip flexion in the swing phase. New walkers lack the cushioning knee flexion movement which occurs in mature walkers in early stance. This may be due to difficulty controlling eccentric muscle activity. Several months after achieving heel strike, the early knee flexion is apparent in the stance phase (Sutherland *et al.* 1980).

Walking is a complex multisegment action, and for physiotherapists whose role is to analyse, measure and train walking in disabled infants and children, it is necessary to have an understanding of the kinematics, kinetics and muscle activation patterns in normal gait. There have been a very large number of biomechanical studies of gait, but there are several texts that serve as an introduction to the topic (Winter 1979, 1987; Inman *et al.* 1981).

Certain aspects of the biomechanics of normal walking appear to be particularly critical and Saunders and colleagues (1953) have identified what they called the 'biomechanical necessities' of walking. Carr and Shepherd (1987a) have proposed a similar list of essential components for the purposes of training (see Chapter 3). These components are principally kinematic paths of body parts and angular displacements. This emphasis on the kinematics is not to ignore the importance of being able to compare kinetic information, which deals with the forces producing the segmental movement. The value of this approach, however, is that, in the clinic, gait analysis will usually take the form of an observational analysis and it is only the kinematic elements of the movements that are directly observable. The kinetics and muscle activation patterns have to be inferred from the paths of body parts and angular displacements.

The development of prehension

The neonate at rest typically holds the hands fisted and the arms flexed. When asleep or being fed the hands are open. However, if the head and trunk are supported, the infant will spontaneously reach out the hand towards an object. The arm and hand are coupled in that, as the arm is extended, there is a tendency for the hand to open and when the arm is flexed the hand tends to close (von Hofsten 1982). This synergistic motion is also seen in the Moro reflex in which arm extension and hand-opening are followed by flexion and hand-closing, and in the traction response (Twitchell 1970).

The evidence is that neonatal arm movements are not necessarily random, which has been the traditional belief (White *et al.* 1964). Neonates make extensive arm movements and, in reaching away from their body, appear to be more effective when the infant fixates a target than when it looks elsewhere or closes the eyes. When von Hofsten (1982) videotaped newborns well-supported in a specially designed seat, he found that the arm was aimed closer to the target when the infants looked at the target than when they did not. Others have found evidence of directed arm movements towards the mouth. Butterworth (1986) noted that the mouth was open significantly more often before and throughout arm movement when the hand reached the mouth than when it did not. Furthermore, when the hand touched another part of the face first, the infant held the head still while the hand moved towards the mouth rather than getting the mouth to the hand via the rooting reflex.

Although the neonate reaches towards an object, it is not grasped, but an involuntary grasp can be elicited by placing a finger across the palm and applying gentle traction against the fingers. This grasp can be maintained for a short time and is strong enough to support the body weight if the infant is lifted from the bed. A change from the earlier reaching synergy is seen in the 2-month-old infant, who reaches towards an object very vigorously with arm extended but hand fisted (von Hofsten and Lindhagen 1979; von Hofsten 1984). By 3 months, when looking at the object, the infant opens the hand when reaching and the number of reaching attempts increases considerably (von Hofsten 1984).

The neonate's arm movements seem to be under some visual control, as it has been found that when the infant fixates an object, arm movements are aimed closer to the object than when the eyes are shut or looking elsewhere (von Hofsten 1982). Around 3 months the visual system is developing binocularity, visually guided grasping is developing and the infant watches the hands as they are moved into the visual field. Binocular sensitivity develops rapidly between 3 and 5 months of age (Fox *et al.* 1980; Birch *et al.* 1982).

Early reaching is not smoothly controlled. However, by 6 months an adult-like pattern is evident, consisting of the two elements described by Jeannerod (1984). First, there is the fast ballistic part of the movement (the transportation phase) which gets the hand to the vicinity of the object to be grasped, then the slower movement to the object during which fine adjustments are made, probably under visual control. Jeannerod studied reaching in young adults, and described the transportation component as the movement of the hand between starting position and object. The second element he termed the manipulation component, in which the grip was formed by movements of the fingers and thumb which began at the start of arm movement. The pattern of the transportation component was shown as an inverted U-shape as the hand lifted off the support, inscribing an arc before lowering on to the object. The pattern of the hand shaping was an initial increase in grip size followed by a decrease to a grip size a little larger than required for the object. Wing and Fraser (1983) found that only movement of the index finger appeared to contribute to grip formation, the position of the thumb remaining invariant throughout the movement towards the object. Infants as young as 5 months are able to supinate their hand once they have grasped the object (Fig. 2.22), but they do not reach out with the hand oriented in anticipation until a little later.

At around 3–4 months, when hand-opening is no longer stereotypically linked to reaching (arm extension) and visual binocularity is developing, the infant spends a considerable period of time watching the hands as they are moved in the visual field (White *et al.* 1964). This experience probably is critical to enable the infant to

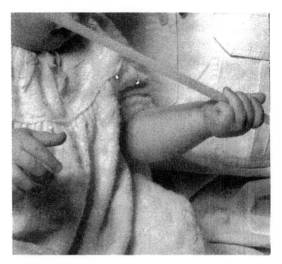

Figure 2.22 She supinates and pronates the rod once it has been grasped.

master the visually guided grasping phase of reaching. Vision assumes an increasingly important role in manipulation (Lasky 1977).

A critical element of reaching to grasp involves the orientation of the hand to fit the object (Iberall *et al.* 1986; Rosenbaum *et al.* 1990) and infants as young as 5 months have been shown to orient the hand appropriately before it reaches the object (von Hofsten and Fazel-Zandy 1984). Another critical feature of reaching to grasp is the ability to open the hand to fit the object size (Jeannerod 1981). By monitoring the distance between thumb and index finger with an optoelectronic technique during reaching, infants have been shown to adjust the opening of the hand relative to the object size by 9–13 months of age (von Hofsten and Ronnquist 1988). The adjustment was not, however, as well-organized as in adults, as the infants opened the hand more fully during the approach phase than do adults. Infants under 9 months do not appear to vary hand aperture according to the size of the object (Fig. 2.23). Young infants will not approach an object with an appropriate hand and arm orientation, nor will they vary this once the object is touched when what is to be done with the object is unclear (Fig. 2.24).

Precise timing between hand and object is critical to effective manipulation and requires visual control. The ability to time hand closure in relation to object position appears to be present in infants as young as 5 and 6 months (von

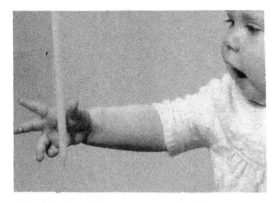

Figure 2.23 Grasp aperture is too wide and components of the hand are not aligned appropriately for the object's characteristics.

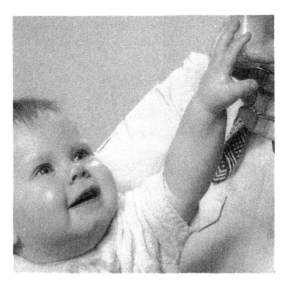

Figure 2.24 The infant reaches out for the glass of juice but cannot orient the hand appropriately to grasp it.

Hofsten and Ronnquist 1988). In these young infants, however, the hand closed when the object was touched, while in infants aged 13 months the grasping action started before touch. Data from several studies (e.g. Laszlo and Bairstow 1980) suggest that during the late preschool period, non-visual means of controlling manipulation are well-developed. Where younger children depend to a large extent on visual control, children aged 4–5 years appear to have increased kinaesthetic control.

Some ability to judge the speed with which an object is moving and to estimate its location in space – essential abilities for ball-catching, for example – appear to be present at an early age. Von Hofsten and Lindhagen (1979) found that infants as young as 18 weeks could reach for, intercept and catch quite rapidly moving (30 cm/s) objects. They were able to reach for and catch moving objects at the time when they had mastered reaching for stationary objects. Since this is a rather surprising finding, it is relevant to examine details of the methodology used by the investigators. The fact that the experimental set-up was organized to optimize the infant's chances of success provides a useful lesson for physiotherapists working with disabled infants. The infants in the study were semireclined in a seat which allowed free movement of the arms while supporting the head and trunk. The object was brightly coloured and of graspable size and shape. It moved across the baby's field of vision at a distance of 12 cm from the eyes and therefore would have been easier to pick up by young infants, with their limited visual acuity.

There are few studies of the development of bimanual activities (Fagard 1987), yet one of the challenges to the infant is to coordinate two hands in interacting with objects, which requires that the two hands act virtually as one unit in terms of temporal, spatial and muscle relationships (Figs 2.25–2.27).

Development of oral function, speech and communication

The normal neonate demonstrates several reflexive behaviours which seem to have a survival role. The *rooting reflex* is elicited by a touch to the corner of the mouth and stimulates the infant to seek the nipple. The *gag reflex*, present throughout life, is elicited by touch to the soft palate and prevents fluid and food from being aspirated. The young infant demonstrates a reflexive *suckling–swallowing* which is different from both sucking and swallowing in older infants and adults. A stimulus to the hard palate is followed by the tongue moving forwards and under the finger or teat, triggering off a rhythmic sucking action. Sucking patterns can be either extinguished or enhanced by such factors as light, loud noises and specific schedules of fluid delivery during feeding (Siqueland and

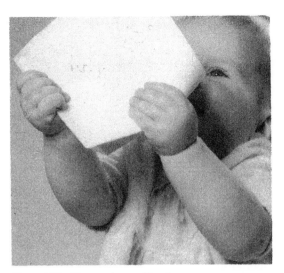

Figure 2.25 Bimanual use of hands.

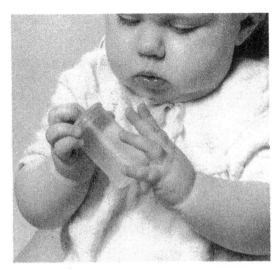

Figure 2.27 Learning to pass the object from hand to hand. Note the inappropriate alignment of components of the hand.

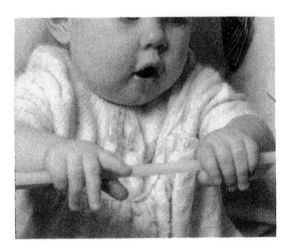

Figure 2.26 Bimanual use of hands in a different task.

DeLucia 1969; Sameroff 1970). The mechanisms of sucking, swallowing and breathing in infants are described by several authors (Logan and Bosma 1967; Sameroff 1970; Bosma 1972).

The subsequent development of tongue movement, of mature swallowing, of chewing and of coordination of respiration and swallowing enable the child to eat a greater variety of food, and to drink from a cup or straw without choking. It is also thought that the development of control over oral musculature, particularly of lips and tongue, for eating and drinking enables the development of coordinated movements for speech.

A baby starts to babble and then to talk depending on the opportunities offered for communication. This has been considered one of the reasons for the relatively poor early speech development in twins, since they mainly talk to each other (Luria and Yudovich 1959). Babies in institutions are known to be slow to babble. An infant may vocalize as early as 4–6 weeks, making small throaty sounds. By 12 weeks, these sounds are made as a means of deliberate communication and with obvious pleasure. The infant laughs at 3–4 months. By 8 months, repetitive sounds such as 'da-da' are made but at irrelevant moments. This babbling is a prelude to speech and adults instinctively reinforce it by making babbling sounds back to the infant. At 12 months, the infant knows one or two words, although in a stimulating environment the vocabulary may be greater.

It is interesting to consider the association between vocalization and movement in infancy. Vocalization tends to be associated with movement and the infant may reach a crescendo of babbling and jerky bouncing movements, vocalization and movement seeming to reinforce each other. In the older child, speech is used in play to reinforce action, and the child can be heard describing aloud the story behind the game being played.

Crying has been shown to improve lung function in the first few days of life (Long and Hull

1961). It is also the earliest form of vocal communication, triggered off by hunger, cold and pain. The stages of preverbal and verbal communication are described in detail by Sheridan (1964) and include smiling, frowning, nestling and pushing away as well as crying. In the first few weeks, crying takes on a cyclic form and it is difficult to console the infant by the usual methods. At this stage parents worry that the crying represents a failure in their nurturing, not realizing that is usually self-limiting and unavoidable. However, the tension engendered by their anxiety seems to communicate itself to the baby who may cry even more.

Development of the preterm infant

An infant born before term can survive after 25 weeks' gestational age if temperature and nutrition are adequate. A more rational use of oxygen (ensuring that it does not cause either ocular damage or mental retardation), monitored by frequent blood gas estimations, reduces the risks usually associated with prematurity. Nevertheless, the more advanced the infant's maturity, the better the chance of surviving in good condition. The infant matures similarly (there are some differences) whether *in utero* or in an incubator. At 41 weeks the neurological status is approximately the same as that of a full-term infant. The development of preterm infants appears related to biological age until approximately 18 months of age and correction for gestational age is generally considered necessary during infancy for purposes of developmental assessment (Forslund and Bjerre 1989).

The posture of preference is often used as an indicator of maturity in preterm infants (Dargassies 1977; Amiel-Tison 1968; Dubowitz and Dubowitz 1981). Preterm infants typically appear floppy (Forslund *et al.* 1989; Touwen *et al.* 1988), lying in extension in the supine position, rather than in the flexed position of the full-term neonate. There have been reports of preterm babies assuming the flexed posture over time (e.g. Dargassies 1977; Dubowitz and Dubowitz 1981). However, in one study of 15 low-risk infants between 32 and 36 weeks postmenstrual age, no dominant posture of preference was found and no correlation between posture of preference and post-menstrual age (Vles *et al.* 1989). Similar findings had been

reported in another small group of low-risk infants by Prechtl and colleagues (1979). The different findings between studies might be the result of the populations studied. The study of Dubowitz and Dubowitz (1981), for example, included neurologically abnormal infants. Vles and coworkers (1989) suggest that since low-risk healthy preterm infants show no clearly dominant preference for one particular posture in supine, the presence of a persistent posture may be an indication of abnormality.

Infants born prematurely are generally considered to be at risk for developmental delay and CNS dysfunction due to immaturity of the nervous system. The question is also raised as to whether premature infants lack readiness for extrauterine existence (Bennett *et al.* 1981; Piper *et al.* 1985).

Although there are several studies of the movement patterns of infants born prematurely, most investigations have been qualitative, reporting such variables as frequency and movement duration (e.g. Dargassies, 1977; Hines *et al.* 1980). The infant tends to be somnolent and floppy, often demonstrating tremorous, shaky movements of the arms. The Moro reflex and placing reactions are usually present, the latter from 32 weeks. The development of the premature infant, based on observational studies, is described in detail by Dargassies (1968). Carter and Campbell (1975) described the progress of one premature infant, born at 34 weeks, for the first 8 weeks of extrauterine life.

Increased extension of the lower limbs (called by some authors 'hypertonicity') is commonly considered to be a characteristic of preterm motor behaviour in the first 12 months (Dubowitz and Dubowitz 1981; Bottos and Stefani 1982; Touwen and Hadders-Algra 1983; McGrew *et al.* 1985). Its significance is the subject of considerable debate and it has been reported to have little or no apparent effect on subsequent development (Touwen and Hadders-Algra 1983) apart from a likelihood of toe-walking (Georgieff *et al.* 1986). However, it has also been suggested to limit mobility by decreasing the infant's variability of response (McGrew *et al.* 1985) and to lead to initial (but not long-term) deviances in walking (Bottos and Stefani 1982). This extensor muscle activity is said to be typical of a 28 to 30-week fetus and as due to the infant no longer being constrained in the uterus (Dubowitz and Dubowitz 1981). An interesting explanation is offered by Touwen and Hadders-Algra (1983), who point out that, since the preterm infant is predominantly nursed in extension in supine, and has relatively weak musculature, muscle growth may occur favouring the extended position. Following on from this view, it is possible that, since any movement the infant is capable of will involve extensor muscles contracting at relatively short lengths, it is possible that the tension-generating capacity of the flexor and extensor muscles will develop specifically to reflect the predominant lengths of the muscles. The characteristic extension of the infant and child who was preterm may, if this was the case, indicate the development of an adaptive muscle imbalance with the extensor muscles generating greatest force in their shortened range, and the flexor muscles contracting only weakly in the lengthened range.

There have been few biomechanical studies of the movements of preterm infants. One exception is Heriza's study of the organization of kicking in preterm infants, in which she used video analysis to determine kinematic variables, including sequencing of flexion and extension onsets at hip, knee and ankle, amplitudes and velocities of segmental angular displacements (Heriza 1988a). This was the first study to utilize these experimental methods with preterm infants and enabled a comparison of the results from these infants with a group of full-term infants (Heriza 1988b).

The Heriza study of infants born between 34 and 36 weeks' gestational age, who were in the low-risk category, showed that these infants had highly organized leg movements that changed little between birth and 40 weeks post gestational age. When the movements of these infants were compared with the full-term infants, Heriza found that all the infants showed a close temporal and spatial synchronization between the lower limb joints, indicating that movement topography was similar whether infants were premature or full-term. The full-term infants did, however, kick more than the preterm. The full-term infants were also more flexed, that is, did not kick out into as much extension as the full-term infants.

The major changes that occurred over time in these infants were decreases in amplitude and peak velocity of joint angular displacements. Heriza suggested that these results sup-

port the view that movement emerges as a result not only of a pattern of neuromuscular activations but also out of gravitational, reactive and inertial forces. Morphological factors such as limb mass and length, muscle properties such as extensibility and muscle strength may, therefore, be responsible for the changes noted and not only neural maturation.

It is not known whether at-risk or neurologically impaired infants would show the same kinematic movement patterns. Future studies should be designed to answer these questions, since such information would have diagnostic relevance. Kinematic investigations could also be designed to study the organization of joint angular displacements and the relationship between the joints of the lower limb before and after early intervention to improve lower limb movement.

Social and environmental effects on motor development

As Hopkins and Westra (1988) point out, motor development has been considered a maturational phenomenon distinct from environmental influences, particularly for everyday actions such as sitting and walking. The importance of environmental effects and experience on motor development is, however, revealed by comparative studies of development in a range of different cultures (Bril 1986). These studies have largely involved ecological and anthropological observations. Child-rearing and training practices from birth onwards have been shown to influence rates of motor development, particularly in the first year or 18 months of life.

This information is of significance to physiotherapists, not just in terms of increasing our understanding of different cultures, which is important for physiotherapists involved with infants from cultures different from their own. More importantly, it shows what *training* and *practice* can accomplish in infants and is, therefore, of great significance to physiotherapists working towards increasing the skill of disabled children in such critical actions as reaching in sitting and standing, walking and manipulating objects. Another implication from this research is that culturally unsuitable items should be excluded during testing.

The long-held view that infants will develop despite specific environmental influences (Buhler 1935) is now being challenged and many studies have illustrated the differences in rate of motor development across different cultures. Furthermore, it appears that in the Euro-American culture from which the original subjects in the development of scales such as the Bayley were taken, there have also been changes, with modern infants achieving motor milestones ahead of the traditional norms (Gesell *et al*. 1940; Capute *et al*. 1985).

The so-called precocity of infants in different cultures can usually be reduced to precocity in specific motor actions rather than an overall precocity. For example, babies of African descent have been shown to be ahead of Caucasian babies specifically in sitting, standing alone and walking (Super 1976; Konner 1977; Hopkins and Westra 1988). That specific handling practices or training of specific actions should affect these actions is not surprising given the evidence elsewhere of the effects of specific training on muscle strength and motor learning (e.g. Rasch and Morehouse 1957; Sale and McDougall 1981). Motor development is, in a sense, the result of learning, and skill in actions, even such everyday actions as reaching out in sitting and walking, could be expected to improve with practice. The opportunity for practice is made available to infants by their parents, whether by particular cultural practices (for example, being carried on the mother's back while she works), the environment or by specific training (e.g. optimizing sitting behaviour).

Cross-cultural and intracultural studies increase our understanding of the roles played by practice and training, parental handling and the environment and provide insights for physiotherapists working clinically with the objective of optimizing motor performance in movement-disabled infants and children.

Infants in the Yucatán, Mexico, have been found to be ahead of their North American peers in manipulative skills, for example using a fine pincer grasp before the age of 9 months (Solomons and Solomons 1975). These infants are rarely placed on the floor, perhaps due to the floor being cool tiles or earth (depending on socioeconomic level) or perhaps the tradition of cleanliness in this group. They are, however, relatively slow to walk and the investigators point out that there is little for an unsteady infant to hold on to in many of the houses.

Japanese children under 1 year in Okinawa have been noted to develop actions which require the ability to bear weight through the lower limbs earlier than children in Tokyo (Ueda 1978). Infants of African descent appear to be precocious in comparison to Caucasian infants in controlling antigravity muscle activity and therefore advanced in gaining control of the head and trunk in vertical postures such as sitting and standing. Kenyan Kipsigi infants and San infants in the Kalahari desert of Botswana have been shown to be advanced in actions that were subject to formal instruction and could be practised, namely sitting and walking (Super 1976; Konner 1977). The Kenyan babies' mothers believed it was important to train sitting and they set up the conditions for this by scooping out a hole in the soil into which the infant was sat. Caesar (1976) showed that postural development (head control) in Dutch neonates was influenced by maternal handling.

There have been relatively few *intracultural studies* in which different child-rearing practices are investigated for the same cultural group. However, Lagerspetz and colleagues (1971) have shown that infant crawling could be facilitated by particular exercise and Zelazo and colleagues (1972) that neonatal stepping is susceptible to training.

In another study, Hopkins and Westra (1988) showed the effects of formalized exercise and handling on motor development in a study of babies born to Jamaican mothers in England. The infants were divided into two groups according to whether or not their mothers had given them a specific routine of exercise and handling traditional among Jamaican families. By 1 month of age, the infants who were exercised had better control of the head when pulled to sitting from supine than the other infants. By 6 months, the exercised group were superior at independent sitting and were more advanced when held in standing. There was no difference between the two groups in manipulation or crawling. Jamaican mothers place particular emphasis on their infant's ability to sit alone. At 3–4 months infants are sat propped up against a cushion that is gradually removed as the baby shows the ability to sit upright. In addition, stepping is elicited early.

McGraw, in her study of twins (1935), practised crawling and walking with one twin,

Johnny, but not with the other, Jimmy. Interestingly, Jimmy crawled before Johnny, and there was no difference in the age at which the two walked. However, the style of early walking appeared to be influenced by the practice.

It may be, therefore, that although providing an infant or child with the opportunity to practise will enable the child to make use of inherent abilities, such practice is unlikely to accelerate the process of maturation.

Effects of parental expectations

Parents seem to have clear expectations regarding the attainment of major motor milestones such as the onset of independent sitting and walking (Hopkins and Westra 1989). That these expectations may guide parental behaviour during child-rearing is an important consideration for a physiotherapist who may require to modify some aspects of parental behaviour for the purpose of training specific motor actions in a disabled infant. For example, a parent who believes that taking weight through the feet too early will cause the infant to develop bowing of the legs may be reluctant to help the infant practise standing and stepping.

In a study comparing Jamaican and English mothers whose babies were born in England, Jamaican mothers' predictions of the onset of independent sitting and walking in their 1-month-old infants were significantly earlier than those of English mothers (Hopkins and Westra 1989). Furthermore, the actual ages at which these events subsequently were attained were also significantly earlier in the Jamaican group (mean age of sitting: 6 months; of walking: 11 months), supporting earlier studies which found African infants to be precocious in these actions. Whereas the Jamaican mothers were better at predicting sitting age, the English mothers were better at predicting crawling age. When asked about their preferred choice for seeking information about child-rearing, the Jamaican women cited their own mothers and family members, whereas the English women gave reading material as their first choice. These findings are interesting in that they suggest that, for one generation of immigrants at least, traditional theories of child-rearing and development are resistant to social change.

Summary

This chapter examines some of the traditional views of motor development based on observational studies of infants and children and compares them with the findings from studies of developmental biomechanics, acquisition of motor skill and the child-rearing practices of different cultural groups. An up-to-date understanding of the changes that occur as skill develops provides a background for therapeutic intervention. Although information related to the approximate ages at which marked changes occur has some value, information related to performance of common actions provides a guide to analysis and training of disabled infants. The gradual increase in investigative studies of motor performance and the insights gained about the effects of parental expectations on quality of performance from child-rearing studies enable us to develop new and more informed methods of physiotherapy intervention.

References

Abitbol, M.M. (1993) Quadrupedalism and the acquisition of bipedalism in human children. *Gait & Posture*, **1**, 189–195.

Amiel-Tison, C. (1968) Neurological evaluation of the maturity of newborn infants. *Arch. Dis. Child.*, **43**, 89–93.

Basmajian, J.V. (1977) Motor learning and control. *Arch. Phys. Med. Rehabil.*, **58**, 38–41.

Bayley, N. (1969) *The Bayley Scales of Infant Development.* New York: The Psychological Corporation.

Belenkii, V.E., Gurfinkel, V.S. and Paltsev, R.I. (1967) On the elements of voluntary movement control. *Biofizika*, **12**, 135.

Bennett, F.C., Chandler, L.S. and Robinson, N.M. (1981) Spastic diplegia in premature infants: etiologic and diagnostic considerations. *Am. J. Dis. Child.*, **135**, 732–736.

Berger, W., Quintern, J. and Dietz, V. (1985) Stance and gait perturbations in children: developmental aspects of compensatory mechanisms. *Electroencephalogr. Clin. Neurophysiol.*, **61**, 385–395.

Bernstein, N. (1967) *Coordination and Regulation of Movements.* New York: Pergamon.

Birch, H.G. and Lefford, A. (1963) Intersensory development in children. *Monogr. Soc. Res. Child Dev.*, **28**, 2–27.

Birch, E.E., Gwiazda, J. and Held, R. (1982) Stereoacuity development for crossed and uncrossed disparities in human infants. *Vision Res.*, **22**, 507–513.

Bobath, B. (1971) *Abnormal Postural Reflex Activity Caused by Brain Lesions.* London: Heinemann.

Bobath, K. and Bobath B. (1964) The facilitation of normal postural reactions and movements in the treatment of cerebral palsy. *Physiotherapy*, **50**, 8, 246.

Bosma, J.F. (1972) Form and function in the infant's mouth and pharynx. In: *Third Symposium on Oral Sensation and Perception*, edited by J.F. Bosma. Springfield, IL: Charles C. Thomas.

Bottos, M. and Stefani, D. (1982) Postural and motor care of the premature baby. *Dev. Med. Child Neurol.*, **24**, 706–707.

Bouisset, S. and Zattara, M. (1981) A sequence of postural movements precedes voluntary movements. *Neurosci. Lett.*, **22**, 263–270.

Bower, T.G.R., Broughton, J.M. and Moore, M.K. (1970) The coordination of visual and tactual input in infants. *Percept Psychophys.*, **8**, 51.

Bradley, N.S. (1990) Animal models offer the opportunity to acquire a new perspective on motor development. *Phys. Ther.*, **70**, 12, 776–787.

Breniere, Y., Do, M.C. and Bouisset, S. (1987) Are dynamic phenomena prior to stepping essential to walking? *J. Mot. Behav.*, **19**, 1, 62–76.

Breniere, Y., Bril, B. and Fontaine, R. (1989) Analysis of the transition from upright stance to steady state locomotion in children with under 200 days of autonomous walking. *J. Mot. Behav.*, **21**, 1, 20–37.

Bril, B. (1986) Motor development and cultural attitudes. In: *Themes in Motor Development*, edited by H.T.A. Whiting and M.G. Wade. Dordrecht: Martinus Nijhoff.

Bruner, J.S. (1973) Organisation of early skilled action. *Child Dev.*, **44**, 1–11.

Buhler, C. (1935) *From Birth to Maturity*. London: Kegan Paul.

Butterworth, G. (1986) Some problems in explaining the origins in movement control. In: *Motor Development in Children. Problems of Coordination and Control*, edited by M.G. Wade and H.T.A. Whiting. Dordrecht: Martinus Nijhoff, pp. 23–32.

Butterworth, G. and Hicks, L. (1977) Visual proprioception and postural stability in infancy: a developmental study. *Perception*, **6**, 255.

Caesar, P. (1976) *Postural Behavior in Newborn Infants*. Leuven: Acco.

Capute, A.J., Shapiro, B.K., Palmer, F.B., Ross, A. and Wachtel, R.C. (1985) Normal gross motor development: the influences of race, sex and socio-economic status. *Dev. Med. Child Neurol.*, **27**, 635.

Carr, J.H. and Shepherd, R.B. (1987a) *A Motor Relearning Programme for Stroke*, 2nd edn. Oxford: Butterworth-Heinemann.

Carr, J.H. and Shepherd, R.B. (eds) (1987b) *Movement Science, Foundations for Physical Therapy in Rehabilitation*. Oxford: Butterworth-Heinemann.

Carr, J.H. and Shepherd, R.B. (1990) A motor learning model for rehabilitation of the movement-disabled. In: *Key Issues in Neurological Physiotherapy*, edited by L. Ada and C. Canning. Oxford: Butterworth Heineman.

Carter, R.E. and Campbell, S.K. (1975) Early neuromuscular development of the premature infant. *Phys. Ther.*, **55**, 12, 1332.

Cavagna, G.A. (1977). Storage and utilization of elastic energy in skeletal muscle. *Exerc. Sport Sci. Rev.*, **5**, 89–129.

Clark, J.E. and Phillips, S.J. (1987) The step cycle organisation of infant walkers. *J. Mot. Behav.*, **19**, 4, 421–433.

Connolly, K.S. (1973) Factors influencing the learning of manual skills by young children. In: *Constraints on Learning*, edited by R.A. Hinde and J. Stevenson-Hinde. London: Academic Press.

Connolly, K. and Stratton, P. (1968) Developmental changes in associated movements. *Dev. Med. Child Neurol.*, **10**, 49–56.

Cordo, P.J. and Nashner, L.M. (1982) Properties of postural adjustments associated with rapid arm movements. *J. Neurophysiol.*, **47**, 287.

Dargassies, S. S.A. (1968) *The Development of the Nervous System in the Foetus*. Geneva: Nestlé.

Dargassies, S. St-Anne (1977) *Neurological Development in the Full-Term and Premature Infant*. New York: Elsevier Science.

Delacato, C.H. (1966) *Neurological Organization and Reading*. Springfield, IL: Charles C. Thomas.

De Vries, J.I.P., Visser, G.H.A. and Prechtl, H.F.R. (1982) The emergence of fetal behavior: 1. Qualitative aspects. *Early Hum. Dev.*, **7**, 301–322.

De Wit, G. (1972) Optic versus vestibular and proprioceptive impulses measured by posturometry. *Agressologie.*, **13**, 75–79.

Dubowitz, V. and Dubowitz, L. (1981) *The Neurological Assessment of the Preterm and Full-Term Infant*. Philadelphia, PA: J.B. Lippincott.

Eckersley, P. and King, L. (1993) Treatment systems. In: *Elements of Paediatric Physiotherapy*, edited by P.M. Eckersley. London: Churchill Livingstone, pp. 323–341.

Fagard, J. (1987) Bimanual stereotypes: bimanual coordination in children as a function of movements and relative velocity. *J. Motor Behav.*, **19**, 3, 355–366.

Fentress, J.C. (1981) Order in ontogeny: relational dynamics. In: *Behavioral Development: The Bielefeld Interdisciplinary Project*, edited by K. Immelmann, G.W. Barlow, I. Petrinovich *et al.* Cambridge: Cambridge University Press.

Flament, D., Hall, E.J., Lemon, R.N. and Simpson, M. (1990) The development of cortically evoked responses in infant Macaque monkeys studied with electromagnetic brain stimulation. *J. Physiol.*, **426**, 105.

Fog, E. and Fog, M. (1963) Cerebral inhibition examined by associated movements. In: *Minimal Cerebral Dysfunction. Clinics in Developmental Medicine 10*, edited by M. Bax and R.C. MacKeith. London: Heinemann.

Forslund, M. and Bjerre, I. (1989) Follow-up of preterm children 1. Neurological assessment at 4 years of age. *Early Hum. Dev.*, **20**, 45–66.

Forssberg, H. (1985) Ontogeny of human locomotor control. 1: Infant stepping, supported locomotion, and transition to independent locomotion. *Exp. Brain Res.*, **57**, 480–493.

Forssberg, H. and Wallberg, H. (1980) Infant locomotion: a preliminary movement and electromyographic study. In: *Children and Exercise IX*, edited by K. Berg and B.O. Eriksson. Baltimore, MD: University Park Press, pp. 32–40.

Forssberg, H. and Nasher, L.M. (1982) Ontogenetic development of posture control in man: adaptation to altered support and visual conditions during stance. *J. Neurosci.*, **2**, 545–552.

Fox, R., Aslin, R.N., Shea, S.L. and Dumais, S.T. (1980) Stereopsis in human infants. *Science*, **207**, 323–324.

Gahery, Y. and Massion, J. (1981) Coordination between posture and movement. *Trends Neurosci.*, **4**, 199.

Gentile, A.M. (1987) Skill acquisition: action, movement, and neuromotor processes. In: *Movement Science. Foundations for Physical Therapy in Rehabilitation*, edited by J.H. Carr and R.B. Shepherd. Rockville, MD: Aspen.

Georgieff, M.K., Bernbaum, J.C., Hoffman-Williamson, M. and Daft, A. (1986) Abnormal truncal muscle tone as a useful early marker for development delay in low birth weight infants. *Pediatrics*, **77**, 659–663.

Gesell, A. (1928) *Infancy and Human Growth*. New York: Macmillan.

Gesell, A., Halverson, H., Thompson, H., Castner, B., Ames, L. and Amatruda, A. (1940) *The First Five Years of Life*. New York: Harper and Row.

Gibson, J.J. (1979) *The Ecological Approach to Visual Perception*. Boston, MA: Houghton Mifflin.

Glencross, D.J. (1977) Control of skilled movement. *Psychol. Bull.*, **84**, 14–29.

Green, E.M. and Nelham, R.L. (1991) Development of sitting ability, assessment of children with a motor handicap and prescription of appropriate seating systems. *Prosthet. Orthot. International*, **15**, 203–216.

Gregoire, L., Veeger, P.A., Huijing, P.A. and van Ingen Schenau, G.J. (1984) Role of mono- and biarticular muscles in explosive movements. *Int. J. Sports Med.*, **5**, 301–305.

Halverson, H.M. (1931) Study of prehension in infants. *Genet. Psychol. Monogr.*, **10**, 107–285.

Halverson, H.M. (1933) The acquisition of skill in infancy. *J. Genet. Psychol.*, **43**, 3–48.

Hein, A. (1974). Prerequisite for development of visually guided reaching in the kitten. *Brain Res.*, **71**, 259–263.

Held, R. and Hein, A. (1976) Movement produced stimulation in the development of visually guided behavior. *J. Compar. Physiol. Psychol.*, **37**, 87–95.

Heriza, C.B. (1988a) Organisation of leg movements in preterm infants. *Phys. Ther.*, **68**, 9, 1340–1346.

Heriza, C.B. (1988b) Comparison of leg movements in preterm infants at term with healthy full-term infants. *Phys. Ther.*, **68**, 11, 1687–1693.

Higgins, J.R. and Spaeth, R.K. (1972) Relationship between consistency of movement and environmental condition. *Quest*, **17**, 61–69.

Hines, R.B., Minde, K., Marton, P. *et al.* (1980) Behavioral development of premature infants: an ethological approach. *Dev. Med. Child Neurol.*, **22**, 623–632.

Hirschfeld, H. (1992) Postural control: acquisition and integration during development. In: *Movement Disorders in Children*, edited by H. Forssberg and H. Hirschfeld. Basel: Karger, pp. 199–208.

Holt, K.S. (1977) *Developmental Paediatrics Perspectives and Practice*. London: Butterworth.

Hopkins, B. and Westra, T. (1988) Maternal handling and motor development: an intracultural study. *Genet. Soc. Gen. Psychol. Monogr.*, **114**, 379.

Hopkins, B. and Westra, T. (1989) Maternal expectations of their infants' development: some cultural differences. *Dev. Med. Child Neurol.*, **31**, 384.

Iberall, T., Bingham, G, and Arbib, M.A. (1986) Opposition space as a structuring concept for the analysis of skilled hand movements. *Exper. Brain Res. Suppl.*, **15**, 153.

Inman, V.T., Ralston, H.J. and Todd, F. (1981) *Human Walking*. Baltimore, MD: Williams & Wilkins.

Jeannerod, M. (1981) Intersegmental coordination during reaching at natural objects. In: *Attention and Performance IX*, edited by J. Long and A. Badderley. Hillsdale, NJ: Erlbaum, pp. 153–169.

Jeannerod, M. (1984) The timing of natural prehension movement. *J. Mot. Behav.*, **26**, 3, 235–254.

Jensen, J.L., Thelen, E. and Ulrich, B.D. (1989) Constraints on multi-joint movements: from the spontaneity of infancy to the skill of adults. *Hum. Mov. Sci.*, **8**, 393–402.

Katona, F. (1989) Clinical neurodevelopmental diagnosis and treatment. In: *Challenges to Developmental Paradigms: Implications for Theory, Assessment, and Treatment*, edited by P.R. Zelazo and R. Barr. Hillsdale, NJ: Lawrence Erlbaum, pp. 167–187.

Kelso, J.A.S. and Clark, J.E. (eds) (1982) *The Development of Movement Control and Co-ordination*. New York: John Wiley.

Kelso, J.A.S. and Tuller, B. (1984) A dynamical basis for action systems. In: *Handbook of Cognitive Neuroscience*, edited by M.S. Gazzaniga. New York: Plenum.

Kelso, J.A.S., Putnam, C.A. and Goodman, D. (1983) On the space–time structure of human interlimb co-ordination. *Q. J. Exp. Psychol.*, **35A**, 347–375.

Kidd, G., Lawes, N. and Musa, I. (1992) *Understanding Neuromuscular Plasticity. A Basis for Clinical Rehabilitation*. London: Edward Arnold, p. 102.

Konner, M. (1977) Maternal care and infant behavior and development among the Kalahari Desert San. In: *Kalahari Hunter Gatherers*, edited by R. Lee and I. deVore. Cambridge, MA: Harvard University Press.

Kuypers, H.G.J.M. (1982) A new look at the organisation of the motor system. *Prog. Brain Res.*, **57**, 381–404.

Lagerspetz, K., Nygard, M. and Strandvik, C. (1971) The effects of training in crawling on the motor and mental development of infants. *Scand. J. Psychol.*, **12**, 192.

Lasky, R.E. (1977) The effect of visual feedback of the hand on the reaching and retrieval behaviour of young infants. *Child Dev.*, **48**, 112–117.

Laszlo, J.I. and Bairstow, P.J. (1980) The measurement of kinesthetic sensitivity in children and adults. *Dev. Med. Child Neurol.*, **22**, 454–464.

Lee, W. (1980) Anticipatory control of postural and task muscles during rapid arm flexion. *J. Mot. Behav.*, **12**, 185–196.

Lee, D.N. and Aronson, E. (1974) Visual proprioceptive control of standing in human infants. *Percept. Psychophys.*, **15**, 529.

Lee, D.N. and Lishman, J.R. (1975) Visual proprioceptive control of stance. *J. Hum. Movement Stud.*, **1**, 87–95.

Leonard, E.L. (1990) Early motor development and control: foundations for independent walking. In: *Gait in Rehabilitation*, edited by G.L. Smidt. New York: Churchill Livingstone.

Lestienne, F., Soechting, J. and Berthoz, A. (1977) Postural readjustments induced by linear motion of visual scenes. *Exper. Brain Res.*, **28**, 363–384.

Logan, W.J. and Bosma, J.F. (1967) Oral and pharyngeal dysphagia in infancy. *Pediatr. Clin. North Am.*, **14**, 47.

Long, E.C. and Hull, W.E. (1961) Respiratory volume flow in the crying newborn infant. *Pediatrics*, **27**, 373.

Luria, A.R. and Yudovich, F.I. (1959) *Speech and Development of Mental Processes in the Child*. London: Staples Press.

McGraw, M.B. (1935) *Growth: A Study of Johnny and Jimmy*. New York: Appleton-Crofts.

McGraw, M.B. (1945) *The Neuromuscular Maturation of the Human Infant*. New York: Columbia University Press.

McGrew, L., Catlin, P.A. and Bridgford, A. (1985) The Landau reaction in fullterm and preterm infants at 4 months of age. *Dev. Med. Child Neurol.*, **27**, 161–169.

Milani-Comparetti, A. (1980) Pattern analysis of normal and abnormal development: the fetus, the newborn, the child. In: *Development of Movement in Infancy*, edited by D.S. Slaton. Chapel Hill, SC: University of Southern Carolina Press.

Moss, S.C. and Hogg, J. (1983) The development and integration of fine motor sequences in 12- to 18-month-old children: a test of the modular theory of motor skill acquisition. *Genet. Psychol. Monogr.*, **107**, 145–187.

Nashner, L.M. (1982) Adaptation of human movement to altered environments. *Trends Neurosci.*, **5**, 358–361.

Nashner, L.M. and Woollacott, M. (1979) The organisation of rapid postural adjustments of standing humans: an experimental–conceptual model. In: *Posture and Movement*, edited by R.E. Talbot and D.R. Humphrey. New York: Raven Press.

O'Connell, A.L. (1972) *Understanding the Scientific Basis for Human Movement*. Baltimore, MD: Williams & Wilkins.

Oddsson, L. and Thorstensson, A. (1986) Fast voluntary trunk flexion movements in standing: primary movements and associated postural adjustments. *Acta Physiol. Scand.*, **128**, 341–349.

Peiper, A. (1963) *Cerebral Function in Infancy and Childhood*. New York: Consultants Bureau.

Perin, B. (1989) Physical therapy for the child with cerebral palsy. In: *Pediatric Physical Therapy*, edited by J.S. Tecklin. Philadelphia, PA: J.B. Lippincott, pp. 68–105.

Piper, M.C., Kunos, J. and Willis, D.M. (1985) Effect of gestational age on neurological functioning of the very low-birthweight infant at 40 weeks. *Dev. Med. Child Neurol.*, **27**, 596–605.

Prechtl, H.F.R., Fargel, J.W., Weinmann, H.M. and Bakker, H.H. (1979) Postures, motility and respiration of low-risk pre-term infants. *Dev. Med. Child Neurol.*, **21**, 3–27.

Rasch, P.T. and Morehouse, L.E. (1957) Effect of static and dynamic exercise on muscular strength and hypertrophy. *J. Appl. Physiol.*, **11**, 29–34.

Reed, E.S. (1982) An outline of a theory of action systems. *J. Mot. Behav.*, **14**, 98–134.

Roberton, M.A. (1978) Stages in motor development. In: *Motor Development: Issues and Applications*, edited by M.C. Ridenour. Princeton, NJ: Princeton Books.

Robson, P. (1984) Prewalking locomotor movements and their use in predicting standing and walking. *Child: Care Health Dev.*, **10**, 317–330.

Rosenbaum, D.A., Vaughan, J., Barnes, H.J., Marchak, F. and Slotta, J. (1990) Constraints on action selection: over-hand versus underhand grips. In: *Attention and Performance*, edited by M. Jeannerod. Hillsdale, NJ: Erlbaum, pp. 321–342.

Rosenbloom, J. and Horton, M. (1971) Maturation of fine prehension in young children. *Dev. Med. Child Neurol.*, **13**, 3.

Sale, D. and McDougall, D. (1981) Specificity in muscle strength training: a review for the coach and athlete. *Can. J. Appl. Sports Sci.*, **6**, 87–92.

Sameroff, A.J. (1970) Changes in the non-nutritive sucking response to stimulation during infancy. *J. Exp. Child Psychol.*, **10**, 112.

Saunders, J.B., Inman, V.T. and Eberhart, H.D. (1953) The major determinants in normal and pathological gait. *J. Bone Joint Surg.*, **35-A**, 543–558.

Shepherd, R.B. and Carr, J.H. (1991) An emergent or dynamical systems view of movement dysfunction. *Aust. J. Physiother.*, **37**, 1, 4–5, 17.

Shepherd, R.B., Crosbie, W.C. and Squire, T. (1994) The contribution of the ipsilateral leg to postural adjustment during fast voluntary reaching in sitting. *J. Biomech.*, **27**, 742.

Sheridan, M.D. (1964) Disorders of communication in young children. *Monthly Bull. Min. Health Lab. Serv.*, **23**, 20.

Shirley, M.M. (1931) *The First Two Years: A Study of Twenty-five Babies. Vol. 1 Postural and Locomotor Development*. Minneapolis: University of Minnesota Press.

Shumway-Cook, A. and Woollacott, M. (1985) The growth of stability: postural control from a developmental perspective. *J. Motor. Behav.*, **17**, 131.

Siqueland, E.R. and DeLucia, C.A. (1969) Visual reinforcement of non-nutritive sucking in human infants. *Science*, **165**, 1144.

Solomons, G. and Solomons, H.C. (1975) Motor development in Yucatecan infants. *Dev. Med. Child Neurol.*, **17**, 41.

Sparrow, W.A. and Zrizarry-Lopez, V.M. (1987) Mechanical efficiency and metabolic cost as measures of learning a novel gross motor task. *J. Motor Behav.* **19**, 240–264.

Super, C.M. (1976) Environmental effects on motor development: the case of 'African infant precocity'. *Dev. Med. Child Neurol.*, **18**, 561.

Sutherland, D.H., Olshen, R., Cooper, L. and Woo, S.L.Y. (1980) The development of mature gait. *J. Bone Joint Surg.*, **62A**, 336–353.

Thelen, E. (1983) Learning to walk is still an 'old' problem: a reply to Zelazo (1983). *J. Motor Behav.*, **15**, 99–137.

Thelen, E. (1986) Treadmill-elicited stepping in seven-month-old infants. *Child Dev.*, **57**, 1498–1506.

Thelen, E. and Cooke, D.W. (1987) Relationship between newborn stepping and later walking: a new interpretation. *Dev. Med. Child. Neurol.*, **29**, 380–393.

Thelen, E. and Fisher, D.M. (1982) Newborn stepping: an explanation for a 'disappearing reflex'. *Dev. Psychology*, **18**, 760–775.

Thelen, E. and Lockman, J.C. (eds) (1993) Special section: developmental biodynamics: brain, body, behavior connection. Child Develop., **64**, 4, 953–1173.

Thelen, E., Fisher, D.M., Ridley-Johnson R. and Griffin N.J. (1982). Effects of body build and arousal on newborn infant stepping. *Developmental Psychobiology*, **15**, 5, 447–453.

Thelen, E., Kelso, J.A.S. and Fogel, A. (1987) Self-organising systems and infant motor development. *Dev. Rev.*, **11**, 39–65.

Todor, J.I. and Lazarus, J.C. (1986) Exertion level and the intensity of associated movements. *Dev. Med. Child Neurol.*, **28**, 205–212.

Touwen, B.C.L. and Hadders-Algra, M. (1983). Hyperextension of neck and trunk and shoulder retraction in infancy – a prognostic study. *Neuropediatrics*, **14**, 202–205.

Touwen, B.C. and Prechtl, H.F. (1970) *The Neurological Examination of the Child with Minor Nervous System Dysfunction*. Clinics in Developmental Medicine 38. London: SIMP with Heinemann Medical.

Touwen, B.C.L., Hadders-Algra, M. and Huisjes, J.H. (1988) Hypotonia at 6 years in prematurely-born or small-for-gestational-age children. *Early Hum. Dev.*, **17**, 79–88.

Twitchell, T.E. (1970) Reflex mechanisms and the development of prehension. In: *Mechanisms of Motor Skill Development*, edited by K.J. Connolly. London: Academic Press.

Ueda, R. (1978) Child development in Okinawa compared with Tokyo and Denver, and the implications for developmental screening. *Dev. Med. Child Neurol.*, **20**, 657.

Vles, J.S.H., Kingma, H., Caberg, H. *et al.* (1989). Posture of low-risk preterm infants between 32 and 36 weeks postmenstrual age. *Dev. Med. Child Neurol.*, **31**, 191–195.

von Hofsten, C. (1982) Eye–hand coordination in newborns. *Dev. Psychology*, **18**, 450.

von Hofsten, C. (1984) Developmental changes in the organisation of pre-reaching movements. *Dev. Psychology*, **20**, 378.

von Hofsten, C. and Lindhagen, K. (1979) Observations on the development of reaching for moving objects. *J. Exp. Child Psychol.*, **28**, 158.

von Hofsten, C. and Fazel-Zandy, S. (1984) Development of visually-guided hand orientation in reaching. *J. Exp. Child Psychol.*, **38**, 208.

von Hofsten, C. and Ronnquist, L. (1988) Preparation for grasping an object: a developmental study. *J. Exp. Psychol: Hum. Percept. Perform.*, **14**, 610–621.

Wade, M.G. and Whiting, H.T.A. (eds) (1986) *Motor Development in Children: Aspects of Coordination and Control*. Dordrecht: Martinus Nijhoff.

Walshe, F.M.R. (1923) Certain tonic or postural reflexes in hemiplegia with special reference to the so-called 'associated movements'. *Brain*, **1**, 46, 1–37.

Whitall, J., Clark, J.E. and Phillips, S.J. (1985) Interaction of postural and oscillatory mechanisms in the development of interlimb coordination of upright bipedal locomotion. Paper presented at North American Soc. for the Psych. of Sport and Phys. Activity. Long Beach, Mississippi.

White, B.L., Castle, P. and Held, R. (1964) Observations on the development of visually-directed reaching. *Child Dev.*, **35**, 349–364.

Whiting, H.T.A. and Wade, M.G. (eds) (1986) *Themes in Motor Development*. Dordrecht: Martinus Nijhoff.

Wickstrom, R.L. (1983) *Fundamental Motor Patterns*. Philadelphia: Lea & Febiger.

Wilson, J.M. (1991) Cerebral palsy. In: *Pediatric Neurologic Physical Therapy*, edited by S.K. Campbell, 2nd edn. New York: Churchill Livingstone.

Wing, A.M. and Fraser, C. (1983) The contribution of the thumb to reaching movements. *Q. J. Exp. Psychol.*, **35A**, 297–309.

Winter, D.A. (1979) *Biomechanics of Human Movement*. New York: John Wiley.

Winter, D.A. (1983) Biomechanical motor patterns in normal walking. *J. Motor Behav.*, **15**, 302–330.

Winter, D.A. (1987) *The Biomechanics and Motor Control of Human Gait*. Waterloo, Ontario: University of Waterloo Press.

Wolff, P.H., Gunnoe, C.E. and Cohen, C. (1983) Associated movements as a measure of developmental age. *Dev. Med. Child Neurol.*, **25**, 417–429.

Woollacott, M.H. (1986) Postural control and development. In: *Themes in Motor Development*, edited by H.T.A. Whiting and M.G. Wade. Dordrecht: Martinus Nijhoff.

Wynn-Parry, C.B. (1966) *Rehabilitation of the Hand*, 2nd edn. London: Butterworth.

Zattara, M. and Bouisset, S. (1986) Chronometric analysis of the posturo-kinetic programming of voluntary movement. *J. Motor Behav.*, **18**, 215–225.

Zelazo, P.R. (1983) The development of walking: new findings and old assumptions. *J. Motor Behav.*, **15**, 99–137.

Zelazo, P.R., Zelazo, N.A. and Kolb, S. (1972) 'Walking' in the newborn. *Science*, **176**, 314.

Zernicke, R.F. and Schneider, K. (1993) Biomechanics and developmental neuromotor control. *Child Develop.*, **64**, 982–1004.

Further reading

Adolph, K.E., Eppler, M.A. and Gibson, E.J. (1993) Crawling versus walking infants' perception of affordances for locomotion over sloping surfaces. *Child Develop.*, **64**, 1158–1174.

Berger, W., Discher, M., Trippel, M., Ibrahim, I.K. and Dietz, V. (1992). Developmental aspects of stance regulation, compensation and adaptation. *Exp. Brain Res.*, **90**, 610–619.

Bower, T. (1966) The visual world of infants. *Sci. Am.*, **215**, 80.

Bower, T.G.R. (1976) Repetitive processes in child development. *Sci. Am.*, **235**, 38–47.

Bushnell, E.W. and Boudreau, J.P. (1993) Motor development and the mind: the potential role of motor abilities as a determinant of aspects of perceptual development. *Child Develop.*, **64**, 1005–1021.

Connolly, K. (1975) Movement action, skill. In: *Movement and Child Development*, edited by K.S. Holt. London: Heinemann.

Gatev, V. (1972) Role of inhibition in the development of motor co-ordination in early childhood. *Dev. Med. Child Neurol.*, **14**, 336.

Gesell, A. and Ilg, F.L. (1937) *Feeding Behaviour of Infants*. Philadelphia, PA: J.P. Lippincott.

Gesell, A. and Ilg, F.L. (1949) *Child Development*. New York: Harper & Row.

Gordon, I.J. (1973) *Baby Learning Through Baby Play*. London: Sidgwick and Jackson.

Huror, J.R. (1991) Rethinking primate locomotion: what can we learn from development? *J. Motor Behav.*, **23**, 3, 211–218.

Illingworth, R.S. (1975) *The Development of the Infant and Young Child*, 6th edn. Edinburgh: Livingstone.

Isaacs, N. (1961) *The Growth of Understanding in the Young Child. A Brief Introduction to Piaget's Work*. London: Ward Lock.

Lemon, R.N., Bennett, K.M. and Werner, W. (1991) The cortico-motor substrate for skilled movements of the primate hand. In: *Tutorials in Motor Neuroscience*, edited by J. Requin and G.E. Stelmach. Amsterdam: Kluwer Academic Publishers, pp. 477–495.

Roberton, M.A. and Halverson, L.E. (1988) The development of locomotor coordination: longitudinal change and invariance. *J. Motor Behav.*, **20**, 3, 197–241.

Robinson, R.J. (1969) *Brain and Early Behaviour*. London: Academic.

Rorke, L.B. and Riggs, H.E. (1969) *Myelination of the Brain in the Newborn*. Philadelphia, PA: J.P. Lippincott.

Rosenbloom, J. and Horton, M. (1971) Maturation of fine prehension in young children. *Dev. Med. Child Neurol.*, **13**, 3.

Schneider, K., Zernicke, R.F., Ulrich, B.D., Jensen, J.L. and Thelen, E. (1990) Understanding movement control in infants through the analysis of limb intersegmental dynamics. *J. Motor Behav.*, **22**, 4, 493–520.

Sheridan, M.D. (1968) *The Developmental Progress of Infants and Young Children*. London: Ministry of Health.

Van Blankenstein, M., Welbergen, U.R., de Haas, J.H. (1975) *The Development of the Infant*. London: Heinemann.

3

Training motor control and optimizing motor learning

Introduction

The aim of physiotherapy of the individual who has a lesion affecting any part of the neuromusculoskeletal system, such as following birth trauma or head injury, associated with developmental disability or acquired musculoskeletal problem or disease, is to enable that individual to function as effectively as possible in everyday life. This means that the movement-disabled individual must attempt to gain or regain effective motor performance in at least such essential everyday actions as standing up, walking, reaching in sitting and standing, and manipulation.

The first section of this chapter contains a brief review of some of the factors known to be necessary for the learning of movement and the acquisition of skill. It is followed by a section in which the training of everyday actions is discussed in relation to infants and children with movement disability.

It has been proposed that physiotherapy for individuals with movement dysfunction should be based on research data and theoretical concepts in the burgeoning areas of science which have to do with human movement (Carr and Shepherd 1987a, b). The movement-related material from such fields as neuroscience, biomechanics, motor learning, cognitive and ecological psychology and muscle biology make up the broad area called human movement science (Shepherd 1987). The impetus for this proposal came from the fact that scientific knowledge about human movement and its control was increasing due both to the development of technology enabling the collection of data-based descriptions of movements such as walking (e.g. Winter 1987) and to changes in emphasis in motor control research to the study of real-life movements (e.g. Jeannerod 1981; Johansson and Westling 1990). It is particularly relevant to relate physiotherapy practice to scientific findings about the characteristics of real-life movement. Up until recently, physiotherapy practice, certainly in regard to disorders of neural mechanisms, has been based solely on clinical experience and neurophysiological concepts developed out of *in vitro* investigations of the muscle and nerve or single joint movements.

Although the concept of developing a movement science framework for physiotherapy has been illustrated principally in regard to the motor problems following stroke, such a concept has equal value where motor problems result from other lesions, in any age group and in any part of the neuromuscular system. At whatever age the individual needs to gain effective motor performance, individuals should be considered active learners in a process of habilitation or rehabilitation designed to promote the learning or relearning of effective motor behaviour. Infants and young children whose motor dysfunction has been present since birth or earlier have to learn how to organize the body parts in order to achieve a particular goal. If we use Gentile's (1987) division of goal-directed

behaviour into investigative and adaptive behaviour, the infant has to develop the ability to
position body parts in the way that best enables
relevant information from the environment to
be picked up (*investigative behaviour*) so there
can be the required interaction with the environment. In order to develop the ability to interact in a flexible manner with the environment,
the infant has to learn to adapt previously
learned behaviours and skills to new challenges
as they arise (*adaptive behaviour*).

A major purpose of this chapter is to show
how everyday actions can be trained in disabled
infants and young children in much the same
way as they are trained in able-bodied children
and adults. Sitting, standing, standing up, walking, reaching and manipulation may seem an
odd choice of actions to train in infants since
our perspective of what movements infants need
to perform is strongly influenced by traditional
views of motor development. Nevertheless, two
factors should be kept in mind when considering how best to train motor behaviour in disabled infants. The first is the rather obvious fact
that the major objective of any infant is to be
able to function effectively as an adult. The
inherent ability to perform similar movement
patterns to mature activities and the ability to
solve problems is, however, present from birth
and even earlier, as has been discussed in
Chapter 2. The second factor to consider is
the probability that a disabled infant
(particularly one with a severe neural dysfunction) may develop only a limited repertoire of
actions and that practice in infancy should be
concentrated on those actions that will best
equip the infant to function as an adult.

It is very likely, for example, that in severely
disabled children, time should not be devoted to
the training of crawling, since crawling is both
complex and relatively less important than
standing and walking. The view that crawling
has some important causative relationship to
walking can no longer be upheld given the differences in the biomechanical interactions and
muscle activity patterns. Such time would be
better spent in giving the infant practice of
moving about in the two erect postures (sitting
and standing) most critical for everyday life.
Early emphasis on erect body positions is probably particularly important in severely disabled
infants, enabling them to learn the necessary
orienting behaviours that enable them to
explore and attend to their environment and

develop their ability to formulate goals out of
what they sense.

In this section, the training of individual
actions, such as standing up, walking and
reaching is based on biomechanical models of
these actions. These models are in an ongoing
state of development dependent upon new
research findings that give more insight into
these actions. Standing up is one action about
which a good deal more has become known in
the last 5 years (Carr and Shepherd 1990).
Although there have been some investigations
of the changes occurring from newborn to
mature performance in many actions, at this
time comparatively little is known about the
development of mature motor performance –
not enough to give us models for analysis and
training. Nevertheless, it is evident that infant
performance is similar to mature performance
in many ways and it may not be too inaccurate
to base training of infants on biomechanical
models worked out from studies of adults
until more is known about the critical changes
which occur during the development of mature
performance.

The methods used in training infants and
young children are also similar to those already
shown to be effective in promoting motor learning and in increasing motor skill in non-
disabled subjects. The techniques used include
instruction, goal identification, auditory and
visual feedback, manual guidance and practice
(for review, see Gentile 1987).

Methods of intervention take into account
movement biomechanics, muscle characteristics and environmental context as well as the
underlying pathology and dyscontrol processes. They consist of methods of lengthening
muscles, activating muscles, strengthening muscle groups and promoting synergic activity
between muscles. All training is task- and context-specific; that is to say the child practises a
particular desired action in a variety of different
environmental contexts. If it is not possible to
practise the whole action, exercise may need to
be given which is related to some part of the
action. In terms of dyscontrol processes, we
still know very little, and physiotherapists are
in the prime position to investigate the changes
to movement control arising out of pathological
and recovery processes.

As an illustration of the application of this
model, let us look at how the action of standing up from the crouch position would be

trained in an infant (Fig. 3.1a). In this figure, the infant is held supported in crouch with his body weight through the feet, heels down. This position has an added advantage of lengthening calf muscles, which have a strong tendency to become short and stiff when the ankles are not actively moved through full range. The infant is encouraged to stand up (Fig. 3.1b and c). He may need to be moved passively into standing to give him the idea of the movement. He may get the idea if presented with an attractive object held just out of reach. When he performs the action, he receives both verbal feedback and the object. The infant in this action is practising an essential function of the lower limbs, using the ground (support surface) and lower limb muscles to propel the body into standing. He is learning to control his lower limb extensor muscles in a synergic manner, to generate and time the appropriate amount of muscle force. If he continues to practise this action as he grows and gets heavier, he will also be gaining the necessary strength in the muscles for effective performance of the action. When he is able, he should practise the action independently, using his hands for support initially, so that he can develop the postural activation patterns associated with independence in the action. Practice of this action should result in him having the ability to extend the lower limbs in the extension phase of standing up from a seat. However, to do the entire action effectively he will also need to practise specifically, since sit-to-stand involves linking a pre-extension phase in which the upper body flexes forwards at the hips before the lower limb extension phase.

Motor learning

Basic motor actions appear to mature as a result of interactions between central nervous system (CNS) maturation, growth, and the environment, as described in the previous chapter. The child builds on basic actions, acquiring skill in performing everyday actions as well as the actions involved in sport, recreation and work. Annett (1971) defined skill as any human activity which becomes better organized and more effective as the result of practice. Learning a motor skill requires, according to Singer (1980), monitored practice, motivation, awareness of goal, and a knowledge of results.

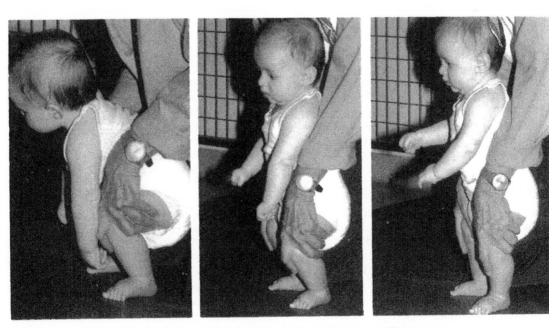

Figure 3.1 Aged 3 months. Infant with left hemiplegia practising crouch-to-stand with support.

Motor learning and control are said to depend more on the progressive inhibition of unwanted muscular activity than on the activation of additional motor units (O'Connell 1972; Basmajian 1977). Unnecessary muscle activity is characteristic of both infant and adult as they strive to gain control over a new action. This is also the case for the disabled individual. The excessive muscle activity seen in infants and children as they struggle to control an arm for reaching, a hand for holding a cup, or attempt to stand without holding on, is likely to represent in part a lack of skill as well as the effects of the brain lesion. Much of the training of action in infants and children, as with adults, consists of teaching the child to cut down excessive muscle activity, eliminate inappropriate muscle activity – in other words to match force generation and the pattern of muscle activation to the needs of the task. This is quite a different approach to one in which the therapist handles the child to inhibit abnormal tone and facilitate more normal movement, as is done in neurodevelopmental or Bobath therapy. Although inhibition of excessive muscle activity by handling does appear to affect muscle activity or tone, and may be useful in a severely mentally retarded and hyperreflexic infant or child, for movement to be controlled requires that the individuals themselves are able to activate their muscles effectively. That is to say, for volitional and effective interactions with the environment, an individual, no matter what age, has to be able to control actively and independently the contraction of muscles and the movements of body segments.

Some techniques to promote motor learning are described below. The reader should refer to Gentile (1987) for an overview of this topic. In paediatric physiotherapy, techniques may need to be modified according to the child's age or ability to comprehend.

Feedback

Feedback gives information about the environment and our relationship with it, usually in relation to a particular goal. Feedback is information derived from internal and external sources via eyes, ears, labyrinths, skin and muscle. It gives knowledge of performance and results.

The physiotherapist uses verbal feedback as a training technique in the clinic to provide reinforcement in the attainment of a goal: 'Yes, you did it', and to give information related to performance, 'Try again – this time push down more through your left foot'. With small infants, such feedback needs to be modified according to the infant's capacity to understand and a smile or a hand clap can be enough to show an infant what should be repeated. Since feedback is essential to learning, the therapist should avoid using positive feedback – 'Good' – when it is inaccurate, and instead confine its use to situations in which it will encourage the child to repeat a successful or nearly successful performance. That is, there should not be a mismatch between the consequence of an action and the feedback. For example, when a child can see that a goal – 'Pick up the glass' – has not been achieved, it is meaningless if the therapist (as coach) says 'Good'. One of the advantages of having infants and children practise goal-directed actions with objects is that visual and tactile feedback gives the child evidence of the success or otherwise of the attempt. Bruner (1973) suggested that, in the infant's growth of competence, there are three central themes: intention, feedback and the patterns of action which mediate between them.

Biofeedback Augmented sensory feedback utilizes visual or auditory feedback to give objective information related to some aspect of performance. A major advantage in children with movement dysfunction is the fact that they can practise relatively independently, with some supervision from therapist or parent, and gain pleasure and a sense of achievement from their own intended actions. One potential use for biofeedback devices is the use of training stations, where children can spend a period of time practising different functional actions. Feedback devices described in the literature include limb load monitors or pressure switches to detect force through a lower limb in walking (Seeger *et al.* 1981; Seeger and Caudrey 1983) or sit-to-stand (Engardt *et al.* 1993); head position trainers to monitor head position (Harris 1971; Wooldridge and Russell 1976; Leiper *et al.* 1981; Walmsley *et al.* 1981; Malouin *et al.* 1985); electrogoniometers to monitor joint angle (Flodmark 1986) and pressure-sensitive switches to monitor the position of body parts (Bertoti and Gross 1988).

Biofeedback is not a substitute for motor training but an adjunct. It would probably be optimally effective when combined with training of specific actions and when it is withdrawn gradually so that the individual learns to perform the action using internal feedback mechanisms. The withdrawal of the device is not necessarily followed by a continuation of the desired behaviour (e.g. Wooldridge and Russell 1976; Seeger *et al.* 1983; Bertoti and Gross 1988), that is, the ability to generalize a newly learned skill to different environments. This may be remedied by a gradual withdrawal of the device and the realization by the child that there are important benefits to be gained from the improved performance during the feedback training. If the cessation of biofeedback is not followed up either by refresher sessions with the physiotherapist or by the continuation of an exercise and stretching programme at home, then carry-over cannot really be expected in children with severe motor control problems. Seeger and Caudrey (1983) comment that children who did not maintain gains after a period of walking with a pressure-sensing device under the heel had short ankle plantarflexors and did not continue with stretching or with physiotherapy after cessation of biofeedback. Flodmark (1986) used a goniometric device as a joint position trainer to aid children to control the angle of the knee in mid-stance of walking. The author comments that feedback devices seem most effective for children who have a good attention span and are well-motivated.

If biofeedback is given without an analysis of the nature of the motor problem and without the provision of an appropriate training programme, it is unlikely to be of any benefit. For example, one study (Bertoti and Gross 1988) investigated the effect on sitting posture of a pressure-sensitive switch placed in the back-rest of a seat. When the children sat with the upper trunk in contact with the switch, a video film was turned on. Although the children were very motivated, since they enjoyed the film, and the feedback was immediately effective, there was no evidence of any carry-over effect once the feedback was withdrawn. Interestingly, in this study, the functional level of sitting of the 5 children with cerebral palsy (CP), diplegia or quadriplegia, aged 3–5 years was reported in terms of floor sitting. Prior to the study, the children sat on the floor with upper trunk flexed and head extended. This posture was taken to mean the children had poor trunk control. However, children with CP typically find floor-sitting very difficult for a number of reasons. For example, short hamstring and hip adductor muscles will result in flexed knees and extended hips as the short muscles tilt the pelvis in a backwards direction (i.e. extend the hips) in this position. The flexion of the lumbar and thoracic spine and the extension of the neck are adaptations, enabling the body mass to be brought forwards over the base of support; that is, preventing the child from falling backwards (see Fig. 5.5). In children with this problem, floor-sitting should be avoided; after all, learning to move about when sitting on a seat and learning to use muscle activity of the upper body over the base of support (thighs and feet) for making postural adjustments are more relevant to function than floor-sitting. In addition, when sitting on a seat, the child may learn easily to sit erect (see Fig. 8.8).

Future developments of electronic devices to provide feedback and motivation should enable children to enjoy performing exercise programmes designed to increase strength and control of specific muscle groups and to improve physical fitness. Devices need to be developed to monitor reaching and manipulative actions and appropriate devices for training young infants need to be developed. The potential of electronic devices in motor training has not yet been realized. This may be partly because of the emphasis in paediatric physiotherapy on the therapist handling the infant or child to inhibit unwanted muscle activation and facilitate automatic responses, rather than the child being encouraged to be an active and independent participant in training.

Goal identification

Not only is it important to identify clearly the goal of an action, it seems that the goal, if it is to be pursued with enthusiasm, needs to be perceived as worthwhile and meaningful to that individual. Tasks which have goals which are directed towards controlling one's physical interaction with objects or persons in the immediate environment seem to have more meaning than goals which are directed at movement for its own sake. The first type of task is termed concrete, the second abstract.

Deficiencies in performance of an abstract task (such as abducting the thumb) and a concrete task (abducting a thumb in order to grasp a glass) have been noted in adults following stroke. As a result, it has been proposed that training of motor-disabled individuals should involve the practice of concrete tasks in which the individual achieves a particularly difficult action by attempting to control an interaction with an object in the environment (Carr and Shepherd 1987b). The effectiveness of practice of more concrete tasks has been shown to improve coordination of movement in adults after stroke (Lee and Young 1986; Ada and Westwood 1992) and in individuals with Parkinson's disease (Frischer 1989).

Van der Weel and colleagues (1991) have recently described an experiment in which the performance on a concrete task was compared to an abstract task which required the same action, pronation and supination of the forearm. The subjects were 9 children with CP of hemiplegic distribution aged between 3 and 7 years and a group of non-disabled children. The authors found with the CP children that movement range was significantly greater for the concrete task (beating two drums by alternately supinating and pronating) than for the abstract task in which the children were asked to supinate and pronate the forearm as far as they could. Whereas the non-disabled children showed no difference between these two simple tasks, the CP children showed a significant increase in the range of both supination and pronation in the concrete task. Interestingly, supination range increased by more than 20%, yet it is supination that is a particularly difficult movement to perform in many individuals with brain dysfunction.

In explanation, the authors point out that movement is not an independent process but an integral part of an act. The extent and quality of movement depend on how much practice the individual has in performing the action, how interested the person is and the quality of information available. Concrete tasks are associated with more information from the environment than abstract tasks. The drum in this experiment would have provided visual, auditory and tactile information about the child's relationship with it and the children received relevant information about the attainment of the goal (feedback). The abstract task would have depended primarily upon proprioceptive inputs about sense of muscle effort and limb configuration. This is particularly relevant given that

children with hemiplegia have been found to have proprioceptive deficits (e.g. Lee *et al.* 1990).

A similar result was found in patients with joint and peripheral nerve injuries (Leont'ev and Zaporozhets 1960), who were able to reach higher when they attempted to grasp an object compared to when they were asked to reach as high as they could.

Demonstration and instruction

Just as in any sports training, demonstration of the action and instructions on the major points to concentrate on are important teaching tools in the clinic. Demonstration can be given by the therapist (see Fig. 3.20a) or by a videotape of either the desirable performance or the child's own performance. In the latter case, it may be preferable to edit the videotape and show the child only his or her best performance of the action being learned (Dowrick 1983). Instruction should be kept to a minimum in order to avoid overloading the child with information.

Manual guidance

There are said to be two types of manual guidance used in training – passive movement and spatiotemporal constraint or physical restriction (Holding 1965, 1970; Newell 1981). During training in the clinic, passive movement may involve placing a limb in a position that enables a movement to take place (see Fig. 8.4) or moving a limb to give an idea of the action required – that is, the goal and the spatiotemporal characteristics of the action.

Spatial constraint may involve holding part of a limb stable, constraining the action spatially while the infant or child has only to control part of the limb (see Figs 3.9 and 3.19). As more control is gained, the physical restraint is reduced, increasing the number of degrees of freedom to be controlled. Manual guidance can be replaced by verbal feedback or object-mediated guidance.

Newell (1981) considers that this latter type of manual guidance decreases the likelihood of the learner making serious errors and developing bad habits. However, he also points out that, provided fundamentally inappropriate actions (which would include adaptive movements) that would hinder learning are prevented, errors of execution in spatiotemporal details of the action may be beneficial to learning.

Practice

Practice of an action is a necessary prerequisite for acquiring skill in that action. What is practised needs to be relevant, meaningful and desirable. One of the advantages of task-specific training is that it enables the infant or child to see the advantages of becoming skilled. Ability to stand up, for example, means that walking becomes a real possibility; learning to reach out and grasp a toy means it can be played with. Practice may involve performing in a closed environment if the child has difficulty activating muscles and controlling force production. However, practice should take place as soon as possible in an open environment whenever this is relevant to the particular action.

Practice with many repetitions is required:

1 to enable a movement pattern to be learned;
2 to enable that pattern to be modified as necessary according to environmental and other demands (i.e. to develop flexibility of performance); and
3 to strengthen the muscles specifically for that action.

Actions can be practised in their entirety or broken down into their component parts (Singer 1980). However, practice of the entire action is generally considered preferable to practice of a part of an action, since an action is more than the sum of its parts. Practice of a component of an action may be necessary in the clinic to prevent repetition of a fundamentally inappropriate action.

Attentiveness is a necessary part of practice and improved performance has been found to be associated with improved attention (Diller 1970). For small infants, practice has to be accomplished by organizing the environment to force the required motor behaviour (see Fig. 3.27). Eye contact between child and therapist encourages attentiveness. However a reminder to watch the object may be necessary when a child is easily distractible.

Particular cues may enable more effective practice. Fitts (1963) proposed three stages in learning a skill – cognitive, associative and automatic. Cognitive cues are used, therefore, in the early stage of training with the objective of practice enabling the child to make the transition from cognitive cues to more automatic ones. Although it may appear difficult to use cognitive cues with young infants, visual and verbal cues can be used to guide movement and to reward performance.

Environmental modification

Since the environment plays a significant role in modulating motor performance, specific aspects of the environment can be utilized to channel and direct the motor output in training. Similarly, if an action is too difficult for an infant with movement dysfunction, some feature of the environment can be modified to make the task possible without too much physical struggle. For example, seat height can be increased to enable an infant with poor control over lower-limb extensor muscles (particularly the quadriceps) to practise standing up and sitting down. The way in which the interaction with the environment takes place can be altered to take account of an individual's dyscontrol. For example, the child could practise sitting down (an eccentric contraction of lower-limb extensors) independently, receiving some physical guidance to stand up again (concentric activity), since the eccentric action may be easier to control than the concentric.

The environment can be altered to prevent unwanted actions from occurring and to set up a joint alignment that ensures that the muscles contract at the length required. For example, in young infants and severely disabled children, the environment may be modified to provide constraint. A seat may need to be modified to prevent undesirable actions (see Fig. 5.13). The objective in this example was to prevent the child's head from falling sideways, enable his neck flexor muscles to contract with his head erect face forward, and to enable him to pay attention, develop visual perception, particularly of horizontality and verticality, and to practise tracking objects.

Unwanted reflex actions can also be extinguished by environmental modification which physically prevents the reflexive movement from occurring. Lee and colleagues (1985) found that using a simple device (a foam headpiece) to prevent the occurrence of a asymmetrical tonic neck reflex (ATNR) in an 11-year-old girl with CP and profound mental retardation was effective not only in extinguishing the unwanted reflex action but also in improving food intake. The investigators established that the ATNR occurred with the highest frequency at lunch-time, when the child was being fed. The child's head was, therefore, restrained in the device during lunch. During the study, the investigators took simple measures such as the number of occurrences of the ATNR. The headpiece was gradually cut down to make it less restrictive until the ATNR no longer occurred during lunch periods. Prior to this intervention, the teacher would use verbal requests to keep the head centred and physical guidance to bring the head back to the midline. As the authors point out, reinforcement of the wanted behaviour (head centred with no ATNR) occurred due to the child's ability to ingest more food.

The environment can also be organized to optimize an infant's ability to perform difficult actions. Figure 3.27 shows a 6-month-old infant with hemiplegic CP, who had a virtually immobile and unused left upper limb. Under normal environmental conditions, she would use only her unaffected hand for playing with objects presented to her. When desirable objects were positioned so that they were unobtainable by the unaffected hand, she started to reach out with her affected hand.

Visual monitoring of performance

Vision appears to dominate touch in certain circumstances. The way an object feels is affected by its appearance, but not the reverse (Rosenbaum 1991). Furthermore, it appears from several reported observations that subjects are unable to distinguish visually between their own and another person's hand provided the other hand moves in synchrony with the subject's. This dominance of vision leads Rosenbaum (1991) to suggest that, in physical rehabilitation, someone trying to gain control over a limb may be helped by seeing an image of the limb with greater mobility than it really has.

Self-modelling is an approach that promotes behavioural change by observing oneself on videotapes that show only the desired behaviours (Dowrick 1983). It is not certain whether disabled children would acquire skill more by observing their own errors during performance or by observing edited videotapes of their optimal performance. However, a study described by Dowrick (p. 111) suggests that observing optimal performance can be effective under certain circumstances. A 6-year-old girl with CP walked easily over smooth surfaces but was intimidated by obstacles such as kerbs and stairs. She was videotaped in her attempts to walk on surfaces just beyond the limits of her capability, and was given considerable reinforcement to produce an optimal performance. The videotape was edited and the best performances were extracted and duplicated to make a 2-minute best-performance self-model tape. She was shown the tape three times a week for 3 weeks. At the end of this period she was able to step over all the original obstacles without assistance and her skills generalized into negotiating other obstacles.

Motor training

In this section, the training of some individual actions will be considered in the following format: first, a *model of the action* will be defined using information about the biomechanics of the action derived from investigative studies. This will include a *list of essential components* (Carr and Shepherd 1987a) which has been set up to provide a simplified model for analysis and training. The essential components comprise what appear to be the major observable kinematic features of the action, principally linear paths of body parts and angular rotations/displacements. These features have been selected not because the kinematics of an action are the most critical features, but because they are observable and therefore of assistance to therapists analysing performance in the clinic. In fact, as Winter (1987) points out, the major features of an action have to do with muscle activation patterns and the forces produced – the kinematics are the result of force production. Although these components form a useful guide for the clinic, the therapist has to understand enough about the underlying kinetics and muscle activation patterns to be able to deduce the possible sources of any discrepancy in the paths of body parts and angular rotations.

Second, the *common problems seen in the performance of the action* by individuals with movement dysfunction will be described. These problems arise from the dyscontrol characteristics associated with the underlying pathology but also from the system's capacity for adaptation or compensation.

Third, illustrations will be given of *methods of training the action* in infants and children when the movement pattern is absent or not effective.

Sit-to-stand

Developing the ability to stand up is essential to the independent performance of other actions such as walking which require the ability to get into standing (Carr and Shepherd 1990). Standing up requires the ability to extend the lower-limb joints (knees, hips and ankles) over a fixed base of support (the feet). Lower-limb extension appears to be an innate movement pattern, since it has been observed in the fetus and at birth (see Fig. 2.8). This ability to use the lower limbs to propel the body mass away from the support surface is an important feature of standing up, needing only the addition of upper-body flexion at the hips to bring the body mass forwards over the feet and the ability to balance the body throughout the action.

It is the author's view that standing up from crouch and from sitting on a seat should be practised by very small infants if they demonstrate or are at risk of developing movement dysfunction (see Figs 3.1 and 3.9). Propulsion, support and balance are the major attributes of the lower limb. The action of extending and flexing the lower limbs over a fixed base of support is part of several everyday actions, standing up and sitting down, stance phase of walking, walking up and down stairs, and the initial phase of jumping and hopping. Practice of extending the lower limbs from crouch then flexing them back into crouch provides exercise of an apparently innate pattern which, if it is not exercised in early infancy, may be lost. Lack of practice of this movement pattern in many children is eventually associated with short calf muscles and short hip and knee flexors – a situation which will make it mechanically impossible to do the action. Standing up from crouch and from a seat, if considered solely from a mechanical point of view, are exercises that provide an active stretch to the calf muscles, a muscle group which tends in relatively immobile/inactive infants to become very short. Of course, the

effect is magnified because the inactivity is present in combination with growth.

The literature on motor development has typically described the infant's developing ability to stand up from the floor and, therefore, from a crouched position. Standing up from a seat is not generally discussed. One reason may be that in the population of children usually observed in developmental studies, there may have been little opportunity for the children to stand up from seats that relate to their height and they usually have to clamber up and down from adult-sized chairs. There appear to have been no published studies of standing up in young children, although there is at least one in progress (see Fig. 3.2), and it is only recently that the adult movement pattern has been investigated. It is not known, therefore, if and in what ways young children vary in performance compared to adults.

A child is unlikely to stand up independently without using the hands for support until postural adjustments in standing have developed sufficiently for independent standing to be maintained. The major differences between children and adults may lie in the ability to control the horizontal momentum of the body mass produced by the pre-extension phase upper-body flexion at the hip and to coordinate this flexion with the onset of the lower-limb extension phase. Standing up requires the ability to maintain balance while moving the body mass from over one large base of support – the thighs and feet – to a small one – the feet. Generating linear and angular momentum sufficient to perform this translatory movement is potentially destabilizing. The young child who first attempts this action from a small seat will have to learn not only how to generate and control muscle forces but also how to harness the interactional effects of segment rotations so that the action eventually becomes well-balanced and energy-efficient.

Description of the activity

Standing up can be divided into a pre-extension and an extension phase (Shepherd and Gentile 1994), the change occurring at the time the thighs leave the seat (thighs-off). In the *pre-extension phase*, in which the initial or starting posture is formed, one critical action required is a movement of the feet to a position behind an imaginary perpendicular line drawn down from the knees. This positions the feet so that the activation of lower-limb extensor muscles in the extension phase will generate the backwards horizontal component of ground reaction forces essential to propel the body mass forwards. This foot position also limits the distance which the body mass needs to be moved forwards (Shepherd and Koh 1994). Having positioned the feet, the upper body is swung forwards at the hips, the shoulder tracing a path horizontally, then vertically, with some overlap around the time the thighs leave the seat (Fig. 3.2). The velocity of the trunk flexion causes the thighs to move forwards, this movement taking place at the knee (flexion) and ankle (dorsiflexion) joints. The overlap between horizontal and vertical movement of the shoulder path shows that the horizontal movement of the body mass is transferred into a vertical movement with no pause; the pre-extension and extension phases forming one continuous movement. There is some experimental support for the proposal that hip angular momentum and horizontal momentum of the body are transferred into vertical momentum (Shepherd and Gentile 1994; Schenkman *et al.* 1990). This means that the movement forwards of the body, by angular displacement at the hip (flexion) and ankle (dorsiflexion) in the

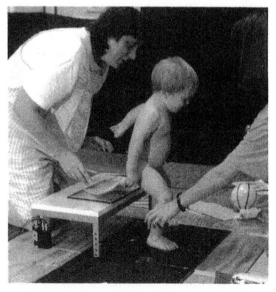

Figure 3.2 Aged 12 months, independent sit-to-stand: extension phase just after thighs-off. Taken during data collection for a study on the development of sit-to-stand. Note the forceplate, height-adjustable seat and start switch to record thighs-off. (Courtesy of B. Duffy.)

pre-extension phase, has an effect on the upcoming extension phase.

In the *extension phase*, the knees start to extend at thighs-off, followed by extension at the hips, then by plantarflexion at the ankles. Hip and knee extension have a linear relationship throughout this phase (Canning *et al.* 1985). Extensor moments of force at the three lower-limb joints peak around thighs-off. Support moment of force, which is a summation of the three joint moments (Winter 1980), also peaks at this time, at approximately four to five times body mass (Shepherd and Gentile 1994). Thighs-off is, therefore, the time at which the leg extensor muscles must be strongly active in order to lift the body mass vertically into the standing position.

Essential components (Carr and Shepherd 1987a) can be considered as:

1 Foot placement.
2 Flexion of trunk forwards at hips with extended spine, and a horizontal movement forwards of the knee with ankle dorsiflexion.
3 Knee, hip and ankle extension.

Sitting down is not described here in detail; however, the kinematic movement pattern virtually mirrors standing up. Sitting down requires eccentric muscle activity rather than concentric and, since it lacks the facilitating effect of vigorous trunk flexion, the part of the movement just before the body mass is lowered on to the seat requires considerable muscle strength and control. There have been virtually no published studies of sitting down so biomechanical details are not available.

The position is similar with regard to *standing up from crouch* in that there have been few reports of the action (Murray *et al.* 1967). It is probably, however, similar to the phase of the vertical jump that precedes lift-off, and the vertical jump has been investigated in many studies (Hay 1975; Gregoire *et al.* 1984). The major distinction between the initial phase of the vertical jump (and probably crouch-to-stand) and the extension phase of standing up is the different sequence of joint extension onsets (vertical jump: hip, knee, ankle; sit-to-stand: knee, hip, ankle), reflecting the fact that standing up requires a shift from one base of support to another while the jump takes place over the one base of support.

Motor dysfunction

There are several motor control *problems* which may interfere with the ability to stand up:

1. Difficulty generating force with lower-limb extensor muscles (hip, knee extensors, ankle plantarflexors), if severe, will make it impossible for a child to stand up from a seat (Fig. 3.3). Adduction and internal rotation at the hips (Fig. 3.4) may be a way of gaining more effective lower-limb extension or may be due to short and overactive adductor muscles.

2. If the feet are not moved back sufficiently, subsequent lower-limb extension will propel the child backwards instead of forwards and upwards (Fig. 3.5). The problem will be magnified if the amplitude and velocity of upper-body flexion at the hips are inadequate since the body mass has to be moved a greater distance forwards. Inability to place the foot appropriately can be due to shortness of the soleus muscle which will prevent the ankle being dorsiflexed. Even a small amount of soleus shortening will create a problem in standing up as the ankles must dorsiflex well beyond the plantigrade position. Similarly, if calf muscles are hyperreflexic to stretch, the feet cannot be placed

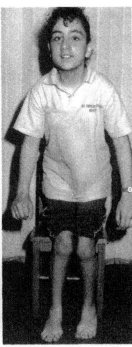
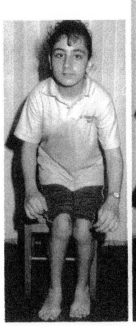

Figure 3.4 Girl with diplegic cerebral palsy can, after a period of specific training, stand up independently without using her hands for support. Note the adduction and internal rotation of her hips.

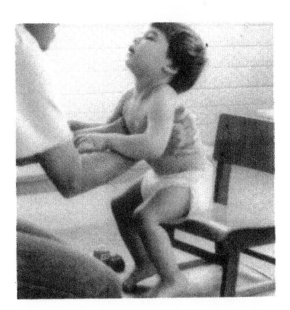

Figure 3.3 Boy with diplegic cerebral palsy attempting to stand up. He is unable to stabilize his feet on the floor and to generate sufficient force in his lower limb extensors to stand up without assistance.

back and the shanks cannot move forwards (Fig. 3.6).

3. Failure to move the upper body sufficiently far forward by thighs-off, at which point the body mass should be over the feet (Carr and Gentile 1994), will cause the propulsive extension force to propel the body backward (Fig. 3.5).

4. If the child flexes the upper body forwards then stops before the extension phase, the natural effect of the momentum created by the large trunk segment is absent and the extension phase will start from zero momentum. There is evidence that there may be some energy cost in this case as the extension phase is prolonged and a high value of extensor force is produced throughout a large proportion of the phase (Shepherd and Gentile 1994).

In response to these problems, the child will utilize the typical *adaptive motor behaviours* seen in all age groups:

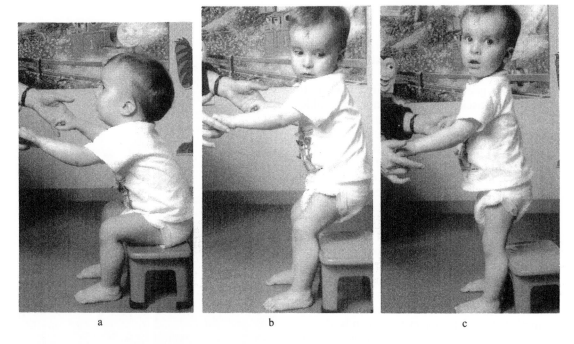

a   b   c

Figure 3.5 Boy with diplegia cannot stand up independently. (a) He has not moved his feet back. (b) He has started extending his hips before his body mass is forwards over his feet. (c) In standing, body mass is still too far back (note insufficient extension at hips and dorsiflexion at ankles).

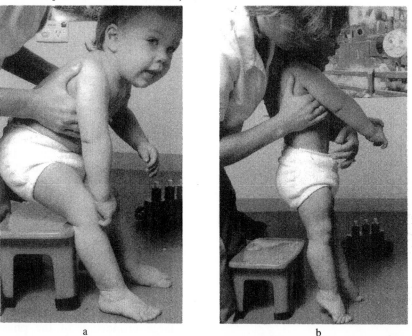

a   b

Figure 3.6 This little boy with cerebral palsy can only stand up with assistance. (a) His feet are too far forwards at the start of the movement and he has not moved the shank segments forwards at the ankles (dorsiflexion). (b) As a result, his body mass is behind the base of support in standing. Note that he has generated excessive force in the plantarflexor muscles and is standing on his toes.

1 If muscle weakness is unilateral, the child may stand up by generating force principally through the intact leg. The body mass will be seen to shift laterally at thighs-off.

2 If lower limb extensor force is inadequate, the child may use the hands to push up from the seat to assist in moving the body mass forward or may swing the arms forwards and upwards to aid the horizontal and vertical propulsion (Fig. 3.7). Habitual use of the hands or arms will prevent the child from developing the ability to transfer horizontal momentum to vertical momentum.

Training

Standing up is practised from a seat which is of appropriate size for the individual child. The seat should be flat and not sloped backwards. The initial position imposed by this type of seat increases any difficulty the child has in standing up since the thighs have to be rotated forwards a greater distance than if the seat is flat. Initially, the height of the seat should be chosen depending on the child's ability to generate the necessary force with lower-limb extensor muscles. If considerable muscle weakness is present or if lower limb control is poor, the child may find it easier to practise from a higher than normal seat since this is known to require less force production (Burdett *et al.* 1985).

Since practice is usually required in order to develop the necessary strength in the muscles involved and also to enable the child to learn the movement pattern, the seat should not have arms. The presence of chair arms in the child's environment will facilitate the use of the hands to push the body up into standing. It is important during training that practice of an action encourages flexibility, as the goal of training is for the individual to be able to perform the action from a variety of different seats and in combination with other goals or actions, such as standing up to walk away or standing up while holding on to a plate. However, with children who

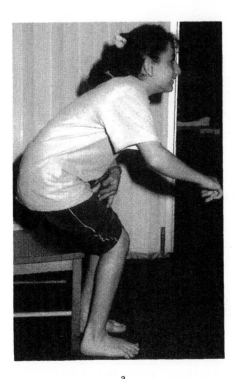 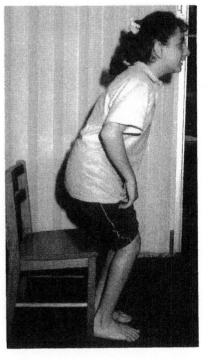

a b

Figure 3.7 (a, b) Independent sit-to-stand. In (a) it is apparent that she may have used the arms to assist in bringing the body mass forwards and to augment the production of vertical momentum at thighs-off.

have a great deal of difficulty controlling the action, it is probably inevitable that the action be practised first in a relatively closed environment.

Training is aimed at giving the child *practice* in standing up and sitting down with a pre-scribed number of repetitions. *Repetition* is necessary for two principal reasons – to opti-mize learning and to strengthen the muscles for this specific action. Emphasis during prac-tice is on ensuring that the essential components form part of the action (Fig. 3.8). However, it is necessary for the child to practise the whole action in order to develop the necessary timing of segmental rotations. As skill develops in the action, timing will become more precise since the child is learning how to utilize the charac-teristics of the segmental linkage. Effective tim-ing will optimize the intersegmental transfer of power and minimize the energy requirements.

In initial practice sessions, the child may ben-efit from a *demonstration* of the action or from being moved passively through the action, in order to give the idea of the movement required. However, if possible, with optimum seat selection and manual guidance from the therapist or parent, the child should stand up in response to some desirable goal (Fig. 3.9).

Some *manual guidance* will usually be required to ensure appropriate foot placement. The shoulders can be guided along the normal path, the foot or feet held in contact with the ground by pressure downwards along the line of the shank, the knees guided forwards to ensure sufficient ankle dorsiflexion (Figs 3.8 and 3.9). Fixing the foot to the ground may be necessary to ensure that when the quadriceps muscles are activated, the thigh will be moved on the shank and not the reverse. In other words, if the foot is not fixed to the floor (either by muscle activa-tion or by manual guidance by the therapist), quadriceps activation will extend the shank on the thigh and the foot will slide forwards and lift off the floor. This movement has been described as due to spasticity; it may, in many cases, however, be due to an inability to time

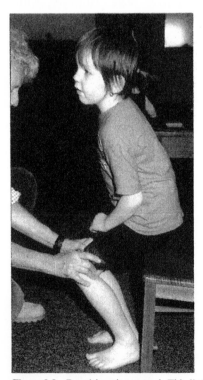 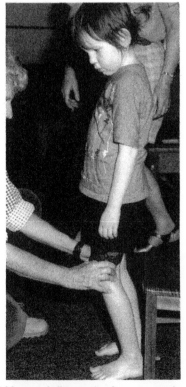

Figure 3.8 Practising sit-to-stand. This little girl has cerebellar ataxia after a traumatic brain injury. The therapist assists by holding the knees forwards at the start of the movement so the child has only to control the thigh and trunk segments. Pushing down through the shanks ensures a fixed base of support over which the lower limb and upper body segments rotate into extension.

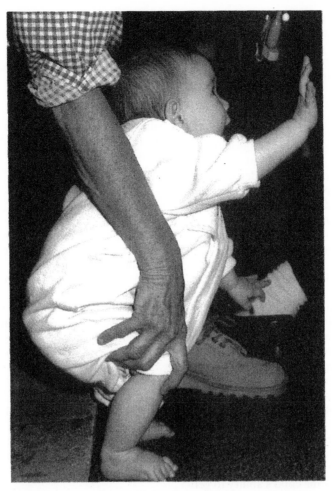

Figure 3.9 Young infant with developmental delay practising sit-to-stand. She is encouraged to move by holding a toy just out of reach. The therapist assists the movement by fixing the feet to the floor and ensuring appropriate alignment of shank segments.

muscle contractions for the action, together with inappropriate segmental alignment.

When manual guidance is given to the knee, care has to be taken that the knee is not passively extended too early in the movement sequence. The knee does not fully extend until the end of the movement. To put it another way, the ankles remain in dorsiflexion until well after thighs-off, probably in order to keep the body mass centred over the base of support. Whoever assists the child should not be so close that his or her presence impedes the movement forwards of the shoulders. The shoulders and head move forwards towards the knees and impeding this movement will prevent the child from standing up (and also from sitting down).

The best method of giving a child *feedback* about performance will depend on the individual child, but particularly on the age of the child. Augmented feedback using electronic devices can be used to give information about the presence of or amount of pressure through the feet. Auditory feedback can be given by pressure-sensitive devices under the feet which are connected to an auditory signal. Visual feedback of pressure through the feet via an interesting display may encourage the older child to practise. An older child may enjoy concurrent video or computerized feedback about performance, matching performance against an ideal performance. Video replay is also a useful way to explain to an older child where performance needs improvement. Matching the shape of the movement against an ideal will probably be one of the most effective learning tools; however, such devices have yet to be developed for the clinic.

The major route to learning how to stand up and sit down is through practice of the action in order to improve the biomechanical characteristics of the action. However, in order to enable practice, many disabled children will need *exercises designed to address specific control problems*. If a child has difficulty sustaining extensor muscle activity, stopping the stand-up movement at various points in the extension phase may be useful. Stopping the movement and reversing for a few degrees can help the child develop control over changing from concentric to eccentric muscle activity. Doing repetitive step-ups on a small box (see Fig. 3.20b) will increase strength in the lower-limb extensor muscles. The calf muscles may need to be lengthened to enable the feet to be placed appropriately for standing up (see Fig. 3.21). All exercises and stretches are followed immediately by practice of standing up and sitting with, if necessary, the environment modified to optimize practice conditions.

Modification of the environment may involve increasing the height of the seat to decrease force requirements. As the child's ability to generate force improves, the seat is lowered. In this way, seat height is used to add progressive resistance to the leg extensor muscles and strengthen them.

For some children, placing the arms on a table in front will provide some support so the child can concentrate on the lower-limb extension and not have to attend also to the need to move the upper body forwards and balance. The child should not be encouraged to pull into standing by using a parent's hands or the furniture, particularly if this is done with the feet forward and minimal use of the legs (see Fig. 3.5). As soon as possible, the child should practise without using the hands either for support or to assist in pushing the body mass vertically, since an essential feature of standing up is the concurrent postural adjustment that occurs throughout the action. The muscles which make these adjustments are particularly those distal muscles that link the shank to the foot.

Crouch-to-stand

Figure 3.1 illustrates how this action can be practised by a young infant. In an infant with hemiplegia, the action can be guided to ensure weight-bearing through the affected leg (Fig. 3.10). The feet may have to be held on the floor in crouch or in standing so that the feet support the body mass if the infant persists in lifting them up (Fig. 3.11). Arch supports may be necessary if the foot rolls into a valgus position.

Walking

Just as standing up is essential to independence, so also is walking. The principal substitute for walking is propelling a wheelchair and, although this is preferable to not being able to get about at all, individuals who must use this substitution miss out on the considerable versatility of walking. Normally infants watch others walk around them and try very hard to match their performance, despite many falls.

There is a very large body of literature on the biomechanics and control of normal walking (e.g. Saunders *et al.* 1953; Bernstein 1967; Inman, Ralston and Todd 1981; Winter 1987). There have also been several studies investigating the characteristics of gait in the presence of neuromusculoskeletal dysfunction in children.

Description of the activity

For ease of analysis in the clinic, walking can be divided into a stance and a swing phase. There is also a brief double-support phase when both feet are on the support surface.

In the stance phase of walking, the lower limb's principal functions are support, balance and propulsion, together with absorption of energy:

1   *Support*: the upper body is supported by the prevention of lower-limb collapse.
2   *Balance*: of the whole body over a fixed base of support (i.e. the foot in stance phase).
3   *Propulsion*: generation of mechanical energy to enable the appropriate forwards velocity of the body.
4   *Absorption*: of mechanical energy for both shock absorption and to decrease the body's forwards velocity.

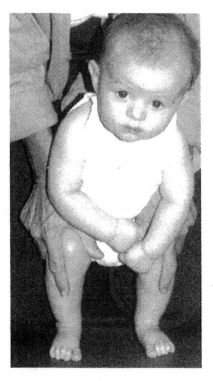

Figure 3.10 Practising crouch-to-stand. This infant with left hemiplegia is being encouraged to practise with weight through the left leg.

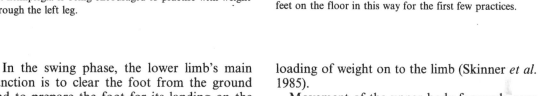

Figure 3.11 It was necessary with this infant.to hold the feet on the floor in this way for the first few practices.

In the swing phase, the lower limb's main function is to clear the foot from the ground and to prepare the foot for its landing on the support surface:

5   *Trajectory*: control of foot and knee paths through swing to heel strike.

These five functions are, according to Winter (1987), the main functions that must be performed in effective walking.

The *stance phase* begins at heel strike and, after foot contact, is characterized by extension of the hip and dorsiflexion at the ankle as the body moves forwards over the fixed foot. At heel strike, the ankle plantarflexes to bring the foot in contact with the ground. Early in the phase, there is a small flexion movement at the knee, the so-called yield of the knee. The knee functions in this way to smooth the path of the centre of gravity (Saunders *et al.* 1953) and, since the knee flexion occurs with quadriceps activity, to act as a shock absorber for the

loading of weight on to the limb (Skinner *et al.* 1985).

Movement of the upper body forwards over the stance hip is associated with some internal rotation at the hip. The pelvis is prevented from dropping down more than a few degrees (on average 5°, according to Saunders *et al.* 1953) on the swing side, probably by activity of the hip abductor muscles of the stance leg and the lateral flexors of the lumbar spine. Activation of the hip abductors would also prevent the pelvis from shifting too far laterally. This lateral shift is normally only about 4–5 cm (Saunders *et al.* 1953). Knee extension during mid-stance seems an important factor in preventing an excessive shift, due to the abduction of the tibia relative to the femur which occurs when the knee is extended and the femur is adducting at the hip (Saunders *et al.* 1953).

Since the body is moving over the fixed foot in stance phase, it is not surprising that the muscles linking the foot to the shank play a critical role in body translation. The tibialis anterior and long toe flexors show increased activity at the start of stance phase. Although this muscle activity will control the plantarflexion that places the foot on the floor after heel strike, it also rotates the shank forwards over the heel. At the start of single support, dorsiflexion at the ankle accounts for the forwards progression of the body over the foot.

The effect of muscle activation when linked segments rotate over a fixed distal segment is quite different from what one might expect from reading anatomical texts, in which lower-limb muscle function is described in relation to segmental rotations when the foot is free to move. For example, the quadriceps are active early in the stance phase to prevent the limb from collapsing into flexion but also to bring the thigh forwards over the shank (Skinner *et al.* 1985) and, therefore, to aid in the progression of the whole body forwards over the foot.

As another example, the restraining action of the plantarflexors as they prevent the collapse of the shank forwards makes an essential contribution to stability of the ankle, the tension required to prevent collapse being two to three times body weight (Skinner *et al.* 1985). Although the knee is extended in the last part of stance phase, the extension cannot be brought about by the quadriceps since these are inactive at this stage. It has been suggested, therefore, that the extension is maintained by extrinsic forces, with some contribution from the plantarflexors, which make an essential contribution to the stability of the knee as well as to the ankle (Sutherland 1966).

Towards the end of the stance phase, while the hip is still extending, the knee starts to flex and the ankle to plantarflex (heel-off). Investigation of the kinetics of this phase shows that the calf muscles cause a rapid ankle plantarflexion which generates a major propulsive power burst just before toe-off (Winter 1987). Extension of the hip appears to be essential in setting up the conditions both for the propulsive push-off and for the initiation of the swing phase of that leg (Pearson 1976).

The *swing phase* begins at toe-off, with ankle plantarflexion, knee flexion and hip extension, and is characterized initially by hip flexion with the knee flexed, then by extension at the knee and dorsiflexion at the ankle prior to heel strike. The pelvis drops down slightly on this side and the flexion at the knee effectively 'shortens' the swinging leg, enabling the foot to take a forwards path without contacting the ground (Eberhart *et al.* 1965).

Some rotation of the pelvis at the hip occurs in the horizontal plane and is countered by thoracic rotation. The magnitude of the pelvic rotation is typically small, some 4° on either side of the central axis (Saunders *et al.* 1953), although it varies with stride length (Murray *et al.* 1964). Sagittal plane rotation (anterior and posterior pelvic tilting) occurs through a mean excursion of 3°, with the maximum anterior tilt occurring just before heel strike and the maximum posterior tilt early in stance phase (Murray *et al.* 1964).

Essential components

Saunders and colleagues (1953) described what they called the 'biomechanical necessities' of walking. These kinematic features are:

1 Pelvic rotation occurring at each hip joint.
2 Pelvic tilt downwards on the side opposite to the weight-bearing limb.
3 Knee flexion in early stance.
4 Foot mechanism.
5 Knee mechanism.
6 Lateral horizontal shift of the pelvis.

The essential components as described by Carr and Shepherd (1987a) form the kinematic pattern of walking which can be used to compare a patient's performance with normal performance, since they are readily observable:

Stance phase
1 Extension at the hip and dorsiflexion at the ankle to move the body forwards.
2 Lateral horizontal shift of pelvis (approximately 4–5 cm in total).
3 Flexion at knee (approximately 15°) initiated on heel strike, followed by extension, then flexion prior to toe-off. Plantarflexion at the ankle towards the end of the phase.

Swing phase
1 Flexion at the knee (with the hip initially in extension).
2 Lateral pelvic tilt downwards (approximately 5°) in the horizontal plane at toe-off.
3 Flexion of hip.
4 Rotation of pelvis forwards on swinging leg.

The biomechanics of *walking up and down steps* is described by several authors (Joseph and Watson 1967; Townsend *et al.* 1978; Andriacchi *et al.* 1980). Although it is discussed briefly in this section as an action involving the lower limbs in support, balance and propulsion, it is mechanically different from level walking in terms of ranges of joint movement, muscle activity and magnitude of joint forces (Andriacchi *et al.* 1980).

In walking up steps, concentric lower limb extensor activity raises the body mass vertically; in walking down steps, the body mass is lowered by eccentric muscle activity. The extent of movement at the knee joint in stance phase is greater than in walking, being from full extension to approximately 90° in both climbing and descending (Shinno 1971). Knee extensor muscles have to generate much larger forces than in level walking. Quadriceps muscle strength is, therefore, particularly critical to the activity since the body mass must be raised or lowered by one limb.

An essential feature of walking up steps is the ankle dorsiflexion and knee flexion which occur after the foot has been placed on the step. These movements bring the body mass forwards over the front foot to a point where extension of the hip, knee and ankle of this leg will propel the body along a vertical inclination. In contrast, when descending, the body mass is kept back over the supporting leg as the extensor muscles of this leg contract eccentrically to lower the body mass.

Motor dysfunction

Infants and children with lesions of the neuro-musculoskeletal system which affect the ability to walk can be considered as forming two groups–those who have never walked and those who have. This is probably an important distinction, since the problems associated with gait dysfunction in the young cerebral-palsied child who has never developed a mature walking pattern will be different in certain respects from those of a child of 10 who has had a head injury or who has developed rheumatoid arthritis.

The analysis of an abnormal walking pattern is very complex, yet physiotherapists must do this in the clinic in order to be able to plan an appropriate training programme for infants and children with disability. The task is made more difficult by the paucity of biomechanical studies of the abnormal walking pattern in disabled children.

In most clinics, physiotherapists have to make their analyses qualitatively via observation. In the future, therapists will need to have access to quantitative biomechanical measures from movement analysis laboratories attached to rehabilitation centres.

Some findings related to normal gait in children are described later in this section. There are, however, several mechanical problems that commonly interfere with the ability to walk, irrespective of the age of the individual and the underlying pathological mechanisms. In general, it will be problems associated with the stance phase that will interfere most. Maintenance of the stance phase requires extensor muscle activity to prevent the support leg from collapsing, preparatory and ongoing muscle activity to balance the body as the body mass is moved forwards, extensibility of muscles, particularly hip flexor and calf muscles, to allow the body to move forwards over the foot and, finally, the ability to generate force, particularly in calf muscles, in order to propel the body forwards.

The major problems in the *stance leg* are:

1 Inability to extend the hip due to decreased length of hip flexors and/or calf muscles (Fig. 3.12) or hip flexors and adductors (Fig. 3.13).
2 Absence of the 'yield' of the knee which normally occurs early in stance due to weakness or paralysis of knee extensors with lack of control of eccentric activity and shortness of the soleus muscle which will hold the shank back and, therefore, the knee extended.
3 Excessive lateral horizontal shift of the pelvis, associated with an excessive downwards tilt on the side of the swinging leg (Fig. 3.14). This occurs with weakness of lower limb extensors and of the hip abductors.
4 Lack of plantarflexion at the ankle at heel-off/toe-off at the end of stance phase due to weakness or decreased length of calf muscles.
5 Knee flexion may occur in mid to late stance phase due to weak plantarflexor muscles which will result in the uncontrolled shank moving forwards at the ankle.

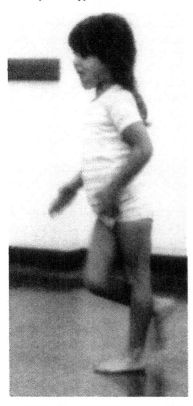

Figure 3.12   Girl with left hemiplegia. Note the alignment of the left leg in stance phase: lack of hip extension and ankle dorsiflexion. In this case, the shank is prevented from moving forwards at the ankle by short calf muscles.

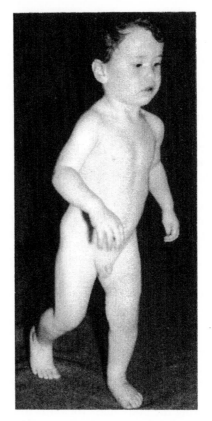

Figure 3.13   Boy with diplegic cerebral palsy. Note the internally rotated hip and valgus foot on the left.

In addition, children with disordered motor control will have difficulty balancing over one foot and also in double-support phase.

The major problems in the *swing leg* result mainly from the above dysfunctions since the stance phase normally sets up the optimal conditions for swing. They are:

1   Lack of knee flexion and, therefore, the inability to clear the foot from the ground, which may be due to lack of hip extension (movement of the body forward over the foot) in stance and to loss of force generated by calf muscles at push-off. Weakness of hamstrings or lack of control resulting in an inability both to extend the hip may aggravate the problems. Lack of knee flexion may also be due to shortness or increased stiffness of rectus femoris muscle, which will cause the knee to begin extending prematurely.

2   Lack of knee extension and ankle dorsiflexion in the last part of the swing phase will result in the foot being set down flat or toe first, instead of heel first. This is commonly due to short hamstring or calf muscles, although it will also occur when knee extensors and ankle dorsiflexors are paralysed. Where both lower limbs are involved, knee extension and ankle dorsiflexion may not occur in the swinging leg if the stance leg does not extend sufficiently.

Data-based studies, largely on children with CP, help elucidate the performance and control deficits in children with neural lesions. The rhythm, sequencing and timing of segmental rotations may be abnormal even when muscle activity is present. In addition, coactivation of leg muscles is reported as a characteristic of abnormal gait in children with CP (Knutsson 1980; Dietz and Berger 1983). It has been sug-

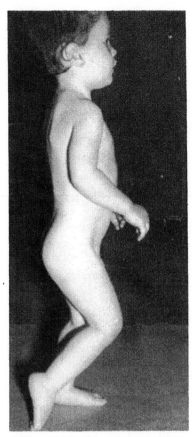

Figure 3.14 This view shows the lack of hip extension at the beginning of swing phase on the right. In stance phase on the left leg, the left hip abductors and right trunk muscles do not control the pelvis at the left hip and the pelvis drops down on the right. As a result, more hip flexion is needed to swing the right leg through.

gested that coactivation may alter the biomechanical characteristics of a limb, its capacity for absorbing and storing energy (Harrison and Kruze 1987).

Angle-angle (hip-knee) diagrams (Grieve 1968) have been used to compare abnormal motor patterns with normal in children with CP. One study (de Bruin *et al.* 1982) reported such abnormalities as reduced hip and knee motion, knee flexion at stance initiation, and hyperextension of the knees at the end of stance phase.

Another study (Norlin and Odenrick 1986) used a computerized gait analysis system to study the gait of 50 children with CP. The children showed reduced walking speed and stride length, longer stance and double support phases than normal.

Energy cost of walking can be higher than normal, as has been shown in children with diplegia (Adler and Black 1986). Studies of mechanical energy used in walking by CP children provide a global measure of energy cost and can identify the movement component responsible for abnormal energy cost. (Olney *et al.* 1987). For example, higher than normal energy costs were attributed by Olney and colleagues to very low levels of kinetic energy and poor patterns of exchange between potential and kinetic energy of the upper body (head, arms and trunk).

Considerable attention has been directed to the deficits occurring at the ankle joint in stance phase, that is, between shank and foot segments (e.g. Berger *et al.* 1982, 1984; Hoffer and Perry 1983; Olney *et al.* 1990). One study of power curves in CP children (Olney *et al.* 1990) reported a low level of power generated by the ankle plantarflexors. This concurs with results of other studies in which plantarflexor activity during stance was found to be lower than normal in children with CP (Berger *et al.* 1982, 1984; Lai *et al.* 1988). Berger and colleagues (1984) found that CP subjects showed an increase in tension in the Achilles tendon that did not equate with plantarflexor activation. This increased tension was said to be due to mechanical changes in muscle fibres themselves. They found no influence of pathological reflex activity in the gastrocnemius. This finding is supported by the work of Tardieu and colleagues (Tardieu *et al.* 1982a,b). The reduced amount of work done at the ankle may be responsible for the larger amount of work done at the hip (Olney *et al.* 1990), illustrating the importance of control between the fixed foot segment and the segment above. In a study of toe walking by Tardieu and colleagues (Tardieu *et al.* 1989), the authors showed that two mechanisms have the potential to cause toe walking: excessive contraction of triceps surae and contracture. This study illustrates the importance of understanding the mechanism underlying motor performance deficits in planning intervention. Physiotherapy would involve training control of the foot shank segment during stance, increasing the force output of calf muscles at the length where this output is required for the action and decreasing it at other lengths; with the addition of serial casting in the case of contracture.

In response to motor control and muscle length problems, the child will utilize certain typical *adaptive motor behaviours*. The behaviours listed below are the observable ones. It is not possible at the present time to do other than make an educated guess about the underlying mechanisms since the lower limb joints are controlled by both mono- and biarticular muscles. In addition, muscles do not affect only the joints they span. Figure 3.12 shows, for example, how shortness of the soleus muscle will affect not only the ankle joint alignment but also the alignment of knee and hip. The complexity of muscle action in a multisegment system, particularly when the foot is fixed, is only briefly referred to in some anatomy texts (e.g. Kapandji 1970), and it is only relatively recently that investigations have been carried out into muscle function in multijoint actions such as jumping (e.g. Gregoire *et al.* 1984; van Ingen-Schenau, 1989).

1   Lack of hip extension and ankle dorsiflexion may be compensated for by taking a short step with the swinging leg. The ability to bring the body mass forward over the foot is normally dependent on these two joint displacements.
2   Lack of control of the muscles which control knee position in stance may be associated with two adaptive behaviours – the knee either extends (or hyperextends) and remains extended or it is held in a few degrees of flexion throughout stance (Winter 1987; Butler *et al.* 1992) (Figs 3.13 and 3.14).
3   A child may hitch the pelvis up on the side of the swinging leg in response to a lack of knee flexion at the end of stance–beginning of swing, in order to clear the foot from the ground.
4   Difficulties with postural adjustments may result in a wide-based double support. There are two ways of increasing the base of support: the swing foot may be set down too far to the side and/or the foot is set down with the hip in external rotation. The arms may be held abducted as an additional method of restoring balance. If a child feels unable to walk without falling over, the hands will be used to gain stability in order to compensate for the lack of postural muscle activations in the lower limbs. The child may be aided in this compensa-

tory behaviour by the provision of a walking aid, which is sometimes essential but can prevent the child from developing balance while walking.
5   Speed of walking may be altered by the presence of some element of dyscontrol. The child may walk rather fast, which probably makes it easier to balance (Winter 1987). This is common in children with cerebellar lesions after head injury. Alternatively, walking may be abnormally slow.

Training

A child will develop the ability to walk only by practising the activity. The timing relationships between segmental rotations are critical to effective gait and can only be learned through *practice* of the activity itself. Early walking, present in the normal neonate, can be practised and maintained with guidance and support from the child's parents. For walking to become independent, however, the child has to be able to stand and move about in standing without falling over. In other words, postural adjustments, brought about primarily by distal leg muscles, must develop in standing for a child to be able to take independent steps. The major emphasis in training for independent walking for both infant or child, is, therefore, on assisted/supported walking and practice of moving about in standing. Support for walking is withdrawn as soon as possible and, in standing, use of the hands for support should be discouraged as soon as the infant or child has some control.

Training infant standing and stepping

Given the importance of the erect posture to the development of visuomotor and vestibulomotor function, more emphasis than is usual in current practice should be placed on supported standing and stepping from the first few days after birth in any infant who is at risk of developmental delay. In addition, organizing the neonate and young infant's environment to encourage kicking may influence the infant's potential for walking, since the muscle synergy of kicking has been shown to be similar to newborn stepping (Thelen and Fisher 1982; Thelen and Cooke 1987; Heriza 1988).

Standing The infant can be given practice of standing by parents (Fig. 3.1c). It should be clear to them that the way in which the infant stands – that is, the alignment of body segments – has to be carefully monitored. Specifically, the infant's feet should be flat on the support surface and the body inclined slightly forwards at the ankles with hips extended. The feet should be a few centimetres apart. The rationale for this posture lies in the predicted typical dysfunction and adaptations that can develop over time in infants with neural lesions – a tendency to plantarflex the ankles and stand on the toes, associated with shortening of the calf muscles. In the standing position, the infant can practise flexing the legs into crouch and standing up, keeping the heels on the ground (Fig. 3.1). It may be necessary to stand the infant in small plantar moulds that prevent the feet from rolling over into a pronated position.

If the infant cannot keep the knees extended, standing should still be practised but with *leggings* to keep the knees straight and enable the person giving support to concentrate on other aspects of the standing posture (see Fig. 8.5).

Stepping Stepping will be present in most infants for a short period after birth, and when it is, parents can be taught how to give the infant practice in order to reinforce the stepping action. Since the infant will grow and become heavier, practice should be continued through infancy, as it appears that practice of bearing weight through the lower limbs in stepping enables the leg muscles to maintain the necessary strength for this action (Thelen and Fisher 1982). Unfortunately, infants at risk of developmental delay are not always referred to physiotherapy and this potentially useful means of training walking is made very difficult by the secondary changes, both neural and mechanical, which will have occurred by the time the child is referred.

Parents should understand, as with standing practice, that certain abnormal aspects of walking which may develop, particularly in the neurologically impaired infant, must be discouraged. The parents should have a clear idea that what the infant practises is what will be become 'learned' or habitual. Crossing one leg over the other and walking on the toes in particular should be discouraged. Muscle extensibility or length must be maintained as the infant grows, otherwise when certain muscles are held short they will cause unwanted mechanical effects which will interfere with the normal walking and standing pattern. For example, short hip flexors prevent hip extension; short calf muscles prevent the shank (and body mass) moving forwards at the ankle; short hip adductor muscles affect step length.

Training walking in older infants and children

In general, walking can be trained using the guidelines described by Carr and Shepherd (1987a) for adults, since mature walking is what the infant aspires to. Furthermore, the child over 4 or 5 years, if he or she has walked before the lesion, will have already developed a mature walking pattern (Sutherland *et al.* 1980). This means that the child has to be given the opportunity to walk and will usually need to do specific exercises to increase strength and control in muscles required to generate force at particular stages in the gait cycle and to improve postural adjustments in stance and double support phase. A treadmill provides an opportunity to practise under challenging and interesting conditions. The moving belt maximizes the extent of hip extension, thereby setting up one of the necessary conditions for the swing phase of that leg (Fig. 3.15). Treadmill walking has been shown to be effective in training walking in adults following stroke (Malouin *et al.* 1992).

Infants normally *walk sideways* around the furniture just before walking independently. This action probably enables them to develop postural adjustments as they experiment with taking their hands off the support to reach for toys. Walking sideways is a useful exercise for the disabled infant also. Since, unlike walking forward or backwards, the knees are kept relatively extended, an infant who is having difficulty controlling the lower limbs in standing can wear wraparounds (see Fig. 8.5) during practice. This modification to the practice conditions may make independent practice possible.

All infants need *support* for their early attempts at walking before they are able to walk independently. Although disabled infants will also need support, the physiotherapist should ensure this support is withdrawn gradually when the infant can stand independently. Support can be given by the parents holding

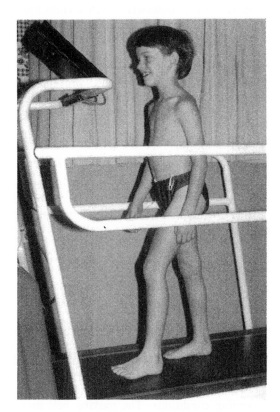

Figure 3.15   Practising on the treadmill with feedback about distance walked and time taken. This boy has right hemiplegia. (Courtesy of the Royal Far West Hospital, Sydney, Australia.)

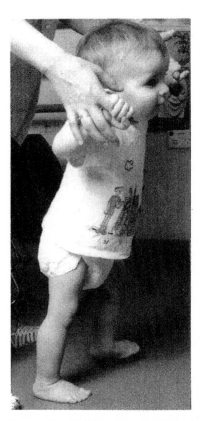

Figure 3.16   Walking practice with assistance.

the infant's hands as they would do with their non-disabled child (Fig. 3.16). If this is not sufficient or if it provokes unwanted adaptations to the walking pattern, support can be given at the shoulders and upper trunk as in the walking facilitation technique devised by Bobath (Bobath and Bobath 1964; Fig. 3.17). Some children, for example those with lesions of the spinal cord, are dependent on more substantial methods of support if they are to stand and progress on their feet. Such methods will be discussed in the relevant chapters.

Some form of *orthosis* may be needed to enable independent walking to be trained. In children with spina bifida cystica, for example, an orthosis which prevents the lower limb from collapsing will be critical in the absence of lower limb extensor power. In children with brain lesions, the issue is more controversial and it is possible that there may be an incongruity between the goals of training and the design

of the orthosis. For example, an orthosis designed to aid ankle dorsiflexion may be less effective in helping a child produce an efficient walking pattern than exercises and walking training designed to lengthen shortened calf muscles and train control of the lower limb as it moves over the fixed foot.

The effect of an orthosis on a child's walking can be measured in terms of physiological parameters such as heart rate (e.g. Mossberg *et al.* 1990) or biomechanical variables (e.g. Butler *et al.* 1992).

Exercises designed to address specific control problems will usually have to be practised. Strength and control of propulsion and support over a fixed foot can be practised by step up and down exercises (Figs 3.18 and 3.19). These require the ability to generate concentric force in the lower limb extensors while keeping the body weight forward over the foot, then the ability to switch from a concentric to an

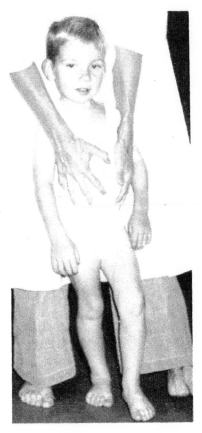

Figure 3.17 Facilitated walking. The therapist assists with weight shift and rotates the upper body on the stance hip. Assistance is withdrawn as the child gets the idea of the action required.

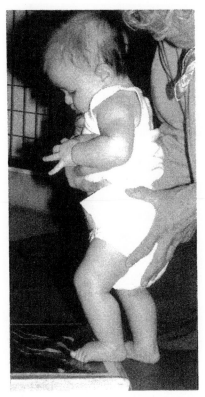

Figure 3.18 Infant with left hemiplegia practising stepping up and down on a small wooden block with therapist support. Reaching for a toy can be used to encourage the action.

eccentric mode of contraction to lower the body weight. Stepping up and down sideways requires a different synergic relationship between hip extensors and abductors (Fig. 3.20).

Standing on a block, the child can practise lowering the heels (which stretches the calf muscles) and raising the heels to the plantigrade position (which strengthens the calf muscles from the fully extended length to mid-length; Fig. 3.21). This is a suitable exercise for children with neural lesions who have a tendency to develop short stiff calf muscles in the presence of hyperreflexia and neural dyscontrol. This mechanical, peripheral component of spasticity results in calf muscles which have structurally adapted to a shortened length and which generate tension at this short length. This exercise (and other similar exercises) both ensures optimal muscle length as well as train-

ing the muscles to generate force in the range from full dorsiflexion to plantigrade. This range is necessary for the end-of-stance phase in walking as well as walking up and down stairs and standing up and sitting down. The exercise should probably be practised routinely by any infant or child in whom shortness and stiffness can be predicted since, at the very least, prevention of this peripheral component of hypertonus sets up an internal environment which enables the child to improve performance.

Exercises may have to be set up to stimulate the contraction of a muscle or to strengthen a weak muscle group. The position in which muscles are strengthened may not be of any consequence in the early stage of training, since such exercises are designed to get weak or inactive muscles to generate more force, for much the same reason that one goes to a gymnasium.

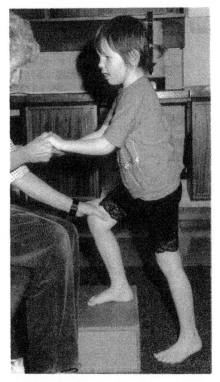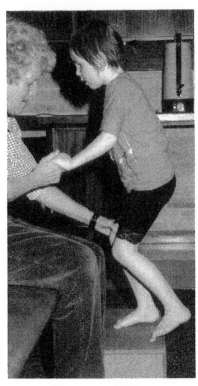

Figure 3.19   Girl with cerebellar ataxia practises stepping up and down to increase strength and control of lower-limb extensor muscles. She needs support for this exercise as her balance is poor.

However, for muscles to be able to generate the necessary force in the synergy required for stance phase of walking or for walking up steps, it is clear that these actions must themselves be practised repetitively.

Modification of the environment

The environment may need to be modified to enable a child to correct abnormalities in the gait pattern. The therapist needs to recognize the movement component interfering with effective walking by comparing the child's performance against a normal model of essential components. For example, if a child has difficulty with hip and knee flexion in swing phase, walking can be practised over an obstacle course, with the obstacles placed so the child has to step over them. If a child places the feet too closely together, walking can be practised with each foot on one side of a plank. If a child walks with a wide base, practice can be encouraged with a narrower base by the child

walking within a boundary outlined on the floor (Fig. 3.22). Such modifiers assist by giving feedback about error. Their main benefit, however, is probably in forcing or driving the required action.

Reaching and manipulation

It can probably be said that the arm functions principally in order to get the hand to the action, that reaching is the major action of the arm and interaction with the environment the major purpose of the hand. However, the arms are also yoked into the postural system (Gentile 1987). When balance is compromised, the arms have a stabilizing function and, if balance is lost, the hands are used to form a new base of support. Unless the body is in a fully supported position, any reaching action in sitting or standing is preceded and accompanied by postural adjustments. These ensure that the body segment alignment is appropriate to the upcoming perturbation which will be caused by the arm

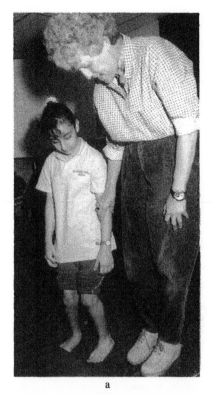 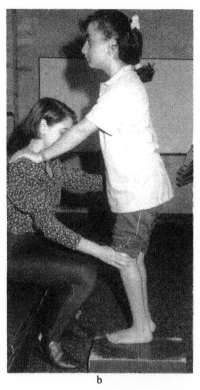

a   b

Figure 3.20 In (a) the therapist shows how the exercise is done; in (b) the girl practises with maximum repetitions in blocks of three. She should take her hands from the therapist's shoulders when she thinks she has her balance.

movement. Postural adjustments associated with body movement towards the object also allow an extension of the reach, effectively enlarging the attainable part of the environment.

It is evident that the arm and hand function as a single unit in reaching and manipulation, enabling the individual to interact with objects and people in the environment. The individual both responds to environmental demands and imposes intentions upon the environment. In many actions involving reaching, the upper body also becomes part of the single coordinated unit, movement of the upper body functioning to increase the reaching distance. Unless the body is supported during reaching, arm movement will require postural adjustments for the action to be controlled. In standing, postural adjustments have been shown to occur prior to arm movement in order to prevent arm movement from destabilizing the body. These postural adjustments are brought about by muscle activation and usually result in some alteration in segmental alignment (e.g.

Bouisset and Zattara 1981). Pre-arm movement postural activity has also been reported in sitting during fast pointing (Shepherd *et al.* 1993). Due to the important informational role of vision in reaching and manipulation, eye and head movement will also play a critical part in enabling a coordinated movement to take place (Biguer *et al.* 1982).

That the arm and hand function as a single coordinated unit is remarkable given the number of components in the unit and the complexity of human manipulative actions. The unit is made up of many joints and muscles (monoarticular, biarticular and multiarticular), with many degrees of freedom which must be constrained or utilized if reaching and manipulative activities are to be coordinated.

Description of the activity

Normal newborn infants have been shown to be able to reach in different directions towards objects (Bower *et al.* 1970; von Hofsten 1982).

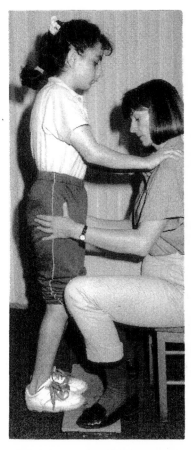

Figure 3.21 Practising an exercise for actively stretching calf muscles and increasing strength and control of calf muscles from their lengthened position to mid-range. The therapist is reminding her to keep her hips extended in order to confine movement to the ankles.

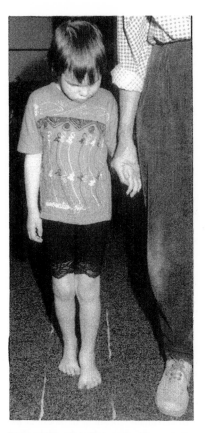

Figure 3.22 This little girl with cerebellar ataxia is learning how to walk with a narrower base of support. She needs some support at first.

By the end of the first 4–5 months, infants can predict the future position of moving objects and reach to catch them (von Hofsten and Lindhagen 1979). It has been shown that infants a few days old will not reach for objects that are out of reach (Bower 1974) and at 5 months they will not reach for objects longer than an arm's length away. It has been shown in adults that the reaching action slows just before contact with the object (Jeannerod 1984), and in infants this component has been demonstrated by 5 months of age (von Hofsten 1979). Infants younger than 9 months may not orient their hands appropriately for objects in anticipation of contact, even though they are capable of pronating and supinating their forearms. Before that age, at around 5 months, they will orient their forearms so the palm of the hand is correctly positioned to grasp a bar held vertically or horizontally, but only after having contacted the bar (Lockman *et al.* 1984).

Reaching to grasp

According to Jeannerod's investigations (Jeannerod 1984), reaching can be divided into two stages – a *transportation component*, in which the hand moves quickly to the vicinity of the target, and a *manipulation component* when final adjustment to the grasp apertures is made just prior to grasp.

Support for the suggestion that the arm and hand function as a single unit comes from the finding that the hand starts to open for grasp at the start of the reaching action (Jeannerod 1981). Jeannerod filmed his subjects as they reached for objects of various sizes lying on the surface of a table. The grasp aperture (the distance between thumb and index finger) increased throughout the transport phase, reaching a maximum before contact and around the time the transport movement started to decelerate. The grasp size then decreased as the hand neared the object. When under visual control, the distance between the two grasp components (thumb and index finger) was a little greater than necessary for the size of the object and reflected the size of the object. This distance was increased when visual control was removed.

A study of a single subject (Wing and Fraser 1983) suggests that the thumb plays a role in guiding the transport component of reaching. During the final approach phase in a reaching task, the closing of the hand from peak aperture was largely due to movement of the finger with very little thumb movement. The authors suggested that, since the position of the thumb relative to the line of approach to the object remained invariant, the thumb stabilization provided a focus for visual monitoring of the movement of the relationship between grasp aperture and object size.

Evidence of the effect of environmental context and the individual's intention on reaching and grasping comes from a study in which the orientation of the hand was shown to vary according to what was to be done with the object once it was grasped (Iberall *et al.* 1986). When subjects were asked to tap the end of the dowel on the table top, approach and grasp were different from when they were asked to shake the dowel up and down.

When the hand contacts the object, grasp comes under tactile feedback control. This information is used to monitor the friction quality of the object and its weight, enabling muscle force to be adjusted according to the slip or load force required (Johansson and Westling 1990).

Manipulation

The hand is the principal means by which the individual interacts with people and objects in the external environment. The anatomical structure of the hand and the nature of cortico-motoneuronal connections to hand muscles (Kapandji 1970; Landsmeer 1976; Smith 1981; Muir 1985; Lemon *et al.* 1990) allow a large number of combinations of joint rotations and a vast array of movement possibilities. Even in

relatively simple tasks, there may be a variety of different configurations of the hand segments and it has been shown in the limited number of studies available that the intention as well as the object itself affect the approach and grasp as well as the manipulation (Iberall *et al.* 1986).

Many actions involve interactions between an object and the thumb and index finger as the object is grasped and manipulated. These actions require the thumb to abduct and rotate and the index finger to flex so that their pulps contact the object. Force is effectively exerted on the object primarily by the long flexor muscles of thumb and index finger, and stabilization of each bone is achieved by both joint geometry and intrinsic musculature (Spoor 1983). The force produced on the index finger by the thumb is countered by the first dorsal interosseus muscle. The force produced on the mobile carpometacarpal joint of the thumb is constrained by activity of all the thenar muscles (Chao *et al.* 1989). As in any other part of the segmental linkage, force applied to one segment will affect segments sometimes quite far distant from the original force, and motor control mechanisms must take these segmental interactions into account. With the hand, the combination of small mobile segments and a rich array of muscles means that the complexity of these interactional forces, even though they may be small, is considerable. The lumbrical and interossei muscles, for example, exert axial rotary moments of force which are balanced by other appropriate muscles (Lemon *et al.* 1991). Interestingly, it appears that for a given task, although similar muscle groups are active, the degree of activity and the relative contributions of muscles differ.

Essential components

Part of the complexity of hand movement arises out of the potential of so many degrees of freedom and from the different possibilities inherent in the physical interaction between intention and object. It is, however, possible to identify certain components of movement, or combinations of components which are present in many otherwise different tasks.

Reaching forward

1 Flexion at the shoulder in some external rotation.

2 Opening of the hand aperture between thumb and fingers.
3 Extension of wrist.
4 Pronation–supination appropriate to object orientation.

Grasping
1 Extension of the fingers and abduction of the thumb during reach.
2 Closure of fingers and thumb around object.

Manipulation
1 Flexion and extension at metacarpophalangeal joints of fingers.
2 Abduction and conjunct rotation of thumb at the carpometacarpal joint.
3 Flexion and conjunct rotation at the metacarpophalangeal joint of the fifth finger.
4 Independent finger flexion and extension.

These movement components are essential at some stage and in various degrees in many tasks. Since there are very few studies of even the kinematics of hand movement in the performance of everyday actions, it is necessary for the physiotherapist in the clinic to study the normal performance of each action which needs to be trained, attempting to identify which components appear to be critical.

As an example, when individuals hold a knife and fork, apart from the position of the index fingers on the implements enabling force to be directed downwards and the flexed wrist position, observation of the palmar surface makes it clear that crucial to any pressure downwards through the knife and fork is the ability to hold the implements firmly against the palm. Although probably critical to effective use of cutlery, this latter component requires the long finger flexor muscles to generate force while held at a very short length, at which the muscle's capacity to generate force is limited by its structure. This component also requires that the long finger extensors are able to lengthen to the extent necessary.

Motor dysfunction

There have been few investigations of the dyscontrol characteristics in reaching and manipulation in disabled individuals. Although there are considerable methodological difficulties in investigating muscle activity in tasks involving the hand, kinematic analyses and analyses of force production between hand segments and the object being manipulated increase our understanding of the motor dysfunction in children with lesions of the neuromusculoskeletal system.

Observable problems with *reaching to an object* include deviations from a normal path, deficiencies in speed of movement and poor timing of contact with an object. Significantly slower hand movements in affected compared to unaffected hand have been shown in children with hemiplegic CP (Brown *et al.* 1987). The hand may not open until it nears the object and it may not be oriented to grasp the object appropriately in terms of its characteristics (e.g. shape) and what is to be done with it.

Path deviations may be caused by inability to combine, for example, glenohumeral joint flexion with external rotation and a deficiency in supination (Fig. 3.23). The hand path may be relatively appropriate but the elbow will be abducted away from the body.

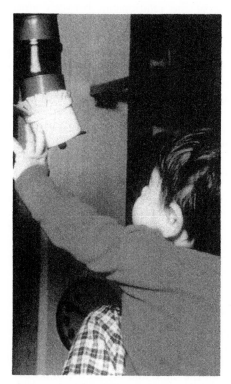

Figure 3.23 This object is too big to grasp so is of little value in training reaching to grasp. For this little boy with left hemiplegia, an object could be used that would require a more supinated forearm, since this is the aspect of the approach phase of reaching that needs training.

Movement speed may be too slow or too fast; the movement may be jerky and lack the smooth acceleration–deceleration profile seen in controlled movement. Poor timing of contact may result in the hand knocking into the object or closing before the object is reached.

Lesions affecting the motor cortex or corticomotoneuronal projections seem to be followed by a loss or clumsiness of fine finger control (Lough *et al.* 1984; Fig. 3.24). Abnormal posturing of the hand may vary from a persistent finger flexion despite the ability to extend the fingers (see Fig. 3.28b) to wrist flexion, pronation and ulnar deviation (Fig. 3.25). While in normal children contact with an object is followed immediately by a grasp, in infants with a brain lesion, as was shown in one recent study, the fingers of the affected hand may remain extended after contact and the child may be able to manage only a clumsy grasp (Jeannerod 1986).

As demonstrated in Jeannerod's study, an infant with hemiplegia may not use the affected hand until the other hand is immobilized. There is considerable evidence from monkey experiments and from studies and observations of adults and children with hemiplegia that restraint of the unaffected arm is associated with increased use of the affected arm. This will be discussed below as a possible training

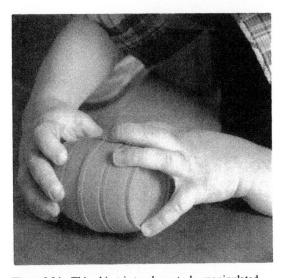

Figure 3.24 This object is too large to be manipulated accurately by the child, who has poor control of his fingers. A smaller object would enable him to practise (see Fig. 3.28).

strategy in infants with hemiplegia and children with acquired hemiplegia.

Training

Therapy for motor impaired infants and children has typically addressed upper-limb function in terms of fine motor skills (by which is meant grasping and manipulation) and support (e.g. through the hands or forearms in prone, sitting). Reaching as such is not often discussed in the clinical literature, although the therapist is very likely in practice to include reaching in a child's therapy programme (e.g. Blaskey 1989; Wilson 1989). Similarly, methods of testing upper-limb function test manipulation and support functions and not reaching (e.g. Burns *et al.* 1989).

The relatively recent investigations of the development of reaching (see Chapter 2) and of the movement characteristics of adult reaching and grasping provide information of considerable value to paediatric clinical practice (Ada *et al.* 1994). For example, given the evidence from studies of reaching development, it can be inferred that in infants with motor impairment, training of active reaching to grasp can commence earlier than has typically been the case in clinical practice. With motor-disabled infants, it has often been assumed that reaching and grasping cannot be expected to occur until an infant develops control of the head and sitting balance. It has further been assumed that development of the ability to support the body through the arms (in the prone position, for example) is a necessary prerequisite for reaching, since shoulder control is necessary for hand use, motor development taking place from proximal to distal. In infants whose motor disability is the result of a brain lesion, however, gaining control over neck, trunk and proximal limb muscle activation may take a considerable period of time. Following from the above assumptions, physical and occupational therapy may concentrate principally on the infant gaining head control and the ability to weight-bear through the arms, and very little on reaching towards objects. In addition, the long-standing therapeutic emphasis on facilitating the infant's automatic response to therapist-imposed perturbations (e.g. Bobath 1967; Perin 1989) may mean that the infant gets little practice in actively engaging with the environment using vision and hands.

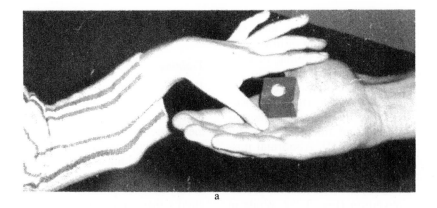

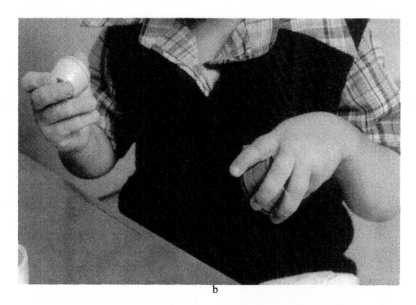

Figure 3.25   (a) The final phase of reaching to grasp is accomplished with the wrist flexed and excessive extension of the metacarpophalangeal joints. (b) Note the left hand. Holding the wrist in a flexed position makes it difficult to generate appropriate force to grasp the toy.

The absence of head control and of sitting balance should not be a deterrent to early training since, as von Hofsten has shown, neonates are able to attempt reaching towards an object if certain conditions are met. For example, the infant must be supported in a semireclined position; the object should be attractive, graspable and within visual range (Fig. 3.26). In addition, the young infant may see the object more clearly when it moves across the visual field than when it is stationary (von Hofsten and Lindhagen 1979).

The benefits of early practice include the opportunity to develop eye–hand and object–hand coordination, oculomotor control and an awareness of the possibilities offered by interactions with the environment. However, the training of very young infants needs to give consideration to the constraints placed upon normal young infants as well as the essential aspects of reaching and manipulation to which particular attention should be given. It may be that the opportunity to practise reaching towards an object is critical in infancy if con-

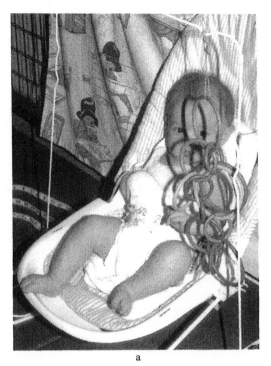
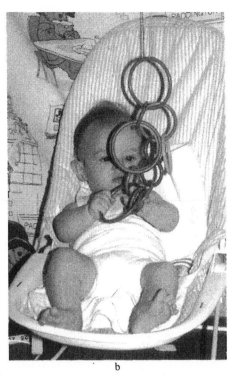

a   b

Figure 3.26 (a) Restraining the unaffected arm and positioning graspable objects on the side of the affected arm encourage use of the arm in this infant with left hemiplegia. (b) When the restraint is removed, the infant is encouraged to use the hands bimanually.

trol over the upper limbs for functional activities is to be acquired by an infant with a disability affecting movement.

In developing control over the linked segments of the upper limb, infants must develop the ability to match their motor performance to the characteristics of objects within their environment. They learn to judge whether or not an object must be picked up in one or both hands; how the hand should be oriented to match the object and what is to be done to it; whether all or only some of the fingers are needed in order to grasp the object. In reaching, infants have to learn to control for direction and distance. They have to gain the ability to judge the distance over which they can successfully reach, which means knowing the length of the arm and the distance over which body movements will extend that reach. Of particular importance in development, therefore, is gaining the ability to use vision to guide hand movement and to provide both information about the environment with which the infant must interact and feedback about movement performance. In addition, the infant must learn to incorporate the necessary postural adjustments into reaching and manipulation in upright positions such as sitting and standing.

Certain research findings suggest a dominance of vision over touch. In one study, subjects watched through a window what they thought was their own hand but was instead the experimenter's hand seen through a mirror (Rock and Harris 1967). As a result of these findings and others, Rosenbaum (1991) suggests a training strategy for the disabled which involves the patient seeing an image of the limb with greater mobility than it actually has.

Limb movement may need to be forced if one limb is effectively paralysed and one is not, as in hemiplegia from a brain lesion or brachial plexus lesion. Taub and others (Taub 1980; Chapman and Wiesendanger 1982) have shown with both deafferented and hemiplegic monkeys that a paralysed or insensate arm would be left to hang by the side when there was one effective upper limb. However, when the intact limb was restrained and the monkey given some training to use the affected limb with feedback reward, the affected limb became functional. Promising results have been reported with both adults after stroke (Ostendorf and Wolf 1981; Wolf *et al.* 1989; Taub *et al.* 1993) and children (Schwartzman 1974). However, more investigation is needed to establish the optimal timing and method for such intervention. Nevertheless, the functional outcome for infants with unilateral impairment can be so severe that using some form of restraint to the unaffected upper limb in such infants is probably justified, if performed under conditions of strict monitoring. Restraint can be achieved by enclosing the unaffected arm within the infant's clothing (Fig. 3.26), or the arm can be wrapped to the side. In addition, training can also be planned to ensure that an object can only be reached by reaching with the affected arm (Fig. 3.27).

It is only relatively recently that it has been recognized that motor performance is governed to a considerable extent by objects and their 'affordances' (Gibson 1977). That is to say, objects offer possibilities for interaction. When we reach out for an object, the movement pattern reflects the object's position in relation to the body and its orientation, and what we are intending to do with it (Iberall *et al.* 1986; Rosenbaum *et al.* 1990). As with motor training in adults, objects should be chosen, there-

fore, not only for their inherent interest and usability but also for the options they offer for hand orientation (see Figs 10.5–10.7). For example, if a child has difficulty controlling the orientation of the hand and limb during reach and reaches persistently with the shoulder internally rotated and the forearm pronated, an object should be chosen that demands a relatively externally rotated and supinated approach. Toys and objects can be chosen and games played that actively encourage the action with which the infant has difficulty. If a child is offered toys which can be grasped in many different ways, the movement pattern used by the child will reflect the options provided by the lesioned system and will probably be the easiest one (see Figs 3.23 and 10.3). Toys and objects need to be specially chosen to enable practice to take place without a struggle. Tasks should on the whole be challenging but not impossible.

It is necessary to train bimanual actions since the two upper limbs work cooperatively in most everyday functions (Fig. 3.28). For example, unscrewing a jar involves coordinating opposing forces between lid and jar. There has recently been considerable experimental interest in bimanual actions (Kelso *et al.* 1979; Martenuik *et al.* 1984; Castiello *et al.* 1993). One experiment showed that when a subject

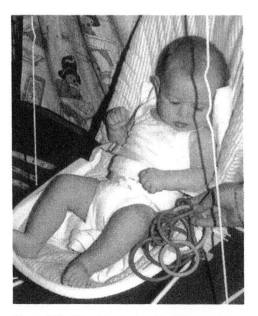
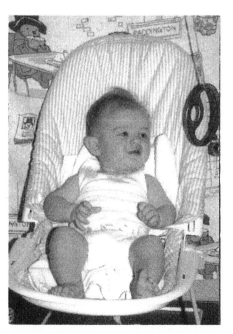

Figure 3.27   The object is placed in different positions so it can only be reached with the affected arm.

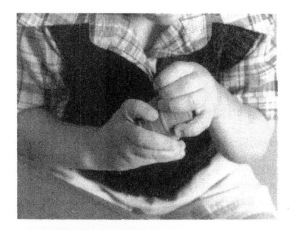

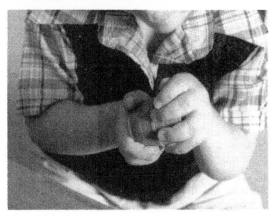

Figure 3.28 Bimanual tasks are necessary to encourage the forces generated by the two hands to be matched to the object characteristics. This child is experimenting with the best way to configure the fingers to achieve the goal.

ing the trunk may need to wrap around the shoulders to encourage shoulder flexion rather than abduction.

Reaching and manipulation should be practised in positions which optimize performance. For example, using the upper limbs in floor-sitting may be difficult for a child with poor lower-limb control and adaptive muscle changes (Fig. 3.29). In this position, the arms are needed principally for support. Sitting at a table, however, will make it possible for a child to develop skill in reaching and manipulative tasks (Fig. 3.30).

In reaching to grasp and manipulate, the grasp aperture forms from the start of the

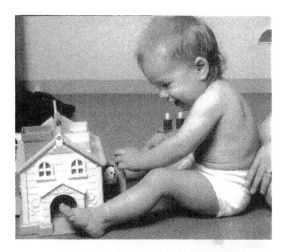

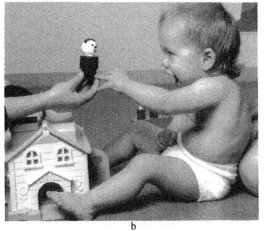

b

Figure 3.29 (a) This child cannot flex the hips sufficiently and has difficulty making postural adjustments in sitting. (b) When she reaches up for a toy, she falls backwards as she cannot make the necessary anticipatory adjustments.

holds a ball and lets it drop into a cup held by the other hand, the grip force of the cup hand increases in anticipation of the ball's impact (Johansson and Westling 1988). Practice of games like this is aimed at improving visual and tactile processing as well as preparatory and ongoing adjustments to grip force.

Modification of the environment

With a motor-disabled infant, additional support may need to be given in order that reaching is possible and the angular displacements and hand path will be optimal. For example, when the infant is supported in a seat (see Fig. 5.13), the head may need to be supported so it does not fall to one side; the back-rest support-

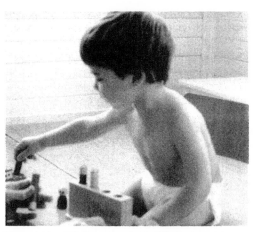

Figure 3.30 This boy, who had difficulty practising reaching when sitting on the floor (see Fig. 5.5), is able to concentrate on manual tasks when seated on a chair at a table.

reach and, as the hand nears the object, this aperture is slightly greater than the size of the object (Jeannerod 1981). The thumb plays a critical part in establishing the size of the grasp aperture (Wing and Fraser 1983; Wing *et al.* 1986) and allowing the manipulation of objects within the hand. In infants and children with problems activating and controlling hand musculature, the thumb typically lies in an adducted position and web space soft tissues rapidly become short. In training such children, it may be necessary to support the thumb in a small splint so that the carpometacarpal joint is maintained in abduction and opposition. The splint will serve to maintain passively the extent of the grasp aperture so that, in an immobile infant, the soft tissues between thumb metacarpal and index metacarpal will not shorten. If the splint is designed so that some active abduction of the thumb away from the splint is possible, the splint may, when worn during training sessions, promote activity in the thumb muscles. A single case study (Goodman and Bazyk 1991) showed with a 4-year-old child with CP that wearing an opponens splint for 6 hours a day and all night for a 4-week period resulted in significant improvement in active range of movement and in some functional tasks.

To train the opening phase of the grasp, it may be necessary not only to support the thumb and train thumb abduction and opposi-

tion, but also to train wrist extension. Wrist extension and finger metacarpophalangeal joint extension work together with thumb abduction to develop the necessary grasp aperture.

Balancing in sitting and standing

The ability to balance while moving about in sitting and standing is critical to effective daily life. Movement of one body segment involves movement of other segments since our bodies are composed of linked segments. Even the smallest movements, including taking a deep breath, looking up or around the room and reaching for an object, require the ability to balance the linked body segments over a fixed base of support. In sitting on a seat, the base of support comprises the feet (on the floor) and the thighs; in standing, the feet form the base of support.

Balancing the body mass while moving about is achieved by muscular activations called postural adjustments, which are known to occur before a self-initiated focal limb movement (e.g. reaching out to grasp an object) as well as during the movement. In this situation, postural adjustments occur to set up the segmental linkage in such a way that, when the arm is raised forwards towards the object, the body is kept steady and well-balanced. All self-initiated actions are preceded by these preparatory or anticipatory postural muscle activations. Under other circumstances, when sitting on a train or standing on a boat, for example, postural adjustments occur principally in response to unexpected support surface perturbations. That is why we often have to hold on to a support so that the unexpected movement of the floor does not throw us off balance. Even under these circumstances, we may use vision to predict the upcoming perturbation and make preparatory adjustments accordingly. When we are practised at making these judgements, we may not need to hold on as the boat moves about under us.

Interestingly, it appears that the postural muscle activations are specific both to the action and to the context in which that action is taking place. Furthermore, muscles act as postural muscles according to the environmental conditions prevailing at the time. For example, if we are holding on to a stable object when the support surface on which we are standing unexpectedly moves, the biceps brachii can function as a postural muscle, preventing us from losing balance. If we are holding on to an object which unexpectedly moves, muscles linking the shank to the fixed foot will be active to prevent us falling (Cordo and Nashner 1982).

Muscles close to the base of support seem particularly critical to our maintenance of a balanced body when we are moving and when we are standing still. In sitting on a seat with the feet on the floor, the leg muscles are active when we reach out, both before the arm starts to move and during the movement (Shepherd *et al.* 1993). Some of this muscle activity, which is linked closely to the arm muscle activity, prevents us from overbalancing as we reach out. Activity of the muscles in the legs and of those which link the upper body with the thighs enables us to move our body mass about over the base of support within a certain perimeter. If we move our body mass beyond this perimeter, we will fall off the seat and make a new base of support with our hands.

In standing, the situation is similar, only the muscle activity is different since in this position the base of support is different. Again there is a perimeter beyond which we cannot move the body mass without taking a step (i.e. making a new base of support) or falling. The area in which we can maintain balance while moving has been referred to as the 'region of reversibility' (Nashner and McCollum 1985).

The development of postural adjustments associated with self-initiated movement is dependent first upon neural maturation and then upon the practice of actions in particular contexts. The young infant, however, is able from early in life to move body segments in response to certain stimuli and externally imposed body movements. Many of these responses demonstrate an ability to orient the body in some way and many illustrate the infant's apparently innate ability to appreciate changes in the body's relationship to gravity and changes to the alignment of segments. For example, when the newborn infant is held in standing and the body mass is tilted forwards, the infant will step. When the infant is moved from sitting backwards towards supine, the head will be held vertical for a large part of the way, apparently until the neck muscles can no longer generate sufficient force.

Many of the movements of young infants appear to be related to keeping the head erect. For example, placed in prone or supported in ventral suspension, an infant will raise the head. Moved about in the air, an infant will lift the head and body sideways, backwards, forwards, depending on the direction the body is tilted. The young infant's postural adjustments appear, therefore, to be principally concerned with the righting of the head and body in response to externally imposed movement. These adjustments are traditionally termed body-righting or head-righting reactions and they probably represent early attempts to respond to the effects of gravity. Interestingly, the infant from quite early in life is able to override these reactions if something catches the attention. For example, it may be impossible to elicit a Landau response in ventral suspension if the infant's attention is captured by an object on the floor or a person off to one side.

Similarly, the reactions to externally imposed body movement which occur over a base of support, such as in sitting or standing, called equilibrium reactions, probably represent the body's attempt to prevent displacements from causing the body to overbalance.

Movement dysfunction

Infants and children seen in paediatric practice with lesions resulting in balance dysfunction can be considered as forming two groups – those who have previously developed postural adjustments and those who have not. The typical problems seen include lack of righting reactions in infants and poor postural adjustments over a fixed base of support in older infants and children.

In infants, righting reactions are assessed as an indication of the infant's ability to respond to externally imposed movement of the body. This involves moving the infant about and observing the responses, comparing them to normal performance at different ages (see Appendix 1).

In older infants and children, postural adjustments are analysed in sitting and standing during self-initiated movements. This involves, for example, observing the child's performance while reaching forwards, sideways, down to the floor, to grasp or touch an object; while looking up at the ceiling, turning to look behind; and during walking. In children whose motor control deficits are the result of an acute lesion occurring beyond the time that postural adjustments would have matured, performance can be compared in general with that of an adult. In younger children, deficits in performance can be expected due to immaturity, and the analysis needs to be weighed against the typical performance at various ages. This is problematic at present due to a relative lack of knowledge about the changes occurring in normal children as they mature. However, as more knowledge is gained, so can the clinical analysis becomes more complete.

The ability of children to respond to support surface perturbations and to other, therapist-imposed, perturbations (equilibrium reactions) can also be analysed. The former can be measured using electromyograms and kinematic analysis, although this is not a reality in most clinics at the moment. The value of analysing equilibrium reactions is uncertain. The information provided is similar to that provided by testing righting reactions, that is, the ability of the child to move body parts to ensure the body's centre of mass remains within a secure perimeter when an external destabilizing force is being applied to the body.

The typical problems seen in infants range from absence of any response to body movement due to apparent muscle weakness of cortical origin, to a stereotyped response which does not vary. In the former case, the infant hangs like a rag doll when held up by the tester (see Fig. 5.1). In the latter case, seen, for example, in severely mentally retarded infants with microcephaly, the righting reactions are immediate, stereotyped and persistent. The infant is not attracted towards any environmental stimuli and does not demonstrate the flexibility of response seen in the normal infant. An infant with severe hyperreflexia and hypertonia may demonstrate no ability to respond to imposed positional changes, remaining stiff and immobile, typically with legs extended and abducted and arms flexed.

The infant who starts off being very flaccid with little muscle activity usually develops the ability to respond to externally imposed displacements of the body, although much later than normal infants. However, most infants and children with congenital and traumatic brain injury will usually have problems making postural adjustments to self-initiated actions as part of a generalized motor control problem. The most commonly seen problems include:

1   Inability to make effective preparatory adjustments when in sitting or standing. This may be due to poor timing of muscular contractions but is also seen in children who have had no experience of moving about independently in either of these positions. This problem results in an inability to move about without falling or staggering.
2   Difficulty with ongoing postural adjustments due to poor timing of muscular contractions, poor grading of force output and, as above, is seen in children who have not learned to put together postural adjustments with focal limb movements.
3   Children with cerebellar lesions demonstrate uncoordinated movement called dyssynergia and dysmetria or ataxia. These terms translate, as far as balance is concerned, into an inability to put together in a coordinated manner the segmental rotations or joint displacements of which a motor act is composed (i.e. dyssynergia) and an inability to grade muscle force production so that linear and angular displacements are of the amplitude and velocity required for a particular action. The observable feature of this problem is the tendency to over- or undershoot the goal (i.e. dysmetria). These problems result in excessive postural sway in quiet standing, a tendency to overbalance when the child reaches for an object, and motor performance that lacks a smooth execution.

Since postural adjustments are a critical part of any active volitional movement, the problems described above will be evident in anything the child attempts to do, whether in walking, stair-climbing, getting up from the floor to standing, or sitting down.

In response to these problems, children with poor balance utilize *adaptive motor behaviours* in a similar way to adults (Carr and Shepherd 1987b; Shepherd 1992). The range of mechanically possible adaptive movements has not been the subject of much investigation. However, it is likely that the behaviours listed below represent the most commonly observed.

1   *Widening the base of support*. This is achieved by sitting or standing with the

legs apart. In standing, the legs may be externally rotated as well as apart. The child may walk with feet too widely spaced and may not be able to stop in double-support phase without externally rotating the legs to increase the base of support still further. If the perimeter within which the child can safely move is very small, the child may also take a step prematurely when looking around or reaching out for a toy. In sitting, the child may bend fowards to reach for a toy rather than sideways, since the latter involves shifting over a narrower base of support (Fig. 3.31).

2 *Using the hands for support*. The child may hold on to a stable object such as a chair or table, or clutch on to an adult. This strategy may be encouraged by the use of parallel bars for standing or walking practice.

3 *Holding the body stiffly*. This is a common problem seen in children with cerebellar lesions who typically experience difficulty in controlling even small amounts of postural sway in standing. However, it is also common in any child who is afraid of falling or who has poor control over the muscles

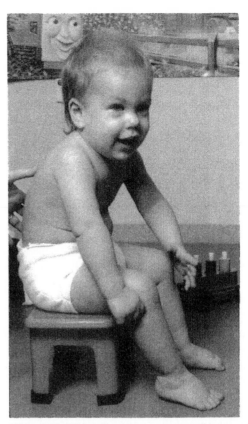

Figure 3.32 This infant has not yet learned how to sit on a seat using the feet as part of the base of support. He should practise reaching forwards and sideways, looking around, for example, in order to develop the postural adjustments necessary for balanced sitting. He could play with toys on a table in front of him as part of training.

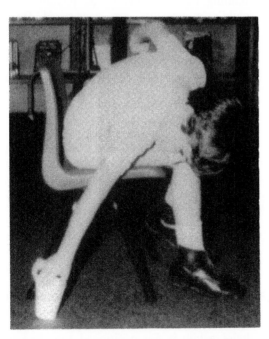

Figure 3.31 With poor control over postural adjustments when he moves laterally, the boy picks up the glass by flexing forwards at the hips instead of bending down sideways.

linking upper body to lower limbs and difficulty using the feet to balance (Fig. 3.32). It is seen, for example, in the mentally retarded child who resists any attempt to encourage movement of the body mass beyond a certain limited point. A child may not even permit an adult passively to shift the body away from a set position.

In analysing children's motor performance and in planning appropriate intervention, it is critical to recognize the difference between primary problems of balance (e.g. absence of preparatory adjustments, difficulty timing muscle activity) and the secondary adaptive behaviour which is the child's way of coping with an underlying motor control problem. Secondary adaptation of soft tissues, including muscle shortening and weakness from disuse, needs also to be recognized. Intervention should be directed towards the underlying motor problem with training incorporating means of preventing or avoiding adaptive behaviour, as described below. Where adaptive behaviour or soft tissue changes have already become established, it will be necessary to correct these as part of training. For example, it may be necessary to incorporate calf muscle lengthening into the child's programme so that the body movement associated with reaching forwards can be accomplished by dorsiflexion at the ankle. If a child has developed adaptive behaviours in reaching when sitting on the floor, it may be necessary to make a radical change in the environment by having her sit on a stool (see Fig. 8.8). Severe soft tissue shortening may need to be corrected by serial casting (see p. 148).

Training

The development of postural adjustments that enable the body to be balanced during movement is tied, as is all motor development, to the maturation of the nervous system. However, it is unlikely that these adjustments will develop in a particular position until the infant is placed in or can independently assume that position, no doubt because of the context-specificity of these adjustments. Similarly, adjustments are unlikely to develop as part of a specific action until that action is practised.

These points require of course to be confirmed by biomechanical studies. Nevertheless, given the results so far on the nature of postural adjustments in adults, it is reasonable to accept these ideas for the time being and to utilize them in the training of movement in infants and children who must develop or regain the ability to balance the body while moving (changing the alignment of the segmental linkage).

Training to improve a child's balance and ability to move about effectively takes into account the following issues:

1 *Postural adjustments are task- and context-specific.* To improve the ability to sit requires that the child be placed in sitting and given exercises and games to play which encourage reaching away from the body (Fig. 3.30) and moving around over the base of support. Similarly, for the acquisition of balanced standing the child has to practise performing different activities in standing (Fig. 3.33).

Contrary to some clinical practice, balance does not have to develop in one position before another. Although normal infants typically become more proficient moving about in sitting before standing, this reflects limits imposed by immaturity. Disabled children, particularly those with brain deficits, but also those with spinal cord dysfunction and limb deficiency, will be slow to gain motor control, and there is no reason why therapy should be organized along sequential lines. It is necessary to consider that postural adjustments are learned along with the actions they support and that the acquisition of skill involves the opportunity to practise the muscle activations which make up particular actions.

2 *Adaptive motor behaviour should be prevented* since, if it becomes learned or habitual, the child will subsequently have to unlearn the behaviour in order to function effectively in daily life. For example, the base of support should be relatively narrow and the child should be prevented from adopting a wide-based stance and from holding on. For this to be possible, the child's movements are progressed from those which require the body mass to be moved only a small distance, such as looking up to the ceiling or taking a deep breath, to movements such as reaching to arm's length, which require the centre of body mass to move towards the limits of stability.

In order for balanced sitting to be gained, for example, training may be better done with the child sitting on a small seat with the feet on the floor, or on a parent's knee with the feet on a solid surface than sitting on the floor. Sitting on a seat avoids the tendency of the child to adopt a wide base of support with legs widely abducted (see Fig. 8.1). It also encourages the use of the feet for support and balance – a critical feature of many functional actions which is slow to develop in many disabled children.

3 *Vision provides exproprioceptive information* critical to balance. It may be easier for a toddler to balance in standing if the adult helping him is not positioned too close in front, providing a looming effect which can cause the child to fall backwards. Visual feedback can provide a means of training

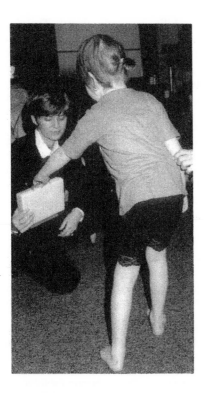
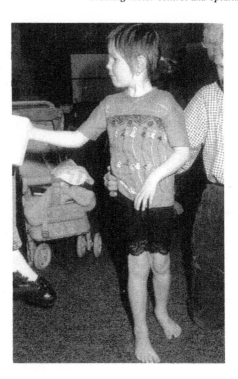
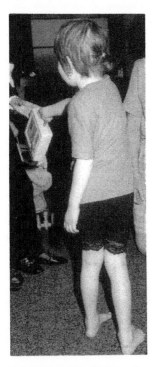
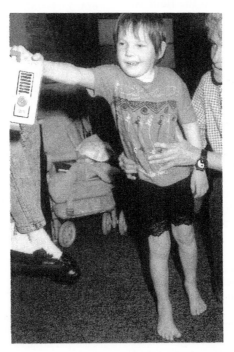
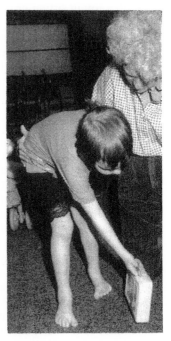

Figure 3.33   This child practises reaching for objects in different positions with different bases of support. The most difficult, because it is so narrow, is with one foot in front of the other. She needs support initially.

balanced movement over either a sitting or standing base of support for an older child. Computerized devices give feedback on a screen of the position of the centre of pressure as the child moves about and make practice interesting and fun. Outlining footprints on the floor is a way of providing information and motivation to a child who tends to adopt a wide-based stance either in standing or while walking.

Modification of the environment

Some methods of modifying the environment to ensure the appropriate movement have been described above. For example, training balanced sitting on a small seat may be more effective in the long term than allowing the infant to become 'stuck' in long sitting, unable and unwilling to sit on a seat or to move out of the sitting position. A seat may be modified to encourage active use of the legs for support while moving about in sitting (e.g. with straps to hold the feet in contact with the floor).

Practice should always provide a challenge while still allowing the possibility of success. For example, if a child does not have sufficient balancing ability to reach down to the floor to pick up a toy in sitting or standing, the toy can be placed on a box, in this way decreasing the amount of body mass displacement and weight shift. As the child improves, the toy can be placed progressively nearer to the floor.

Summary

This chapter comprises an introduction to the concept of training to develop or promote skill in the performance of critical everyday actions in infants and children. Although it has been assumed by approaches to physiotherapy such as neurodevelopmental therapy that young infants can only respond to facilitation techniques employed by the therapist, there is evidence that from birth the normal infant is prepared to make those active interactions with the environment that an immature visual and motor system permit.

The emphasis in the chapter is on the use of techniques to promote motor learning, such as verbal and visual feedback, demonstration and environmental modification, according to the child's age or ability to comprehend. Training involves practice of self-initiated activity, the infant or child learning to activate muscles to perform the biomechanical components of the action and to incorporate the postural adjustments which form an integral part of the action. For training to be successful, the musculoskeletal system needs to be flexible and soft tissues must be prevented from adaptively shortening. Where an infant is unable to respond to externally imposed perturbations, specific experience of these perturbations may need to be incorporated.

References

Ada, L. and Westwood, P. (1992) A kinematic analysis of recovery of the ability to stand up following stroke. *Aust. J. Physiother.*, **38**, 135.

Ada, L., Canning, C., Carr, J.H., Kilbreath, S.L. and Shepherd, R.B. (1994) Task-specific training of reaching and manipulation. In: *New Perspectives in the Control of the Reach to Grasp Movement*, edited by K.M.B. Bennett and U. Castiello. Oxford: Elsevier Science Publishers.

Andriacchi, T.P., Andersson, G.B.J., Fermier, R.W., Stern, D. and Galante, J.O. (1980) A study of lower-limb mechanics during stair-climbing. *J. Bone Joint Surg.*, **62A**, 5, 749–757.

Annett, J. (1971) Acquisition of skill. *Br. Med. Bull.*, **27**, 266.

Basmajian, J.V. (1977) Motor learning and control. *Arch. Phys. Med. Rehabil.*, **58**, 38–41.

Berger, W., Quintern, J. and Dietz, V. (1982) Pathophysiology of gait in children with cerebral palsy. *Electroencephalogr. Clin. Neurophysiol.*, **53**, 538–548.

Berger, W., Horstmann, G. and Dietz, V. (1984) Tension development and muscle activation in the leg during gait in spastic hemiparesis: independence of muscle hypotonia and exaggerated stretch reflexes. *J. Neurol, Neurosurg Psychiatry*, **47**, 1029–1033.

Bernstein, N. (1967) *Coordination and Regulation of Movement*. New York: Pergamon.

Bertoti, D.B. and Gross, A.L. (1988) Evaluation of biofeedback seat insert for improving active sitting posture in children with cerebral palsy. A clinical report. *Phys. Ther.*, **68**, 7, 1109–1113.

Biguer, B., Jeannerod, M. and Prablanc, C. (1982) The coordination of eye, head and hand movements during reaching at a single visual target. *Exp. Brain Res.*, **46**, 301–304.

Blaskey, J. (1989) Head trauma. In: *Pediatric Neurologic Physical Therapy*, edited by S.K. Campbell. New York: Churchill Livingstone, pp. 213–250.

Bobath, B. (1967) The very early treatment of cerebral palsy. *Dev. Med. Child Neurol.*, **9**, 4.

Bobath, B. and Bobath, K. (1964) The facilitation of normal postural reactions and movements in the treatment of cerebral palsy. *Physiotherapy*, **50**, 246.

Bouisset, S. and Zattara, M. (1981) A sequence of postural movements precedes voluntary movement. *Neurosci. Lett.*, **22**, 263–270.

Bower, T.G.R. (1974) *Development in Infancy*. San Francisco: Freeman.

Bower, T.G.R., Broughton, J.M. and Moore, M.K. (1970) The coordination of visual and tactual input in infants. *Percept. Psychophys.*, **8**, 51.

Brown, J.K., van Rensburg, F., Walsh, G., Lakie, M. and Wright, G.W. (1987) A neurological study of hand function in hemiplegic children. *Dev. Med. Child Neurol.*, **29**, 287–304.

Bruner, J.S. (1973) Organisation of early skilled action. *Child Dev.*, **44**, 1–11.

Burdett, R.G., Habesevich, R., Pisciotta, J. and Simon, S.R. (1985) Biomechanical comparison of rising from two types of chairs. *Phys. Ther.*, **65**, 8, 1177–1183.

Burns, Y.R., Ensbey, R.M. and Norrie, M.A. (1989) The neuro-sensory motor development assessment part 1: development and administration of the test. *Aust. J. Physiother.*, **35**, 3, 141–150.

Butler, P.B., Thompson, N. and Major, R.E. (1992). Improvement in walking performance of children with cerebral palsy: preliminary results. *Dev. Med. Child Neurol.* **34**, 567–576.

Canning, C., Carr, J.H. and Shepherd, R.B. (1985) A kinematic analysis of standing up. In: *Proceedings of Australian Physiotherapy Association Conference*, Brisbane.

Carr, J.H. and Gentile (1994) The effect of arm movement on the biomechanics of standing up., *Hum. Movt. Sc.*, **13**, 175–193.

Carr, J.H. and Shepherd, R.B. (1987a) *A Motor Relearning Programme for Stroke*. Oxford: Butterworth-Heinemann. 2nd Edition.

Carr, J.H. and Shepherd, R.B. (1987b) A motor learning model for rehabilitation. In: *Movement Science Foundations for Physical Therapy in Rehabilitation*, edited by J.H. Carr and R.B. Shepherd. Rockville, MD: Aspen.

Carr, J.H. and Shepherd, R.B. (1990) A motor learning model for rehabilitation of the movement-disabled. In: *Key Issues in Neurological Physiotherapy*, edited by L. Ada and C. Canning. Oxford: Butterworth-Heinemann.

Castiello, M.B., Bennett, K. and Stelmach, G.E. (1993) *Behav. Brain Res.* in press.

Cerny, K. (1984) Pathomechanics of stance. Clinical concepts for analysis. *Phys. Ther*, **64**, 12, 1851–1859.

Chao, E.Y.S., An, K.N., Cooney, W.P. and Linscheid, R.L. (1989). *Biomechanics of the Hand*. Singapore: World Scientific Publishing, pp. 31–72.

Chapman, C.E. and Wiesendanger, M. (1982) Physiologic and anatomical basis of spasticity. *Physiother. Canada*, **34**, 125–136.

Cordo, P.J. and Nashner, L.M. (1982) Properties of postural adjustments associated with rapid arm movements. *J. Neurophysiol.*, **47**, 287.

de Bruin, H., Eng, P., Russell, D.J. *et al.* (1982) Angle-angle diagrams in monitoring and quantification of gait patterns for children with cerebral palsy. *Am. J. Phys. Med.*, **61**, 4, 176–192.

Dietz, V. and Berger, W. (1983) Normal and impaired regulation of muscle stiffness in gait: a new hypothesis about muscle hypertonia. *Exp. Neurol.*, **7**, 9, 680–687.

Diller, L. (1970) Psychomotor and vocational rehabilitation. In: *Behavioral Change in Cerebrovascular Disease*, edited by A.L. Benton. New York: Harper & Row, pp. 81–116.

Dowrick, P.W. (1983) Self-modelling. In: *Using Video*, edited by P.W. Dowrick and S.J. Biggs. London: John Wiley.

Eberhart, H.D., Inman, V.T. and Bresler, B. (1965) The principal elements in human locomotion. In: *Human Limbs and their Substitutes*, edited by P.F. Klopstag and D.P. Wilson. New York: McGraw Hill, pp. 437–471.

Engardt, M., Ribbe, T. and Olsson, E. (1993) Vertical ground reaction force feedback to enhance stroke patients' symmetrical body-weight distribution while rising/sitting down. *Scand. J. Rehabil. Med.*, **25**, 41–48.

Fitts, P.M. (1963) Factors in complex skill learning. In: *Training Research and Education*, edited by R. Glaser. Pittsburgh: University of Pittsburgh Press.

Flodmark, A. (1986) Augmented auditory feedback as an aid in gait training of the cerebral palsied child. *Dev. Med. Child Neurol.*, **28**, 147–155.

Frischer, M. (1989) Voluntary vs. autonomous control of repetitive finger tapping in a patient with Parkinson's disease. *Neuropsychology*, **27**, 1261–1266.

Gentile, A.M. (1987) Skill acquisition: action, movement, and neuromotor processes. In: *Movement Science Foundations for Physical Therapy in Rehabilitation*, edited by J.H. Carr and R.B. Shepherd. Rockville, MD: Aspen, pp. 93–154.

Gibson, J.J. (1977) The theory of affordances. In: *Perceiving, Action and Knowing: Towards an Ecological Psychology*, edited by R. Shaw and J. Bransford. Hillsdale, NJ: Erlbaum, pp. 67–82.

Goodman, G. and Bazyk, S. (1991) The effects of a short thumb opponens splint on hand function in cerebral palsy: a single subject study. *Am. J. Occup. Ther.*, **45**, 8, 726–731.

Gregoire, L., Veeger, H.E., Huijing, P.A. and van Ingen Schenau, G.J. (1984) Role of mono- and biarticular muscles in explosive movements. *Int. J. Sports Med.*, **5**, 301.

Harris, F.A. (1971) Inapproprioception: a possible sensory basis for athetoid movements. *Phys. Ther.*, **51**, 761–770.

Harrison, A. and Kruze, R. (1987) Perturbation of a skilled action II. Normalising the responses of cerebral palsied individuals. *Hum. Mov. Sc.*, **6**, 133–159.

Hay, J.G. (1975) Biomechanical aspects of jumping. In: *Exercise and Sports Sciences Review*, edited by J.H. Wilmore and J.F. Keogh. New York: Academic Press, 135–161.

Heriza, C.B. (1988) Organisation of leg movements in pre-term infants. *Phys. Ther.*, **68**, 9, 1340–1346.

Hoffer, M.M. and Perry J. (1983) Pathodynamics of gait alterations in cerebral palsy and the significance of kinetic electromyography in evaluating foot and ankle problems. *Foot Ankle*, **4**, 128–134.

Holding, D.H. (1965) *Principles of Training*. London: Pergamon.

Holding, D.H. (1970) Learning without error. In: *Psychology of Motor Learning*, edited by L.E. Smith. Chicago, IL: Athletic Institute.

Iberall, T., Bingham, G. and Arbib, M.A. (1986) Opposition space as a structuring concept for the analysis of skilled hand movements. Exper. Brain Res. Supplement 15, 153.

Inman, V.T., Ralston, H.J. and Todd, F. (1981) *Human Walking*. Baltimore, MD: Williams & Wilkins.

Jeannerod, M. (1981) Intersegmental coordination during reaching at natural visual objects. In: *Attention and Performance IX*, edited by J. Long and A. Baddeley. Hillsdale, NJ: Erlbaum.

Jeannerod, M. (1984) The timing of natural prehension movements. *J. Motor Behav.*, **16**, 235.

Jeannerod, M. (1986) The formation of the finger grip during prehension: a cortically-mediated visuo-motor pattern. In: *Themes in Motor Development*, edited by H.T.A. Whiting and M.G. Wade. Dordrecht: Martinus Nijhoff.

Johansson, R.S. and Westling, G. (1988) Coordinated isometric muscle commands adequately and erroneously programmed for the weight during lifting tasks with precision grip. *Exp. Brain Res.*, **71**, 59–71.

Johansson, R.S. and Westling, G. (1990) Tactile afferent signals in the control of precision grip. In: *Attention and Performance*, edited by M. Jeannerod. Hillsdale, NJ: Erlbaum.

Joseph, J. and Watson, R. (1967) Telemetering electromyography of muscles used in walking up and down stairs. *J. Bone Joint Surg.*, **49-B**, 774–780.

Kapandji, I.A. (1970) *The Physiology of the Joints, vol. 1: Upper limb*. Edinburgh: Churchill Livingstone, pp. 146–203.

Kelso, J.A.S., Southard, D.L. and Goodman, D. (1979) On the nature of human interlimb coordination. *Science*, **203**, 1029–1031.

Knutsson, E. (1980) Muscle activation patterns of gait in spastic hemiparesis, paraparesis and cerebral palsy. *Scand. J. Rehabil. Med. Suppl.*, **7**, 47.

Lai, K.A., Kuo, K.N. and Andriacchi, T. (1988) Relationship between dynamic deformities and joint movements in children with cerebral palsy. *J. Pediatric Orthop.*, **9**, 690–695.

Landsmeer, J.M.F. (1976) *Atlas of Anatomy of the Hand*. Edinburgh: Churchill Livingstone.

Lee, D.N. and Young, D.S. (1986) Gearing action to the environment. In: *Generation and Modulation of Action Patterns*, edited by H. Heuer and C. Fromm. Heidelberg: Springer.

Lee, D.N., Daniel, B.M., Turnbull, J. and Cook, M.L. (1990). Basic perceptuo-motor dysfunctions in cerebral palsy. In: *Attention and Performance XIII: Motor Representation of Control*, edited by M. Jeannerod. Hillsdale, NJ: Erlbaum.

Lee, J.M., Mahler, T.J. and Westling, D.L. (1985) Reducing occurrences of an asymmetrical tonic neck reflex. *Am. J. Mental Deficiency*, **89**, 6, 617–621.

Leiper, C.I., Miller, A., Lang, J. *et al.* (1981) Sensory feedback for head control in cerebral palsy. *Phys. Ther.*, **61**, 512–518.

Lemon, R.N., Mantel, G.W.H. and Rea, P.A. (1990) Recording and identification of single motor units in the free to move primate hand. *Exp. Brain Res.*, **81**, 95–106.

Lemon, R.N., Bennett, K.M. and Werner, W. (1991) The cortico-motor substrate for skilled movements of the primate hand. In: *Tutorials in Motor Neuroscience*, edited by J. Requin and G.E. Stelmach. Amsterdam: Kluwer Academic Publishers, pp. 477–495.

Leont'ev, A.N. and Zaporozhets, A.V. (1960) *Rehabilitation of Hand Function*. London: Pergamon.

Lockman, J.J., Ashmead, D.H. and Bushnell, E.W. (1984) The development of anticipatory hand orientation during infancy. *J. Exp. Child Psychol.*, **37**, 176–186.

Lough, S., Wing, A.M., Fraser, C. and Jenner, J.R. (1984) Measurement of recovery of function in the hemiparetic upper limb following stroke: a preliminary report. *Hum. Movt. Sci.*, **3**, 247–256.

Malouin, F., Gemmell, M., Parrot, A. and Dutil, R. (1985) Effects of auditory feedback on head position training in young children with cerebral palsy: a pilot study. *Phys. Can.*, **37**, 3, 150–156.

Malouin, F., Potvin, M., Prevost, J., Richards, C.L. and Wood-Dauphinee, S. (1992) Use of an intensive task oriented gait programme in a series of patients with acute cerebrovascular accident. *Phys. Ther.*, **72**, 781–793.

Martenuik, R.G., MacKenzie, C.L. and Baba, D.M. (1984) Bimanual movement control: information processing and interaction effects. *Q. J. Exp. Psychol.*, **36a**, 335.

Mossberg, K.A., Linton, K.A. and Friske, K. (1990) Ankle-foot orthoses: effect on energy expenditure of gait in spastic diplegic children. *Arch. Phys. Med. Rehabil.*, **71**, 490–494.

Muir, R.B. (1985) Small hand muscles in precision grip. In: *Hand Function and the Neocortex*, edited by A.W. Goodwin and I. Darien-Smith. Berlin: Springer-Verlag, pp. 155–174.

Murray, M.P., Drought, A.B. and Kory, R.C. (1964) Walking patterns of normal men. *J. Bone Joint Surg.*, **46-B**, 2, 335–360.

Murray, M.P., Seireg, A. and Scholz, R.C. (1967) Center of gravity, center of pressure, and supportive forces during human activities. *J. Appl. Physiol.*, **23**, 831.

Nashner, L.M. and McCollum, G. (1985) The organisation of human postural movements: a formal basis and experimental synthesis. *Behav. Brain Sci.*, **8**, 135–172.

Newell, K.M. (1981) Skill learning. In: *Human Skills*, edited by D.H. Holding. New York: John Wiley, pp. 203–226.

Norlin, R. and Odenrick, P. (1986) Development of gait in spastic children with cerebral palsy. *J. Pediatric Orthop.*, **6**, 678–680.

O'Connell, A.L. (1972) *Understanding the Scientific Basis for Human Movement*. Baltimore, MD: Williams & Wilkins.

Olney, S.J., Costigan, P.A. and Hedden, D.M. (1987) Mechanical energy patterns in gait of cerebral palsied children with hemiplegia. *Physical Therapy*, **67**, 1348–1354.

Olney, S.J., MacPhail, H.E., Hedden, D.M. and Boyce, W.F. (1990) Work and power in hemiplegic cerebral palsy gait. *Physical Therapy*, **70**, 431–438.

Ostendorf, C.G. and Wolf, S.L. (1981) Effect of forced use of the upper extremity of a hemiplegic patient on changes in function. *Phys. Ther.*, **61**, 1022–1028.

Pearson, K. (1976) The control of walking. *Sci. Am.*, **Dec.**, 72–86.

Perin, B. (1989) Physical therapy for the child with cerebral palsy. In: *Pediatric Neurologic Physical Therapy*, edited by S.K. Campbell. New York: Churchill Livingstone.

Rock, I. and Harris, C.S. (1967) Vision and touch. *Sci. Am.*, **216**, 5, 96–104.

Rosenbaum, D.A. (1991) *Human Motor Control*. New York: Academic Press.

Rosenbaum, D.A., Vaughan, J., Barnes, H.J., Marchak, F. and Slotta, J. (1990) Constraints on action selection: overhand versus underhand grips. In: *Attention and Performance XIII*, edited by M. Jeannerod. Hillsdale, NJ: Erlbaum, pp. 321–342.

Saunders, J.B.D.M., Inman, V.T. and Eberhart, H.D. (1953) The major determinants in normal and pathological gait. *J. Bone Joint Surg.*, **35A**, 3, 543–558.

Schenkman, M., Berger, R.A., Riley, P.O., Mann, R.W. and Hodge, W.A. (1990) Whole-body movements during rising to standing from sitting. *Phys. Ther.*, **70**, 638–651.

Schwartzman, J. (1974) Rehabilitation of infantile hemiplegia. *Am. J. Phys. Med.*, **53**, 75.

Seeger, B.R. and Caudrey, D.J. (1983) Biofeedback therapy to achieve symmetrical gait in children with hemiplegic cerebral palsy: long-term efficacy. *Arch. Phys. Med. Rehabil.*, **64**, 160–162.

Seeger, B.R., Caudrey, D.J. and Scholes, J.R. (1981) Biofeedback therapy to achieve symmetrical gait in hemiplegic cerebral palsied children. *Arch. Phys. Med. Rehabil.*, **62**, 364–368.

Shepherd, R.B. (1987). Movement science and physiotherapy: deriving implications for the clinic. In: *Proceedings of World Confederation Physical Therapy*, Sydney.

Shepherd, R.B. (1992) Adaptive motor behaviour in response to perturbations of balance. *Physiother. Theory Pract.*, **8**, 137–143.

Shepherd, R.B. and Carr, J.H. (1991) An emergent or dynamical systems view of movement dysfunction. *Aus. J. Physiother.*, **37**, 4–5.

Shepherd, R.B. and Gentile, A.M. (1994) Sit-to-stand: functional relationship between upper body and lower limb segments. *Hum. Movt. Sc.*, in press.

Shepherd, R.B., Crosbie, J. and Squire, T. (1993) The contribution of the ipsilateral leg to postural adjustment during fast voluntary reaching in sitting. In: *Proceedings of the XIVth ISB International Congress of Biomechanics*, Paris.

Shepherd, R.B. and Koh, H-P. (1994). Some biomechanical consequences of varying foot placement in sit-to-stand in young women. *Scand. J. Rehabil. Med.*, in press.

Shinno, N. (1971) Analysis of knee function in ascending and descending stairs. *Med. Sport*, **6**, Biomechanics 11. pp. 202–207.

Singer, R.N. (1980) *Motor Learning and Human Performance*, 3rd edn. New York: Macmillan.

Skinner, D.R. Antonelli, D., Perry, J. and Lester, D.K. (1985) Functional demands on the stance limb in walking. *Orthopedics*, **8**, 355–361.

Smith, A.M. (1981). The coactivation of antagonist muscles. *Can. J. Physiol. Pharmacol.*, **59**, 733–747.

Spoor, C. (1983) Balancing a force on the finger tip of a two-dimensional finger without intrinsic muscles. *J. Biomechanics*, **16**, 497–504.

Sutherland, D.H. (1966) An electromyographic study of the plantar flexors of the ankle in normal walking on the level. *J. Bone Joint Surg.*, **48A**, 1, 66–71.

Sutherland, D.H., Olshen, R., Cooper, L. and Woo, S.L.Y. (1980) The development of mature gait. *J. Bone Joint Surg.*, **62A**, 336–353.

Tardieu, C., Huet de la Tour, E., Bret, M.D. and Tardieu, G. (1982a) Muscle hypoextensibility in children with cerebral palsy: 1. Clinical and experimental observations. *Arch. Phys. Med. Rehabil.*, **63**, 97–102.

Tardieu, C., Huet de la Tour, E., Colbeau-Justin, P. and Lespargot, A. (1982b). Muscle hypoextension in children with cerebral palsy 11. Therapeutic implications. *Arch. Phys. Med. Rehabil.*, **63**, 103–107.

Tardieu, C., Lespargot, A., Tabary, C. and Bret, M.D. (1989) Toe walking in children with cerebral palsy: contributions of contracture and excessive contraction of triceps surae muscle. *Phys. Ther.*, **69**, 656–662.

Tardieu, G., Tardieu, C., Colbeau-Justin, P. and Bret, M.D. (1982) Effects of muscle length on an increased stretch reflex in children with cerebral palsy. *J. Neurol., Neurosurg. Psychiatry*, **45**, 348–352.

Taub, E. (1980) Somatosensory deafferentation research with monkeys: implications for rehabilitation medicine. In: *Behavioral Psychology in Rehabilitation Medicine: Clinical Implications*, edited by L.P. Ince. Baltimore, MD: Williams & Wilkins, pp. 371–401.

Taub, E., Miller, N.E., Novack, T.A., Cook, E.W., Fleming, W.C., Nepomuceno, C.S., Connell, J.S. and Crago, J.E. (1993) Technique to improve chronic motor deficit after stroke. *Arch. Phys. Med. Rehabil.*, **74**, 347–354.

Thelen, E. and Cooke, D.W. (1987) Relationship between newborn stepping and later walking: a new interpretation. *Dev. Med. Child Neurol.*, **29**, 380–393.

Thelen, E. and Fisher, D.M. (1982) Newborn stepping: an explanation for a 'disappearing' reflex. *Dev. Psychol.*, **18**, 760–775.

Townsend, M.A., Lainhart, S.P. and Shiavi, R. (1978) Variability and biomechanics of synergy patterns of some lower-limb muscles during ascending and descending stairs and level walking. *Med. Biol. Eng. Comput.*, **16**, 681–688.

van Ingen-Schenau, G.J. (1989) From rotation to translation: constraints on multijoint movements and the unique action of bi-articular muscles. *Hum. Movt. Sc.*, **8**, 423–442.

van der Weel, F.R., van der Meer, A.L. and Lee, D.N. (1991) Effect of task on movement control in cerebral palsy: implications for assessment and therapy. *Dev. Med. Child Neurol.*, **33**, 419–426.

von Hofsten, C. (1979) Development of visually-guided reaching: the reaching phase. *J. Hum. Movement Stud.*, **5**, 160–178.

von Hofsten, C. (1982) Eye–hand coordination in newborns. *Dev. Psych.*, **18**, 450.

von Hofsten, C. and Lindhagen, K. (1979) Observations on the development of reaching for moving objects. *J. Exp. Child Psychiatry* **28**, 158.

Walmsley, R.P., Crichton, L. and Droog, D. (1981) Music as a feedback mechanism for teaching head control to severely handicapped children: a pilot study. *Dev. Med. Child Neurol.*, **23**, 739–746.

Wilson, J. (1989). Cerebral palsy. In: *Pediatric Neurologic Physical Therapy*, edited by S.K. Campbell. New York: Churchill Livingstone.

Wing, A.M. and Fraser, C. (1983) The contribution of the thumb to reaching movements. *Q. J. Exp. Psychol.*, **35A**, 297–309.

Wing, A.M., Turton, A. and Fraser, C. (1986) Grasp size and accuracy of approach in reaching. *J. Motor Behav.*, **18**, 245–260.

Winter, D.A. (1980) Overall principle of lower limb support during stance phase of gait. *J. Biomech.*, **13**, 302–330.

Winter, D.A. (1987) *The Biomechanics and Motor Control of Human Gait.* Waterloo, Ontario: University of Waterloo Press.

Wolf, S.L., LeCraw, D.E., Barton, L.A. and Jann, B.B. (1989) Forced use of hemiplegic upper extremities to reverse the effect of learned non-use among chronic stroke and head injured patients. *Exp. Neurol.*, **104**, 125.

Wooldridge, C.P. and Russell, G. (1976) Head position training with the cerebral palsied child: an application of biofeedback techniques. *Arch. Phys. Med. Rehabil.*, **57**, 407–414.

Further reading

Field, J. (1976) The adjustment of reaching behaviour to object distance in early infancy. *Child Dev.*, **47**, 304–308.

Thelen, E. (1985) Developmental origins of motor coordination: leg movements in human infants. *Dev. Psychobiol.*, **18**, 1–22.

Section II

Neurological disorders

4 Maturational, pathophysiological and recovery processes in the CNS

5 Cerebral palsy

6 Acute brain injury

7 Minimal brain dysfunction: learning disability, attention deficit disorder, clumsiness

8 Mental retardation: cognitive impairment and developmental delay

9 Infections of the nervous system

10 Brachial plexus lesions in infancy

4

Maturational, pathophysiological and recovery processes in the CNS

Introduction

Section II describes the disorders of movement which result from abnormal development of or interference with the nervous system. In children, the commonest sites of these disorders are the brain and the spinal cord. The peripheral system may be involved in certain hereditary diseases which will result in poor motor development, but in children this system is not commonly subject to trauma. Nevertheless, a child who falls over with a glass in his hand may sustain a median or ulnar nerve lesion as would an adult, a child with a complicated supracondylar fracture may suffer a Volkmann's ischaemia of the nerves and muscles in the forearm, and an infant may sustain a brachial plexus lesion during a difficult birth.

The poliomyelitis virus may destroy anterior horn cells in the spinal cord. Guillain–Barré's syndrome is an acute polyneuritis of uncertain origin and peripheral neuropathy may also result from such factors as vitamin deficiency or lead poisoning. Failure of the spinal cord of the embryo to develop normally causes malformation of the spinal cord as occurs in spina bifida cystica.

Cerebral palsy is a broad term indicating abnormal development of or injury to the fetal or infant brain, and the area involved may be relatively circumscribed and confined to the cerebral cortex in its motor or sensory parts, to the cerebellum or the basal ganglia, or more generalized and involving many areas in the brain. Trauma may occur to the brain due to accident, with motor vehicle accidents being an ever-increasing cause. In these cases the damage tends to be more generalized than specific. Infection may cause an encephalitis or a meningitis which injures the brain in a diffuse manner. Genetic factors may cause a baby to be born with Down's syndrome or with a developmental disorder which results in cognitive impairment and clumsy movement. Microcephaly results in considerable cognitive impairment and motor disability through the failure of the skull (and brain) to develop adequately. An abnormal increase in cerebrospinal fluid or a failure of its absorption results in hydrocephalus which, if uncontrolled, leads to sensorimotor disorders and intellectual retardation. Tumours developing within the brain or spinal cord will cause symptoms depending upon the area involved. Cerebrovascular accident or stroke may occur as a result of occlusive vascular disease or congenital anomalies, such as aneurysms or vascular malformations.

This chapter comprises three sections. In the first, the development of the nervous system in terms of its growth and maturation is described for its explanatory value in terms of motor development. Second, the pathophysiological processes associated with brain dysfunction are discussed in terms of the major dyscontrol characteristics in an attempt to clarify the clinical signs observed in infants and children. In the final section, research findings related to the process of central nervous system (CNS) recovery and adaptation after brain lesion, principally in animals, are described. It is reasonable to assume that the infant's experiences following a neural lesion, that is, what movements the infant practises and how the environment mediates those movements, might affect recovery and adaptive processes. Animal studies lend considerable support to this concept.

The maturation of the nervous system

The development of the nervous system through the fetal and embryonic periods is briefly outlined in Table 4.1. A period of rapid brain growth, called the brain growth spurt, begins in mid-gestation. However, 85% of brain growth takes place postnatally. Certain periods involve more active growth than others, and the brain is thought at these times to be particularly sensitive to changes in the environment and to internal influence, thus demonstrating its plasticity (Timiras 1972; Dobbing 1974).

At birth the part of the brain posterior to the precentral sulcus is better developed than the part anterior to it. The convolutions of the brain are partly developed. The cerebral cortex of the full-term neonate is only half its eventual adult thickness. The increase in thickness will result from an increase in size of nerve cells and sprouting of their processes. The dendritic processes of cortical neurons begin to develop a few months before birth but are still rudimentary in the brain of the newborn. During the first year of postnatal life, these dendritic processes develop to establish their connections with other neurons.

The cerebral capillaries are relatively permeable at birth. Therefore, in infants with jaundice, serum bilirubin may penetrate the brain, damaging the basal ganglia.

It is interesting to note that the ascending afferent fibres in the spinal cord are relatively well-myelinated at birth, while the descending corticospinal tracts and the white matter of the cerebral and cerebellar hemispheres are to a large extent unmyelinated. The descending motor tracts do not become fully myelinated until years 1 and 2. The olfactory tracts are unmyelinated, the optic tracts partly and the remainder of the cranial nerves are well-myelinated. The early myelination of the cranial

nerves is related to the infant's well-developed ability to suck and swallow. The cerebellum itself is immature and remains relatively immature until the child is 2 years old.

At 6 months of age, when the infant is gaining more cortical control over her activities, the frontal and temporal lobes are becoming more mature, most of the tracts in the spinal cord are well-myelinated, and the optic nerve is completely myelinated. The immaturity of the cerebellum at this stage can be demonstrated by the infant's lack of control over attempted grasping (Dekeban 1970).

Myelination commences near the nerve cell and spreads along the fibre (Hamilton *et al.* 1972). The pattern of myelination in the brain follows a predictable sequence, starting in the brain stem and cerebellum and progressing to the cerebrum (McArdle *et al.* 1987). All structures in the spinal cord, brainstem and cerebellum are myelinated by 2 years and the peripheral nerve roots by 3 years. By 5 years myelination of all cerebral structures seems to be completed and, from the development point of view, in a 6-year-old has reached its optimum (Dekeban 1970).

Although the maturation of the nervous system is little understood, there appears to be a direct relationship between the development of myelination within the nervous system and the development of neural function, and a stimulus to myelination seems to occur from activity within the various systems. Certainly it appears that tracts may become myelinated at approximately the same time as they become functional. Fibres appear to be able to conduct impulses before they have developed myelin but these impulses are conducted at a slower pace.

Function and experience appear to play an important role in postnatal maturational mechanisms (Bishop 1982). Postnatal changes in spinal motoneurons, for example, are correlated with function and behavioural change in kittens (Huizar *et al.* 1975). Neurons in the cerebral cortex develop dendritic spines as they mature and the growth of these receptor structures on pyramidal cells can be influenced by the animal's environment. Rats raised in an enriched environment have a higher density of dendritic spines than rats raised in an impoverished environment (Globus *et al.* 1973). This information provides some insights into the need to address in physiotherapy the relatively

Table 4.1 The development of the central nervous system

	Structure	Function
Week 2	*Blastocyst* (future embryo and placenta), embedded in the uterine mucosa, begins its specific development	
Week 3	Ectoderm thickens to form *neural plate* Neural plate develops *neural groove* *Neural crest* cells form Neural groove deepens → formation of *neural folds*	
Week 4	Fusion of neural folds → *neural tube* Neural tube dilates → *forebrain vesicle* *midbrain vesicle* *hindbrain vesicle* Remainder of tube elongates → *spinal cord* Neural crest cells differentiate into various sensory and autonomic ganglia	Heart beats
Week 5	Forebrain and hindbrain vesicles divide Their cavities form lateral, third and fourth *ventricles* and *aqueduct of Sylvius* *Cerebral hemispheres* begin to expand	
Week 6	*Thalamus* indicated *Cerebellum* appears *Cerebral commissures* appear Motor and sensory nuclei of *cranial nerves* IX–XII originate in medulla oblongata Capillary system formed (*cerebral vascular system*)	
Week 8	*Corpus striatum* differentiates into *caudate nucleus* and *lentiform nucleus* Lentiform nucleus divides into *putamen* and *globus pallidus* Expansion of cerebral hemisphere → overlapping of mid- and hindbrain Formation of *frontal, temporal* and *occipital lobes* *Spinal cord* same length as vertebral column Development of *sense organs* progressing *Meninges* (pia, arachnoid, dura mater) are distinct *Brain* has a human appearance	First reflex arc functional Reflex responses to tactile stimulation Irritation of upper lip → withdrawal of head Neck and trunk movement
Week 10	*Corpus callosum* appears and connects right and left cerebral hemispheres *Epithalamus, thalamus* and *hypothalamus* developing from forebrain	Spontaneous movements observable and stereotyped Tactile stimulation of lips → swallowing movement
Week 12	*Vermis* and *cerebellar hemisphere* recognizable *Anterior commissure* develops and connects right and left cerebral hemispheres *Taste buds* appear *Inner ear* developing adult configuration	Less stereotyped movements becoming more individuated Movements increase in force Mouth opening and closing Chest muscles contract
Week 14	*General sense organs* (pain, temperature, deep pressure and tactile endings, chemical endings, neuromuscular spindles and neurotendinous end organs) begin to differentiate	Tactile stimulation of face → head turning, contraction of contralateral trunk muscles, trunk extension, rotation of pelvis to other side
Week 16	Characteristic folia of adult *cerebellum* gradually develop Three small apertures (f. of *Luschka* and f. of *Magendie*) appear → *free passage* of CSF between ventricles and subarachnoid space Cervical *spinal cord* developing *myelin* Cervical and *lumbar enlargements* form	Tongue movements Abdominal muscles contract
Week 20	Main components of middle and external *ear* have assumed adult form *Pacinian corpuscles* appear *Muscle spindles* in almost all muscles *Golgi endings* and rudimentary *joint endings* present	Effective but weak grasp Protrusion and pursing of lips Contraction of diaphragm Sucking
Week 24	*Myelination* in brain begins in *basal ganglia, pons, medulla, midbrain* *Spinal cord* extends to S1 vertebra Posterior columns *myelinated* Vestibulospinal, reticulospinal tracts *myelinated*	Temporary respirations if born
Week 28	*Cerebral* and *cerebellar connections* myelinated *Spinocerebellar, spinothalamic tracts* myelinated	Permanent respiratory movements established on birth Eye sensitive to light Maintained grasp Olfactory perception
Final 12 weeks	Differentiation of some *sense organs* completed *Taste buds* reach functional maturity	Reflex mechanisms for sucking, swallowing well-established

From Carr, J.H. and Shepherd, R.B. (1980) *Physiotherapy in Disorders of the Brain*. London: Heinemann.

impoverished environment (in terms of sensorimotor experiences) of the infant immobilized by a brain lesion.

Pathophysiological processes and dyscontrol characteristics

It is likely that the effects of a lesion of the nervous system differ according to the maturational state of that system. If interference to the brain due, for example, to teratogens, infections or genetic effects occurs early in gestation, there will be interference with cell production and migration. It has until relatively recently been assumed that fewer deficits arise if brain damage is sustained during infancy than comparable damage in childhood. This view is currently being questioned. Goldman (1974) proposed that maturational status of lesion site, functional status of remaining system, lesion size and experience prior to the lesion may be critical variables affecting the extent of deficit or sparing. In an immature system, deficits may appear at a time when the lesioned area would normally assume its functions (Milner 1974).

Since the structure and physiology of the preterm infant's brain are significantly different from that of a full-term infant, it is not surprising that the effects of a brain lesion in a very premature infant appear to differ from those in the full-term infant (Pape and Wigglesworth 1979; Stewart *et al.* 1987). The preterm infant is at risk of having retarded myelination due to the effects of hypoxic-ischaemic haemorrhage or intra-cranial haemorrhage (McArdle *et al.* 1987).

It appears that considerable reorganization of cerebral cortical and subcortical circuitry may occur when CNS damage occurs prenatally (Goldman-Rakic 1980). In the young child, however, the cerebral hemispheres have already become more committed to function.

In this section, common dyscontrol characteristics associated with lesions of the upper motor neuron system, cerebellum and basal ganglia are briefly described. As indicated above, there is increasing evidence that the age at which brain lesions occur influences the physiological mechanisms and resulting dyscontrol characteristics. It is also becoming increasingly evident that the experience of the infant or child

and the state of the muscular system have critical influences on both physiological mechanisms and dyscontrol characteristics.

The prevailing theories of the mechanisms underlying motor dysfunction in brain-damaged infants and children, which have had considerable influence on therapeutic strategies, are related to the disruptive effects of abnormal reflexes on motor control and motor performance (e.g. Brain 1977; Bobath 1980; Mountcastle 1980). More recent evidence suggests, however, that abnormalities in the descending motor commands and not abnormal reflex activity may be the major deficit underlying motor dysfunction (Sahrmann and Norton 1977; Neilson and McCaughey 1982; Vaughan *et al.* 1988). In other words, inappropriate voluntary muscle activity appears to be the principal basis of movement abnormalities rather than involuntary muscle contractions (Vaughan *et al.* 1988).

Dyscontrol characteristics associated with upper motor neuron lesions

The so-called upper motor neuron (UMN) syndrome is seen following lesions that damage the corticofugal pathways (including the pyramidal tract) at any level, whether cortex, internal capsule, brainstem or spinal cord. The syndrome itself is considered a clinically useful concept (Burke 1988); patients with lesions at different levels present with different intensities of reflex phenomena and different degrees of muscle dyscontrol.

It is typical to classify the dyscontrol characteristics as either positive or negative (e.g., Jackson 1958; Landau 1980; Burke 1988), although it is probably only the negative features that result from the pyramidal lesion, with the positive features arising from involvement of the parapyramidal fibres (Shahani and Young 1980; Burke 1988). The major negative features are weakness and loss of dexterity. The positive features are all exaggerations of normal phenomena and include abnormal posturing, increased proprioceptive reflexes producing spasticity and, in the case of spinal cord injury, exaggeration of exteroceptive (cutaneous) reflexes of the limbs.

The following classification is from Burke (1988):

Negative features

1 Shock.
2 Weakness.
   (a) Loss of strength of voluntary muscle action.
   (b) Fatigability.
3 Loss of dexterity.
   (a) Loss of fractionation of movement.
   (b) Slowing of rate of voluntary contraction.
   (c) Withdrawal of tonic descending activity that maintains excitability of spinal motoneurons and interneurons.

Shock is an acute response to an abrupt lesion and in children may be seen following a cerebrovascular accident or head injury. It is likely that infants who suffer an acute episode in the perinatal period also show signs of the shock to the CNS. Shock is demonstrated by paralysis and profound hyporeflexia. Paralysis may range from dense flaccidity involving all muscle groups with complete areflexia to a state in which cutaneous responses (Babinski) are evident, tendon jerks are present but depressed, and residual strength is present in certain muscles.

Weakness is due to a loss of strength of voluntary muscle action or a depression of motor function. Clinically this is called *hypotonus*. Both weakness and loss of dexterity are due to insufficient descending fibres converging on the final motoneuron population either to coordinate complex movements by graded muscle activation or to bring motoneurons to the necessary discharge frequency (Landau 1980). All muscles may be involved after a lesion of acute onset. In the recovery phase, or with lesions of less abrupt onset, the degree of weakness differs for different muscle groups. As the pyramidal tract is the executive pathway for volitional goal-directed movement, the main deficiency, according to Burke (1988), seems to be in those muscles that normally act as prime movers in voluntary movement. Muscles of shoulder and elbow may be less involved than hand muscles. It has been shown in adult stroke patients that, contrary to clinical belief, the elbow extensors are not necessarily weaker than flexors (Colebatch and Gandevia 1986). In the lower limbs, weakness may be greater in the flexors of hip, knee and ankle than in the extensors.

Loss of manual dexterity is an inevitable consequence of pyramidal tract injury and is due to:

1 a loss of fractionation of movement; that is, the inability to make independent movements with individual muscle groups – a problem thought to reflect the specificity of corticomotor connections established by many pyramidal axons;
2 a slowing of the rate of voluntary muscle contraction, which is thought to be due to a loss of inputs from fast large pyramidal tract neurons to the spinal motoneurons.

This is a major problem in patients with severe pyramidal tract dysfunction and some loss of dexterity can be expected, even with mild dysfunction.

Positive features

1 Abnormal posturing.
2 Exaggerated proprioceptive reflexes (hyperreflexia or spasticity).
   (a) Claspknife phenomenon.
   (b) Exaggerated tendon reflexes.
   (c) Clonus.
3 Exaggerated cutaneous reflexes.
   (a) Flexor withdrawal reflex.
   (b) Extensor, flexor spasms.
   (c) Babinski response.

The classic *abnormal postures* seen in some children with brain lesions (see Figs 5.2 and 5.3) may reflect a dystonia rather than, as commonly believed, spasticity (Burke 1988). Abnormal postures appear not to be due to overactivity in spinal reflex circuits since they are not abolished by posterior root section (Denny Brown 1966). The abnormal posture is unlikely to result from hyperreflexia since it continues in the absence of movement, and the necessary stimulus to demonstrate spasticity is velocity-dependent movement (Herman 1970; Burke and Lance 1973). Posturing may, however, be due to excessive supraspinal drive, with spinal motoneuron roots sensitive to change in that drive. For example, the posture may reverse when the individual's orientation in space is changed (Denny Brown 1966), presumably in this case due to an alteration in vestibular input. It has been pointed out that, since these postures are not due to spasticity, they are unlikely to respond to treatment designed to treat spasticity (Burke 1988).

In young children, it may be fruitful to clarify experimentally a distinction between:

1 Abnormal postures due to well-practised and learned adaptive patterns of behaviour, together with impoverished motor experiences.
2 Postures due to adaptive length changes in muscles.
3 Postures due to neural events (dystonia).

Increased exaggerated proprioceptive reflexes produce the disorder termed *spasticity*, and manifested as tendon jerk hyperreflexia and a velocity-dependent resistance to passive movement (Carr *et al*. 1994). The more rapid the stretching movement, the greater the increase in resistance. It should be noted that slow passive movements may not elicit any reflex contraction.

The *claspknife phenomenon* is also velocity-dependent and caused by a build-up of reflex resistance. It may be evident in the elbow flexors and knee extensors and is felt on passive movement of the limb to produce a catch-and-give sensation. *Exaggerated tendon jerks*, tested with a percussion hammer, represent a synchronized reflex response generated by abrupt mechanical disturbance. *Clonus* is set in train by an abrupt passive stretch or tendon percussion.

Exaggerated cutaneous reflexes (flexor withdrawal and flexor and extensor spasms) are a manifestation of a severely damaged spinal cord. Babinski or extensor plantar response (flexion of the great toe) is unequivocally associated with dysfunction of the pyramidal tract (Phillips and Porter 1977). This response is elicited by a firm pressure along the lateral plantar surface of the foot.

Muscle tone

Normal tone is said to be a slight constant tension of healthy muscles, so that when the limbs are handled or moved passively, they offer a small resistance to displacement (Kandel and Schwartz 1985); in other words, the degree of resistance offered to passive movement. It has long been believed, as the previous sentence indicates, that normal tone depends on

a low-grade tonic contraction of low-threshold motoneurons maintained by activity in stretch reflex pathways. Clinically, hypotonus has been taken to represent decreased activity in reflex circuits, hypertonus by increased activity, with either decreased or increased fusimotor drive (Rushworth 1960). These views, however, may be based on a false premiss (Burke 1988), since normal resting-state muscle tone does not appear to depend on neural mechanisms. There is no background motor unit activity present in a relaxed normal subject. Furthermore, fusimotor overactivity cannot by itself produce spasticity (Burke *et al*. 1976). Fusimotor dysfunction is instead more likely to contribute to the negative features, for example loss of dexterity, than to the positive (Burke 1988). Normal resistance to passive movement is determined by several factors: physical inertia of the limb; mechanical-elastic factors (compliance of muscle tendon and connective tissue); and reflex muscle contraction (Katz and Rymer 1989). Some resistance to passive movement can occur in normal individuals, although its presence may reflect an individual's inability to relax and allow the limb to be moved.

Tone is typically tested in the clinic by passive movement of a joint or limb (e.g., the Ashworth scale, Ashworth 1964), with no account taken by the examiner of the velocity of the movement. Any reduction in resistance to passive movement after a CNS lesion is called *hypotonus*. Similarly, the term *hypertonus* or *spasticity* is used to describe an increased resistance to passive movement of a joint or limb. However, since for tonic reflex activity to be evoked movements must be performed sufficiently fast, any resistance felt by the clinician to relatively slow passive movement may be due in large part to decreased compliance in the soft tissues (Herman 1970; Dietz *et al*. 1981). Nevertheless, any resistance to passive movement is – in most cases erroneously – taken by clinicians to reflect the level of excitability of the components of the segmental stretch reflex arc due to increased fusimotor drive, and, therefore, the 'spastic' manifestation of the neural lesion.

It is essential in planning intervention aimed at improving motor control and performance to clarify the underlying dysfunction and this involves keeping up to date with developments in science. It has generally been considered in physiotherapy, as it has in medicine, that it is the positive features of the UMN syndrome, the hyperreflexia and hypertonus (resistance to passive stretch), that are the major barriers to functional movement (Paine and Oppé 1966; Brain 1977; Swaiman and Jacobson 1986; Bobath 1990). Many treatment methods have been developed to inhibit these features, including medications and reflex inhibitory techniques (Bobath 1980; Levitt 1982) and the assumption has been that inhibition of spasticity will lead to an improvement in function. However, there is no clinical or experimental evidence to support this assumption (Corston *et al.* 1981; Neilson and McCaughey 1982; Landau 1988; Richards *et al.* 1991; Guiliani 1991). Rather, research findings support the view that movement dysfunction is principally caused by the loss of muscle strength and control. However, studies of the effects of medication have shown that hyperreflexia is not the major barrier to gaining functional movement (Nathan 1969; Landau 1974; McLellan 1977) and it is now considered that the negative symptoms constitute the major barrier to functional movement (Landau 1974; Neilson and O'Dwyer 1981; Burke 1988). In addition, one investigation of cerebral palsied subjects showed that when they were trained to control their tonic stretch reflex activity, they still could not learn to perform a novel motor task (Neilson and McCaughey 1982). Hence, directing treatment at inhibiting hyperreflexia can probably not be expected to result in improved motor function.

If the physiotherapist views resistance to passive movement as having a purely neural cause then intervention will be directed towards the neural system. Reflex inhibiting movements in neurodevelopmental therapy are based on this premiss. However, once scientific endeavour makes it clear that one premiss is false and investigations support an alternative one, then it becomes necessary to develop and test different intervention strategies based on this new premiss. For example, research results suggest that the clinically perceived increased resistance to passive movement in patients with brain dysfunction may be to some extent the result of mechanical factors affecting muscle (Dietz *et al.* 1981). In addition, lack of compliance in muscles (resistance to passive movement) which have shortened has been reported to be highly correlated with the clinical sign of hypertonus (Perry 1980). Given this information, treatments are designed to prevent loss of extensibility in soft tissues (Ada and Canning 1990).

Hypertonus

Hypertonus has been defined as characterized by a velocity-dependent increase in tonic stretch reflexes resulting from hyperexcitability of the stretch reflexes (Lance 1980). This increased tone may be the result of changes intrinsic to muscle or altered reflex properties (Katz and Rymer 1989). The results of electromyogram studies on walking in children with spasticity or rigidity (Berger *et al.* 1982; Dietz and Berger 1983; Hufschmidt and Mauritz 1985) support the view that muscle fibre changes are partly responsible for the clinical sign of hypertonus, although exact pathophysiological mechanisms remain unknown.

One contribution to muscle tone is the intrinsic stiffness of muscle. Muscle stiffness can be estimated by examining the tension elicited when a joint is moved through a given range at varying velocities (Partridge and Benton 1981). Increased mechanical stiffness in muscle would appear as increased resistance to passive movement and be responsible for the clinical sign of hypertonus (Katz and Rymer 1989).

Velocity-dependent hyperreflexia will contribute to hypertonus but exactly how is not understood. The current view is similar to that of Landau in the 1960s, that spastic hyperreflexia has its origins in a disturbance of reflex circuits within the spinal cord. This will be reflected in increased excitation of the alpha motoneuron, without necessarily implying that therein lies the primary problem (Burke 1988). Increased excitation of the spinal motoneurons may be associated with adaptations occurring in the nervous system itself. It has been suggested, for example, that the slow time course for the development of spasticity following stroke in adults suggests that plastic changes in synaptic connections may contribute to the development of hyperreflexia (Chapman and Weisendanger 1982). Adaptive changes such as new synaptic connections through axonal sprouting could occur as a response to denervation; pre- or postsynaptic elements may become abnormally sensitive to remaining afferent input; there may be a change in the normal pattern of synaptic use, with previously inactive synapses becoming active.

As electrophysiological and biomechanical studies of patients with brain dysfunction provide increasing information about mechanisms underlying the motor dysfunction, it appears that, whether hyperreflexia develops or not, it is the negative features that constitute the major defects in function, not the positive (Burke 1988).

There is also the possibility that the individual's own efforts to move in the presence of the negative factors (muscle weakness or depressed motor activity) and positive factors (hyperexcitability of proprioceptive reflexes) associated with the brain lesion may be a factor in the development of muscular imbalance and abnormal patterns of movement synergies. When an individual attempts a goal-directed action, the movement pattern which emerges will reflect the best that can be done in the circumstances, given the state of the neuromuscular system and the dynamic possibilities inherent in the multi-segment linkage (Shepherd and Carr 1991). The exaggerated force generated by some muscles as the individual struggles to perform an approximation of the action required may be a significant factor in the development of the typical picture of spastic cerebral palsy.

It may also be that, since initial attempts at movement in infancy are relatively random and position-dependent, the same muscles are constantly being activated. Together with this, the relative immobility of the brain-damaged infant may mean that certain muscles (depending on the positions habitually experienced) contract only when held short while others contract only when lengthened. The typical posture of infants with cerebral palsy may reflect to a large extent the effects of this mechanism and be responsible for the typical picture of the infant in supine, of adducted shoulders and hips and extended, adducted legs.

The relationship between the neural lesion and muscle adaptability

Skeletal muscle has been shown, largely in animal studies, to be very adaptable, altering its structure (length, volume, cross-sectional area) in response to changes in the operating conditions (Tabary *et al.* 1976, 1981). Muscle also adapts during growth and development and these changes appear to be due to the demands of increasing bone growth and body weight, as well as to the active use of the muscles (Koning *et al.* 1987). In other words, the structural characteristics of muscle are determined by the conditions of use (O'Dwyer *et al.* 1989). Studies of mice have shown that gastrocnemius muscle grows as fast as bone in normal mice and half as fast in spastic mice (Ziv *et al.* 1984). As Lieber (1986) points out, skeletal muscle represents a classic biological example of the relationship between structure and function.

Changes in muscle length occur through the addition or subtraction of sarcomeres. The number of sarcomeres has been shown to alter in response to imposed immobility, changing according to whether a muscle is positioned in a shortened or a lengthened position. The regulation of sarcomere number appears to be determined by the length imposed on a muscle rather than its tension (Huet de la Tour *et al.* 1979). When a muscle is immobilized in a shortened position, the sarcomeres are less than their optimal length for tension generation and the muscle responds to this by decreasing the number of sarcomeres. This occurs particularly if the muscle is able to contract (Tabary *et al.* 1981). Fibre length is thereby shortened to suit the muscle's new functional length (Williams and Goldspink 1973, 1978). Muscle adaptation has been shown to be particularly rapid when muscle shortening is brought about by electrically induced muscle activation (Tabary *et al.* 1981).

When muscle is immobilized in a lengthened position, its response in younger animals has been shown to be different from that occurring in older animals. In the young, an initial brief increase in sarcomere number is followed by a decrease in number and muscle fibre length is thereby decreased (Tardieu *et al.* 1977). Overall muscle length is obtained by a relative lengthening of the tendon.

Adaptive increases in connective tissues have been found to occur in shortened muscle in the early stages of immobilization before a significant loss of sarcomere numbers can be seen. In children, an alteration in the orientation of collagen fibres relative to muscle fibres may be a factor in the hypoextensibility of a muscle (Goldspink and Williams 1979; Williams and Goldspink 1984) rather than an increase in connective tissue itself (Tardieu *et al.* 1982).

Muscle contracture in children with cerebral palsy, which is very common and seems to occur quite rapidly, is due to decreased muscle length and a decrease in the number of sarcomeres as well as a decrease in extensibility. One cause of the contracture in infants with brain lesion is said to be a failure of muscle growth brought about by a lack of full stretch to the spastic muscle (Ziv *et al.* 1984). That is, stretch induces growth (Holly *et al.* 1980). Muscle contracture appears to occur in response to prolonged abnormal function. This includes the immobility imposed on the individual by such negative features as the inability to initiate voluntarily or control muscle activation. There is also a tendency to generate force involuntarily in response to stimulation of hyperreflexic proprioceptive reflexes and, in some infants, in response to vestibular inputs elicited by positioning. This involuntary muscle activity seems to be strongest in muscles held at a shortened length.

Muscles may be held persistently at certain lengths (immobilized) due to the immobility caused by the negative features of the brain lesion, although in some children abnormal dystonic posturing and hypersensitivity of the tonic stretch reflexes may also play a part. The immobility caused by these *neural factors* is one cause of muscular and connective tissue adaptation in which the length of the soft tissues is effectively altered. These *mechanical factors*, together with the neural factors, will alter muscle extensibility and result in the resistance to passive stretch or stiffness we call hypertonus.

Length-associated changes have an effect on both passive and active properties of muscles. The *passive properties* affected are length and stiffness. Not only do muscles lose sarcomeres and become shorter (Williams and Goldspink 1978), when immobilized in a shortened position, they also become stiffer (Goldspink and Williams 1979). Stiffness is the ratio of passive tension developed to the amount of lengthening of the muscle when it is stretched (Gordon 1990).

The most significant changes in *active properties* (significant in terms of the functional sequelae) occur when muscles are held lengthened. These muscles cannot generate tension when the muscle is in its inner range since the myofilaments are maximally overlapped before that range is reached. For example, the anterior tibial muscles, as antagonists to shortened calf muscles, may not be able to generate tension with the foot in dorsiflexion. Conversely, once the calf muscles have been lengthened (e.g. by serial casting), they may not be able to generate tension when the foot is in dorsiflexion.

Isometric tension of muscles fibres also varies as a function of sarcomere length (Gordon *et al.* 1966). Many studies suggest that spastic contracture is the result of a complex process involving degenerative changes, including atrophy, as well as an alteration of passive and contractile muscle properties (Hufschmidt and Mauritz 1985).

The information we have at present suggests that the focus of therapeutic intervention should shift from an emphasis on inhibiting the abnormal positive features associated with the brain lesion. Intervention should instead focus on:

1 *Maintenance of soft tissue extensibility* by:
   (a) functional exercises to promote active lengthening and activation of both agonists and antagonists at the lengths necessary for function, and
   (b) positioning to optimize effective motor performance (see Fig. 3.27) and prevent length-associated changes in soft tissue.

For example, practice of crouch-to-stand or sit-to-stand (see Figs 3.1, 3.9) may be effective in maintaining the functional length of calf muscles as well as optimizing the ability of anterior and posterior tibial muscles to generate force at the necessary lengths for these actions.

Should the infant tend to exaggerate plantarflexion by going on to the toes instead of keeping the feet flat on the floor, the movement can be guided manually so that the infant performs only the first part of the action (see Fig. 3.1b) In addition, the infant can be positioned during the day to minimize the possibility of muscles shortening and maximize the opportunity for goal-directed movement. It is not known for what period of the day muscles need to be either held at an optimal length or actively stretched. However, it has been suggested that it may be as long as 14 hours out of the 24 (Tardieu *et al.* 1987).

Those muscles predisposed to shortening because of the natural resting position of the limbs are, in particular in the upper limb, the shoulder adductors and internal rotators, forearm pronators, long finger flexors and thumb adductors; and in the lower limb, hip adductors, rectus femoris and calf muscles.

Where soft tissue shortening has already occurred, passive lengthening through serial casting (see Chapter 5) may be necessary, combined with exercises to promote active lengthening.

2 *Gaining optimal motor control (i.e. control of force generation)* by task- and context-specific training (see Chapter 3).

In infants, this may involve positioning or casting to prevent muscles generating force in a stereotyped manner, for example, repetitively contracting at a short length. In children, as in adults, exercises and practice of functional actions need to be planned to encourage the appropriate application of muscle force. Feedback can be given electronically or mechanically by toys and objects in order to discourage muscle activity (Neilson and McCaughey 1982; Malouin *et al.* 1986; Richards and Malouin 1992), whether this be unnecessary force or force generated by inappropriate muscles. The objective should be to help the child learn to gain control over muscle activity in the context of task-related activity rather than the therapist 'inhibiting' unwanted muscle activity. It is probable that motor training that is specific to an action, with practice under natural environmental and task conditions, will assist the child to optimize neural control in the presence of brain lesions. Training is directed at the behavioural consequences of the central lesion, providing a means of measuring outcome of intervention in a meaningful way (e.g., Ada and Westwood, 1992; Richards and Malouin 1992). The assumption underlying task-specific training is that training a child to improve performance of relevant actions provides a stimulus to the system to re-adjust and learn a pattern of neuromotor activity relevant to the child's goals. Rather than emphasizing the 'preparation' for function as in the Bobath approach (Maystone 1992) the child is encouraged to ˙gain control during the practice of meaningful actions. Studies on neural recovery mechanisms in animals and humans suggest the possibility that intensive training positively affects recovery processes (Travis and Woolsey 1956; Taub 1980; Held 1987; Visintin *et al.* 1989; Malouin *et al.* 1992).

A subject with quadriplegic cerebral palsy has, for example, been shown to achieve skill in performing an arm swinging task, both perturbed and unperturbed, decreasing muscular reactivity to stretch as skill increased (Harrison and Kruze 1987). The authors suggested that training renders 'spastic performance' more normal, decreasing muscle activity in certain muscles and eliminating excessive antagonistic involvement.

Dyscontrol characteristics associated with lesions of the cerebellum

The cerebellum contains complete motor and sensory representations of the body, yet lesions do not produce either weakness or disorders of perception. The major disorder appears to be an inability to regulate movement. The patient seems to have little control over movement trajectories, that is, the programmed use of muscle force in relation to its rate of change (Brooks 1986). Lesions affect the ipsilateral side of the body, lateral lesions affecting the limbs and vermal lesions the trunk. In childhood, lesions may be associated with stroke, tumour, head injury and, rarely, cerebral palsy.

The cerebellum plays a critical role in the adaptation, learning and skilled execution of motor actions (Brooks 1986). It seems to play a large part in the coordinated execution of the motor intention and as such has a regulatory role, controlling the timing and patterning of muscles activated during movement.

Although the cerebellum is involved in the regulation of muscle tone and the initiation and coordination of voluntary movements, it is still unclear how it is involved in the coordination of movements. The neocerebellum may be involved in the planning and initiation of movement. This area receives input from the frontal association areas of the cerebral cortex. The intermediate parts of the cerebellum may be involved in moment-to-moment control. The cerebellum may, therefore, spare us from having to think out every movement of a limb and enable us to act automatically.

The cerebellum may be involved in compensating for disorders of the cerebral cortex or in learning new motor routines. This view is supported by the loss of previously regained function when a cerebellar lesion follows on at some time after a cerebral lesion.

The cerebellum is involved, therefore, in the regulation of movement, the initiation and control of voluntary movement, moment-to-moment control, and possibly in compensating for disorders of the cerebral cortex and learning new routines (Kandel and Schwartz 1985).

The distinctive *signs* of cerebellar lesions were described by Gordon Holmes early in the century (Holmes 1939) and reflect the role of the cerebellum in movement control. These signs are:

1 *Dyssynergia or ataxia.* The lack of coordination is manifested in a combination of motor control deficits, including:
   (a) *Inaccurate range and direction or dysmetria*, characterized by excessive extent of movement or overshooting (hyper-metria) or deficient extent of movement (undershooting). This is evidenced in walking, by irregular foot placements, and in reaching for an object, by over- or undershooting in the final part of the approach phase.
   (b) *Uncontrolled amplitude of force production*, which is seen during manipulation of objects, but which also produces the dysmetria.
   (c) *Decomposition of movement* is a lack of smooth sequential performance of various components due to errors in the timing or sequencing of components in a movement pattern. Movements appear jerky. This characteristic is particularly noticeable when the individual changes direction.
   (d) *Dysdiadochokinesia* is an irregular pattern of movement seen when the person performs rapid alternating movements. The child tends to perform such movements slowly and deliberately and only with considerable concentration.
2 *Hypotonia.* One sign linked to cerebellar dysfunction is an abnormal extensibility of muscle on passive movement, so that the amplitude of passive wrist extension, for example, is greater than normal. This sign is said to indicate an increased compliance of muscle (Burke 1988).
3 *Rebound phenomenon or lack of check*, that is, the inability of a rapidly moving limb to stop. The limb overshoots and may rebound excessively. This lack of control over braking (antagonistic) muscle activity is seen, for example, at the end of swing phase in walking, when the forward swinging leg is uncontrolled and also in pointing. The limb

movement appears to be braked by the non-muscular structures at the joint rather than by antagonistic muscle activity. Fast movements are particularly impaired because of the braking difficulties, but slow movements are also difficult to control.
4 *Tremor.* This is an oscillatory movement about a joint due to alternating contractions of agonists and antagonists. It occurs with movement of the limb and is most marked at the end of the movement – *terminal* or *intention tremor*. A truncal tremor (*titubation*) may be present when the patient is standing or sitting. A cerebellar tremor is not a true tremor but a tendency to make corrections that are too large, resulting in overshooting and the need to reverse direction. This is particularly noticeable in the terminal stage of reaching, when the hand normally slows and adjusts grasp aperture to pick up the object.
5 *Dysarthria.* A disorder of speech articulation. Symbols of speech are normal but mechanical aspects of speech are impaired. Speech is slurred and slow with prolonged syllables, called scanning speech.
6 *Nystagmus.* Seesaw rhythmical movement of the eyes is a sign of vestibular dysfunction and may be present with a lesion involving the flocculonodular lobe.
7 *Disturbances of balance* (see Fig. 3.33) are seen in the ataxic gait, and in increased postural sway in standing. Walking is characterized by a wide base of support, which is compensatory, an excessive sway and arm movement.

The above signs result in poor control of motor actions and can be summarized as: errors of rate, range, direction and force; lack of modulation of movement and excessive motion or, alternatively, a voluntary restriction of motion (a compensatory phenomenon); poor control over postural adjustments which are normally interrelated with voluntary movement; loss of fluidity of motion, that is, poor timing and patterning of the synergic components with motor tasks being broken down into their components.

Training of specific actions when a child has any of the above dyscontrol characteristics is as described in Chapter 3. Specific attention is paid to analysing the control deficits during performance of activities and these form the basis for planning intervention.

Take for example a child who has difficulty controlling the lower-limb extensor muscles while walking up and down stairs. Stepping up can be practised with the child stopping the movement at various points and reversing from a concentric to an eccentric contraction (see Figs 3.18 and 3.19). This type of exercise may help the child improve the ability to reverse direction. Stepping down can be practised to improve the ability to brake movement caused by body weight.

Dyscontrol characteristics associated with lesions of the basal ganglia

In infants and children, basal ganglia disorder is characterized by excessive activity and involuntary movements (athetosis, chorea) and abnormal involuntary posturing (dystonia; see Fig. 5.4). Intended motor actions are degraded into movements of inappropriate amplitude and postures of inappropriate duration (Brooks 1986).

There is evidence that poor functional performance is due to abnormal voluntary motor control rather than to involuntary movements (Neilson and O'Dwyer 1984). It has been shown by O'Dwyer and Neilson (1988) that poor control is reflected in abnormalities in the spatiotemporal patterns of muscle activity. They propose that the selection of muscles to be inhibited or activated and the timing of the contraction of each muscle relative to the contraction of other muscles are poorly controlled in athetoid subjects.

It has been shown that an increased level of muscle activity appears to be a primary abnormality in athetoid subjects in both arm movements (Hallett and Alvarez 1983) and speech movements (O'Dwyer and Neilson 1988). An increased amount of lip muscle activity has been reported in response to an expected external perturbation (Abbs and Gracco 1984).

There might be several reasons for this unnecessary muscle activity. Increased muscle activity has been noted in the early phase of motor skill learning in able-bodied subjects, and has been suggested to reduce the extent of movement error (Humphrey and Reed 1983). Increased levels of muscle activation have also been suggested to occur as part of increased tonic coactivation of agonist and antagonist muscles, serving to increase the stiffness of body segments (Houk *et al.* 1981). It appears evident from both clinical observation and research findings (O'Dwyer and Neilson 1988) that individuals with athetoid cerebral palsy may increase muscle activity around a joint in order to minimize the deviations of movement which arise out of their poor control of muscle activity as well as their involuntary muscle activity.

Harris (1971) suggested that athetoid movements may arise from defective sensory feedback from the moving limb. He considered the problem to be a control system failure, in which faulty feedback from peripheral sense organs, which does not accurately represent limb position, may cause the instability seen in individuals with athetosis.

It has recently been proposed that the primary abnormality underlying the motor impairment in individuals with mixed spastic–athetoid cerebral palsy is related to problems with perceptual–motor integration; that is, patients are unable to learn the relationships between the motor commands to muscles and the resulting perceptual consequences of the movement (Vaughan *et al.* 1988; Neilson *et al.* 1990). Such a deficit in motor learning would result in poor movement control rather than an inability to move.

The training of motor control in infants and children with involuntary movements or dystonic spasms presents considerable difficulty. In general, training strategies and exercises designed to improve performance of functional actions are as described in Chapter 3. It appears of major importance to attempt to minimize the dystonic posturing in infants by guiding the parents in what positions the infant should avoid. For example, if the infant demonstrates involuntary extension movements of the head and trunk in supine (see Fig. 5.2), then this position should be avoided. The infant may need to sleep in a hammock-type bed (see Fig. 5.14). The child's head may need to be restrained in a collar or similar for periods of the day to enable the development of visuomotor control (see Fig. 5.13). Intervention aims ultimately to enable the child to function independently, but in many children with severe disability, independence may only be achieved in an electric wheelchair. An older child can be encouraged to participate with the therapist in working out, often by trial and error, the best solutions to the motor problems.

Recovery processes after brain injury

There is increasing evidence that the CNS is capable of significant structural and functional changes in response to injury. Much of the research done has been on animals. Nevertheless, it is likely that similar mechanisms exist in the human brain. In this section, the findings related to recovery in animal studies are reviewed briefly. The reader may need to consult the suggested readings for more detailed information.

The issue of recovery processes is of particular interest to physiotherapists since the major objective of therapy is to optimize the functional potential of individuals with brain lesions. Research which reports the outcome of particular strategies in animals is of interest since it may provide information for the testing of hypotheses in humans, which would subsequently be of relevance to the building of rehabilitation programmes. Such research, in addition, supports the view that what happens after a brain lesion, the environment in which intervention takes place and the type of intervention can affect outcome.

There are numerous theories about the *nature of recovery processes*:

1 *Diaschisis* infers that a brain injury is followed by a period of shock which affects a wider area of the brain than the actual lesion. Therefore, as the system recovers from this effect, some previously absent functions reappear.
2 Target neurons develop *supersensitivity* to neurotransmitters, enhancing their ability to function and producing a degree of recovery. This response to damage may provide a molecular basis for
3 *Vicariation or equipotentiality*. This theory proposes that undamaged parts of the nervous system may take over functions previously subserved by damaged areas of the system.
4 *Axonal sprouting* (synaptogenesis), involving regrowth of damaged axons or sprouting of undamaged axons to take over vacated synaptic sites, has been found in experimental animals (Marx 1980). How successful this sprouting is in forming functional connections is thought to depend on such factors as the characteristics of the lesion and the environment (Cotman and Nieto-Sampedro 1982; Held 1987). Little is known of this phenomenon, but it has also been suggested that axonal sprouting may be responsible for harmful effects such as the slow development of hyperreflexia following stroke (Chapman and Weisendanger 1982). It is possible that, in the absence of appropriate experience, new pathways may be maladaptive (Whishaw *et al.* 1984).
5 The theory of *compensation* suggests that functions subserved by the damaged area of brain may recover but are mediated by different means. It is not at all clear just what this means, but it has been suggested that such compensation, if it occurs, may prevent the recovery of the original function (Le Vere and Le Vere 1982).

One line of experimental work of particular interest to physiotherapists is the study of the *effect of environmental stimulation* on normal animals and following brain lesions. Studies of normal animals have shown that those which were housed in enriched environments (in the company of other animals, with a variety of objects to manipulate) had better problem-solving skills than animals housed in impoverished conditions (Finger 1978). Brain changes have been found in rats which correlated with environmental enrichment (Rosenweig *et al.* 1973; Walsh and Cummins 1975), with greater cortical thickness and weight, increased glial proliferation and density of dendritic processes. It has further been shown that neural changes may persist following withdrawal of stimulation (Camel *et al.* 1986).

It has been suggested (Walsh and Cummins 1975) that environmentally induced changes may be due in part to increased arousal brought about by a novel stimulus or one which had significance to the animal. The arousal would be associated with increased electrocortical activity and this would result in increased metabolism, facilitating brain changes. Synapse renewal is considered to occur in response to a change in neural activity (brought about, for example, by environmental changes), which causes either an increase or a decrease in firing patterns (Cotman and Nieto-Sampedro 1982). Of possible relevance to human rehabilitation is that, in Walsh's rat experiments, anatomical and chemical changes peaked early during the enrichment period (Walsh 1981).

Similar results have been found after brain lesions. Rats placed in an enriched environment after a brain lesion have been found to have superior task performance to rats in an impoverished non-learning environment (Wills and Rosenweig 1977; Isseroff and Isseroff 1978; Held *et al.* 1985). It is not certain whether enrichment causes a generalized increase in learning or whether it is specific to the experience available in the environment. Experiments with rats following a hippocampal lesion seem to support the latter view (Pacteau *et al.* 1989). The rats who were housed in an enriched environment following the lesion performed better on a task which resembled that environment. It is also not certain whether some areas of the brain have a greater potential for plasticity than others. Hippocampus and cerebral cortex seem to show a greater potential for synaptogenesis than, for example, sensory relay nuclei (Cotman and Nieto-Sampedro 1982).

Evidence from these animal studies suggests, as Walsh (1981) has proposed, that an interesting line of investigation would involve determining what types of input would be the most effective in optimizing recovery following brain lesions. It appears from his work that active exploration of objects may be critical. In proposing radical changes to the process of rehabilitation and to the environment in which it takes place, Carr and Shepherd (1987a, b) have suggested that structuring the environment to facilitate active exploration, together with early practice of actions such as standing up, reaching out for objects in sitting and standing, grasping and manipulating different objects may be the most effective method of re-establishing function. The emphasis in this approach is on providing a rehabilitation framework that maximizes the individual's active and self-initiated interaction with the environment.

Effect of age on recovery processes

Of major concern to physiotherapists who work with infants and children is whether or not recovery after a brain lesion in the immature infant brain is similar to that of older children and adults whose maturation processes are more advanced.

Age has been considered to be important in the takeover of function previously subserved by damaged areas of brain (vicariation). A widely held view has been that the young brain recovers better from lesions than the adult brain by virtue of its greater plasticity (Kennard 1940; Goldman 1971). This view arose from the idea that localization of cortical function is poorly defined in infants and that functions can be taken over by areas of cortex not normally assigned to them. In other words, if the brain lesion occurs during early development, an uncommitted area may substitute for a damaged one. This view has since been challenged (Isaacson 1975; St James-Roberts 1979). Although young lesioned animals in the early studies appeared to make good recoveries (Goldman 1971), subsequent investigation has shown that deficits emerged when these monkeys were older (Goldman 1974). The substitute area's commitment seemed to result in an impairment of its own intended function at a later time, resulting in a delayed appearance of deficits.

The environment and specific experiences have been shown to affect brain structure in baby animals and it is generally accepted that experience and the resultant shaping of cortical response properties are critical, in vision at least, if neuronal receptive fields are to develop the degree of specificity required for normal function (Singer 1982). The lack of specific experiences and activities has also been shown to affect structure, development and function in young animals. There is experimental evidence that training (exercise) can improve functional recovery after a neural lesion and that this may be due to preventing deterioration of the neuromuscular system (Yu 1980).

It has been established that retinal signals control the development of specific receptive fields in the striate cortex (Singer 1982). Kittens deprived of sight of their forelimbs during locomotion have been found to lack the ability to learn a latch-release task. Monocular visual deprivation in kittens leads to profound effects on the functional capability of occipital cortex neurons. Recovery has been recorded even after prolonged absense of stimulation, suggesting that afferent optic fibres compete for synaptic space on intact cortical neurons (Timney and Mitchell 1979). Deprivation of auditory stimulus is associated in mice with poor development of the brainstem auditory neurons (Webster and Webster 1979). Kolb and Elliot (1987) showed that rearing rats with neonatal brain injury in an enriched environment resulted in an increase in cortical thickness.

There is some evidence that experience-dependent maturation of sensory functions is gated by attentional mechanisms (Singer 1982). Strabismic kittens (which are unable to fuse signals from two eyes into a single image) are said to develop in a similar way to humans. When they alternate the use of their eyes, both eyes develop normal monocular vision; if they always suppress the same eye, that eye becomes amblyopic (Jacobson and Ikeda 1979). Whichever of the two occurs, the majority of cortical neurons lose their binocular connections (Hubel and Wiesel 1965).

Studies of young animals have demonstrated the presence and effects of synaptogenesis following a lesion. Sectioning of the pyramidal tract in baby hamsters is followed by regrowth of severed axons via a new pathway, this regeneration occurring in an apparently functionally useful way (Grobecker and Pietsch 1979). Sprouting of corticospinal terminals has been found to occur after neonatal hemispherectomy and unilateral section of the pyramidal tract, the resulting collaterals crossing the cord and terminating ipsilateral to the lesion (Gomez-Pinilla *et al.* 1986). Redirection of fibre projections in the cerebral cortex of prenatally brain-damaged primates has also been demonstrated (Goldman 1978; Goldman-Rakic 1980) and considerable functional recovery has been noted in primates after unilateral pyramidotomy. Such functional recovery may result from branching of ipsilateral corticospinal projections from the undamaged motor cortex to motoneurons of the distal hand muscles (Kucera and Wiesendanger 1985).

Evidence of reorganization of central motor pathways has been found in a study of the hand and forearm muscles of children with hemiplegic cerebral palsy (Farmer *et al.* 1991). The 4 children in this study demonstrated mirror movements in excess of those found in a group of normal children, and cross-correlational analysis indicated that the right and left motoneuronal pools of these children shared common synaptic inputs, suggesting that axonal sprouting had occurred. The short latency responses recorded from distal hand muscles following magnetic brain stimulation were consistent with transmission via fast-conducting corticospinal tract axons. Since the responses

were bilateral following focal magnetic stimulation of the intact motor cortex, the intact corticospinal tract must have innervated ipsilateral as well as contralateral hand motoneurons. Whether these changes would have occurred during fetal life or postnatally is not known.

It is not certain what clinical implications can be drawn from this research. However, it seems likely that what the infant or child experiences and practises could affect both maturational and recovery processes as they involve the neuromuscular system. If this is so, then intervention should commence early, it should provide challenge and variety, it should encourage active participation, and prevent immobility and its sequelae. Since what the infant practises is probably critical, motor training and exercise should be specific to the action being learned. Therapeutic effort should be concentrated on training functional actions: reaching and manipulation for the upper limbs, support, balance and propulsion for the lower limbs.

Summary

The first section of this chapter includes a brief overview of processes involved in the maturation of the nervous system through the fetal and embryonic periods. Such information draws attention to the vulnerability of the brain in the pre- and perinatal period. Pathophysiological processes and the characteristics of a disordered system are outlined in the middle section as a means of elucidating the mechanisms of motor dyscontrol which result in the movement disorders seen in brain lesions. This information, together with research findings related to recovery and adaptive processes, is critical to the evaluation of motor problems and the development and testing of hypotheses related to therapeutic and training strategies.

References

Abbs, J.H. and Gracco, V.L. (1984) Control of complex motor gestures: orofacial muscle responses to load perturbations of lip during speech. *J. Neurophysiol.*, **51**, 4, 705–723.

Ada, L. and Canning, C. (1990) Anticipating and avoiding muscle shortening. In: *Key Issues in Neurological Physiotherapy*, edited by L. Ada and C. Canning. Oxford: Butterworth-Heinemann.

Ashworth, B. (1964) Preliminary trial of carisoprodol in multiple selerosis. *Practitioner*, **192**, 540–542.

Berger, W., Quintern, J. and Dietz, V. (1982) Pathophysiology of gait in children with cerebral palsy. *Electroencephalogr. Clin. Neurophysiol.*, **53**, 538–548.

Bishop, B. (1982) Neural plasticity 2: postnatal maturation and function-induced plasticity. *Phys. Ther.*, **62**, 8, 1132–1143.

Bobath, B. (1990) *Adult Hemiplegia Evaluation and Treatment.* 3rd edn. Oxford: Butterworth-Heinemann.

Bobath, K. (1980) *A Neurological Basis for the Treatment of Cerebral Palsy.* Philadelphia, PA: JB Lippincott.

Brain, W.R. (1977) *Brain's Diseases of the Nervous System*, 8th edn. Oxford: Oxford University Press.

Brooks, V.B. (1986) *The Neural Basis of Motor Control.* New York: Oxford University Press.

Burke, D. (1988) Spasticity as an adaptation to pyramidal tract injury. In: *Advances in Neurology, 47: Functional Recovery in Neurological Disease*, edited by S.G. Waxman. New York: Raven Press.

Burke, D. and Lance, J.W. (1973) Studies of reflex effects of primary and secondary spindle endings in spasticity. In: *New Developments in Electromyography and Clinical Neurophysiology*, vol. 3, edited by J.E. Desmedt. Basel: Karger, pp. 475–495.

Burke, D., Hagbarth, K.E. Lofstedt, L. and Wallin, B.G. (1976) Responses of human muscle spindle endings to vibration of non-contracting muscles. *J. Physiol.*, **261**, 673–693.

Camel, J.E., Withers, G.S. and Greenough, W.T. (1986) Persistence of visual cortex dendritic alterations induced by post-weaning exposure to a 'superenriched' environment in rats. *Behav. Neurosci.*, **100**, 810–813.

Carr, J.H. and Shepherd, R.B. (1982) *Physiotherapy in Disorders of the Brain.* Oxford: Butterworth-Heinemann.

Carr, J.H. and Shepherd, R.B. (1987a) *A Motor Relearning Programme for Stroke*, 2nd edn. Oxford: Butterworth-Heinemann.

Carr, J.H. and Shepherd, R.B. (1987b) (Eds) *Movement Science. Foundations for Physical Therapy in Rehabilitation.* Oxford: Butterworth-Heinemann.

Carr, J.H., Shepherd, R.B. and Ada, L. (1994). Spasticity: Research findings and implications for intervention. *Physiotherapy*, in press.

Chapman, C.E. and Weisendanger, M. (1982) Physiologic and anatomical basis of spasticity: review. *Physiother. Can.*, **34**, 125–136.

Colebatch, J.G. and Gandevia, S.C. (1986) The distribution of muscular weakness in upper motor neuron lesions affecting the arm. *Brain*, **112**, 749–763.

Corston, R.N., Johnson, F. and Goodwin-Austen, R.B. (1981). The assessment of drug treatment of spastic gait. *J. Neurol., Neurosurg. Psychiatry*, **44**, 1035–1039.

Cotman, C.W. and Nieto-Sampedro, M. (1982) Brain function, synapse renewal and plasticity. *Annu. Rev. Psychol.*, **33**, 371–401.

Dekeban, A. (1970) *Neurology of Early Childhood.* Baltimore, MD: Williams & Wilkins.

Denny Brown, D.B. (1966) *The Cerebral Control of Movement.* Liverpool: Liverpool University Press.

Dietz, V. and Berger, W. (1983) Normal and impaired regulation of muscle stiffness in gait: a new hypothesis about muscle hypertonia. *Exp. Neurol.*, **79**, 680–687.

Dietz, V., Quintern, J. and Berger, W. (1981) Electrophysiological studies of gait in spasticity and rigidity: evidence that altered mechanical properties of muscle contribute to hypertonia. *Brain*, **104**, 431–449.

Dobbing, J. (1974) The later development of the brain and its vulnerability. In: *Scientific Foundations of Paediatrics*, edited by J.A. Davis and J. Dobbing. London: Heinemann.

Farmer, S.F., Harrison, L.M., Ingram, D.A. and Stephens, J.A. (1991) Plasticity of central motor pathways in children with hemiplegic cerebral palsy. *Neurology*, **41**, 1505–1510.

Finger, S. (1978) Environmental attenuation of brain-lesion symptoms. In: *Recovery from Brain Damage*, edited by S. Finger. London: Plenum Press.

Globus, A., Rosensweig, M.R., Bennett, E.L. *et al.* (1973) Effects of differential experience on dendritic spine counts in rat cerebral cortex. *J. Comp. Physiol. Psychol.*, **82**, 175–181.

Goldman, P.S. (1971) Functional development of the prefrontal cortex in early life and the problem of neuronal plasticity. *Exp. Neurol.*, **32**, 366–387.

Goldman, P.S. (1974) An alternative to developmental plasticity: heterology of CNS structures in infants and adults. In: *Plasticity and Recovery of Function in the Central Nervous System*, edited by D.G. Stein, J.J. Rosen and N. Butters. New York: Academic Press, pp. 149–174.

Goldman, P.S. (1978) Neuronal plasticity in primate telencephalon. Anomalous projections induced by prenatal removal of the frontal cortex. *Science*, **202**, 768–770.

Goldman-Rakic, P.S. (1980) Morphological consequences of prenatal injury to the primate brain. *Prog. Brain Res.*, **53**, 3.

Goldspink, G. and Williams, P.E. (1979) The nature of the increased passive resistance in muscle following immobilization of the mouse soleus muscle. *J. Physiol.*, **289**, 55.

Gomez-Pinilla, F., Villablanca, J.R., Sonnier, B.J. and Levine, M.S. (1986) Reorganisation of pericruciate projections to the spinal cord and dorsal column nuclei after neonatal or adult hemispherectomy in cats. *Brain Res.*, **385**, 342–355.

Gordon, J. (1990) Disorders of motor control. In: *Key Issues in Neurological Physiotherapy*, edited by L. Ada and C. Canning. Oxford: Butterworth-Heinemann, pp. 25–50.

Gordon, A.M., Huxley, A.F. and Julian, F.J. (1966) The variation in isometric tension with sarcomere length in vertebrate muscle fibres. *J. Physiol. (Lond.).*, **184**, 170.

Grobecker, D.B. and Pietsch, T.W. (1979) Regrowth of severed axons in the neonatal central nervous systems: establishment of normal connections. *Science*, **205**, 1158.

Guiliani, C.A. (1991) Dorsal rhizotomy for children with cerebral palsy: support for concepts of motor control. *Phys. Ther.*, **71**, 248–259.

Hallett, M. and Alvarez, N. (1983) Attempted rapid elbow flexion movements in patients with athetosis. *J. Neurol. Neurosurg. Psychiatry*, **46**, 745–750.

Harris, F.A. (1971) Inapproprioception: a possible sensory basis for athetoid movements. *Phys. Ther.*, **51**, 761–770.

Harrison, A. and Kruze, R. (1987) Perturbation of a skilled action II. Normalising the responses of cerebral palsied individuals. *Hum. Mov. Sci.*, **6**, 133–159.

Held, J. (1987) Recovery of function after brain damage: theoretical implications for therapeutic intervention. In: *Movement Science. Foundations for Physical Therapy in Rehabilitation*, edited by J.H. Carr and R.B. Shepherd. Oxford: Butterworth-Heinemann, pp. 155–177.

Held, J.M. (1987) Recovery of function after brain damage. In: *Movement Science. Foundations for Physical Therapy in Rehabilitation*, edited by J.H. Carr and R.B. Shepherd, Maryland: Aspen Publishers, pp. 155–177.

Held, J.M., Gordon, J. and Gentile, A.M. (1985) Environmental influence on locomotor recovery following cortical lesions in rats. *Behav. Neurosci.*, **99**, 678–690.

Herman, R. (1970) The myotatic reflex: clinico-physiological aspects of spasticity and contracture. *Brain*, **93**, 273–312.

Holly, R.G., Barnett, J.G., Ashmore, C.R., Taylor, R.G. and Mole, P.A. (1980) Stretch induced growth in chicken wing muscles. *Am. J. Physiol.*, **238**, C62–71.

Holmes, G. (1939) The cerebellum of man. *Brain*, **62**, 1–30.

Houk, J.C., Rymer, W.Z. and Crago, P. (1981) Dependence of dynamic response of spindle receptors on muscle length and velocity. *J. Neurophysiol.*, **46**, 143–166.

Hubel, D.H. and Wiesel, T.N. (1965) Binocular interaction in striate cortex of kittens reared with artificial squint. *J. Neurophysiol.*, **28**, 1041–1059.

Huet de la Tour, E., Tabary, J.C., Tabary, C. and Tardieu, C. (1979) The respective roles of muscle length and muscle tension in sarcomere number adaptation of guinea-pig soleus muscle. *J. Physiol.*, **75**, 589–592.

Hufschmidt, A. and Mauritz, K.H. (1985) Chronic transformation of muscle in spasticity: peripheral contribution to increased tone. *J. Neurol. Neurosurg. Psychiatry*, **48**, 676–685.

Huizar, P., Kuno, N. and Miyate, Y. (1975) Differentiation of motoneurones and skeletal muscles in kittens. *J. Physiol. (Lond.)*, **252**, 465–479.

Huizar, P., Kuno, N. Miyate, Y., Tardieu, C. *et al.* (1987) For how long must the soleus muscle be stretched each day to prevent contracture? *Develop. Med. Child Neurol.*

Humphrey, D.R. and Reed, D.J. (1983) Separate cortical systems for control of joint movement and joint stiffness: reciprocal activation and coactivation of antagonist muscles. *Adv. Neurol.*, **39**, 347–372.

Isaacson, R.L. (1975) The myth of recovery from early brain damage. In: *Aberrant Development in Infancy*, edited by N.R. Ellis. London: Wiley.

Isseroff, A. and Isseroff, R. (1978) Experience aids recovery of spontaneous alternation following hippocampal damage. *Physiol. Behav.*, **21**, 469–472.

Jackson, J.H. (1958) Selected writings. In: *John Hughlings Jackson*, edited by J. Taylor. New York: Basic Books.

Jacobson, S.G. and Ikeda, H. (1979) Behavioural studies of spatial vision in cats reared with convergent squint. Is amblyopia due to arrest in development? *Exp. Brain Res.*, **34**, 11–26.

Kandel, E.R. and Schwartz, J.H. (eds) (1985) *Principles of Neural Science*, 2nd edn. New York: Elsevier/North Holland.

Katz, R.T. and Rymer, W.Z. (1989) Spastic hypertonia: mechanisms and measurement. *Arch. Phys. Med. Rehabil.*, **70**, 144–155.

Kennard, M.A. (1940) Relation of age to motor impairment in man and in sub-human primates. *Arch. Neurol. Psychiatry*, **44**, 377–397.

Kolb, B. and Elliot, W. (1987) Recovery from early cortical damage in rats. II. Effects of experience on anatomy and behaviour following frontal lesions at one or five days of age. *Behav. Brain Res.*, **26**, 47–56.

Koning, J.J. de, Molan, H.F. van der, Woittier, R.D. and Huijing, P.A. (1987) Functional characteristics of rat gastrocnemius and tibialis anterior muscles during growth. *J. Morphology*, **194**, 75–84.

Kucera, P. and Wiesendanger, M. (1985) Do ipsilateral corticospinal tract fibres participate in functional recovery following unilateral pyramid lesions in monkeys? *Brain Res.*, **348**, 297–303.

Lance, J.W. (1980) Pathophysiology of spasticity and clinical experience with baclofen. In: *Spasticity: Disordered Motor Control*, edited by R.G. Feldman, R.R. Young and W.P. Koella. Chicago, IL: Year Book.

Landau, W.M. (1974) Spasticity: the fable of a neurological demon and the emperor's new therapy. *Arch. Neurol.*, **31**, 217–219.

Landau, W.M. (1980) Spasticity: what is it? What is it not? In: *Spasticity: Disordered Motor Control*, edited by R.G. Feldman, R.R. Young and W.P. Koella. Chicago: Year Book Medical Publishers, pp. 17–24.

Landau, W.M. (1988) Parables of palsy, pills and PT pedagogy: a spastic dialectic. *Neurol.*, **38**, 1496–1499.

Latash, M.L., Penn, R.D., Corcos, D.M. and Gottlieb, G.L. (1989) Short-term effects of intrathecal baclofen in spasticity. *Exper. Neurol.*, **103**, 165–172.

Le Vere, N.D. and Le Vere, T.E. (1982) Recovery of function after brain damage: support for the compensation theory of the behavioral deficit. *Physiol. Psychol*, **10**, 165.

Levitt, S. (1982) *Treatment of Cerebral Palsy and Motor Delay*, 2nd edn. Philadelphia, PA: Blackwell Scientific.

Lieber, R.L. (1986) Skeletal muscle adaptability. 1: Review of basic properties. *Dev. Med. Child Neurol.*, **28**, 390–397.

McArdle, C.B., Richardson, C.J., Nicholas, D.A. *et al.* (1987). Developmental features of the neonatal brain: MR imagery 1 Gray-white matter differentiation and myelination. *Radiol.*, **162**, 223–229.

McLellan, D.L. (1977) Co-contraction and stretch reflexes in spasticity during treatment with baclofen. *J. Neurol. Neurosurg. Psychiatry*, **40**, 30–38.

Malouin, F., Potvin, M., Prevost, J., Richards, C.L. and Wood-Dauphinee, S. (1992) Use of intensive task-oriented gait training program in a series of patients with acute cerebrovascular accidents. *Phys. Ther.*, **72**, 781–793.

Malouin, F., Trahan, J., Parrot, A. and Gemmel, M. (1986) Comparison of two strategies of biofeedback withdrawal in head position training in cerebral palsy children. *Physiother. Can.*, **38**, 337–342.

Marx, J.L. (1980) Regeneration in the central nervous system. *Science*, **209**, 378.

Maystone, M.J. (1992) The Bobath concept – evaluation and application. In: *Movement Disorders in Children*, edited by H. Hirschfeld and H. Forssberg. Basel: Karger, pp. 1–6.

Milner, B. (1974) Sparing of language functions after early unilateral brain damage. *Neurosci. Res. Prog. Bull.*, **12**, 213–217.

Mountcastle, V.B. (1980) *Medical Physiology*, 14th edn. St Louis, MO: Mosby.

Nathan, P.W. (1969) Treatment of spasticity with perineural injections of phenol. *Dev. Med. Child Neurol.*, **11**, 384.

Neilson, P.D. and McCaughey, J. (1982) Self-regulation of spasm and spasticity in cerebral palsy. *J. Neurol. Neurosurg. Psychiatry*, **45**, 320–330.

Neilson, P.D. and O'Dwyer, N.J. (1981) Pathophysiology of dysarthria in cerebral palsy. *J. Neurol., Neurosurg. Psychiatry*, **44**, 1013–1019.

Neilson, P.D. and O'Dwyer, N.J. (1984) Reproducibility and variability of speech muscle activity in athetoid dysarthria of cerebral palsy. *J. Speech, Hearing Res.*, **27**, 502–517.

Neilson, P.D., O'Dwyer, N.J. and Nash, J. (1990) Control of isometric muscle activity in cerebral palsy. *Dev. Med. Child Neurol.*, **32**, 778–788.

O'Dwyer, N.J. and Neilson, P.D. (1988) Voluntary muscle control in normal and athetoid dysarthric speakers. *Brain*, **111**, 877–899.

O'Dwyer, N.J., Neilson, P.D. and Nash, J. (1989) Mechanisms of muscle growth related to muscle contracture in cerebral palsy. *Dev. Med. Child Neurol.*, **31**, 543–547.

Pacteau, C., Einon, D. and Sinden, J. (1989) Early rearing environment and dorsal hippocampal ibotenic acid lesions: long term influences on spatial learning and alternation in the rat. *Behav. Brain Res.*, **34**, 89–96.

Paine, R.S. and Oppé, T.T. (1966) *Neurological Examination of Children*. London: Heinemann Medical.

Pape, K. and Wigglesworth, J.S. (1979) *Haemorrhage, Ischaemia and the Perinatal Brain. Clinics in Developmental Medicine*, no. 69–70. Philadelphia, PA: J.B. Lippincott.

Partridge, L.D. and Benton, L.A. (1981) Muscle, the motor. In: *Handbook of Physiology, Section I: Nervous System. Vol. 2: Motor Control*, edited by V.B. Brooks. Bethesda, MD: American Physiological Society.

Perry, J. (1980) Rehabilitation of spasticity. In: *Spasticity: Disordered Motor Control*, edited by R.G. Feldman, R.R. Young and W.P. Koella. Chicago, IL: Year Book, p. 87.

Phillips, C.G. and Porter, R. (1977) *Corticospinal Neurones. Their Role in Movement*. New York: Academic Press.

Richards, C.L. and Malouin, F. (1992) Spasticity control in the therapy of cerebral palsy. In: *Movement Disorders in Children*, edited by H. Hirschberg and H. Forssberg. Basel: Karger pp. 217–224.

Richards, C.L., Malouin, F., Dumas, F. and Wood-Dauphinee, S. (1991) New rehabilitation strategies for the treatment of spastic gait disorders. In: *Adaptability of Human Gait*, edited by A.E. Patla. New York: Elsevier, pp. 387–411.

Rosenweig, M.R., Bennet, E.L. and Diamond, M. (1973) Effects of differential experience on dendritic spine counts in rat cerebral cortex. *J. Comp. Physiol. Psychol.*, **82**, 175–181.

Rushworth, G. (1960) Spasticity and rigidity: experimental study and review. *J. Neurol. Neurosurg. Psychiatry*, **23**, 99–118.

St James-Roberts, I. (1979) Neurological plasticity, recovery from brain insult, and child development. *Adv. Child Dev. Behav.*, **14**, 253.

Shahani, B.T. and Young, R.R. (1980) The flexor reflex in spasticity. In: *Spasticity: Disordered Motor Control*, edited by R.G. Feldman, R.R. Young and W.P. Koella. Chicago: Year Book Medical, pp. 287–295.

Sahrmann, S.A. and Norton, B.J. (1977) The relationship of voluntary movement to spasticity in the upper motor neuron syndrome. *Ann. Neurol.*, **2**, 460–465.

Singer, W. (1982) The role of attention in developmental plasticity. *Hum. Neurobiol.*, **1**, 41–43.

Stewart, A.L., Reynolds, E.O.R. and Hope, P.L. *et al.* (1987) Probability of neurodevelopmental disorders estimated from ultrasound appearance of brains of very preterm infants. *Dev. Med. Child Neurol.*, **29**, 3.

Swaiman, K.F. and Jacobson, R.I. (1986) Developmental abnormalities of the central nervous system. In: *Clinical Neurology*, vol. 4, edited by A.B. Baker and R.J. Joynt. Philadelphia, PA: Harper & Row.

Tabary, J.C., Tardieu, C., Tardieu, G., Tabary, C. and Gagnard, L. (1976) Functional adaptation of sarcomere number of normal cat muscle. *J. Physiol.*, **72**, 277–291.

Tabary, J.-C., Tardieu, C., Tardieu, G. and Tabary, C. (1981) Experimental rapid sarcomere loss with comcomitant hypoextensibility. *Muscle Nerve*, **4**, 198–203.

Tardieu, C., Tarbary, J.C., Tabary, C. and Huet de la Tour, E. (1977) Comparison of the sarcomere number adaptation in young and adult animals. Influence of tendon adaptation. *J. Physiol.*, **73**, 1045–1055.

Tardieu, C., Huet de la Tour, E., Bret, M.D. and Tardieu, G. (1982) Muscle hypoextensibility in children with cerebral palsy: 1. Clinical and experimental observations. *Arch. Phys. Med. Rehabil.*, **63**, 97–102.

Tardieu, C., Lespargot, A., Tabary, C. and Bret, M.D. (1987) For how long must the soleus muscle be stretched each day to prevent contracture? *Dev. Med. Child Neurol.*, **30**, 3–10

Taub, E. (1980) Somatosensory deafferentation research with monkeys: implications for rehabilitation medicine. In: *Behavioral Psychology in Rehabilitation Medicine: Clinical Applications*, edited by L.P. Ince. Baltimore: Williams and Wilkins.

Timiras, P.S. (1972) *Developmental Physiology and Aging*. New York: Macmillan.

Timney, B. and Mitchell, D.E. (1979) Behavioral recovery from visual deprivation: comments on the critical period. In: *Developmental Neurobiology of Vision*, edited by R.D. Freeman. NATO Advanced Studies Institutes, A-27. New York: Plenum Press.

Travis, A.M. and Woolsey, C.W. (1956) Motor performance of monkeys after bilateral, partial and total cerebral decortications. *Am. J. Phys. Med.*, **35**, 273–310.

Vaughan, C.W., Neilson, P.D. and O'Dwyer, N.J. (1988) Motor control deficits of orofacial muscles in cerebral palsy. *J. Neurol. Neurosurg. Psychiatry*, **51**, 534–539.

Visintin, M. and Barbeau, H. (1989) The effects of body weight support on the locomotor pattern of spastic paretic patients. *Canad. J. Neurol. Sc.*, **16**, 315–325.

Walsh, R. (1981) Sensory environments, brain damage, and drugs: a review of interactions and mediating mechanisms. *J. Neurosci.*, **14**, 129–137.

Walsh, R. and Cummins, R.A. (1975) Mechanisms mediating the production of environmentally induced brain changes. *Psychol. Bull.*, **82**, 986–1000.

Webster, D.B. and Webster, M. (1979) Effects of neonatal conductive hearing loss on brain stem auditory nuclei. *Ann. Otol. Rhinol. Laryngol.*, **88**, 684.

Whishaw, I.Q., Zaborowski, J. and Kolb, B. (1984) Post-surgical enrichment aids adult hemidecorticate rats on a spatial navigation task. *Behav. Neural Biol.*, **42**, 183–190.

Williams, P.E. and Goldspink, G. (1973) The effect of immobilization on the longitudinal growth of striated muscle fibres. *J. Anat.*, **116**, 45–55.

Williams, P.E. and Goldspink, G. (1984) Connective tissue changes in immobilized muscle. *J. Anat.*, **138**, 343–350.

Wills, B. and Rosenweig, M.R. (1977) Relatively brief environment aids recovery of learning capacity and alters brain measures after post-weaning brain lesions in rats. *J. Comp. Physiol. Psychol.*, **91**, 33–50.

Yu, J. (1980) Neuromuscular recovery with training after central nervous system lesions: an experimental approach. In: *Behavioral Psychology in Rehabilitation Medicine: Clinical Applications*, edited by L.P. Ince. Baltimore, MD: Williams & Wilkins, pp. 402–419.

Ziv, I., Blackburn, N., Rang, M. and Koreska, J. (1984) Muscle growth in normal and spastic mice. *Dev. Med. Child Neurol.*, **26**, 94–99.

Further reading

Conel, J.L. (1939) *The Postnatal Development of the Human Cerebral Cortex, Vol. I: The Cortex of the Newborn*. Cambridge, MA: Harvard University Press.

Davidoff, R.A. (1992) Skeletal muscle tone and the misunderstood stretch reflex. *Neurol.*, **42**, 951–1009.

Garrod, D.R. and Feldman, J.D. (eds) (1981) *Development in the Nervous System*. New York: Cambridge University Press.

Hamilton, W.J., Boyd, J.D. and Mossman, H.W. (1972) *Human Embryology Prenatal Development of Form and Function*. Cambridge: Heffer.

Jacobson, M. and Hunt, K. (1973) Origins of neuronal specificity. *Sci. Am.*, 26–35.

Kelly, A.M. and Rubenstein, N.A. (1980) Why are fetal muscles slow? *Nature*, **288**, 266.

Lovely, R.G., Gregor, R.J., Roy, R.R. and Edgerton, V.R. (1986) Effects of training on the recovery of full weight-bearing stepping in the adult spinal cat. *Exper. Neurol.*, **92**, 421–435.

Rothwell, J.C., Traub, M.M. and Marsden, C.D. (1980) Influence of voluntary intent on the human long-latency stretch reflex. *Nature*, **286**, 496–498.

Towe, A.L. and Luschei, E.S. (eds) (1981) *Handbook of Behavioral Neurobiology, vol. 5: Motor Coordination*. New York: Plenum Press.

5

Cerebral palsy

Introduction

Cerebral palsy (CP) is the term used to refer to a non-progressive group of brain disorders resulting from a lesion or developmental abnormality in fetal life or early infancy. These disorders are characterized by poor control of movement, adaptive length changes in muscles and, in some cases, skeletal deformity. Disorders of movement are typically differentiated and classified clinically in terms of the part of the body involved (e.g. hemiplegia, diplegia, quadriplegia) and by clinical perceptions of tone and involuntary movement (e.g. spastic, ataxic, athetoid). In some cases the causative factors are known but in many others they are not. The neurophysiological abnormalities underlying the various motor disorders are largely unknown (Brouwer and Ashby 1991).

However varied the aetiological factors may be, the pathological central nervous system (CNS) mechanisms ought not to be progressive. Nevertheless, the clinical features do appear to change as the infant grows older. These changes are probably the result of maturational and adaptive processes and could be expected, therefore, to be affected by the infant's experiences. After birth, the body structure and the system which controls it adapt as a result of the brain lesion, but also as a result of the amount and variety of movements the infant performs. These movements emerge to a large extent as a result of the

motor control deficits, the baby's cognitive abilities and the environment in which the movements take place. That is, as the infant with CNS dysfunction attempts to move about, the movements made reflect not only the motor control and cognitive deficits but also the nature of the dynamic interactions within the musculoskeletal linkage and the demands of the environment. For example, the infant attempts to reach out for a desirable object in the most effective manner possible given the state of the neural system and any soft tissue adaptations. The movement pattern which emerges and which will strengthen with practice reflects the possible biomechanical options for transporting the hand to the object, where the object is, its characteristics (shape, graspability), and what is to be done with it.

Normally, development of the young infant is characterized by learning how to use the dynamic characteristics of linked body segments to achieve particular intentions or goals. It is very likely that these experiences direct to some extent the maturational changes taking place in the nervous system. Since the young infant with motor control deficits moves about in the only way possible given the neural deficits and the environment in which he or she is placed, the position and what movements are practised are important factors. As a result, an infant with CP, when positioned in supine, may demonstrate more activity in the posterior trunk and limb muscles than in the flexors. This muscle activity may be the result of dystonic spasms associated with the brain lesion. However, there may also be a mechanical and functional cause. These muscles may be the easiest to contract in this position, given the demands of gravity and the short resting length of the muscles. Habitual muscle activation patterns, through repetition, become reinforced or learned. In a sense, therefore, the motor control deficits are progressive in that what the infant practises and experiences must affect the development of the CNS and musculoskeletal system. The apparently progressive nature of the motor disability is particularly evident in the first 2 years, and especially in the absence of intervention to encourage more flexible motor behaviour and prevent length-associated changes in muscles.

Since the neural deficits in CP affect many functional systems, these children may experience a variety of problems requiring help and guidance from a number of different health- and education-related fields: neurology, psychology, social work, physiotherapy, speech therapy, occupational therapy, physical education, orthopaedics, orthotics and ophthalmology. It is advisable for individuals in both health and education to have a global view of the functional problems faced by a child with CNS dysfunction, as well as of the child's and family's positive attributes, whether or not these seem at first sight to be relevant to the particular field in which the individual practises. Each disability, whether of speech, manipulation, hearing or balance, is the result of damage to or maldevelopment of the infant's brain, as well as of factors associated with the environment and the infant's experiences, and is, therefore, closely related to the others. To attempt to understand the wide range of problems encountered in these children is a difficult undertaking, particularly in view of the paucity of research into the mechanisms underlying the dyscontrol.

A detailed description of the problems of children with CP and of their management is beyond the scope of this book, and the author, in this chapter and in Chapters 3 and 4, has concentrated on illustrating the way in which the physiotherapist can apply scientific findings related to human movement, its development and its dyscontrol, to the development of clinical motor training strategies.

Historical overview

here have been many systems of treatment developed over the years, by Collis, Phelps, Temple Fay, Bobath (called neurodevelopmental therapy or NDT), Kabat, Knott and Voss (proprioceptive neuromuscular facilitation or PNF), Rood, Petö and Vojta, some of these people working specifically in the field of CP, others working with patients with other neurological abnormalities. These individuals have all made contributions to our understanding of CP. However, as Scrutton and Gilbertson pointed out in 1975, 'one approach to the treatment of these disorders is in a category by itself and not to single it out would be to present an unbalanced picture. The work of Dr and Mrs Bobath challenged the established treatments and influenced physiotherapy more than is often appreciated'.

Most of the above approaches were developed out of clinicians' interpretations of neurophysiological theories of the first half of the century. Techniques were developed principally in an inductive manner in the clinic from trial and error, and theoretical explanations were sought, largely in the neurophysiological literature. Conductive education, developed by Petö, was an exception, having been developed as a method of educating motor-disabled children in all aspects of functional daily life.

Although clinicians have had difficulty demonstrating that improved functional motor performance results from any of these treatment methods, there seems little doubt that relatively intensive active intervention has resulted in more children with CP taking an active part in the world, with fewer relegated to their cots in institutions. The critical question is, however, whether intervention based on more recent research findings in the sciences related to human movement would be more effective than the therapeutic approaches commonly in use today. The dominant approaches to therapy are not built on a readily identifiable theoretical base. In addition, many therapists use a hybridized 'cocktail' of techniques, without systematically measuring outcome as a means of identifying which therapeutic strategies are effective in improving functional performance.

The emergence of a substantial body of knowledge in the broad area which can be called movement science provides an opportunity to re-examine the theoretical concepts underlying the traditional methods in common use today and the techniques of treatment employed (Gordon 1987; Shepherd 1987). Movement science comprises those areas of science which are related to:

1 The kinematics and kinetics of human motor performance (biomechanics).
2 How muscles function and how they adapt to immobility and externally imposed restriction (muscle biology).
3 How humans learn to control movement and acquire skill in specific motor actions (motor learning).
4 The attentional demands of action and the relationship between intention and action (cognitive psychology).
5 The relationship of the environment to behaviour (human ecology or environmental psychology.

(Carr and Shepherd 1987).

It is very likely that new methods of intervention, based more on the concept of task- and context-specific training of motor control rather than therapy, and developed out of more modern theoretical concepts and data-based findings from the sciences related to human movement, may be more effective in optimizing functional motor performance in children with CP. In other words, the increasing focus in scientific research on the study of humans performing 'natural' functional actions allows the clinical scientist to develop and test hypotheses related to clinical problems. There is some evidence in adults following stroke that training of specific actions developed out of hypotheses related to motor control has a positive effect both on the biomechanics of a specific action (Ada and Westwood 1992; Malouin *et al.* 1992) and on functional outcome measured on an assessment scale (Dean and Mackey, 1992). In children with CP, intensity of physiotherapy, including intensive practice of specific actions, has been shown to have a positive outcome (Bower and McLellan 1990). In the future, development and systematic evaluation of feedback devices and systems to enable infants and children to practise on their own will mean that many infants can have the opportunity to achieve an optimum number of repetitions of a desired movement, in this way enhancing both motor control and strength and enabling the development of some skill. Technological and theoretical advances are also providing the opportunities for measuring motor performance and fitness as indicators of the effects of intervention.

There have been two major findings from recent research in the field of motor development that should result in a fresh look at physiotherapy methods (see Chapter 2). Studies of different ethnic groups are revealing the effects of child-rearing beliefs and practices on motor development, raising interesting questions about the effects on infant motor performance of adults' biases toward certain motor actions. In addition, biomechanical studies are demonstrating that the basic pattern of certain everyday actions such as walking and reaching is already present in normal infants at birth. Whether these basic patterns are present in infants with CP needs investigation, as their presence or absence at birth may have to do with the gestational age at which the lesion or maldevelopment occurred.

This chapter is based on the view that there are three major objectives for the physiotherapist working in the field of paediatrics. The first is to develop an understanding, at biomechanical, muscular, neural and behavioural levels, of the child's problems, how they affect the child and family and, as far as possible, their physiological, biomechanical or behavioural cause. The second is to plan and evaluate a training programme, both supervised and unsupervised, which will help the child develop effective motor performance in the essential actions of everyday life. The third is to systematically evaluate the effects of training by measuring the child's performance of functional tasks.

Aetiology

The group of disorders of the CNS known as CP may occur as a developmental defect due to direct inheritance; an inherited vulnerability to other risk factors (Stanley and Alberman 1984); maternal influences such as disease or drug use; placental problems; or as the result of cerebral malformations, prematurity or perinatal factors causing trauma to the infant brain.

Last century, Little attributed CP to difficult birth and prematurity. More recent studies have suggested that low birth weight and severe anoxia at birth are important risk factors; however, the incidence of CP due to these factors is still uncertain. Most of the children in one large study were reported as having neither risk factor (Nelson and Ellenberg 1986). Postnatal factors (such as accidents and infections of the CNS) are also implicated and it is generally considered that the upper age limit for the use of the term CP is approximately 3 years. One study of postnatal factors cited as causative factors infections such as meningitis, encephalitis, measles (62.9%), accidents (22.5%), anoxia from suffocation, near-drowning and post-epilepsy (7.8%), cerebrovascular accidents (4.5%), and malnutrition (2%) (Blair and Stanley 1982).

Low birth weight has been implicated in the development of spastic diplegia. An Australian study reported an incidence of 38.5% of spastic diplegia in very low birth weight infants born between 1977 and 1982 (Kitchen *et al.* 1987). On the whole, studies of the incidence of diplegia in low birth weight infants have reported variable findings, some showing that incidence dropped after the establishment of neonatal intensive care units (Hagberg *et al.* 1973), others finding no decline (Kiely *et al.* 1981). Spastic diplegia is less common in full-term infants.

Pathology

In both premature and full-term infants, pathological mechanisms include selective neuronal necrosis and hypoxic–ischaemic cerebral injury. The latter includes focal and multifocal ischaemic cerebral necrosis. Typical hypoxic–ischaemic lesions in premature infants include haemorrhagic lesions and periventricular leukomalacia; in full-term infants, parasagittal cerebral injury and status marmoratus (Hill and Volpe 1987).

Haemorrhagic lesions

These include subependymal and intraventricular haemorrhages with parenchymal extension or development of haemorrhagic hydrocephalus. These lesions are more common in premature infants of less than 32 weeks' gestation. They originate at the thalamic groove (Volpe 1981) and appear to result from a number of physiological factors specific to preterm newborn infants: a relatively large proportion of total cerebral blood flow perfusing the subependymal capillary bed, fragility of vessel walls and an inability to regulate cerebral blood flow (Wigglesworth 1984).

Hypoxic–ischaemic lesions

Periventricular leukomalacia with or without cyst formation (Volpe 1981; Wigglesworth 1984; Weindling *et al.* 1985) is found at the border zones between the penetrating branches of the major cerebral arteries. It frequently occurs together with haemorrhagic lesions and may result from episodes of hypotension during apnoea in premature infants.

Selective neuronal necrosis, affecting cerebral cortex, thalamus, reticular formation and brain-stem nuclei, *status marmoratus* affecting cerebral cortex and basal ganglia, and *parasagittal cerebral injury* affecting the cerebral cortex and subcortical white matter have all been implicated in spastic quadriplegia with intellectual impairment.

Focal or multifocal ischaemic lesions may be associated with hemiplegia and intellectual impairment. However, the prognosis is said to be good, with most infants making an excellent recovery (Trauner and Manuino 1986). Most cerebrovascular accidents (strokes) in children are caused by impairment of arterial blood flow as a result of thrombosis or embolus (Golden 1987). Subependymal and intraventricular haemorrhage are said to be the most common forms of cerebrovascular disease in preterm infants (Volpe 1979).

Intracranial haemorrhage in full-term newborns is most frequently caused by birth trauma. Injuries are typically severe.

In 1962, Banker and Larroche described *periventricular leukomalacia* as an underlying cerebral lesion in the spastic diplegic form of CP. More recently, computed tomography and ultrasonography of the infant brain have aided in the classification of two types of lesion associated with the typical clinical picture of spastic diplegia, which are found either separately or in combination – periventricular leukomalacia and haemorrhagic lesions.

The pyramidal pathways to the lower limbs traverse the internal capsule close to the lateral ventricles. Both haemorrhagic lesions and periventricular leukomalacia can, therefore, lead to the clinical picture of spastic diplegia in which the lower limbs are principally involved. It has been proposed that of most pathogenetic significance is the occurrence of severe cystic damage to the white matter (de Vries *et al.* 1985). Severity of motor disturbance has been said to be reflected by the extent of abnormality on the computed tomography scan (Kanda *et al.* 1982).

Hyperbilirubinaemia caused by rhesus incompatibility used to be a common cause of the athetoid type of CP, due to insult to the basal ganglia, cerebellum and brainstem nuclei. Improved medical techniques have now made this form of CP very uncommon.

The pathological mechanisms most commonly affecting the cerebellum and causing ataxia include those associated with anoxic episodes, posterior fossa tumours, hydrocephalus, viral infection, haemorrhagic lesions, infarctions and demyelinating disease.

It is very likely that *maldevelopment of the nervous system*, both pre- and postnatally, may play a larger role in the pathogenesis of CP than has previously been understood (Nelson and Ellenberg 1986). For example, the corticospinal pathway may develop abnormally if a lesion of the brain occurs during early postnatal development (Brouwer and Ashby 1991).

It is likely that technological advances will gradually enable a more detailed picture of the pathology associated with CP to emerge. For example, in full-term infants who suffered asphyxia, impairment of blood flow in parasagittal areas has been observed on positron emission tomography (Volpe *et al.* 1985). Computerized tomography (CT) scanning in one study showed the most common abnormalities in a group of children with neurodevelopmental delay were cerebral atrophy and specific structural abnormalities (Lingam *et al.* 1982). In another study (Adsett *et al.* 1985), CT scanning of a group of newborns with evidence of perinatal asphyxia supported the view that scanning is a valuable adjunct to neurological evaluation, providing evidence of the severity of cerebral injury. Magnetic resonance imaging is capable of showing focal white-matter abnormality in the mature brain and, in the immature brain, can assess the status of myelination (Harbord *et al.* 1990).

Pathophysiological mechanisms associated with CNS lesions are outlined in Chapter 4.

Characteristics of types

CP is not a single entity but a group of conditions classified according to the parts of the body involved and by clinical descriptions of tone and involuntary movement. CP is classified for treatment purposes as a means of linking similar characteristics. The classifications used clinically reflect the current poor understanding of the motor control deficits associated with brain dysfunction in CP. The nosology utilized in the clinic is neither uniform nor particularly helpful, since it does not elucidate the underlying control deficits. For example, knowing that a child is classified as spastic suggests that increased tone is the major dyscontrol characteristic interfering with function and has tended to direct intervention towards inhibition in both medical and physical therapy. Such a nomenclature takes no account of the fact that the mechanism underlying hypertonus (or resistance to passive stretch) includes such peripheral factors as length-associated changes in muscle. What is needed for clinical purposes, therefore, is not so much a classification as a method of identifying the nature of the control deficits. For example, knowing that a child has difficulty activating a group of muscles or generating sufficient force specifically for particular actions, or in different contexts, or to sustain force production with muscles at certain lengths would provide a more coherent and specific rationale for the development of particular training strategies.

Nevertheless, until more is understood of the pathological mechanisms and dyscontrol characteristics themselves, a more clinically useful method of classification eludes us.

The common classification according to the perceived clinical signs is:

1   *Spastic* – showing the characteristics of upper motor neuron involvement (e.g. hyperreflexia, abnormal movement patterns, weakness, loss of dexterity).
2   *Athetoid* – showing signs of extrapyramidal involvement, with involuntary movements (athetosis), dystonia, ataxia and sometimes rigidity.
3   *Hypotonic* – showing an often severe depression of motor function and weakness.

4 *Ataxic* – showing signs of cerebellar involvement, with ataxia (e.g. dysmetria). This is said to be rare in CP, being more often associated with head trauma and conditions such as uncontrolled or poorly controlled hydrocephalus.
5 *Mixed lesions* are included, combining characteristics of the spastic, athetoid and ataxic groups.

CP is further categorized, according to the distribution of motor involvement, into *quadriplegia, hemiplegia* and *diplegia*. True monoplegia or triplegia probably never occurs, although some children may appear to fit these categories. It has been reported that follow-up examination in children with one or three limbs involved revealed that the children belonged in one of the three groups (Vining *et al.* 1976), with monoplegia, for example, becoming more obviously hemiplegia or diplegia with the passage of time. Diplegia is characterized by bilateral involvement, primarily of the lower limbs, but is said to include some involvement of the upper limbs.

Description of clinical features

Below is a description of the principal clinical signs.

Hypotonic CP

Severe hypotonus or flaccidity is present in some infants and, although it may persist as muscle weakness and a generalized 'floppiness', it is often transient, subsequently being reclassified as spasticity or athetosis. In the early stages it may be difficult to differentiate between the flaccidity of a CNS lesion and the flaccidity associated with other disorders such as Tay–Sachs disease and Werdnigg–Hoffmann disease. Hypotonus is also seen in premature infants and in infants with Down's syndrome. Some hypotonic infants develop athetosis, with the infant initially demonstrating intermittent tonus fluctuations and apparently involuntary movements, for example, extending the body in what Ingram (1955) called dystonic attacks.

Hypotonus is typically evidenced as extreme floppiness when the infant is picked up and by the infant's inability to generate enough muscle force to move the body segments, particularly against gravity. It is frequently possible for the examiner to produce some muscle activity if sufficient stimulus is given, but the infant may show little spontaneous movement. Even respiratory movements occur more as lateral movements than as elevation of the thorax when the child is in supine, and the child may have some respiratory difficulty, with shallow respirations. The infant may lie with arms and legs abducted, externally rotated and flexed. When pulled to sitting, there is usually a head lag (Fig. 5.1). In prone, protective side turning of the head may be absent and the infant risks suffocation. Held in sitting or standing, the child may be unable to hold the head and upper body erect and when held in standing the lower limbs may collapse into flexion. Kicking may be absent or feeble. Difficulty eating and drinking may be the result of inability to generate sufficient muscle force to suckle and swallow effectively. Feeds may be aspirated, coughing may be ineffective and episodes of respiratory distress are relatively common.

Spastic CP

Resistance to passive movement and abnormal patterns of movement may not be clinically evident in young infants. In some infants it has been noted that tone tends to increase as the infant develops (Bobath and Bobath 1975). Some infants, however, appear markedly spastic even in the first few months. It seems reasonable to hypothesize that these children comprise at least two broad groups. In one group, the initial hypotonus appears to represent the so-called negative features of the upper motor neuron lesion (see Chapter 4). The development of spasticity may illustrate the effects of adaptive neural and mechanical events which reflect the capacities for reorganization of both the CNS and musculoskeletal systems. In this group, the gradual development of hypertonus (resistance to passive stretch) may be in part the result both of changes in the structural and functional properties of the muscles and other soft tissues, as well as neural recovery processes, particularly at spinal level. In the second group, the early appearance of spasticity (perhaps a better term is dystonia) may be a reflection of a severe and extensive brain dysfunction affecting cerebral cortex, mid-brain and spinal cord.

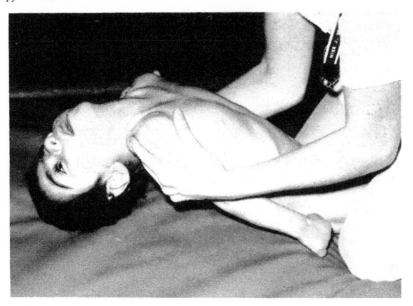

Figure 5.1   Severe head lag in a 'floppy' baby.

An infant with severe spasticity may demonstrate little ability to move in any position. It usually appears that certain muscles of the limbs and trunk contract simultaneously when the child attempts to move, although some groups will usually appear more active than others. In these infants there is considerable resistance to passive movement. When the child is moved from supine to prone some variation in the degree of hypertonus may be evident, apparently due to the influence of the tonic reflexes (tonic labyrinthine and tonic neck reflexes).

The clinical sign called spasticity may result, therefore, from a combination of hyperactive stretch reflexes (hyperreflexia), changes in muscle structure and function, and abnormal muscle activity elicited by changes in head or body position (e.g. tonic neck and labyrinthine reflexes). Even though spasticity is generally considered in the clinic to be the major barrier to the development of more normal motor performance, it is very likely that this is not necessarily so and that in most infants and children the negative features are the major barriers. (See Chapter 4.)

Abnormal patterns of movement have been described in children with spasticity, both at rest and during movement, with a pattern of flexion in the upper limbs and of extension in the lower limbs (Figs 5.2 and 5.3). These movement patterns have been taken to reflect solely the effects of the neural lesion (Bobath 1980). However, in practice there are variations which may reflect the effect of habitual adoption of certain preferred positions, together with adaptive muscle changes (increased muscle stiffness, decreased extensibility), a tendency to time force generation inappropriately (Dietz *et al.* 1981) and adaptive or compensatory motor behaviours. The upper limb may be held flexed at the elbow, wrist and fingers, retracted and depressed at the shoulder girdle, internally rotated and adducted at the shoulder, and pronated at the radioulnar joints. In the lower limb, a pattern of extension may be seen at the hip and knee joints, internal rotation and adduction at the hip, and plantarflexion and inversion of the foot. However, it is not only the limbs which are affected. Excessive muscle activity and muscle shortening involving the limbs must also affect the trunk due to the intersegmental attachments of muscles.

Overactivity and shortening of, for example, latissimus dorsi muscle, with its attachments to the spine, upper limb, shoulder and pelvic girdles, may be responsible for a side flexion posture of the trunk, with the shoulder pulled down and back and pelvis pulled up and back. Overactivity and shortening of hip adductor

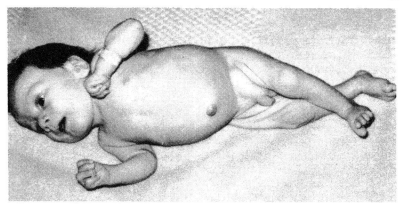

Figure 5.2 Infant with quadriplegic cerebral palsy. Note the flexed arms, extended spine and lower limbs.

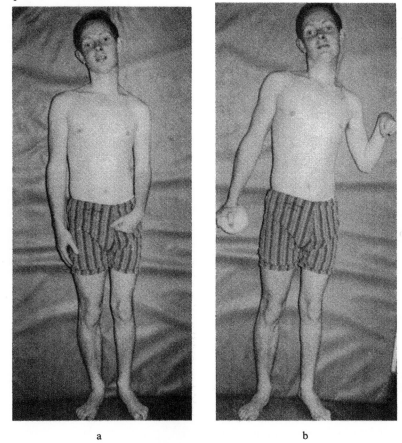

a   b

Figure 5.3 (a) This young man shows the effects of lack of use of the affected side of his body due to a neural lesion several years earlier. (b) When he grasps an object strongly with his unaffected hand, there is an overflow of muscle activity to the flexors of the affected upper limb.

muscles will restrict the active range of flexion and extension at the hip. In some children, any attempts to move tend to be within certain predictable patterns. The child may be able to flex the hip but flexion will typically be accompanied by external rotation and abduction at the hip and dorsiflexion at the ankle. These patterns will be relatively ineffective in achieving particular functional goals.

The child may demonstrate an abnormal amount of muscle activity (*associated movements*) in response to stimuli such as effort, excitement, loss of balance, fear or anxiety (Fig. 5.3b). Associated movements seem to represent a spread of muscle activation similar to that occurring normally when one exerts a lot of force, in opening a jar for example. The pattern in which they occur may well reflect the mechanisms described above. However, some hemiplegic children show 'mirror' movements: grasping of an object in one hand is accompanied by grasping movements in the other hand. These movements appear to be due to a different mechanism (see p. 14).

The child may develop the ability to balance in an erect position by using behavioural adaptations. A diplegic child, for example, may use the arm instead of the leg muscles for postural adjustments in standing by holding on to a firm support. The behavioural adaptations of a child with hemiplegia may also involve the use of the unaffected limbs. However, a child with a severe lesion affecting all four limbs may not develop any ability to move effectively.

Contractures and, eventually, in severely motor- and/or cognitive-impaired infants, *skeletal deformity* develop in the infant if normal muscle length cannot be maintained and if some active control of muscles cannot be gained. Deformity of the skeleton (including skull) can be caused in the first year of life by a combination of prolonged positioning (and gravity), immobility and growth (Fulford and Brown 1976). Contractures probably develop because of an imbalance of muscle activity, lack of active functional movement (providing active stretch), prolonged positioning with muscles held at the one length, and the effect of these on growth. Growth has been shown in animals to depend partly on stretch (Ziv *et al.* 1984). In other words, muscles may develop length-associated changes because of lack of active use or persistent use in one part of a joint's range. The muscles antagonistic to short muscles will lengthen, thereby adding a mechanical disadvantage to the neural disability. The hyperactive muscles continue to shorten and become increasingly stiff, lessening their ability to generate force at the lengths necessary for specific functions.

Despite the inference of the terminology, most infants categorized as spastic have as their major problem inability to activate muscles and control muscle force to produce an intentional movement.

Athetoid CP

Athetosis means without a fixed position and may involve choreiform or writhing movements or a tendency to maintain a fixed dystonic posture. Infants and children with athetosis demonstrate involuntary movements which can occur both at rest and during volitional movement (Fig. 5.4). As infants, typical involuntary movements are trunk and head extension, particularly when in supine. As time passes, if the child is given the opportunity to acquire functional motor actions, it becomes evident that if the child learns to become relatively effective in performing the desired actions, it is by developing behavioural strategies for dealing with the motor dyscontrol. Head turning may be utilized to optimize extension of the arm when reaching. Sit-to-stand and walking may be performed at a fast speed, with the upper limbs used for support and balance.

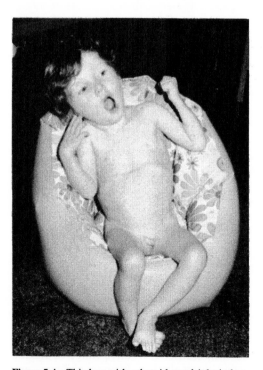

Figure 5.4 This boy with athetoid quadriplegia has involuntary movements which make it difficult to maintain the sitting position.

Control of head position is usually slow to develop and inability to hold the head steady may affect the development of vision and the visual control of actions such as reaching. The inability to hold a steady position and to perform smooth joint displacements makes the development of postural adjustments, reaching and manipulation particularly difficult. Grimacing of the face and difficulty coordinating breathing and swallowing may also be evident, and eating, drinking and vocalization may be impaired.

Joints are often hypermobile and joint dislocations can occur in older children, especially where there are spasms. Persistent asymmetrical posturing with one leg in flexion and adduction predisposes the hip to dislocation. Strong and persistent extension spasms of the jaw can result in subluxation of the temporomandibular joint. Scoliosis is also rather common when there is pronounced muscle imbalance.

Ataxic CP

Ataxia is said to be uncommon in CP and is a more commonly seen associated with hydrocephalus, head injury, encephalitis or cerebellar tumour. The child demonstrates difficulty controlling rate, range, direction and force of movement. Difficulty controlling the velocity and amplitude of movement makes functional actions, such as reaching to an object, inaccurate, and together with difficulty balancing, results in uncoordinated wide-based locomotion with the hands used to provide support. The lack of motor control is particularly evident in the lack of braking of joint displacements which causes a tendency to overshoot.

Functional deficits

The functional deficits reflect not only the neural lesion but also what has been practised and become habitual and the changing state of the system due to growth, disuse and misuse.

Movement dysfunction

Cerebral palsy is characterized by impaired motor control, with the nature of the dyscontrol probably varying according to time, location and extent of the CNS lesion (Eliasson *et al.* 1991). The range of motor disability may vary from almost total paralysis with immobility to relatively mild clumsiness. Some children are so minimally affected as to appear normal until it is realized that their failure to achieve physical and mental equality with their peers is due to brain dysfunction rather than to laziness or mental incompetence. What is called minimal brain dysfunction (see Chapter 7) is frequently associated with some degree of ataxia or clumsiness. However, some children in this group also have specific learning deficits, with difficulty reading and writing, with no apparent motor problems.

The major objective of physiotherapy in CP is to train infants and children with motor dysfunction to perform the essential activities of daily life. To fulfil this objective requires an understanding not only of normal motor performance but also of deficits in functional performance. There are as yet relatively few studies of these deficits in infants and children. Common dyscontrol characteristics which may be seen during the performance of everyday actions are described in Chapters 3 and 4. Below is a brief description of some of the functional deficits associated with CP. The results of several investigations of motor dysfunction are included.

Leg movements in supine

In one of the few descriptive studies of CP, Yokochi and colleagues compared retrospectively the leg movements in supine of diplegic infants and preterm infants subsequently found to have a normal motor developmental outcome (Yokochi *et al.* 1991). Videotape was used to analyse the infants' movements. The authors found that the diplegic babies, aged 3–11 months corrected age, demonstrated a relatively limited repertoire of leg movements compared with the normal group. Only simultaneous flexion and extension of the hips and knees were seen, with occasional isolated hip movements. Isolated knee movements and hip flexion with knee extension were never seen in the infants subsequently confirmed as being diplegic. Their lower-limb movements were stereotyped: a flexor synergy involving hip and knee flexion, hip abduction and external rotation, and ankle dorsiflexion; an extensor synergy involving hip and knee extension, hip adduction and internal rotation, with ankle plantarflexion. In contrast, although the normal infants under 3 months demonstrated simultaneous flexion and extension of the hip and knee, from age 5 months they demonstrated hip flexion combined with knee extension and isolated knee movement. The authors suggested that absence of these latter movements may be a useful diagnostic sign of diplegia.

Reaching and manipulation

Skilled hand movements, involving independent finger movements, usually develop poorly in children with CP. Such children typically learn to grasp with the whole hand, slowly and with excessive force for the task (Twitchell 1959; Brown *et al.* 1987). Impairments are found particularly in reciprocal and rapid alternating movement, in actions requiring fractionation of movement and in bimanual actions.

Deficits in grasping are common and seem to reflect difficulty timing grasp and release, coordinating wrist extensor and long finger flexor muscles for grasping and manipulation, and adapting muscle force to load. Two children with hemiplegia were filmed by Jeannerod (1986) as they reached to grasp a prong from a pegboard. In the child aged 23 months, while contact by the normal hand with the object was followed immediately by a grasp, the fingers of the affected hand remained extended and a clumsy grasp occurred after contact with the object. The other child, aged 5 years, showed a different pattern of grip formation in the affected hand compared to the normal, with abnormal finger posturing and a clumsy grasp. Interestingly, Jeannerod reports that the first child did not use the affected hand until the other hand was immobilized, and then only with difficulty.

Eliasson and colleagues (1991) found with a group of 12 children, aged between 6 and 8 years of age with hemiplegia or diplegia, that they lacked the coordination or coupling between grip force and load force normally achieved by the second year of life. Force generation was excessive in amplitude and the children generated grip force in advance of load force in a similar manner to young children. The authors suggested that the children lacked the ability to use both anticipatory control and sensory feedback. They also suggested that the high grip forces generated may be adaptive – a compensatory mechanism providing a wide safety margin in order to prevent the object from slipping. The authors found that the grip coordination of the diplegic children was better than that of the children with hemiplegia. This view is supported by studies of the different pathological mechanisms of these two types of CP. Although impaired sensory mechanisms may have caused deficits in motor performance, it seems unlikely that an impaired sensory mechanism would have been the main cause of the poor coordination between grip and load force. In a subsequent study of the same children, it was found that they were able to adapt their grip force to the actual weight of the object. This suggests that the timing of force output could be modified, to some extent, by feedback mechanisms (Eliasson *et al.* 1992).

Control of the path of the hand in reaching is often difficult, due to control deficits and lack of extensibility in soft tissues. Forsstrom and von Hofsten (1982) investigated reaching to catch a moving target in a group of children aged between 4 and 11 years with a diagnosis of minimal brain dysfunction. They found that the approach paths were more devious than those of the normal controls. However, by aiming at a point further ahead of the target, the children seemed to take into account their lack of efficiency, and by this strategy caught the ball on most attempts.

Floor-sitting

The typical floor-sitting posture of a child with diplegia involves a flexed trunk, with associated extended neck, the child sitting between internally rotated legs in a W position. When the child attempts to sit with legs out in front, the legs may be flexed at the knees, with the hips insufficiently flexed as the pelvis is forced backwards by short hamstring muscles (Fig. 5.5). Flexing the upper trunk enables the child to bring the body mass sufficiently forwards to allow for balance; without it the child would fall backwards. Difficulty sitting in this position may be largely the result of shortening of ham-

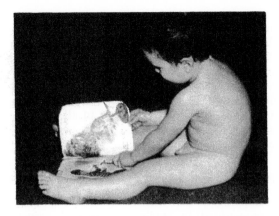

Figure 5.5 This boy with diplegia cannot flex his hips sufficiently to keep his body mass forwards. The flexion of the upper trunk is adaptive, enabling him to sit independently without falling backward.

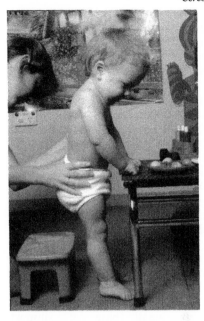

Figure 5.6 In standing, insufficient hip extension and ankle dorsiflexion result in the body mass being too far behind the base of support.

string and hip adductor muscles, plus poor balance due to difficulty controlling the lower limb muscles and muscles linking trunk to lower limbs.

Sitting on a chair

Sitting on a chair may be associated with internal rotation at the hips and difficulty flexing the knees sufficiently to get the feet to the floor. Ankle plantarflexion may prevent the feet from being placed flat on the floor, with the result that the feet cannot be used effectively as part of the base of support, as they normally are. As in floor sitting, the child may sit with hips relatively extended (i.e. lower trunk tilted backwards) and the upper body flexed to compensate (see Fig. 3.32). Balance may be poor due to inability to use one or both legs as an active base of support.

Sit-to-stand

Sit-to-stand, which normally involves extension of the lower limbs over a fixed base (the feet), may be impossible without extensive use of the upper limbs. The diplegic child may pull to standing with feet placed too far forward and plantarflexed, and, as a result, body mass too far behind the base of support (Fig. 5.6). There are no published biomechanical studies of the performance characteristics of CP children during sit-to-stand. However, studies of adults following stroke indicate that typical problems are failure to place the feet (or foot of the affected leg) sufficiently back; decreased amplitude and velocity of trunk flexion at the hip; a pause between trunk flexion and the start of the extension phase; and slowness of movement, the action being performed with less vigour than normal. A recently completed study (McDonald 1994) indicates that children with diplegic CP demonstrate similar problems.

Walking

The muscle coactivation patterns in children with CP have been described as similar to leg muscle activity in stepping newborns (Dietz and Berger 1983); that is, simultaneous flexion at hip and knee and dorsiflexion at the ankle, resulting in a high stepping appearance. Walking may be characterized in children with diplegia by a slow lurching gait with small steps and in children with hemiplegia by uneven step length and a limp. The details of the gait pattern vary according to such factors as muscle length and stiffness and the timing of muscle forces. When calf muscles are short, there will be limited hip extension and ankle dorsiflexion at the end of stance (see Fig. 3.12) with the knees hyperextended throughout most of stance. If hip adductors are short and generate excessive force at this length, the hips during walking will be relatively internally rotated and adducted (see Fig. 3.13). Lack of control over hip extensors and abductors and knee extensors may cause the pelvis to drop downwards on the contralateral side during single support (see Fig. 3.14). The arms, when used for balancing, may be abducted.

Speed of walking may be affected. The child may walk faster than would be normal, reflecting some element of dyscontrol and lack of extensibility of soft tissues. The increased speed may make it easier to balance (Winter 1987) and is seen in children with ataxia, and in diplegic children whose stiff short hip adductor and calf muscles cause them to take small steps with a small base of support. Alternatively, when walking is an effort, speed may be considerably reduced.

Coactivation of leg muscles has been reported as a characteristic of abnormal gait in children with CP (Knutsson 1980; Dietz and Berger 1983). A failure of the normal reciprocal relationship between agonist and antagonist muscles has been reported in voluntary limb movements (Milner-Brown and Penn 1979) and in the stance phase of walking (Dietz and Berger 1983). Coactivation has been proposed to be due to a failure of reciprocal inhibition at the segmental level (Myklebust *et al.* 1982). Another hypothesis, however, is that descending projections to spinal motoneurons may be abnormal (Milner-Brown and Penn 1979; Brouwer and Ashby 1991). Dietz and Berger (1983) suggest that, since it is seen also in the stepping of newborn infants, coactivation reflects an impaired maturation of the neuronal locomotor pattern. Furthermore, this impaired maturation may be due not only to impaired supraspinal influences but also to early structural changes in the peripheral motor system. They note that muscle tension appears to be controlled more by properties of the muscle fibres than by neuronal control, as occurs in normal subjects.

De Bruin and colleagues (1982) used hip–knee angle–angle diagrams to illustrate the gait abnormalities of 3 children with CP. The children demonstrated increased flexion at the knee at the initiation of stance, with the foot

being relatively flat when it made contact with the floor, and decreased knee movement throughout. The degree of hip flexion in swing phase was greater than normal in some children but in one child both hip and knee movement was markedly reduced, probably as a result of muscle contracture. In all children both hips and knees tended to flex and extend concurrently.

Postural adjustments

Interestingly, the deficits in motor control demonstrated in studies of postural adjustments do not correlate well with the clinical diagnosis of hypertonus. In one study, the muscles identified clinically as spastic showed a delayed onset not only in response to support surface perturbations but also to direct stretch input (Shumway-Cook 1989). Nashner and colleagues (1983) found that, despite clinical signs of spasticity (increased resistance to passive stretch), the passive stiffness in response to stretch at the ankle joint was observed to be the same in both spastic and non-spastic limbs.

Deficits in postural adjustments have been reported from several studies. Children with hemiplegia have been shown to have difficulty with the timing of motor responses to support surface perturbations in the affected lower limb (Nashner *et al.* 1983; Shumway-Cook 1989). Muscle onset is frequently delayed. Instability when the centre of mass moves towards the limit of stability may be largely due to this delay in muscle activation onset. The mechanical consequence of delayed muscle activation, even in the presence of a large amplitude electrical signal, is that insufficient torque will be generated across the joints of the affected limb and the necessary movements may be performed by the intact leg, illustrating the adaptive nature of the system.

Abnormal timing of muscle activations is also evidenced by the more proximal muscles being activated before distal muscles when responding to support surface perturbations in standing. This is the reverse of what occurs in children with normal control. Children with hemiplegia have been found to have difficulty organizing anticipatory postural adjustments associated with voluntary arm movement in standing. As in their response to support surface perturbation, muscle onsets occurred in reverse to that found in normal subjects, with the more proximal muscles being activated before the distal muscles.

Children with ataxia show delays in muscle onsets and variability from trial to trial. However, they do not show problems with inter-muscle timing (Nashner *et al.* 1983). Ataxic children have been found to be unable to maintain balance when subjected to conflicting orientation inputs from vision and somatosensory receptors. This suggests the motor control problems may be due to deficits in sensory integration.

Associated deficits

Infants with CP show arrested or delayed motor development and many retain for a longer than normal period *immature motor performance and neonatal reflexive or prefunctional motor patterns*. Many children have other abnormalities, including cognitive/perceptual deficits, deafness, visual defects, dysphagia, seizures, speech and communication disorders. Somatosensory disorders may also be evident.

Connective tissue and muscle contractures have been reported to be considerable in children with CP (Shumway-Cook 1989) and may be a significant part of the mechanism underlying hypertonus (resistance to passive stretch) found clinically. Length-associated changes in muscle and other soft tissues occur, particularly in children who are relatively immobile due to severe motor control deficits and cognitive impairment. However, they will occur in any muscle which is not actively stretched, since muscle length is a reflection of the pattern of muscle use.

Cognitive and perceptual deficits may be relatively common. However, estimation of intelligence in the presence of considerable motor handicap is difficult. Intellectual retardation occurs as a primary defect. However, it may also be secondary to motor and sensory (particularly visual) disability, which restricts the infant's and child's opportunities to learn.

Visual and visuomotor abnormalities are estimated to occur in some 50% of children with CP. A typical problem is poor control of ocular muscles with resulting strabismus. Children with cerebellar dysfunction may demonstrate nystagmus. In general, most eye problems result in a loss of binocular coordination and depth perception. Since vision provides critical inputs for motor control, ocular abnormalities

should be corrected as early as possible in infancy. Central deficits may result in disorders of visual perception. Problems with spatial orientation are sometimes evident and may be the result of a primary deficit or secondary to lack of experience of goal-directed movement.

Deafness is relatively common in athetoid children whose brain lesion is a result of bilirubin encephalopathy. However, now that the cause is correctable, this type of deafness is less common. Auditory deficits are found in other children with CP and may originate centrally, resulting in problems of auditory perception. Children whose brain dysfunction is a result of maternal rubella may lack hearing acuity or have specific frequency deafness.

Speech and learning problems arise from a complex interaction of factors with motor, visuomotor, intellectual and experiential components. Children may have problems of verbal comprehension or expression, or difficulties with articulation, the latter particularly common in children with athetosis or cerebellar lesion. Poor voluntary control of masseter and orbicularis oris muscles has been found in CP adults with dysarthric speech and in the mixed spastic–athetoid group (Vaughan *et al.* 1988). Vaughan and colleagues suggest that the control deficit may have resulted from a failure of perceptuo-motor learning, in which the relationship between motor commands to muscles and perceptual consequences (from speech and eating movements) has not been acquired or learned.

Physiotherapy

The treatment approaches commonly used today were developed four decades ago and reading the clinical literature suggests that there has been little change in physiotherapy for infants and children with CP over that time. The major assumptions underlying the most dominant approach (NDT), for example, include the view that abnormal tone and abnormal movement patterns (spasticity) are the major problems interfering with motor function (Bobath 1972; Bobath and Bobath 1984; Perin 1989; Wilson 1991; Eckersley and King 1993). The principal treatment objectives in NDT remain, therefore, inhibition of spasticity and facilitation of more normal motor patterns, also expressed as a 'preparation for function'

(Maystone 1992). It is assumed that there will be a carryover into more effective functional performance.

Alternatively, in this book, a scientifically-based movement training is described, with clinical practice based upon hypotheses derived from research findings and theoretical perspectives related to human movement. Task-specific training of the infant and child with CP is designed to improve the performance of basic functional actions (walking, standing up and sitting down, reaching and manipulation). Emphasis is on promoting optimal length of soft tissues by positioning, practice of actions which will provide an active stretch to muscles and, when necessary casting (see Chapter 4). This chapter should be read in conjunction with Chapter 2 (issues related to motor development), Chapter 3 (details of training specific actions) and Chapter 4 (description of the dyscontrol problems associated with brain lesions).

Outcome studies

There has been some difficulty in demonstrating the effectiveness of the various physiotherapy approaches to treatment of the past 40 years, although it is apparent that active intervention produces a better outcome in terms of enabling CP children to function as part of the community rather than being institutionalized.

It is doubtful whether many studies have been designed in the field of CP which fulfil criteria critical to establishing whether or not a particular form of intervention is effective. These criteria include:

1 *An indication of the degree of severity of the brain lesion and type of disability.*

It is not always possible to establish exact details of the brain lesion but modern scanning techniques allow for estimation of the site and extent of the lesion. The nature of disability (or potential disability) is also informative, for example the some measure of visual disability, some measure of soft tissue contractures or deformities.

2 *An indication of IQ.*

Assessing IQ in physically or visually handicapped infants is difficult. However, the combination of brain scanning and IQ testing can give in many cases a reasonable estimate of potential intelligence. Any form of intervention is likely to be less effective in promoting motor skill when a motor-disabled child is also severely cognitively impaired.

3 *A clear and detailed description of exactly what therapy was given and for what length of time.* This should include details of what the infant practises at home.

In many studies, therapy may not be described in detail and may not even be categorized broadly as, for example, NDT. However, a categorization such as NDT alone is not satisfactory since the treatment given by various therapists will often vary quite markedly, even though therapeutic objectives may be similar. A clear indication of what treatment was given and for how long enables the reader to consider whether a poor outcome could be the result of inappropriate therapy or insufficient time spent practising.

4 *Methodological considerations, such as appropriate experimental design, suitable measurement instruments, and the posing of valid questions.*

It is common for studies of effectiveness of intervention to be criticized for inadequate research design (Hourcade and Parette 1984; Ottenbacher *et al.* 1986) and in some cases the criticism may be justified. However, it is failure to consider criteria 1–3 above that may also detract from the impact of the findings. That we accept such a state of affairs indicates our lack of understanding that it may not be the provision of physiotherapy as such that is effective or ineffective but that what actually happens within that intervention, what the infant or child practises and repeats, and the capacity of the infant to learn, may be of paramount importance.

What is currently lacking in the clinic is the systematic examination of the details of intervention, with the critical test being of some relevant functional goal, for example, the distance a child can reach in sitting or standing, time taken to walk a certain distance, performance of sit-to-stand, using kinematic and kinetic variables, or physiological measures such as oxygen uptake or heart rate.

In one study that examined the effects of NDT techniques (Laskas *et al.* 1985), dorsiflexor muscle activity was found to improve. Although details of all techniques used were not given, one aspect of therapy mentioned was practice of sit-to-stand. It would be of interest to see if the dorsiflexor muscles would improve their activity as a result solely of the practice of sit-to-stand, without any other intervention. The systematic evaluation of specific interventions would enable ineffective or unnecessary 'techniques' to be dropped in favour of a method of training shown to be critical to success. Sit-to-stand is an action which might optimize the ability of dorsiflexor muscles to contract when shortened. It also provides a stretch to the calf muscles and is a voluntary action initiated by the child. An indication of whether or not the performance of sit-to-stand had improved would have been an effective measure of the effect of training on function.

For physiotherapy to be judged effective or not it should be shown to affect performance of an everyday action. The technological means are available now to determine effectiveness in this way. Rather than searching for ways to measure the small qualitative changes which therapists observe, as sometimes suggested (Lilly and Powell 1990), it is more meaningful to design outcome studies to measure the effects of therapy on performance of everyday actions such as walking, reaching out for an object in standing or sitting, and standing up. Change can be demonstrated using biomechanical measures such as phase plane plots and angle–angle diagrams which give an indication of changes in motor control at one joint or coordination between two joints; measurement of the amplitude of joint displacement and velocity; linear measures of movement of centre of body mass or a particular body part such as the hand (Kluzik *et al.* 1990). Change can also be measured using functional motor scales similar to that designed for stroke (Carr *et al.* 1985; Parker *et al.* 1993). It is not necessarily so that therapy which has small local effects or which merely meets therapy goals will be associated with improved functional performance.

It seems likely that functional outcome for many CP children is not as optimal as it might be. For example, Yokochi and colleagues (1991) reported from their study of a group of 49 diplegic infants that, at 3 years of age, although they could all sit unsupported, none could walk in a stable manner or go up and down stairs.

Most outcome studies have investigated the effects of NDT and conductive education, with a few studies of Vojta's methods. The following section describes some of these results.

NDT

In general, studies of the effects of NDT have had inconclusive results. Some have reported a lack of significant differences between children with CP treated by this approach and children who were not treated or who received different therapy (Wright and Nicholson 1973; d'Avignon *et al.* 1981; Sommerfield *et al.* 1981; DeGangi *et al.* 1983; Lilly and Powell 1990). These studies used both quantitative and qualitative methods: quantitative measures have included motor development scales and biomechanical measures; qualitative methods have utilized descriptive videotape analysis.

In a quantitative review of nine investigations of the efficacy of NDT, Ottenbacher and colleagues (1986) found a small treatment effect. Positive results have been reported by other investigators comparing the results of NDT with a passive range of motion exercises (Scherzer *et al.* 1976), and in a single subject design (Laskas *et al.* 1985). The results of outcome studies after 40 years of NDT practice do not support the continued dominance of this approach, particularly since relevant scientific information is now available to enable physiotherapists to develop more scientifically-based methodologies.

Vojta

Kanda and colleagues (1984) compared the effects of early treatment (mean age 6 months) and late treatment (mean age 16 months) following the approach of Vojta (Vojta 1984). They used photographs, recorded stability of walking and the onset times of crawling, sitting and walking. There was no significant difference between groups. However, the early group comprised a larger number of severely affected infants than the late group, and there were considerable differences in severity of brain lesion as shown by brain scan between infants within both groups.

Conductive education

It has been reported that, of the children who have undergone conductive education at the Petö Institute in Budapest over a period of 4 years from 1985 to 1988 and been discharged, approximately 12% of those attending the

Institute were discharged to normal schools (Robinson *et al.* 1989). Preliminary results from a study of 8 children with CP in England suggest that the children made some progress towards independence in movement, speech and self-help skills (Titchener 1983). The children, who were aged from 8 to 13 years, were given conductive education in a group for 1 hour each day for a period of 7 months by a teacher at a school for the physically handicapped.

Developmental assessment of the infant

It is considered important to evaluate the motor performance of babies who are assumed, because of adverse prenatal or birth history, to be at risk developmentally or neurologically (Köng 1967), as well as those whose feeding difficulties, slow development or apparently dysfunctional motor behaviour make them suspects for a diagnosis of CP or mental retardation.

The criteria for judging normal motor behaviour and development in young babies are not established clearly enough for any assessment of a young baby of less than 3 or 4 months to be conclusive proof of neurological abnormality or normality. Evaluation may give information about the baby's present state but it has uncertain predictive value. Although signs of motor retardation may be present in the early weeks of life, motor dysfunction may not be evident until the baby is a few months old and would normally have attained an increased repertoire of purposeful actions.

Nevertheless, early assessment, even in the neonatal stage, is of value for two particular reasons. It gives information about the baby which can help the parents with their child-rearing, acting as a guide to any specific motor training necessary, and it gives baseline data for charting the progress of infants and studying the predictive value of certain motor behaviours.

In the assessment of both infants and children, it is necessary to discriminate between immature and abnormal motor behaviour. Immature movements are those prefunctional patterns present in early infancy which normally develop into functional actions as the CNS matures and the infant has opportunities to practise. Abnormal movement patterns, however, are patterns which are never present in the normal infant. For example, the neck-righting reflex demonstrates a predictable pattern of motor behaviour which is present until approximately 3 months of age, while a persistent pattern of kicking into adduction, extension and internal rotation of the lower limbs may be an indication of pathology.

Assessment is qualitative or quantitative, depending on the information to be gathered. Qualitative assessment, relying on the observations of a skilled assessor, provides on-the-spot information to enable an analysis of performance and the planning and implementing of a subsequent training strategy. When evidence related to changes in performance is required, some means of quantifying performance must be used. At this time, there is relatively little use in the clinic of such methods of measuring change. It is to be hoped that future paediatric departments will be associated with motor performance laboratories which can provide the necessary biomechanical data related to action. There are, however, simple methods of measuring change such as distance walked or reached, time taken, or step length.

Measurement of aspects of motor performance is critical both to establish the motor behaviours associated with brain lesions (Harris 1991), and as a means of demonstrating the effects of intervention (Fetters 1991) just as in adult physiotherapy (Carr and Shepherd 1987). Motion analysis which provides kinematic (e.g. angular displacements and velocities, linear paths of body parts and their velocities) and kinetic (e.g. joint moments of force, vertical ground reaction forces) details of movement needs to be developed as an essential tool for measurement in paediatric physiotherapy centres.

Currently, physiotherapists use scales such as the Bayley and Denver scales, assessment tools developed by André-Thomas (1960), Milani-Comparetti (1967), Prechtl (1977), Dubowitz and Dubowitz (1981) and the Gross Motor Function Measure (Russell *et al.* 1989). Recently, Chandler and colleagues (Chandler *et al.* 1980) have been developing the Movement Assessment of Infants or MAI which provides information about neuromotor function of infants from birth to 12 months. The scale has been shown to be reliable (Harris *et al.* 1984) and Swanson and colleagues recently reported the predictive validity of the scale (Swanson *et al.* 1992).

A philosophy of early intervention for at-risk or frankly impaired infants may result in some babies whose neurological signs are only transient, and due to delay of maturation or minor brain damage being put on a training programme. These babies may have overcome their problems without intervention (Köng 1967; Illingworth 1970). However, because of the assumption that intervention is more effective if it is begun early in the baby's life, it is generally (although not always) accepted that physiotherapy should commence as early as possible. Early intervention, however, needs to be directed towards helping parents optimize the baby's performance by activities which are in themselves pleasurable for both infant and parent.

Since there is sometimes reluctance to refer infants with signs of impairment early to physiotherapy, it is interesting to consider why early intervention may have advantages over a policy of wait-and-see.

The *reasons for early evaluation and intervention* fall into three groups:

Anatomical

To maintain soft tissue extensibility and optimize the growth and development of the musculoskeletal system (and therefore prevent deformity).

Behavioural

1 To optimize the infant's opportunities to experience active movement and to interact with the environment.
2 To prevent the reinforcement of undesirable and self-limiting adaptive motor behaviours.
3 To ensure that the infant practises goal-related functional motor patterns, since it is known that what is practised is learned.

Physiological

1 To optimize the infant's opportunities to select relevant visual and other sensory inputs and apply them to the control of movement.
2 To affect, and perhaps to drive, the neural maturational and recovery processes.

Active movement and a challenging environment have been shown to have a critical effect upon maturational and recovery processes in animals. For example, active self-initiated movement has been shown to be necessary for the development of visually guided reaching in kittens (Held and Hein 1976). In addition, Piaget (1952) suggested that early motor experiences are essential for the development of cognition in human babies. (See Chapter 4.)

History-taking

The baby's physician takes a detailed history and arranges the necessary tests, which usually include a brain scan. The physiotherapist may in particular note the following details:

1 Family history.
2 Relevant details of pregnancy – trauma, illness, threatened miscarriage, rhesus incompatibility.
3 Details of labour.
4 Baby's condition at birth or Apgar rating (see Appendix 3).
5 Results of brain scan or other imaging process.
6 Relevant details of baby's history since birth.

Observation of motor performance and behaviour

Appendix 2 contains an outline of the type of developmental analysis that is commonly used in the clinic to determine the need for intervention and as a guide to that intervention. Part of the evaluation involves observing the baby's spontaneous movements in supine, prone, and when held in sitting and standing. In addition, nursing the baby gives some clues about the response to being handled. From these observations, the examiner tries to get a general picture of the baby's developmental status.

The assessment is done if possible approximately 2 hours after the baby's last feed. It is difficult to get a realistic impression of the infant's state of development if he or she is hungry and agitated, or well-satisfied and sleepy. On the other hand, as Tronick and Brazelton (1975) point out, seeing a crying or fussing baby enables an evaluation of the baby's coping abilities to be made. The infant should not be assessed while under the influence of certain drugs, particularly muscle relaxants or sedatives.

The effects of child-rearing, cultural and environmental factors on motor development should be acknowledged during evaluation. For example, a baby who is relatively delayed in development of movement control in supine but advanced in prone may spend more time in prone than in supine. If the reverse is the case, the therapist should enquire whether the infant spends much of the day in supine. Chapter 4 provides some guidelines about the different child-rearing practices typical of certain ethnic groups.

One assessment is not sufficient initially, as babies vary from day to day in their responses and behaviour. Two or three assessments should be made over a period of a few days before any conclusions can be drawn. If, after these initial assessments, there is doubt about the baby's condition, training is commenced.

Assessment of response to passive movement

It is doubtful whether clinical evaluation of muscle tone as such provides any reliable information to guide intervention. Nevertheless, an estimate of an infant's responses to handling may provide some information to add to the more critical evaluation of active movement control during intentional and spontaneous actions. An estimate of muscle tone or resis-

tance to passive movement can be obtained by flexing and extending the infant's limbs, and by flexing and extending the head in supine. Very young infants normally demonstrate resistance to extension of both upper and lower limbs, so resistance to flexion may be an indication of neural dysfunction, as may a limb which offers no resistance. In older infants and children, resistance to passive movement may be as much an indication of increased muscle stiffness and length-associated changes as it is of neural state.

In a normal infant, passive flexion of one leg is followed by flexion of the other leg. However, a baby with CP may extend the contralateral leg, adduct, internally rotate it and lift it (Fig. 5.7). Similarly, when both legs are flexed on to the baby's chest and then released they will normally remain flexed on the chest or be lowered. However, in a baby with CP, the legs may extend and adduct, with the feet plantarflexed and the hips internally rotated. In prone, when the knees are passively flexed the normal baby of more than 3 months will keep the pelvis flat until knee flexion is sufficient to stretch rectus femoris and flex the hip. The baby with CP, however, may flex and abduct at the hips as soon as the knee is flexed (Fig. 5.8).

It is commonly assumed that the presence of abnormal patterns of posture and movement is

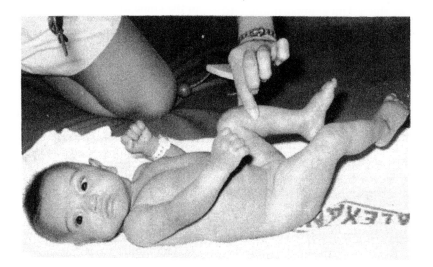

Figure 5.7 Infant with Reye's syndrome. When the left leg is flexed, the right leg lifts from the table and adducts. Note the influence of the asymmetrical tonic neck reflex.

also an indicator of spasticity. However, this may not be so. An abnormal movement pattern, for example, standing with extended, adducted legs and plantarflexed feet, may reflect the development of a habitual pattern of muscle activation which is the result of changes in the muscles themselves, persistent activation of muscles at these lengths, or an imbalance caused by loss of descending inputs to the antagonistic muscles. To explain abnormal motor behaviour solely in terms of abnormal tone is to oversimplify what is complex and as yet little understood.

The presence of reflexes, for example the tonic labyrinthine reflex (see Appendix 1), may dominate the motor behaviour of a baby with severe CP. This reflex originates in the otolinths of the labyrinths. Therefore, it is the position of the head in space which may be considered to determine the distribution of tone throughout the body. In this case, in supine there is a generalized increase in extensor muscle activity, while in prone there is an increase in flexor tone. When this reflex behaviour is dominant the infant cannot raise the head in either supine or prone, and may not be able to roll from one position to the other.

Assessment of oral function

Oral reflexes (see Appendix 1 for details) are tested with the baby in supine or in the physiotherapist's or parent's lap.

The examiner puts a finger inside the baby's mouth and gently moves it between the gums and cheek. A baby with CP may demonstrate marked resistance to passive movement of the tissues. The examiner tests the tongue in a similar manner and watches its movements, as asymmetry and tongue-thrusting are frequently found in babies with CP. The face itself should be observed to check for localized spasms of the muscles around the mouth and nose.

Absence of *vocalization*, which normally begins at 7 weeks and sometimes earlier, may suggest the presence of abnormality. A mentally retarded baby may not develop a varied repertoire of sounds but perseverate on one or two. Crying may also sound abnormal. Illingworth (1970) describes the different types of crying. A baby with CP may not make sounds or may lack a variety of sounds due to poor coordination of oral function with breathing. A speech therapist evaluates the baby's vocalization and attempts at speech.

Feeding

The therapist observes the infant drinking and eating, checking there is adequate lip-sealing around the teat to prevent fluid from escaping. Also checked are the ability to swallow without choking, to take food from a spoon and that the baby swallows without pushing the food from the mouth.

It may not be enough to ask the parents whether or not they are having difficulties feeding the baby. Particularly with a first baby, a mother may accept as normal the difficulties she has with her baby or consider they are her fault.

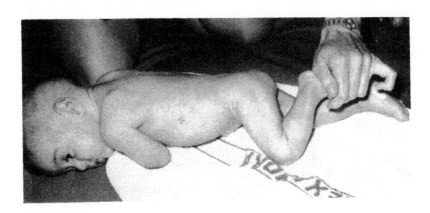

Figure 5.8 Passive flexion of the knee is accompanied by active flexion at the hip.

It is important to find out the answers to the following questions:

1 *How long does it take to feed the baby?* It may take a long time to feed a baby with poor control of oral muscles.
2 *Does the baby push food out of the mouth with the tongue?* This may indicate a tongue thrust, although it is seen in normal babies when they are not hungry, not paying attention or are playing with their food.
3 *Does the baby suckle well?* There may be a weak or absent suckling–swallowing reflex.
4 *Does the baby choke or gag, or vomit after meals?* This, if persistent, may indicate poor control of swallowing, although it may indicate other medical conditions.
5 *Does the baby push the head back when feeding?* A baby with extensor spasms may do this, although so also will an upset cranky baby.
6 *Is the baby able to keep food in the mouth?* Difficulty sealing the lips may be due to poor control over lip closure.

Observing the parent feeding the baby may further clarify any oromotor problems.

Parental inputs to the evaluation process

The physiotherapist or occupational therapist talks to the baby's parents about any difficulties they are experiencing in feeding, dressing, bathing or playing with the baby. Parents of babies with CP frequently notice that the baby is difficult to dress and undress. It may be awkward, for example, to change the nappy because of strong adduction of the legs. The stretch to hyperreflexic hip adductor muscles as the parent adducts the legs may make nappy-changing very difficult.

It is useful to establish some details of the parents' child-rearing practices, for example, the positions the baby is put in during the day. The infant with CP may pose problems for parents, particularly if firstborn and the parents are inexperienced in child-rearing. If the infant is quiet and unresponsive they may worry about their parenting skills; if the infant cries a lot they may feel guilty and uncertain how to act.

The Brazelton Neonatal Behavioral Assessment Scale (Brazelton 1973) is an effective method of evaluating the performance of an infant in the first 30 days and of helping parents understand their baby. This assessment also gives the therapist an understanding of the infant's abilities as well as difficulties.

In summary, it is necessary to observe the baby's development over a period of time, but there are certain signs the physiotherapist should look for in particular: persistent asymmetrical movement or posturing; stereotyped or persistently abnormal movement patterns or dystonia; persistent Moro or Galant reflex beyond the time they are normally elicited; failure to develop the ability to extend the legs and support the body through the feet in standing; failure to reach and interact visually and manually with objects; feeding difficulties, in particular disorders of suckling and swallowing.

Assessment of the older infant and child

Assessment and testing of motor performance

Assessment of the motor function of children older than 6 months should, in this author's view, be concentrated on the performance of those everyday actions essential to effective living: walking, sit-to-stand, self-initiated activities while sitting on a seat and in standing, reaching and manipulation of common objects. Analysis of performance is specific to each action and should, when relevant, involve performing the action in different contexts. The reader should refer to Chapter 3 for models of functional actions, the common elements of abnormal performance and a guide to assessment.

Movement analysis involves comparing the child's performance with a normal model of the action and analysing the underlying dyscontrol characteristics. For example, if a child tries to stand up from a seat without moving the feet back (Figs 3.5 and 3.6), this may be due to:

1 Inextensibility of calf muscles. Ankles must dorsiflex beyond plantigrade for the feet to be placed sufficiently back.
2 Motor control deficits resulting in inappropriate timing and amplitude of muscle forces. The infant has to control hip and knee flexion as well as ankle dorsiflexion in order to move the feet back.
3 Habitual practice of adaptive strategies such as using the hands for support in standing up, or pulling up into standing.

The emphasis in training of sit-to-stand will be organized according to the results of this analysis.

Children normally take some time to develop mature motor performance in everyday actions, especially in walking, balancing and manipulation. There are, however, very few experimental studies examining the developmental process of actions other than walking. Until we have this information, it is possible to match a child's performance against a 'normal' mature model, since adult performance is taken to reflect optimally effective performance. Furthermore, the dynamics of the segmental linkage must be similar in both adult and child. In addition, it is adult performance for which the developing child is aiming.

In analysing *muscle action* during the performance of various actions, the therapist attempts to elucidate the control deficits as the child performs, or attempts to perform, the intended action. For example, in actions involving extension of the lower limbs over fixed feet, sit-to-stand, crouch-to-stand, stepping up and down, stance phase of walking, it may be evident that the child has difficulty performing or controlling these similar actions. It may be hypothesized that the child has difficulty:

1 Generating sufficient force with a particular muscle group (Fig. 5.9).
2 Sustaining the necessary force.
3 Generating force or sustaining force with muscles at different lengths at different phases of the action.
4 Coordinating (timing) a group of muscles appropriately.
5 Moving two limbs in two different patterns (Fig. 5.10).
6 Balancing the body segments throughout the action.

This information helps the physiotherapist to plan a programme for the training of support, balance and propulsion through the lower limbs, concentrating on the motor control deficit (see Chapter 3). Analysing the control deficit in such a way probably provides more useful information than a *manual muscle test* since it is becoming evident that muscle activation and control is specific to the action being performed. Muscle testing provides information only about a muscle's capacity to generate force in a particular context (the testing situation).

It will frequently be necessary to test *range of motion* at a joint. Since the measured range using a goniometer reflects the range of movement obtained by applying a certain (unknown) force to the lengthening muscle, accurate goniometry is more reliably done using a dynamometer (Ada and Canning 1990).

The *measurement of some aspect of motor performance* provides an indication of any changes that have occurred, feedback for child, therapist and parents as to progress made and also generates information of use in planning further intervention. There is evidence that testing an individual on a concrete task is a better indication of that person's ability to move than testing methods which utilize only abstract tasks or passive or therapist-generated movements. Van der Weel and colleagues (1991) have shown that this is so in children with hemiplegic CP. An abstract task is one in which movement is produced for its own sake (e.g. reaching forwards with the hand), whereas a concrete task involves controlling a physical interaction with the environment (e.g. reaching out to pick up a glass of water).

In the van der Weel study, 9 children with hemiplegia aged between 3 and 8 years and 12 normal controls had to:

1 hold a drumstick while the experimenter pronated and supinated the forearm;
2 hold the stick and actively rotate the forearm in both directions as far as they could; and
3 beat two drums by alternately pronating and supinating the forearm.

Tasks 1 and 2 were abstract; task 3 was concrete. Movement range for the CP children was significantly greater for the concrete task than for the abstract, with no difference found for the other children.

Sensory testing

Sensory testing is performed once the child is old enough to cooperate with simple test procedures. Sensation is tested since the problems of movement that many of these children experience may be related to poor attention to and interpretation of sensory inputs. The aspects of sensation particularly relevant to the disorders of movement in CP children are vision,

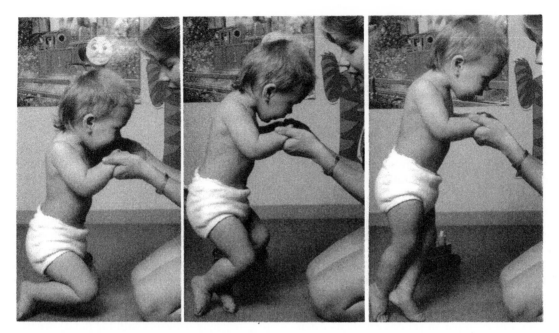

Figure 5.9 When this child is assisted to get from kneeling to standing, she does not put one leg in front of the other, but pulls herself up extending the hips, knees and ankles and standing on her toes.

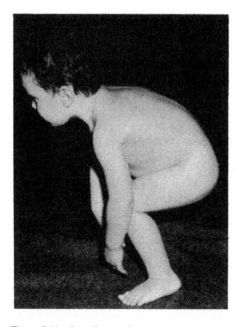

Figure 5.10 Standing up from crouch, this boy has difficulty extending the hips, knees and ankles over fixed feet.

hearing, touch and pressure and proprioception.

Vision is tested by the ophthalmologist and orthoptist; *hearing* by an audiometric laboratory. Tests for *tactile sensation* that incorporate the latest research findings (e.g. those of Johansson and Westling 1990) have not yet been developed. Below are some typical tests used clinically. It should be kept in mind, however, that not only is it essential to have the ability to recognize specific sensations but it is particularly critical that we are able to attend to and select those sensations which are most relevant to what we are doing at any particular time. That is to say, we appear to utilize only those sensory inputs which provide information critical to the control of the action we are performing or the goal on which we are focusing; sensation is itself task- and context-specific. It is this aspect of sensation that cannot at the present time be tested in the clinic, other than by inferring that improvement in the performance of actions reflects improving sensory integration.

Light touch is tested by stroking the skin lightly with a piece of cottonwool. The child's eyes are closed or vision is obstructed.

Stereognosis is the ability to recognize common objects by touch. It involves touch sensation plus the ability to recognize the shape and texture of an object and match it for identification. It is tested by placing an easily recognizable object in the child's hand. The objects chosen will depend on the child's age. Vision is obstructed during the test.

Two-point discrimination is the ability to recognize fine pressure applied to two separate points on the skin simultaneously. It is tested by using a pair of dividers, the two points of which are applied simultaneously to an area such as the palm of the hand. The child, with vision obstructed, is asked to say 'two' or 'one'. The points are moved further together until the child feels only one. A normal 5-year-old can discriminate two points until they are approximately 1 cm apart on the palm of the hand on the dominant hand and 2 cm apart on the non-dominant hand.

Joint position sense indicates awareness of position of a limb or part of a limb in space. It is tested, with the child's vision obstructed, by placing a limb in a position and either asking the child to move the other limb to the same position, or by asking the child whether the limb is bent or straight, up or down.

Tests of perceptual and cognitive function

Some children show dysfunctional motor behaviours that appear not to be due to problems controlling muscle force but which indicate they may have so-called perceptual dysfunctions such as *apraxia* or *visual agnosia* or *unilateral spatial agnosia*. These little understood problems are thought to be due to an inability to process correctly the sensory inputs required for motor behaviour in order for them to be relevant to task and environmental context. Tests are being developed in which an individual's ability to respond to support surface perturbations are analysed under different sensory conditions. Whether or not these tests are of any relevance to actions carried out on stable surfaces during self-initiated actions is unknown.

It may be necessary for a child to have tests of such aspects of comprehension as space and form appreciation, ability to concentrate and other tests of particular cognitive attributes.

Motor training

The overall management of the infant or child with CP involves the interaction of health professionals involved in the areas of speech and communication, and in promoting emotional, psychological and functional independence.

The major goal of any intervention with movement-disabled infants and children is to optimize the child's ability to perform the actions essential to everyday life as effectively and with as little effort as possible. There is now considerable evidence that for an individual to acquire skill in the performance of a particular action, that action has itself to be practised. This is the concept of *task-specific training*. In addition, actions vary according to the contexts in which they are being performed. In order that an individual develops flexibility, that is, the ability to perform an action in a number of different environments, actions need to be practised under different environmental conditions. Hence the concept of *context-specific training*.

Virtually all our actions involve some interaction between ourselves and objects in our immediate environment. This interaction involves a link between our goal or intention and the characteristics of the object itself. That is, when we go to pick up an object, how we shape our hand for grasping it and how we manipulate it within our hand depends not only on the object's characteristics but also on what we are intending to do with the object.

Early training with young infants as well as with older children should be directed in particular towards practice of activities which involve the lower limbs in *support, balance and propulsion*, and the upper limbs in *reaching for and manipulation of objects*. Specific practice of standing and stepping in young infants is, as Leonard (1990) points out, a departure from NDT. It is, however, consistent with the stepping practice normal infants carry out with their parents. Leonard and Zelazo (1988) trained stepping, standing and placing in a group of 4 infants aged 4 months and considered to have abnormal neurological signs. Parents provided daily exercise. After 10 weeks of training, these infants had increased the rate of stepping and standing relative to a control group of infants. This study, and others, provides evidence that task-specific training optimizes the performance of the tasks trained. Katona (1989) has also shown that exercise and opportunity to practise enhance motor function. Van der Weel and colleagues (1991) have shown that arm movements can be augmented in children with CP by practice of concrete as opposed to abstract tasks or passive movement. Studies of adults with brain lesions have shown similar results (Lee and Young 1986; Frischer 1989).

For motor training to be effective, the musculoskeletal system needs to be flexible enough to allow the necessary actions to be performed. Adaptive soft tissue changes occur rapidly in disabled infants and young children where both inactivity and growth are combined. The optimal way of ensuring appropriate length of muscle is through active performance of a variety of different actions. For example, soleus muscle length is maintained at the length necessary for sit-to-stand and crouch-to-stand if these actions are practised under optimal conditions (i.e., with guidance and support where necessary and under typical environmental conditions). That is to say, activity requires muscles to both shorten and lengthen. Passive means of lengthening muscles are commonly advocated as part of therapy, usually when muscles have already shortened. Such methods have been shown to be effective (Tardieu *et al.* 1982; Bertoti 1986). Passive means of lengthening may not, however, carry over into improved motor performance. A single session of stretch to the triceps surae using a tilt table has been shown to decrease spasticity (illustrated by a decreased EMG and mechanical response to passive movement) (Tremblay *et al.* in press). However, this effect was not seen during walking and the typical pattern of early calf muscle activation, remained (Richards *et al.* in press).

As proposed earlier in the chapter, studies are needed to determine the most effective means of improving performance in infants with CP (Leonard and Zelazo 1988; Campbell 1989; Richards *et al.* 1991).

Chapter 3 provides examples of motor training of infants and children with movement dysfunction. Below are some specific areas of physiotherapy intervention not referred to in Chapter 3, and a broad outline of medical and surgical management.

Optimizing oromotor function

Infants with poor control over oral function and consequent problems with eating and drinking require early intervention. In particular, this is aimed at ensuring adequate nutrition, but also preventing abnormal function becoming established and optimizing the infant's chances of developing mature oral function.

Training to reduce abnormal oromotor activity such as a persistent and strong bite reflex, a hypersensitive gag reflex or tongue thrust and to improve the effectiveness of swallowing should be instigated if adequate nutrition is to be obtained. Although they do not appear to have been tested objectively, clinical experience suggests that the techniques developed by Mueller (1977) are effective in improving oromotor control. These are described below, modified according to more recent findings related to normal oral function and methods of optimizing motor control.

To desensitize *hypersensitive lips and cheek* the therapist rubs a finger firmly around the lips, and, as the infant's tolerance improves, the finger is moved into the mouth and around the cheeks and gums. A *persistent bite reflex* may be desensitized by rubbing along the gums. Positive reinforcement is given when the infant does not bite down on the therapist's finger. Where there is *tongue-thrusting*, the finger is pressed firmly down and back on the blade of the tongue, withdrawn immediately and the lips and jaw held closed. Lateral vibration to the tongue with firm pressure downwards may be more effective as a desensitizing technique.

With a *hypersensitive gag reflex*, the infant may not be able to tolerate a finger touching the lips or tongue. Desensitization may be obtained by gently rubbing the finger around the infant's lips, gradually entering the mouth and rubbing along the gums. As tolerance increases, the finger is placed on the tongue firmly and walked back towards the middle of the tongue. Beyond this point a gag would be a normal response.

An infant with *hypotonic oral musculature* may be stimulated to suckle and swallow more effectively if vibration is done on the tongue as described above.

These procedures are carried out by the parent for a few minutes before the baby is fed, when necessary during the feed, and briefly during the day. During feeding, the spoon is pressed down firmly and briefly on the blade of the tongue as the food is put in the baby's mouth. The spoon is withdrawn and the lips and jaw held closed while the baby swallows. Chewing may be encouraged in an older infant by placing a strip of cooked meat between the jaws and holding the jaw lightly closed.

Swallowing is a complex motor act made up of oral, pharyngeal and oesophageal phases (Carr 1979). Swallowing depends on the appropriate external stimulus – food or saliva – contacting the oral and pharyngeal mucosa.

The initial preparation of the saliva or bolus of food is under voluntary control, but once the bolus is positioned for swallowing it sets up a chain of more reflexive movements. In preparation for swallowing, the hyoid bone is elevated, the teeth are occluded, the lips and jaw closed, and the soft palate and uvula raised to seal off the nasopharynx. The lumen of the larynx is narrowed, helping to ensure the saliva is not aspirated.

Swallowing deficits are due to head position, poor control over the tongue and lips and decreased oral sensory awareness (van de Heyning *et al.* 1980). They also occur due to poor attention capacity in children who are cognitively impaired.

Swallowing is encouraged by lip and jaw closure and pressure applied externally to the base of the tongue. However, swallowing is more likely to occur if the infant is given a small amount of food of firm consistency (e.g. cooked fruit), the spoon is withdrawn and the lips and jaws closed and held closed immediately. The head should not be in extension as swallowing and mouth closure are difficult in this position.

It is apparent that there is a difference between solicited and unsolicited swallowing. Kydd and Toda (1962) used strain gauges to measure the pressure exerted by the tongue in swallowing and found that the tongue exerted twice as much pressure with command swallowing than with spontaneous swallowing.

In some children with CP, persistent swallowing deficits result in *drooling* which can become a serious handicap, affecting social acceptance and self-esteem and causing skin rashes. In some children with CP, drooling is the result of oromotor dyscontrol rather than hypersalivation (Ekedahl *et al.* 1974; van de Heyning *et al.* 1980), and is due to ineffective swallowing itself or an inadequate rate of swallowing, allowing saliva to build in the oral cavity.

The problem of drooling is addressed clinically primarily by conservative means, but also by surgery. Conservative treatment includes desensitization of hypersensitive responses (e.g. tongue thrust, hypersensitive bite or gag reflex), swallowing training, behaviour modification (Garber 1971; Drabman *et al.* 1979) and prosthetic devices such as chin cups (Shavell 1977; Harris and Dignam 1980) and lip halters (Nelson *et al.* 1981), and by electromyogram auditory biofeedback (Koheil *et al.* 1987).

Several of these methods have been evaluated and found to be successful in diminishing drooling, for example, behaviour modification (Drabman *et al.* 1979); an auditory reminder plus verbal feedback (Rapp 1980); electromyogram biofeedback from oral musculature (Brown *et al.* 1978; Koheil *et al.* 1987). In one study, chin cups plus oromotor exercises were found to be more effective than exercises alone (Harris and Dignam 1980).

Since the muscles involved in the initial oral phase of swallowing are under voluntary control, it may be appropriate to institute a training programme involving exercises specifically designed to improve the control of lip movements. This should start in infancy, but refresher sessions may be necessary throughout childhood. The principles upon which the training programme is based are those of motor learning or skill acquisition (Gentile 1987). The first stage of learning is cognitive, when the learner gets the idea of the movement. Feedback gives knowledge of results, that is, of the effectiveness of performance, and this can be by verbal praise and by the knowledge that something important has been accomplished (in this case, desirable food has been swallowed rather than drooled). Practice – that is, many repetitions with different types of food as well as fluid – is necessary for learning to take place and control to be gained. Attention to the task during this phase is also essential.

As a test of the effectiveness of any programme of swallowing training or drooling control, the amount of saliva drooled can be measured using a chin cup (Sochaniwskyj 1982; Harris and Dignam 1980). The effect of swallowing training can also be measured by calculating the time taken to eat a given quantity of food.

Vocalizing and breathing control

The physiotherapist helps the development of speech motor control by encouraging the baby to babble and vocalize. The quality of the sounds made can be changed by tapping over the lips or by giving vibrations to the chest. Breathing control may be encouraged by vibrations on expiration and manual pressure on the chest to encourage longer expiration. When the child is older, breathing control can be encouraged by games in which the child tries to bend but not extinguish a candle flame, blow a mobile gently or a ping-pong ball across a table in a controlled manner. Use of a peak flow meter to provide feedback may also be effective.

Parental involvement in intervention

One of the most critical requirements for motor learning to occur is practice. It is doubtful that an infant or child with poor movement control as a result of a CNS lesion or dysfunction will acquire any competence or skill in essential everyday actions if the only practice he or she has is one hour spent with the physiotherapist once or twice a week. The evidence is that many repetitions are necessary for an action to become learned and for the muscles to acquire the strength necessary to carry out the action. It is perhaps not surprising that, despite physiotherapy, some infants become very proficient at performing abnormal or ineffective movements which they practise persistently.

Infants and children practise what movements they can do; they move the best way they can given the possibilities of the musculoskeletal linkage and the environment, and given the state of their neuromuscular system.

The contribution of parents is therefore essential to ensure that the infant or child has the opportunity to practise the actions which are being concentrated on at that time (Figs 5.11 and 5.12). Parents can be helped to set up an environment that 'forces' the action required by preventing unwanted actions or positions (Fig. 5.13). They can be shown how to modify the supine position if in that position the baby habitually extends head and trunk and cannot reach forwards (Fig. 5.14). Parents can be taught the importance of ensuring a prescribed number of repetitions of an action.

With infants, parents may need to be shown how to prevent unwanted movements and encourage the movements to be learned when they are bathing, dressing and carrying the infant, what games to play (Figs 5.15 and 5.16) and with what objects to encourage reaching, grasping and manipulation. They need to understand the actions being trained in order to choose toys or objects that are the right size and shape to be graspable, and those that are most attractive to the infant.

Parents should not be given too many tasks to carry out at home, since they have other responsibilities as well as to the disabled infant. The physiotherapist selects with them one or two actions to concentrate on in train-

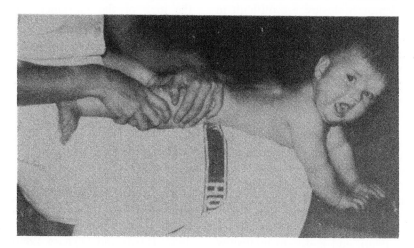

Figure 5.11 Exercises can be organized to strengthen and increase control over muscles – in this case, trunk and hip extensors and arm muscles. The infant has some developmental delay.

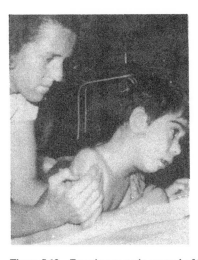

Figure 5.12 Exercises to train control of head and upper trunk extension and weight-bearing through the arms in a boy with athetosis. An interesting visual stimulus facilitates the extension movement.

ing, while encouraging the parents to appreciate the value to the infant's motor development of ensuring that their own handling of the infant and the environment they provide are consistent with the goals at that time. Emphasis is given to actions involving support, balance and propulsion of lower limbs over a fixed foot (feet), reaching and manipulation.

Some clinics give questionnaires to parents to establish what areas of their advice and education are useful and what improvements could be made.

Orthotics

The value of orthotics is a matter for some debate. Some form of splinting may be required by a child to aid in motor training or to lengthen shortened soft tissues (see p. 148). However, there should be a congruence between the goals of training and the rationale behind the design of the orthosis. For example,

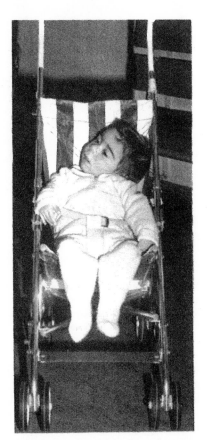 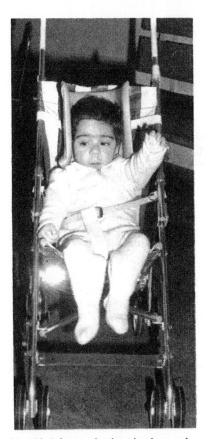

Figure 5.13 Provision of a neck support enables this infant to develop visual control and encourages him to use his arms.

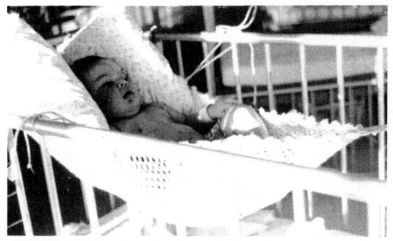

Figure 5.14 A hammock can be used to restrict intermittent spasms or excessive extension in supine. It holds the head centred, encouraging visual development.

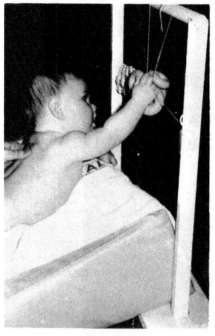

Figure 5.15 Exercising the head, trunk and upper limb extensors by self-initiated and goal-directed actions.

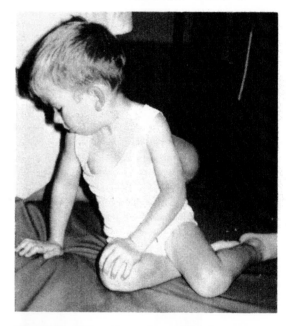

Figure 5.16 Sitting sideways is a position that promotes extensibility of the right-sided lower trunk and leg muscles. Games can be played that involve placing the hands and thighs on marks on the floor.

an orthosis which is designed to hold a joint stable may prevent a child from gaining muscular control of a limb. However, an orthosis may be the only way of enabling a child to sit or stand erect, and, used in walking, an orthosis may result in a more energy-efficient action (e.g. Mossberg *et al.* 1990).

Orthoses can be designed to optimize the ability of muscles to contract at a particular length. For example, a splint designed to hold the thumb abducted at the carpometacarpal joint may optimize an infant's practice of grasping and releasing a toy (see p. 78). Strapping can also be used to alter the direction of a muscle's pull, or to encourage activation with a muscle at a particular length.

Serial casting (e.g. Ada and Canning 1990; Phillips and Audet 1990) is designed progressively to lengthen soft tissues and may be necessary if adaptive changes occur. However, while the child wears the cast and after it is removed, activities need to be practised so the child learns to control actively the agonist and antagonist muscles at their new lengths. Serial casting is described in detail on p. 148.

Medical and surgical management

Pharmacology

Various drugs – in particular baclofen – have been suggested to decrease spasticity and control involuntary movements. The results have been controversial and whether or not there is any measurable functional improvement is not always reported. Side-effects may be deleterious, causing problems ranging from hypotonus and attention deficits to sedation effects. The fact that in some studies little change has been reported in the pattern of functional movements such as walking (Young 1980) indicates that adaptive changes in the mechanical properties of the muscles can be a major cause of movement dysfunction and this will not be affected by spasticity reduction.

Dantrolene sodium has been found to decrease the force of muscle contraction but this is not necessarily followed by functional improvement. Controlled use of baclofen for a short period may be of value in children with marked spasticity without marked soft tissue adaptation, allowing an intensive period of motor training.

Orthopaedic surgery

The current poverty of information about the motor dysfunction associated with CP makes decisions regarding surgery, such as what type and when, very difficult to make. Under certain circumstances surgery may enable a child to participate more actively in motor training. Orthopaedic surgery may be necessary to correct hip dislocation or a severe structural scoliosis (Allen and Ferguson 1982), or to mobilize contracted and inflexible soft tissues.

Surgery to relieve pain and deformity associated with hip dislocation may be necessary in the severely disabled child or adolescent and has been reported to make sitting more comfortable in children who were finding sitting in a wheelchair too painful (McCarthy *et al.* 1988). Hip dislocation occurs in children with severe spasticity or athetosis with severe spasms, and particularly so when the child is also severely mentally retarded and/or immobile. Hip dislocation appears to result from a combination of muscle imbalance and shortness, with anteversion and valgus of the femoral neck contributing. When the hip adductor and iliopsoas muscles adaptively shorten and generate force at this short length, the centre of movement of the hip is transferred from the head of the femur to the lesser trochanter. Anterolateral forces act on the hip capsule causing it to stretch, which leads to the dislocation (Sharrard 1975). Surgical procedures include pelvic osteotomy, adductor release, iliopsoas transfer, femoral resection and arthroplasty.

Orthopaedic surgery is probably only optimally effective if followed by functional training designed to utilize structural gains. Surgery to lengthen contracted soft tissues is more problematic. For example, if a child with diplegia has short calf muscles and if these muscles are capable only of minimal force generation, then lengthening of the tendo Achilles may result in greater range of passive dorsiflexion but a decrease in the muscles' force-generating capacity, since the ratio between the tendon length and muscle belly will not promote a better mechanical advantage. Abnormalities of muscle may contribute to variable outcomes following surgery. For example, according to Castle and colleagues (1979), the status of type II fibres may be an indicator of the quality of neuronal activation of the muscle.

Neurosurgery

Various techniques are utilized including the controversial chronic electrical stimulation of the cerebellum and selective dorsal rhizotomy. Selective dorsal rhizotomy aims to decrease spasticity by separating dorsal and ventral roots from L2 to L5, testing with electromyography to detect an abnormal response to electrical stimulation, then division of those with an abnormal response (e.g. clonus, ipsilateral or contralateral spread to other muscle groups). This technique has been reported to be an effective method of improving walking functions in children with marked spasticity, when followed by intensive physiotherapy (Vaughn *et al.* 1989).

Summary

The infant or child with CP demonstrates the complex effects of a lesion or maldevelopment of the brain. However, other factors combine with the effects of the lesion to augment the functional deficits as the infant matures and grows. These factors include the effects of inactivity and abnormal muscle activity on the flexibility of the musculoskeletal system, and the effects on the neural system of practising a limited and stereotyped repertoire of muscle activations. Physiotherapy for both infant and child is directed towards the specific training of actions such as standing, stepping or walking, sitting, reaching and manipulating, with exercises designed to increase muscular strength and control of movement. The environment is set up to enable the infant or child to practise, and training sessions are set up to maximize the number of repetitions performed and encourage flexibility of action. Methods of measurement are put in place to enable the effects of intervention on performance of functional actions to be tested.

References

Ada, L. and Canning, C. (1990) Anticipating and preventing muscle shortening. In: *Key Issues in Neurological Physiotherapy*, edited by L. Ada and C. Canning. Oxford: Butterworth-Heinemann, pp. 219–236.

Ada, L. and Westwood, P. (1992) A kinematic analysis of recovery of the ability to stand up following stroke. *Aust. J. Physiother.*, **38**, 135.

Adsett, D.B., Fitz, C.R. and Hill, A. (1985) Hypoxic-ischaemic cerebral injury in the term newborn: correlation of CT findings with neurological outcome. *Develop. Med. Child Neurol.*, **27**, 155–160.

Allen, B.L. and Ferguson, R.L. (1982) L-rod instrumentation for scoliosis in cerebral palsy. *J. Pediatr. Orthop.*, **2**, 87.

André-Thomas, Chesni, Y. and Saint-Anne Dargassies, S. (1960) *The Neurological Assessment during the First Year of Life*. London: Heinemann.

Banker, B.Q. and Larroche, J.-C. (1962) Periventricular leukomalacia of infancy: form of neonatal anoxic encephalopathy. *Arch. Neurol.*, **7**, 386–410.

Bax, M. (1987) Aims and outcomes of physiotherapy for cerebral palsy. *Develop. Med. Child Neurol.*, **29**, 689–692.

Bertoti, D.B. (1986). Effect of short leg casting on ambulation in children with cerebral palsy. *Phys. Ther.*, **66**, 1522–1529.

Blair, E. and Stanley, F.J. (1982) An epidemiological study of cerebral palsy in Western Australia 1956–1975, III. Postnatal aetiology. *Develop. Med. Child Neurol.* 24, **5**, 575–585.

Bobath, B. (1972) *Abnormal Postural Reflex Activity Caused by Brain Lesions*. 2nd edn. London: Heinemann Medical.

Bobath, K. (1980) *A Neurological basis for the Treatment of Cerebral Palsy*. Clinics in Developmental Medicine 75. London: Heinemann.

Bobath, B. and Bobath, K. (1975) *Motor Development in the Different Types of Cerebral Palsy*. London: Heinemann Medical.

Bobath, K. and Bobath, B. (1984) The neuro-developmental treatment. In: *Management of the Motor Disorders of Children with Cerebral Palsy*, edited by D. Scrutton. London: Heinemann, pp. 6–18.

Bower, E. and McLellan, D.L. (1990) Effect of increased exposure to physiotherapy on skill acquisition of children with cerebral palsy. *Develop. Med. Child Neurol.*, **34**, 25–39.

Brazelton, T.B. (1973) *Neonatal Behavioral Assessment Scale*. London: Heinemann.

Brouwer, B. and Ashby, P. (1991) Altered corticospinal projections to lower limb motoneurons in subjects with cerebral palsy. *Brain*, **114**, 3, 1395–1407.

Brown, D.M., Nahai, F., Wolf, S. and Basmajian, J.V. (1978) Electromyographic biofeedback in the re-education of facial palsy. *Am. J. Phys. Med.*, **57**, 183–189.

Brown, J.K., van Rensburg, F., Walsh, G., Lakie, M. and Wright, G.W. (1987) A neurological study of hand function in hemiplegic children. *Develop. Med. Child Neurol.*, **29**, 287–304.

Campbell, S.K. (1989) Editorial. *Phys. Occup. Ther. Pediat.*, **9**, 2, 1.

Carr, J.C. (1979) Oral function in infancy – its importance for future development. *Aust. J. Physiother. Paediatric Monograph*. Melbourne: Australian Physiotherapy Association.

Carr, J.H., Shepherd, R.B., Nordholm, L. and Lynne, D. (1985) A motor assessment scale for stroke. *Phys. Ther.*, **65**, 175–180.

Carr, J.C. and Shepherd, R.B. (eds) (1987) *Movement Science. Foundations for Physical Therapy in Rehabilitation*. Oxford: Butterworth-Heinemann.

Castle, M.E., Reyman, T. A. and Schneider, M. (1979) Pathology of spastic muscle in cerebral palsy. *Clin. Orthop.*, **142**, 223.

Chandler, L.S., Andrews, M.S. and Swanson, M.W. (1980) *Movement Assessment of Infants: A Manual*. Rolling Bay, WA: Published by the authors.

d'Avignon, M., Noren, L., and Arman, T. (1981) Early physiotherapy and modum Vojta or Bobath in infants with suspected neuromotor disturbance. *Neuropediatrics*, **12**, 232–241.

Dean, C. and Mackey, F. (1992) Motor assessment scale scores as a measure of rehabilitation following stroke. *Aust. J. Physiother.*, **38**, 1, 31.

de Bruin, H., Eng, P., Russell, D.J. *et al.* (1982) Angle-angle diagrams in monitoring and quantification of gait patterns for children with cerebral palsy. *Am. J. Phys. Med.*, **61**, 4, 176–192.

DeGangi, G.A., Hurley, L., and Lischeid, T.R. (1983) Toward a methodology of the short-term effects of neurodevelopmental treatment. *Amer. J. Occup. Ther.*, **37**, 479–484.

de Vries, L.S., Dubowitz, L.M.S. and Dubowitz, V. *et al.* (1985) Predictive value of cranial ultrasound in the newborn baby: a reappraisal. *Lancet*, **2**, 137.

Dietz, V. and Berger, W. (1983) Normal and impaired regulation of muscle stiffness in gait: a new hypothesis about muscle hypertonia. *Exper. Neurol.*, 7, 9, 680–687.

Dietz, V., Quintern, J. and Berger, W. (1981) Electrophysiological studies of gait in spasticity and rigidity: evidence that altered mechanical properties of muscle contribute to hypertonia. *Brain*, **104**, 431–449.

Drabman, R.S., Crerz, G.C., Russ, J. and Lynd, S. (1979) Suppression of chronic drooling in mentally retarded children and adolescents: effectiveness of a behavioural treatment package. *Behavior Therapy*, **10**, 46–56.

Dubowitz, L. and Dubowitz, V. (1981) *The Neurological Assessment of the Preterm and Full-term Newborn Infant*. London: Heinemann.

Eckersley, P. and King, L. (1993) Treatment systems. In: *Elements of Paediatric Physiotherapy*, edited by P.M. Eckersley. London: Churchill Livingstone, pp. 323–341.

Ekedahl, C., Mansson, I. and Sandberg, N. (1974) Swallowing dysfunction in the brain-damaged with drooling. *Acta Otolaryngolica*, **78**, 141–149.

Eliasson, A-C, Gordon, A.M. and Forssberg, H. (1991) Basic co-ordination of manipulative forces of children with cerebral palsy. *Develop. Med. Child Neurol.*, **33**, 661–670.

Eliasson, A-C, Gordon, A.M. and Forssberg, H. (1992) Impaired anticipatory control of isometric forces during grasping by children with cerebral palsy. *Develop. Med. Child Neurol.*, **34**, 216–225.

Fetters, L. (1991) Measurement and treatment in cerebral palsy: an argument for a new approach. *Phys. Ther.*, **71**, 3, 244–247.

Forsstrom, A. and von Hofsten, C. (1982) Visually directed reaching of children with motor impairments. *Develop. Med. Child Neurol.*, **24**, 653–661.

Frischer, M. (1989) Voluntary vs autonomous control of repetitive finger tapping in a patient with Parkinson's disease. *Neuropsychol.*, **27**, 1261–1266.

Fulford, G.E. and Brown, J.K. (1976) Position as a cause of deformity in children with cerebral palsy. *Develop. Med. Child Neurol.*, **18**, 305–314.

Garber, N.B. (1971) Operant procedures to eliminate drooling behaviour in a cerebral-palsied adolescent. *Develop. Med. Child Neurol.*, **13**, 641–644.

Gentile, A.M. (1987). Skill acquisition. In: *Movement Science Foundations for Physical Therapy in Rehabilitation*, edited by J.H. Carr and R.B. Shepherd. Oxford: Butterworth-Heinemann.

Golden, G.S. (1987) Cerebrovascular disease. In: *Pediatric Neurology. Principles and Practice*, 2, edited by K.F. Swaiman. St Louis: C.V. Mosby Co.

Gordon, J. (1987) Assumptions underlying physical therapy intervention: theoretical and historical perspectives. In: *Movement Science. Foundations for Physical Therapy in Rehabilitation*, edited by J.H. Carr and R.B. Shepherd. Oxford: Butterworth-Heinemann, pp. 1–30.

Hagberg, B., Olow, I. and Hagberg, G. (1973) Decreasing incidence of low birth weight diplegia – achievement of modern neonatal care? *Acta Paediatr. Scand.*, **62**, 199–200.

Harbord, M.G., Finn, J.P., Hall-Craggs, M.A., Robb, S.A., Kendall, B.E. and Boyd, S.G. (1990) Myelination patterns on magnetic resonance of children with developmental delay. *Develop. Med. Child Neurol.*, **32**, 295–303.

Harris, S.R. (1991) Movement analysis – an aid to early diagnosis of cerebral palsy. *Phys. Ther.*, **71**, 3, 215–221.

Harris, M.M. and Dignam, P.F. (1980) A non-surgical method of reducing drooling in cerebral-palsied children. *Develop. Med. Child Neurol.*, **22**, 293–299.

Harris, S.R., Haley, S.M., Tada, W.L. and Swanson, M.W. (1984) Reliability of observational measures of the Movement Assessment of Infants. *Phys. Ther.*, **64**, 471–475.

Held, R. and Hein, A. (1976) Movement produced stimulation in the development of visually guided behavior. *J. Compar. Physiol. Psychol.*, **37**, 87–95.

Hershler, C. and Milner, M. (1980) Angle-angle diagrams in above-knee amputee and cerebral palsy gait. *Am. J. Phys. Med.*, **59**, 165–183.

Hill, A. and Volpe, J.J. (1987) Hypoxic-ischemic encephalopathy of the newborn. In: *Pediatric Neurology. Principles and Practice*, 2, edited by K.F. Swaiman. St Louis: C.V. Mosby Co.

Hourcade, J.J. and Parette, H.P. (1984) Motoric change subsequent to therapeutic intervention in infants and young children who have cerebral palsy: annotated listing of group studies. *Percept. Mot. Skills*, **58**, 519.

Illingworth, R.S. (1970) *The Development of the Infant and Young Child*. London: Livingstone.

Ingram, T. (1955) The early manifestations and course of diplegia in childhood. *Arch. Dis. Child.*, **30**, 85.

Jeannerod, M. (1986) The formation of the finger grip during prehension a cortically-mediated visuo-motor pattern. In: *Themes in Motor Development*, edited by H.T.A. Whiting and M.G. Wade. Dordrecht: Martinus Nijhoff.

Johansson, R.S. and Westling, G. (1990) Tactile afferent signals in the control of precision grip. In: *Attention and Performance*, edited by M. Jeannerod. Hillsdale, NJ: Erlbaum.

Kanda, T., Suzuki, J., Yamori, Y. *et al.* (1982) CT findings of spastic diplegia with special reference to grade of motor disturbance. *Brain Develop.*, **4**, 239.

Kanda, T., Yuge, M., Yamori, Y., Suzuki, J. and Fukase, H. (1984) Early physiotherapy in the treatment of spastic diplegia. *Develop. Med. Child Neurol.*, **26**, 438–444.

Katona, F. (1989) Clinical neurodevelopmental diagnosis and treatment. In: *Challenges of Developmental Paradigms: Implications for Theory, Assessment, and Treatment*, edited by P.R. Zelazo and R. Barr. Hillsdale, NJ: Lawrence Erlbaum Associates Inc.

Kiely, J., Paneth, N., Stein, Z. and Susser, M. (1981) Cerebral palsy and newborn care. 11: Mortality and neurological impairment in low-birthweight infants. *Develop. Med. Child Neurol.*, 23, 650–659.

Kitchen, W.H., Doyle, L.W., Ford, G.W., Rickards, A.L. *et al.* (1987) Cerebral palsy in very low birthweight infants surviving to 2 years with modern perinatal intensive care. *Am. J. Perinatol.*, 4, 29–35.

Kluzik, J., Fetters, L. and Coryell, J. (1990) Quantification of control: a preliminary study of effects of Neurodevelopmental Treatment on reaching in children with spastic cerebral palsy. *Phys. Ther.*, 70, 2, 65–78.

Knutsson, E. (1980) Muscle activation patterns of gait in spastic hemiparesis, paraparesis and cerebral palsy. *Scand. J. Rehabil. Med. Suppl.*, 7, 47.

Koheil, R., Sochaniwskyj, A.E., Bablich, K., Kenny, D.J. and Milner, M. (1987) Biofeedback techniques and behaviour modification in the conservative remediation of drooling by children with cerebral palsy. *Develop. Med. Child Neurol.*, 29, 19–26.

Köng, E. (1967) Early detection and diagnosis of cerebral palsy. *Arch. Ital. Pediat. Pueri Colt.*, 25, 1.

Kydd, W.L. and Toda, J. (1962) Tongue pressure exerted on the hard palate during swallowing. *J. Amer. Dent. Assoc.*, 65, 319–330.

Laskas, C.A., Mullen, S.A., Nelson, D.L. and Willson-Broyles, M. (1985) Enhancement of two motor functions of the lower extremity in a child with spastic quadriplegia. *Phys. Ther.*, 65, 1, 11–16.

Lee, D.N. and Young, D.S. (1986) Gearing action to the environment. In: *Generation and Modulation of Action*, edited by H. Heuer and C. Fromm. Heidelberg: Springer.

Leonard, E.L. (1990) Early motor development and control: foundations for independent walking. In: *Gait in Rehabilitation*, edited by G.L. Smith. New York: Churchill Livingstone, pp. 121–140.

Leonard, E. and Zelazo, P.R. (1988) Play in developmental evaluation. *VIth Biennial Meeting of International Society of Infant Studies*. Washington, D.C.

Lilly, L.A. and Powell, N.J. (1990) Measuring the effects of Neurodevelopmental Treatment on the daily living skills of 2 children with cerebral palsy. *Amer. J. Occup. Ther.*, 44, 2, 139–145.

Lingam, S., Read, S., Holland, I.M., Wilson, J., Brett, E.M. and Hoare, R.D. (1982) Value of computerized tomography in children with non-specific mental subnormality. *Arch. Dis. Childhood*, 57, 381–383.

McCarthy, R.E., Simon, S., Douglas, B., Zawacki, R. and Reese, N. (1988) Proximal femoral resection to allow adults who have severe cerebral palsy to sit. *J. Bone Jt. Surg.*, 70-A, 7, 1011–1016.

McDonald, C. (1994). A biomechanical analysis of sit-to-stand in children with diplegic cerebral palsy. Unpublished Honours thesis.

Malouin, F., Potvin, M., Prevost, J. *et al.* (1992) Use of intensive task-oriented gait training program in a series of patients with acute cerebrovascular accidents. *Phys. Ther.*, 72, 11, 781–793.

Maystone, M.J. (1992) The Bobath concept – evaluation and application. In: *Movement Disorders in Children*, edited by H. Hirschberg and H. Forssberg. Basel: Karger, pp. 1–6.

Milani-Comparetti, A. and Gidoni, E. (1967) Pattern analysis of motor development and its disorders. *Develop. Med. Child Neurol.*, 9, 625–630.

Milner-Brown, H.S. and Penn, R.D. (1979) Pathophysiological mechanisms in cerebral palsy. *J. Neurol. Neurosurg. Psychiat.*, 42, 606.

Mossberg, K.A., Linton, K.A. and Friske, K. (1990) Ankle-foot orthoses: effect on energy expenditure of gait in spastic diplegic children. *Arch. Phys. Med. Rehabil.*, 71, 490–494.

Mueller, H. (1977). Personal communication.

Myklebust, B.M., Gottlieb, G.L. and Penn, R.D. *et al.* (1982) Reciprocal excitation of antagonistic muscles as a differentiating feature in spasticity. *Ann. Neurol.*, 12, 367.

Nashner, L., Shumway-Cook, A. and Marin, O. (1983) Stance posture control in selected groups of children with cerebral palsy: deficit in sensory organisation and muscular coordination. In: *Disorders of Posture and Gait*, edited by W. Bles and T. Brandt. Amsterdam: Elsevier.

Nelson, E.C., Pendleton, T.B. and Edel, J. (1981) Lip halter an aid in drool control. *Phys. Ther.*, 61, 361–363.

Nelson, K.B. and Ellenberg, J.H. (1986) Antecedents of cerebral palsy. Multivariate analysis of risk. *N. Engl. J. Med.*, 315, 81.

Ottenbacher, K.J., Biocca, Z., DeCremer, G. *et al.* (1986) Quantitative analysis of the effectiveness of pediatric therapy: emphasis on the neurodevelopmental treatment approach. *Phys. Ther.*, 66, 1095–1101.

Parker, D.F., Carriere, L., Hebestreit, H., Salsberg, A. and Bar-Or, O. (1993) Muscle performance and gross motor function of children with spastic cerebral palsy. *Develop. Med. Child Neurol.*, 35, 17–23.

Perin, B. (1989) Physical therapy for the child with cerebral palsy. In: *Pediatric Neurologic Physical Therapy*, edited by S.K. Campbell. New York: Churchill Livingstone.

Phillips, W.E. and Audet, M. (1990) Use of serial casting in the management of knee joint contractures in an adolescent with cerebral palsy. *Phys. Ther.*, 70, 8, 521–523.

Piaget, J. (1952) *The Origins of Intelligence in Children*. New York: International University Press.

Prechtl, H. (1977) *The Neurological Examination of the Full-term Newborn Infant*. London: Heinemann.

Rapp, D.L. (1980) Drool control: long-term follow-up. *Develop. Med. Child Neurol.*, 22, 448–453.

Richards, C.L., Malouin, F. and Dumas, F. (in press). Effects of a single session of prolonged plantarflexor stretch on muscle activations during gait in spastic cerebral palsy. *Scand. J. Rehabil. Med.*

Richards, C.L., Malouin, F., Dumas, F. and Wood-Dauphinee, S. (1991). New rehabilitation strategies for the treatment of spastic gait disorders. In: *Adaptability of Human Gait*, edited by A.E. Patla. New York: Elsevier Science, pp. 387–411.

Robinson, R.O., McCarthy, G.T. and Little, T.M. (1989) Conductive Education at the Peto Institute, Budapest. *B.M.J.*, **299**, 1145–1149.

Russell, D.J., Rosenbaum, P.L., Cadman, D.T., Gowland, C., Hardy, S. and Jarvis, S. (1989) The Gross Motor Function Measure: a means to evaluate the effects of physical therapy. *Develop. Med. Child Neurol.*, **31**, 341–352.

Scherzer, A.L., Mike, V. and Ilson, J. (1976) Physical therapy as a determinant of change in the cerebral palsied infant. *Pediat.*, **58**, 47–51.

Scrutton, B. and Gilbertson, M. (1975) *Physiotherapy in Paediatric Practice*. London: Butterworth.

Sharrard, W.J.W. (1975) The hip in cerebral palsy. In: *Orthopaedic Aspects of Cerebral Palsy*, edited by R.L. Samilson. London: William Heinemann, pp. 145–172.

Shavell, A. (1977) Drooling in cerebral palsy. *S. African J. Communic. Dis.*, **24**, 75–88.

Shepherd, R.B. (1987) Movement science and physiotherapy. Deriving implications for the clinic. *Proceedings of 10th WCPT Congress, Sydney*, pp. 6–12

Shumway-Cook, A. (1989) Equilibrium deficits in children. In: *The Development of Posture and Gait Across the Lifespan*, edited by M. Woollacott and A. Shumway-Cook. Columbia, S.C.: Univ. S. Carolina Press.

Sochaniwskyj, A.E. (1982) Drool quantification: non-invasive technique. *Arch. Phys. Med. Rehabil.*, **63**, 605–607.

Sommerfield, D., Fraser, B., Hensinger, R.N. *et al.* (1981) Evaluation of physical therapy service for severely mentally impaired students with cerebral palsy. *Phys. Ther.*, **61**, 3, 338.

Stanley, F. and Alberman, E. (1984) *The Epidemiology of the Cerebral Palsies*. Philadelphia: J.B. Lippincott Co.

Swanson, W., Bennett, F.C., Shy, K.K. and Whitfield, M.F. (1992) Identification of neurodevelopmental abnormality at four and eight months by the Movement Assessment of Infants. *Develop. Med. Child Neurol.*, **34**, 321–337.

Tardieu, G., Tardieu, C., Colbeau-Justin, P. and Lespargot, A. (1982). Muscle hypoextensibility in children with cerebral palsy. Therapeutic implications. *Arch. Phys. Med. Rehabil.*, **63**, 103–107.

Titchener, J. (1983) A preliminary evaluation of Conductive Education. *Physiother.*, **69**, 8, 313–315.

Trauner, D.A. and Manuino, F.L. (1986) Neurodevelopmental outcome after neonatal cerebrovascular accident. *J. Pediatr.*, **108**, 459

Tremblay, F., Malouin, F., Richards, C.L. and Dumas, F. (in press) Effects of prolonged muscle stretch on reflex and voluntary muscle activations in children with spastic cerebral palsy. *Scand. J. Rehabil. Med.*

Tronick, E. and Brazelton, T.B. (1975) Clinical uses of the Brazelton Neonatal Behavioral Assessment Scale. In: *Exceptional Infant* 3, edited by B.Z. Friedlander *et al.* New York: Bruner Mazel.

Twitchell, T.E. (1959) On the motor deficit in congenital bilateral athetosis. *J. Nerv. Ment. Dis.*, **129**, 105.

van de Heyning, P.H., Marquet, J.F. and Creten, W.L. (1980) Drooling in children with cerebral palsy. *Acta Oto-Rhino-Laryng Belgica*, **34**, 691–705.

van der Weel, F.R., van der Meer, A.L.H. and Lee, D.N. (1991) Effect of task on movement control in cerebral palsy: implications for assessment and therapy. *Develop. Med. Child Neurol.*, **33**, 419–426.

Vaughan, C.W., Neilson, P.D. and O'Dwyer, N.J. (1988) Motor control deficits of orofacial muscles in cerebral palsy. *J. Neurol. Neurosurg. Psychiat.*, **51**, 534–539.

Vaughn, C.L., Berman, B., Peacock, W.J. *et al.* (1989) Gait analysis and rhizotomy: past experiences and future considerations. In: *Neurosurgery: State of the Arts Reviews*, 4, 2, edited by T.S. Park, L.H. Phillips and W.J. Peacock. Philadelphia: Hanley and Belfus.

Vining, E.P.G., Accardo, P.J., Rubenstein, J.E. *et al.* (1976) Cerebral palsy, a pediatric developmentalist's overview. *Am. J. Dis. Child.*, **130**, 643.

Vojta, V. (1984) The basic elements of treatment according to Vojta. In: *Management of the Motor Disorders of Children with Cerebral Palsy*, edited by D. Scrutton. London: Blackwell Scientific.

Volpe, J.J. (1979) Intracranial hemorrhage in the newborn: current understanding and dilemmas. *Neurol.*, **29**, 732.

Volpe, J.J (1981) *Neurology of the Newborn*. Philadelphia: W.B. Saunders.

Volpe, J.J., Herscovitch, P., Perlman, J.M. *et al.* (1985) Positron emission tomography in the asphyxiated term newborn: parasagittal impairment of cerebral blood flow. *Ann. Neurol.*, **17**, 287.

Weindling, A.M., Rochefort, M.J., Calvert, S.A., Fok, T-F. and Wilkinson, A. (1985) Development of cerebral palsy after ultrasonographic detection of periventricular cysts in newborn. *Develop. Med. Child Neurol.*, **27**, 800–806.

Wigglesworth, J. (1984) Brain development and its modification by adverse influences. *Clin. Develop. Med.*, **87**, 12–26.

Wilson, J. (1991) Cerebral palsy. In: *Pediatric Neurologic Physical Therapy*, edited by S.K. Campbell. New York: Churchill Livingstone.

Winter, D.A. (1987) *The Biomechanics and Motor Control of Human Gait*. Waterloo, Ontario: University of Waterloo Press.

Wright, T. and Nicholson, J. (1973) Physiotherapy for the spastic child: an evaluation. *Develop. Med. Child Neurol.*, **15**, 146–163.

Yokochi, K., Inukai, K., Hosoe, A., Shimabukuro, S. Kitazumi, E. and Kodama, K. (1991) Leg movements in the supine position of infants with spastic diplegia. *Develop. Med. Child Neurol.*, **33**, 903–907.

Young, J.A. (1980) Clinical experience in the use of baclofen in children with spastic cerebral palsy: a further report. *Scott Med. J. Suppl.*, **1**, 523.

Ziv, I., Blackburn, N., Rang, M. and Koreska, J. (1984) Muscle growth in normal and spastic mice. *Develop. Med. Child Neurol.*, **26**, 94–99.

Further reading

Berger, W., Horstmann, G. and Dietz, V. (1984) Tension development and muscle activation in the leg during gait in spastic hemiparesis: independence of muscle hypotonia and exaggerated stretch reflexes. *J. Neurol. Neurosurg. Psychiatry*, **47**, 1029–1033.

Bruininks, R.H. (1978) *Bruininks-Oseretsky Test of Motor Proficiency: Examiner's Manual*. Circle Pines, MN: American Guidance Service.

Campbell, S.K. (1983) Effects of developmental intervention in the special care nursery. In: *The Advances in Developmental and Behavioral Pediatrics*, edited by M.L. Wolraich and D. Routh. Greenwich, CT: JAI Press, pp. 165–179.

Cole, J. (1989) A review of the effect of early intervention programmes on the developmental status of very preterm, very low birth weight infants. *Aust. J. Physiother.*, **35**, 3, 131–139.

Fetters, L. (1991) Cerebral palsy: contemporary treatment concepts. *Proceedings of IISTEP Conference*. Alexandria, Virginia: Foundation for Physical Therapy.

Goodman, M., Rothberg, A.D., Houston-McMillan, R., Cooper, P.A., Cartwright, J.D. and van der Velde, M.A. (1985) Effect of early neurodevelopmental therapy in normal and at-risk survivors of neonatal intensive care. *Lancet*, 1327–1330.

Hoffer, M.M. and Perry, J. (1983) Pathodynamics of gait alterations in cerebral palsy and the significance of kinetic electromyography in evaluating foot and ankle problems. *Foot Ankle*, **4**, 128–134.

Lee, D.N., Daniel, B.M. and Turnbull, J. (1990) Basic perceptuo-motor dysfunctions in cerebral palsy. In: *Attention and Performance XIII*, edited by M. Jeannerod. Hillsdale, NJ: Erlbaum, pp. 583–603.

Moseley, A. and Adams, R. (1991) Measurement of passive ankle dorsiflexion: procedure and reliability. *Aust. J. Physiother.*, **37**, 3, 175–181.

Norlin, R. and Odenrick, P. (1986) Development of gait in spastic children with cerebral palsy. *J. Pediat. Orthop.*, **6**, 674–680.

Olney, S.J., MacPhail, H.E.A., Hedden, D.M. and Boyce, W.F. (1990) Work and power in hemiplegic cerebral palsy gait. *Phys. Ther.*, **70**, 7, 431–438.

Richards, C.L., Malouin, F. and Dumas, F. (1991) Effects of a single session of prolonged plantarflexor stretch on muscle activations during gait in spastic cerebral palsy. *Scand. J. Rehab. Med.*, **23**, 103–111.

Stuberg, W.A. (1991) Bone density changes in non-ambulatory children following discontinuation of passive standing programs. *Proceedings of American Academy of Cerebral Palsy and Developmental Medicine Conference*. Louisville, KY.

Tardieu, C., Lespargot, A., Tabary, C. and Bret, M.D. (1988) Toe-walking in children with cerebral palsy: contributions of contracture of triceps surae muscle. *Phys. Ther.*, **69**, 8, 656–662.

Wilhelm, I.J. (Ed.) (1993) *Physical Therapy Assessment in Early Infancy*. New York: Churchill Livingstone.

Winters, T.F., Gage, J.R. and Hicks, R. (1987) Gait patterns in spastic hemiplegia in children and young adults. *J. Bone Jt. Surg.*, **69-A**, 437–441.

6

Acute brain injury

Head trauma is a major cause of serious disability and death in childhood. Many children with head trauma recover uneventfully. Others, however, are left with epilepsy, motor disability, and/or learning, behavioural and emotional disorders. Head injuries are seen in children as the result of motor vehicle and bicycle accidents, falls, diving accidents and contact sports. Young children are prone to accidents, partly because of their unawareness of danger, partly because of their immature nervous system, which makes them clumsy and poor at maintaining their balance.

However, they may also be the victims of inadequate protection (seat belts in motor vehicles and bicycle helmets) as well as abuse from parents or care-givers. Acute brain injury at birth accounts for a significant proportion of head injuries in infants (DiRocco and Velardi 1986).

Mechanical forces acting on the cranium may expose the brain to the effects of acceleration (when a stationary head is hit by a solid object such as a ball), deceleration (when the moving head hits a relatively fixed object such as a windscreen or the pavement) or rotation (when a blow is asymmetrical). The latter is a common result in both acceleration and deceleration injuries. Injuries may be focal, diffuse or a mixture of both. Diffuse axonal injury is considered to be due to shearing forces and may only be evident microscopically.

Pathophysiological mechanisms of acute brain injury

The space inside the cranium is occupied by brain tissue, blood and cerebrospinal fluid and the sum of these three volumes is a constant. When a mass such as a haematoma is present, the surrounding tissues are compressed. In other words, an increase in volume by one component leads to a decrease in volume of another component. As space available is finite, increase in mass (for example, haematoma, oedema) will cause an increase in intracranial pressure (Maset *et al.* 1987).

Oxygen and nutrient supply to the brain is dependent upon the integrity of cerebral perfusion (Noah *et al.* 1992). Alterations in perfusion pressure may occur, with high-perfusion pressure causing vasoconstriction and low pressure causing vasodilation. If pressure reaches a critical low, ischaemia results.

The infant's brain is more vulnerable to injury than an adult's and in infants the injury occurs to an immature structure. Rapid changes in neuronal development, myelination and biochemical changes occur significantly within the first 2 years. The effects of the injury on growth and maturational processes are poorly understood (Fletcher *et al.* 1987; Ewing-Cobbs *et al.* 1989). The immediate effects of head injury may be *concussion* (temporary and reversible), *cerebral contusion or laceration* (direct bruising or tearing of tissue) and *intracranial haemorrhage* (from tearing of the middle meningeal artery or its branches), *subdural haematoma* (injury to veins in the subdural space) or *subarachnoid haemorrhage* (commonly accompanying contusion or laceration).

Concussion is a clinical state characterized by transient impairment of consciousness occurring immediately after the injury and lasting from a few seconds to a few hours. The force of the injury is less than that which would produce a fracture of the cranium. Intracranial pressure rises, causing a temporary shearing strain on the brainstem and this causes unconsciousness. Bruce (1990) has hypothesized that the mechanism of concussion is a combination of stretch, shearing injury to white matter plus transient dysfunction of the reticular formation. There is no obvious pathological change in the brain but concussion may be followed by some degree of amnesia. Post-concussion syndrome may occur in some children, with headache, irritability and impaired concentration in older children and inattention and regressive or aggressive behaviour in younger children (Craft 1975). These changes may last for days or months.

Cerebral contusion and laceration Contusion is a bruising of brain tissue caused by a blunt head injury, whereas a laceration is usually caused by a penetrating injury. Contusion of the brain in infants under the age of 5 months appears to cause a morphologically distinct pathology compared to this injury in older children (Lindenberg and Freytag 1969). Infants were severe blunt head trauma typically show gross tears in cerebral white matter with microscopic tears in the outermost cortex. There is frequently widespread involvement of the brain, which is due to the brain's mobility within the relatively rigid cranium. Thus the effects of a blow to one side of the head (coup) may be seen on the opposite side where the brain has hit against that side of the cranium (contrecoup), as well as in the brain stem due to the movement of this confined area against the adjacent bony projections.

Epidural and subdural haemorrhage may occur after relatively mild head injury such as occurs when the infant is severely shaken or suffers a jarring fall.

As well as the effects due directly to the impact on the head, termed primary brain injury, indirect damage to the central nervous system, which is more common than direct cellular damage, can also occur as a result of hypoxia, ischaemia or intracranial hypertension (Noah *et al.* 1992). Secondary brain damage occurs as a result of such intracranial factors as cerebral oedema and extracranial factors such as hypoxaemia or hypotension. Prevention of secondary brain injury is a major goal in management of the head-injured child.

Prognosis

The problems resulting from head trauma in children are basically the same as in adults, but there are some differences. The infant and young child's brain is relatively immature, and although there may be severe signs of brain injury such as decerebrate or decorticate rigidity and long periods of unconsciousness, it has been generally believed that a child will make a better recovery than an adult with a similar injury (Lewin 1966, Fletcher *et al.* 1987). However, studies using sensitive psychometric measures suggest children may have a poorer outcome than adults (Fletcher *et al.* 1987) and other authors have questioned the theory of early brain plasticity (St James Roberts 1979; Ewing-Cobbs *et al.* 1985).

Most children hospitalized after a head injury with loss of consciousness or a cranial fracture recover completely within 24–48 hours. A small number of these children may show postconcussion syndrome or develop post-traumatic epilepsy. Children who have persistent coma and who develop motor dysfunction and cognitive impairment can show improvement for more than 3 years (Richardson 1963). Reviews of outcome include those of Gilchrist and Wilkinson (1979), Jennett and Teasdale (1981), Eiben *et al.* (1984) and Filley *et al.* (1987).

Categories of possible outcome after acute brain injury are listed as:

1 Death.
2 Persistent vegetative state.
3 Severe disability.
4 Moderate disability.
5 Good recovery (Jennett and Bond 1975; Jennett and Teasdale 1981).

The Glasgow Coma Scale (GCS) was devised by Teasdale and Jennett (1974) as a graded measure of motor responsiveness, verbal responsiveness and eye-opening. The best response for each behaviour is recorded and the sum of the grades for each response is taken as an indication of the depth of coma, ranging from 3 (deepest level) to 15. This scale is difficult to apply to infants and young children and there have been attempts to adapt it to this group (e.g. Ewing-Cobbs *et al.* 1989).

The GCS has also been used in attempts to anticipate eventual functional outcome in adults (e.g. Raimondi and Hirschauer 1984) and children (Leurssen *et al.* 1988), although such prognostication is problematic. Bruce (1985) found that children with GCS scores of 6 or better had an 80–90% chance of recovery with independent function and minimal neurological deficit, while with a score of 4 or 5, cognitive and neurological deficits could be anticipated. Length of coma has also been found to be a predictor of outcome (Filley *et al.* 1987). Coma for more than 24 hours has been found to be a predictor of neurological abnormality in children (Brink *et al.* 1980). Another study has shown that almost 100% of children and adolescents whose coma had lasted less than 13 weeks regained independent ambulation (Stover and Zeiger 1975). It has been reported that when coma lasts longer than 3 weeks, some degree of permanent cognitive impairment can be anticipated (Bruce 1985) and IQ score at 1 year post-trauma is reported to relate directly to length of coma (Hoffer *et al.* 1990).

Severity of injury is typically considered the major predictor of motor function outcome. In a study of 26 children who were unconscious for more than 90 days, considerable variability in outcome 2 years after injury was reported (Kriel *et al.* 1988). The two extremes noted were the 6 children who remained in a persistent vegetative state, and the 1 subject who was expected to live independently and be competitively employed. The authors report that the only helpful predictor was the total computed tomography atrophy score.

Factors such as premorbid functional level, family background, presence of cognitive impairment, the nature of motor training and the presence of an environment which encourages motor learning may also be predictive. It is not usual to consider that the type of rehabilitation may affect motor outcome since the lesion itself is considered the most important factor. Nevertheless, it is evident from animal studies (Ogden and Fransz 1971; Black *et al.* 1975; Held 1987) and from studies of motor learning and training in non-disabled humans that the process of rehabilitation (i.e. what the individual practises and for how long) and the environment in which it is carried out may have a significant effect on the extent of recovery of function (Carr and Shepherd 1987b; 1990).

Clinical features

The clinical features depend upon the severity of the trauma and the areas of the brain involved. The early features may include vomiting, restlessness, or drowsiness, developing into unconsciousness, coma or decerebrate rigidity. The later features include problems of motor control, ataxia (dyssynergia, dysmetria), inability to perform rapid movements, difficulty timing force production, spasticity and weakness, visuo-motor dysfunction, distractibility and impairment of memory and concentration, headaches, vertigo or post-traumatic epilepsy (Klonoff *et al.* 1977; Gulbrandsen 1984). Children may develop deficits some time after injury, and this may be due to progressive neurological dysfunction or to difficulty coping with increased demands which occur as the child grows older (Lehr 1989).

In terms of motor dysfunction, the incidence of spasticity (hyperreflexia) and ataxia is said to be very high in children with severe head injury. Ataxia is probably more common than may be recognized by clinicians, although the child may be recognized as being clumsy.

Changes in behaviour and personality may include hyperactivity, distractibility, poor social judgement, impulsivity, emotional lability, low frustration tolerance, temper tantrums and aggression (Ewing-Cobbs and Fletcher 1987; Hoffer *et al.* 1990). Behaviour problems may be severe enough to interfere with rehabilitation. However, they may present the greatest difficulty when the child tries to cope with life at home and at school.

Heterotopic ossification, particularly around shoulders, elbows, hips and knees, may occur in children in prolonged coma. Soft tissue contractures caused by immobility and persistent posturing and compounded by hyperexcitability of the motoneuron pool can occur rather rapidly in unconscious or relatively immobile children and if not prevented will be a significant factor interfering with the regaining of motor control once the child regains consciousness. Soft tissue contracture can be a persistent problem in children with muscle imbalance.

Medical management

The neurological examination includes assessment of alertness, orientation and memory, an ophthalmological examination, testing of sensory and motor function, reflexes, coordination, presence and extent of amnesia. The GCS is commonly used to assess level of consciousness (Jennett and Teasdale 1977). X-ray, computed tomography, magnetic resonance imaging and cranial ultrasonography all play a part in the medical assessment.

The goal of immediate medical management is stabilization and maintenance of vital signs, ensuring adequate oxygen and nutrient delivery to the brain. Medical care is described in detail by Noah *et al.* (1992) and others. Serial monitoring of respiratory rate, blood pressure, pulse rate, temperature, intracranial pressure and level of consciousness is carried out. Intubation and artificial ventilation may be required to prevent repeated episodes of hypoxia and cyanosis (Ellis 1990). Children with acute brain injury are kept as calm and undisturbed as possible. If they are intubated, comatose or chemically paralysed, they are nursed in supine (Noah *et al.* 1992). The head may be kept elevated and in the midline (Mitchell *et al.* 1982), to facilitate cerebral venous return. However, the elevated head position may decrease blood pressure (Rosner and Coley 1986). If coma is prolonged, nasooesophageal feeding will be necessary to ensure adequate fluid intake and nutrition.

Children with head trauma frequently have additional injuries which may include spinal cord injury, brachial plexus injury or fractures of ribs, spine or limb bones. These injuries will further complicate an already complex management and will often have a considerable impact on motor function (Tepas *et al.* 1989).

Physiotherapy management

The major goals of physiotherapy in the early stages after acute brain injury relate principally to *respiratory management*, which may include methods of ensuring clear airways with modified bronchial drainage and assisted breathing exercises, as part of the team involved in preventing secondary brain injury (see Chapter 27; Ellis 1990). Postural drainage typically needs to be modified since the head-dependent position is contraindicated where there is a risk of increased intracranial pressure.

The *prevention of soft tissue contracture* is also an important consideration in the early stages in order that the child's musculoskeletal system is as flexible as possible when motor training can commence. Secondary musculoskeletal complications are known to be associated with a poor functional outcome (Perry 1980). Normal motor performance will not be possible in the presence of muscle length adaptations as these length-associated changes have an adverse effect on both the passive and active properties of the muscles (Gossman *et al.* 1982; Herbert 1988). Soft tissue contractures have been reported as being very common following acute brain injury (Yarkony and Sahgal 1987). Muscles at particular risk of shortening at this stage are hip and knee flexors and ankle plantarflexors, and adductors and flexors of the upper limb. It is very difficult and in many cases impossible to prevent contractures in deeply comatose children. The supine position should be avoided if possible where this position stimulates dystonic posturing. It is doubtful whether passive range of motion exercises have any effect on contracture development in the immobile individual (Williams 1990). However, passive movements of limbs provide an opportunity to make some contact with the child, and the therapist while moving the limbs should talk to the child, describing the movements being done. At times when the level of consciousness improves, making contact in this way may help the child keep in touch with the surroundings. Brief periods of passive stretching appear not to be effective in improving either muscle activation or functional activity (Richards *et al.* 1991). Active exercise, if necessary assisted, should start as soon as possible and the child positioned in sitting and standing as soon as vital signs are stable.

The use of *serial casting* has been shown to be effective in both children (Tardieu *et al.* 1982a; Conine *et al.* 1990) and adults (Booth *et al.* 1983) in correcting contracture of the calf muscles following acute brain injury. Casting applied very early – that is, while the child is still in intensive care – may be instrumental in preventing calf muscle contractures from occurring. There is some evidence that this is so (Barnard *et al.* 1984; Imie *et al.* 1986). Other joints may also require serial casting. The use of a dynamic splint to correct a long-standing contracture of the elbow flexors is described by MacKay-Lyons (1989).

Casting enables a joint to be restrained with imposed lengthening of muscles that are at risk of shortening. Where muscles are already shortened, casts are reapplied periodically as the muscles gradually lengthen. The main features of serial casts are described by Carr and Shepherd (1987a) and Ada and Canning (1990). Casts are applied with minimum padding to ensure a sustained stretch. Care is taken when applying a cast over the ankle joint, that, in producing sufficient force to gain some stretch to the calf, the alignment of the foot is preserved. This is particularly important in infants and small children, whose feet can be easily pushed into a rocker shape by force applied to the forefoot instead of to the ankle joint. Once a cast is applied, motor training should continue, in stance when the calf muscles have been casted, since the maintenance of any muscle-lengthening gained will be dependent upon the child actively preserving muscle length and flexibility. The beneficial effects of casting have been shown to be lost within 6 months of their removal (Watt *et al.* 1986), indicating the importance of the child gaining improved control over muscle activation.

It should be noted that casting may increase the range of joint movement by lengthening either the muscle or the tendon or both (Tardieu *et al.* 1982a and b) but only lengthening of the muscle will increase the range over which the muscle can actively generate tension.

Evaluation of motor performance and motor training

The motor dysfunction of children with acute brain injury has not been subject to much detailed analysis and there is little information relating nature and site of lesion to motor dysfunction and motor outcome (Pang 1985). As in cerebral palsy, the clinical assumption has been that the movement problems derive principally from spasticity, the release of abnormal reflexes and an abnormal postural reflex mechanism (Bobath 1985). This approach has not encouraged an analysis of the effects of the negative features associated with upper motor neuron lesions, such as problems activating muscles, generating and timing force appropriately, or of ataxia and adaptive motor behaviour, upon the performance of everyday actions. Nevertheless, an understanding of the motor performance deficits and of the motor control problems underlying these deficits is critical both as a means of planning motor training and as a way of evaluating change. To add further complexity, the brain injury may occur at a time when motor abilities are not fully matured (Fletcher *et al.* 1987).

Evaluation of motor performance and training for infants and children following acute brain injury follows the same principles as described in Chapter 3. Recent developments in the treatment or training of adults with brain injury have stressed the need for task- and context-specific motor training based on biomechanical models of performance and techniques for promoting motor learning (Carr and Shepherd 1987a and b; 1990). Results of studies with adults following stroke have suggested that this movement-science based approach is effective in normalizing the biomechanics of sit-to-stand (Mungovan and Shepherd 1991; Ada and Westwood 1992), in improving performance on a functional motor scale (Dean and Mackey 1992) and in improving gait (Malouin *et al.* 1992). An emphasis on functional training for children with acute brain injury is also stressed by Blaskey (1992). However, as in physiotherapy for children with cerebral palsy, the treatment approaches in common use, including NDT or Bobath therapy, have neither been shown to be effective in improving motor performance and functional effectiveness (see Chapter 5), nor are they based on an up-to-date scientific foundation (Haley *et al.* 1990).

Analysis of motor performance should include observational analysis of the performance of everyday actions (such as sit-to-stand, walking, reaching, manipulation) and other actions as necessary (e.g. jumping and hopping on one leg). In addition, biomechanical and other measurements are carried out to enable measurement of outcome (e.g. Moseley and Adams 1991). Evaluation of motor proficiency should be carried out in unsupervised as well as supervised situations and should include evaluation of such factors as attention span, memory, ability to plan appropriate motor actions and problem-solving ability (Haley *et al*. 1990). Even if motor performance in actions such as walking, standing up and reaching to grasp an object approximates normal performance, it is the ability to match intention to action, to use judgement and to predict the consequences of an action, which is critical to effective motor performance.

Following head injury, some children have cognitive and behaviour problems which may interfere with the rehabilitation process. Such children may benefit from *attention control training* (Adams 1990). Adams points out that the attentional abilities necessary for normal functioning include the ability to focus attention on a task, to sustain concentration, to shift attention if relevant information is presented and to ignore irrelevant inputs. The following are some training techniques which may be useful.

The child may be helped to focus on the task by making eye contact with the therapist as an aid to concentration, while the task is briefly explained; by reinforcing attention to the task through meaningful feedback (Smith *et al*. 1985); by modifying the task or the environment to ensure some measure of success (see Chapter 3), and by arranging the environment initially to minimize distractions, gradually adding them as the child's attention improves.

Carry-over of improved performance outside the therapy room and practice of the desired action can be obtained by techniques such as covert monitoring (Canning and Adams 1985). With some children who appear not to be aware of their problems or who may be denying them, it is necessary to bring the child's attention not only to the task to be practised but also to the discrepancy between the child's own dysfunctional performance and a functional model (see Gouvier 1987).

Behaviour management techniques are necessary when a child displays either a disruptive or a socially inappropriate behaviour, or if motivation appears low (Adams 1990). As Meyerson and colleagues have pointed out (1967), lack of motivation is the therapist's problem rather than the patient's. Motivation may be enhanced by selecting actions for training that are relevant to the child and which are challenging, yet achievable, and by ensuring that the child receives feedback. However, functional reinforcers may also be needed (Hollon 1973; Lincoln 1981; Adams and Ramsey 1988).

Summary

Acute brain injury is a relatively common cause of death and morbidity in young children and adolescents. The problems which result can be complex and far-reaching, affecting motor and cognitive function, behaviour and personality and, therefore, the overall ability of the child to function effectively, succeed at school and ultimately in the work place. A multidisciplinary team of physicians, surgeons, therapists, psychologists and special educators is necessary for the early and subsequent long-term management of children with problems related to acute brain injury.

In the early stages, the major role of the physiotherapist is in aiding the preservation of effective respiratory function by clearing airways and promoting an efficient breathing pattern. In addition, the physiotherapist plays a critical role in ensuring the flexibility of the musculoskeletal system in order that the child will be able to commence an active training programme as soon as possible. The effect of the brain injury on motor abilities in the long term will depend on the severity of the original lesion and any subsequent secondary brain damage, the brain's capacity for reorganization (which may be related to its maturity at the time of the lesion), the effect of cognitive and behavioural deficits on learning and the quality of motor training and educational programmes during rehabilitation (Haley *et al*. 1990).

References

Ada, L. and Canning, C. (1990) Anticipating and avoiding muscle shortening. In: *Key Issues in Neurological Physiotherapy*, edited by L. Ada and C. Canning. Oxford: Butterworth-Heinemann, pp. 219–236.

Ada, L. and Westwood, P. (1992) A kinematic analysis of recovery of the ability to stand up following stroke. *Aust. J. Physiother.*, **38**, 2, 135–142.

Adams, R. (1990) Attention control training and behaviour management. In: *Key Issues in Neurological Physio-*

therapy, edited by L. Ada and C. Canning. Oxford: Butterworth-Heinemann, pp. 81–97.

Adams, R. and Ramsey, S. (1988) Behaviour management with brain-injured patients: case studies from a rehabilitation centre. In: *Advances in Behavioural Medicine, 5*, edited by J.L. Sheppard. Sydney: Cumberland College Press.

Barnard, P., Dill, H., Eldredge, P. *et al.* (1984) Reduction of hypertonicity by early casting in a comatose head-injured individual. A case report. *Phys. Ther.*, **64**, 10, 1540–1542.

Black, P., Markowitz, R.S. and Cianci, S.N. (1975) Recovery of motor function after lesions in motor cortex of monkeys. *Ciba Found. Symp.*, **34**, 65–83.

Blaskey, J. (1992) Head trauma. In: *Pediatric Neurologic Physical Therapy*, 2nd edn, edited by S.K. Campbell. New York: Churchill Livingstone.

Bobath, B. (1985) *Abnormal Postural Activity Caused by Lesions of the Brain*. Oxford: Butterworth-Heinemann.

Booth, B.J., Doyle, M. and Montgomery, J. (1983) Serial casting for the management of spasticity in the head-injured adult. *Phys. Ther.*, **63**, 1960–1966.

Brink, J.D., Imbus, C. and Woo-Sam, J. (1980) Physical recovery after severe closed head trauma in children and adolescents. *J. Pediatr.*, **97**, 721–727.

Bruce, D.A. (1985) Outcome – does it work? In: *Progress in Pediatric Trauma*, edited by B.H. Harris. Boston: Nobb Hill Press.

Bruce, D.A. (1990) Scope of the problem: early assessment and management. In: *Rehabilitation of the Adult and Child with Traumatic Head Injury*, edited by M. Rosenthal, E.R. Griffith, M.R. Bond *et al.*, 2nd edn. Philadelphia, PA: F.A. Davis.

Canning, C. and Adams R. (1985) Covert monitoring to promote consistency of walking performance: a case study. *Aust. J. Physiother.*, **31**, 152.

Carr, J.H. and Shepherd, R.B. (1987a) *A Motor Relearning Programme for Stroke*, 2nd edn. Oxford: Butterworth-Heinemann.

Carr, J.H. and Shepherd, R.B. (1987b) A motor learning model for rehabilitation. In: *Movement Science. Foundations for Physical Therapy in Rehabilitation*, edited by J.H. Carr and R.B. Shepherd. Rockville, MD: Aspen.

Carr, J.H. and Shepherd, R.B. (1990) A motor learning model for rehabilitation of the movement-disabled. In: *Key Issues in Neurological Physiotherapy*, edited by L. Ada and C. Canning. Oxford: Butterworth-Heinemann.

Conine, T.A., Sullivan, T., Mackie, T. *et al.* (1990) Effect of serial casting for the prevention of equinus in patients with acute head injury. *Arch. Phys. Med. Rehabil.*, **71**, 310–312.

Craft, A.W. (1975) Head injury in children. In: *Handbook of Clinical Neurology*, edited by P.J. Vinken and G.W. Bruyn. Amsterdam: North Holland.

Dean, C. and Mackey, F. (1992) Motor Assessment Scale scores as a measure of rehabilitation outcome following stroke. *Aust. J. Physiother.*, **38**, 1, 31–35.

DiRocco, C. and Velardi, F. (1986) Epidemiology and etiology of craniocerebral trauma in the first two years of life.

In: *Head Injuries in the Newborn and Infant*, edited by A.J. Raimondi, M. Choux and C. DiRocco. New York: Springer-Verlag.

Eiben, C.F., Anderson, T.P., Lockman, L. *et al.* (1984) Functional outcome of closed head injury in children and young adults. *Arch. Phys. Med. Rehabil.*, **65**, 168–170.

Ellis, E. (1990) Respiratory function following head injury. In: *Key Issues in Neurological Physiotherapy*, edited by L. Ada and C. Canning. Oxford: Butterworth-Heinemann.

Ewing-Cobbs, L. and Fletcher, J.M. (1987) Neuropsychological assessment in head injury in children. *J. Learning Disorders*, **20**, 526.

Ewing-Cobbs, L., Fletcher, J.M. and Levin, H.S. (1985) Neuropsychological sequelae following pediatric head injury. In: *Head Injury Rehabilitation: Children and Adolescents*, edited by M. Yivisaker. Boston, MA: College-Hill.

Ewing-Cobbs, L., Miner, M.E., Fletcher, J.M. *et al.* (1989) Intellectual, motor and language sequelae following closed head injury in infants and preschoolers. *J. Pediatr. Psychol.*, **14**, 531–547.

Filley, C.M., Cranberg, L.D., Alexander, M.P. *et al.* (1987) Neurobehavioral outcome after closed head injury in childhood and adolescence. *Arch. Neurol.*, **44**, 194–198.

Fletcher, J.M., Miner, M.E. and Ewing-Cobbs, L. (1987) Age and recovery from head injury in children: developmental issues. In: *Neurobéhavioral Recovery from Head Injury*, edited by H.S. Levin, J. Grafman and H.M. Eisenberg. New York: Oxford University Press.

Gilchrist, E. and Wilkinson, M. (1979) Some factors determining prognosis in young people with severe head injuries. *Arch. Neurol.*, **36**, 355.

Gossman, M.R., Sahrmann, S.A. and Rose, S.J. (1982) Review of length-associated changes in muscle. *Phys. Ther.*, **62**, 12, 1799.

Gouvier, W.D. (1987) Assessment and treatment of cognitive deficits in brain-damaged individuals. *Behav. Mod.*, **11**, 312.

Gulbrandsen, G.B. (1984) Neuropsychological sequelae of light head injuries in older children 6 months after trauma. *J. Clin. Neuropsychol.*, **6**, 257–268.

Haley, S.M., Cioffi, M.I., Lewin, J.E. *et al.* (1990) Motor dysfunction in children and adolescents after traumatic brain injury. *J. Head Trauma Rehabil.*, **5**, 4, 77–90.

Held, J. (1987) Recovery of function after brain damage. In: *Movement Science. Foundations for Physical Therapy in Rehabilitation*, edited by J.H. Carr and R.B. Shepherd. Rockville, MD: Aspen.

Herbert, R. (1988) The passive mechanical properties of muscles and their adaptations to altered patterns of use. *Aust. J. Physiother.*, **34**, 3, 141.

Hoffer, M., Brink, J., Marsh, J.S. *et al.* (1990) Head injuries. In: *Pediatric Orthopedics*, edited by W.W. Lovell and R.B. Winter. Philadelphia, PA: J.B. Lippincott.

Hollon, T.H. (1973) Behavior modification in a community hospital rehabilitation unit. *Arch. Phys. Med. Rehabil.*, **54**, 65.

Imie, P.C., Eppinghaus, C.E. and Boughton, A.C. (1986) Efficacy of non-bivalved and bivalved serial casting on head-injured patients in intensive care. *Phys. Ther.*, **66**, 748.

Jennett, B. and Bond, M. (1975) Assessment of outcome after severe brain damage: a practical scale. *Lancet*, **1**, 480.

Jennett, B. and Teasdale, G. (1977) Aspects of coma after severe head injury. *Lancet*, Apr. 23, 878–881.

Jennett, B., and Teasdale, G. (1981) *Management of Head Injuries*. Philadelphia, PA: F.A. Davis.

Klonoff, H., Low, M.D. and Clark, C. (1977) Head injuries in children: prospective five year follow-up. *J. Neurol. Neurosurg. Psychiatry*, **40**, 1211–1219.

Kriel, R.L., Krach, L.E. and Sheehan, M. (1988) Pediatric closed head injury: outcome following prolonged unconsciousness. *Arch. Phys. Med. Rehabil.*, **69**, 678–681.

Lehr, E. (1989) Community integration after traumatic brain injury: infants and children. In: *Traumatic Brain Injury*, edited by P. Bach-y-Rita. New York: Demos Publications.

Leurssen, T.G., Klauber, M.K. and Marshall, L.F. (1988) Outcome from head injury related to patient's age. *J. Neurosurg.*, **68**, 409–416.

Lewin, W. (1966) *The Management of Head Injuries*. London: Bailliere Tindall & Cassell.

Lincoln, N.B. (1981) Clinical psychology. In: *Rehabilitation after Severe Head Injury*, edited by C.D. Evans. Edinburgh: Churchill Livingstone.

Lindenberg, R. and Freytag, E. (1969) Morphology of brain lesions from blunt trauma in early infancy. *Arch. Pathol.*, **87**, 298.

MacKay-Lyons, M. (1989) Low-load, prolonged stretch in treatment of elbow flexion contractures secondary to head trauma: a case report. *Phys. Ther.*, **69**, 4, 292–296.

Malouin, F., Potvin, M., Prevost, J., Richards, C.L. and Wood-Dauphinee, S. (1992) Use of an intensive task-oriented gait training program in a series of patients with acute cerebrovascular accidents. *Phys. Ther.*, **72**, 11, 781–793.

Maset, A.L., Marmarou, A., Ward, J.D. *et al.* (1987) Pressure–volume index in head injury. *J. Neurosurg.*, **67**, 832–840.

Meyerson, L., Kerr, N. and Michael, J. (1967) Behaviour modification in rehabilitation. In: *Child Development: Readings in Experimental Analysis*, edited by S. Bijou and D. Baer. New York: Appleton-Century-Crofts.

Mitchell, P.H., Ozuna, J. and Lipe, H.P. (1982) Moving the patient in bed: effects on intracranial pressure. *Nurs. Res.*, **30**, 212–218.

Moseley, A. and Adams, R. (1991) Measurement of passive ankle dorsiflexion: procedure and reliability. *Aust. J. Physiother.*, **37**, 3, 175–181.

Mungovan, S. and Shepherd, R.B. (1991) The effect of specific standing up training on functional outcome following stroke. *Proceedings of the 11th WCPT Congress*, London.

Noah, Z.L., Hahn, Y.S., Rubenstein, J.S. *et al.* (1992) Management of the child with severe brain injury. *Prog. Pediatr. Clin. Care*, **8**, 1, 59–77.

Ogden, R. and Fransz, S.I. (1971) On cerebral motor control: the recovery from experimentally produced hemiplegia. *Psychobiology*, **33**, 49.

Pang, D. (1985) Pathophysiologic correlates of neurobehavioral syndromes following closed head injury. In: *Head Injury Rehabilitation: Children and Adolescents*, edited by M. Yivisakar. Boston, MA: College-Hill.

Perry, J. (1980) Rehabilitation of spasticity. In: *Spasticity: Disordered Motor Control*, edited by R.G. Feldman, R.R. Young and K.P. Werner. Chicago, IL: Year Book, pp. 87–99.

Raimondi, A.J. and Hirschauer, J. (1984) Head injury in infant and toddler: coma scoring and outcome scale. *Childs Brain*, **11**, 12–35.

Richards, C.L., Malouin, F. and Dumas, F. (1991) Effects of a single session of prolonged plantarflexor stretch on muscle activations during gait in spastic cerebral palsy. *Scand. J. Rehabil. Med.*, **23**, 103–111.

Richardson, F. (1963) Some effects of severe head injury: a follow-up study of children and adolescents after protracted coma. *Dev. Med. Child Neurol.*, **5**, 471.

Rosner, M.J. and Coley, I.B. (1986) Cerebral perfusion, intracranial pressure, and head elevation. *J. Neurosurg.*, **65**, 636–641.

St James Roberts, I. (1979) Neurological plasticity, recovery from brain insult, and child development. In: *Advances in Child Behavior and Development*, vol. 14, edited by H.W. Reese and L.P. Lyscott. New York: Academic Press.

Smith, J., Henriques, M. and Parsonson, B. (1985) The use of reinforcement procedures in training hand movement of CVA hemiplegic. *Behav. Change*, **2**, 52.

Stover, S.L. and Zeiger, H.E. (1975) Head injury in children and teenagers: functional recovery correlated with duration of coma. *Arch. Phys. Med. Rehabil.*, **57**, 201–205.

Tardieu, C., Huet de la Tour, E., Bret, M.D. *et al.* (1982) Muscle hypoextensibility in children with cerebral palsy: 1. Clinical and experimental observations. *Arch. Phys. Med. Rehabil.*, **63**, 97.

Tardieu, G., Tardieu, C., Colbeau-Justin, P. and Bret, M.D. (1982a) Effects of muscle length on an increased stretch reflex in children with cerebral palsy. *J. Neurol. Neurosurg. Psychiatry*, **45**, 348–352.

Tardieu, G., Tardieu, C., Colbeau-Justin, P. and Lespargot, A. (1982b) Muscle hypoextensibility in children with cerebral palsy: 11. Therapeutic implications. *Arch. Phys. Med. Rehabil.*, **63**, 103–107.

Teasdale, G. and Jennett B. (1974) Assessment of coma and impaired consciousness: a practical scale. *Lancet*, **2**, 81–84.

Tepas, J.J., DiScala, C., Ramenofsky, M.L. *et al.* (1989) Mortality and head injury: the pediatric perspective. *J. Pediatr. Surg.*, **25**, 92–96.

Watt, J., Sims, D., Harckman, F., Schmidt, L., McMillan, A. and Hamilton, J. (1986) A prospective study of inhibitive casting as an adjunct to physiotherapy for cerebral-palsied children. *Develop. Med. Child Neurol.*, **28**, 480–488.

Williams, P.E. (1990) Use of intermittent stretch in the prevention of serial sarcomere loss in immobilised muscle. *Ann. Rheum. Dis.*, **49**, 316.

Yarkony, G.M. and Sahgal, V. (1987) Contractures: a major complication of craniocerebral trauma. *Clin. Orthop.*, **219**, 93–96.

Further reading

Ince, L.P. (1971) *Behavior Modification in Rehabilitation Medicine*. Springfield, IL: Charles C. Thomas.

Jennett, B. (1972) Head injuries in children. *Develop. Med. Child Neurol.*, **14**, 137.

Tardieu, C., Lespargot, A., Tabary, C. and Bret, M.D. (1988) For how long must the soleus muscle be stretched each day to prevent contracture? *Dev. Med. Child Neurol.*, **30**, 3–10.

Todorow, S. (1975) Recovery of children after severe head injury. *Scand. J. Rehab. Med.*, **7**, 93–96.

7

Minimal brain dysfunction: learning disability, attention deficit disorder, clumsiness

There is a group of children whose impairments include one or more of the following deficits: dyslexia (difficulty reading), attentional deficit, learning disability and motoric clumsiness. The motor deficit is variously termed clumsiness, motor impairment and dyspraxia. The term specific motor disabilities has recently been suggested (Lockwood *et al.* 1987). Although these clinical signs denote a brain dysfunction, they cannot usually be ascribed to a specific identifiable lesion. To fit into the category of minimal brain dysfunction (MBD), one or more of these deficits must be present without signs of mental retardation or neural damage (Clements 1966).

The above impairments are sometimes considered as syndromes; Critchley (1981) referred to dyslexia as a symptom complex. Historically, the term MBD was coined because the deficits were seen to be primarily behavioural and therefore, in relation to other disorders, minimal. As more is understood about these deficits, the term MBD is considered by some to be too broad to encompass such varying and specific problems (Shaywitz and Shaywitz 1989).

A great deal has been written about these children over the past few decades, and considerable confusion exists, to some extent due to the varying and confusing terminology used to describe their symptoms. It is also due in part to the difficulty physicians and therapists have in evaluating their problems.

This chapter is an attempt to clarify briefly some of the problems of function which may be found and to suggest some ways of approaching the problems which may be amenable to physiotherapy.

Aetiology and pathogenesis

In the presence of such a variety of abnormalities it is understandable that the aetiology is unknown in the majority of children with MBD. With such a varied picture it is probable that there is a multiple aetiology. The following causative factors have been suggested: organic brain damage (such as caused by anoxia in the perinatal period), dysmaturity, prematurity, delayed maturation, exogenous toxins (e.g. lead), infection, metabolic disorder, genetic transmission, malnutrition and psychogenetic determinants (Illingworth 1968; Wender 1971; Gubbay 1975; Shaywitz and Shaywitz 1989). It has also been suggested that poor coordination is the result of delayed motor development and hence that the child will eventually catch up with peers (Knuckey and Gubbay 1983). The evidence is, however, that this may not be so (Losse *et al.* 1990).

Pathogenesis is uncertain. Neurological and radiological tests have not provided much information. Cerebral anomalies have been reported from neuroanatomical and neuroimaging studies in individuals with dyslexia (e.g. Hier *et al.* 1979; Knuckey *et al.* 1983; Galaburda *et al.* 1985). The findings of one study using positron emission tomography suggest the deficits may be in some cases the sequelae of hypoxic–ischaemic encephalopathy (Lou *et al.* 1984). Pharmacological studies suggest that the brain monoaminergic system may play a central role in the pathogenesis of attention deficit disorder (ADD). It is considered that neurochemical measures may provide more relevant explanations than presently exist.

In the rehabilitation model developed by Carr and Shepherd (1987) and transposed in this present book to the training of motor control in infants and children, the emphasis is on the relationship between the primary neural malfunction, the individual's adaptive motor behaviour and the environment. In MBD, whatever the principal causative factor(s) in terms of the motor deficits, it is very likely that the child's impaired motor performance will also be the result of several factors. These may include adaptive behaviours learned by the child as he or she attempts to perform effectively, and environmental interactions. Larkin and Hoare (1992) propose an interactive model in which environmental deprivation interacts with other causal factors (Fig. 7.1). Secondary factors are seen as exacerbat the initial motor dysfunction.

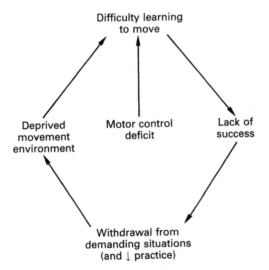

Figure 7.1 An interactive model, demonstrating the possible relationship between causal factors (adapted with permission from Larkin and Hoare 1991).

Diagnosis

There are often difficulties in recognizing the full extent of impairment before the age of 6 or 7 years, when the child's learning difficulty and/or clumsiness become apparent. Diagnosis and assessment are limited by our current knowledge of normal motor control, its development and the nature of dyscontrol processes (see Larkin and Hoare 1992 for discussion). Although there are a large number of tests that purport to give information about movement, few provide much assistance to the planning of intervention. Nevertheless, many of these tests can add considerably to our understanding of the child's movement problems. As in the case of children with cerebral palsy and acute head injury, the development of tests that elucidate the motor control deficits and provide a framework for the development of training strategies depends upon the expansion of research in the area of human movement.

Diagnosis is usually made following the administration of tests which vary considerably from place to place. (See Henderson 1987 and Larkin and Hoare 1991 for a review of assessment batteries.) A neurological examination is routinely carried out in most centres and various interpretations and levels of significance have been placed on the presence of so-called soft neurological signs or neuromaturational signs which are thought to provide evidence of subtle neurological abnormalities. These signs may include choreiform movements (Prechtl and Dijkstra 1960), mirror or overflow phenomena, dysdiadochokinesia, ataxia, and fine and gross motor performance deficits. Interpretation of these signs can be vague and it has been suggested that there are practical and theoretical limitations to such an approach (Shaywitz and Shaywitz 1989). Neuromaturational testing is probably of value for clinicians in providing a structured format for observing children over a period of time. It is necessary to observe how such children respond to direction, how impulsive they are, how they respond to failure and what is the level of persistence at a task.

There is conflicting experimental evidence that a relationship exists between neuromaturational signs and ADD or learning disability (LD). For example, in one study of 35 LD males, 31 exhibited 4 or more neuromaturational signs, compared to 6 of the 32 normal males. However, when IQ was accounted for in the analysis, the normal and LD subjects performed at the same level on most of the measures (Shaywitz *et al.* 1984). One of the problems with identification and assessment of the children can, therefore, be the effect of intelligence level. Intelligence tests (e.g. Wechsler Intelligence Scales for Children–Revised) are usually administered as part of the initial evaluation. Psychometric testing to assess ability and achievement is said to aid the understanding of attentional deficits and their effect on cognitive function.

Tests for finger agnosia, laterality, fine motor function (e.g. rapid sequential finger tapping) and figure drawing may be of value as a guide to intervention, as are tests of such whole-body movements as balancing in standing, heel- and toe-walking, hopping and jumping. There is little evidence that deficits in motor performance are always associated with LD (Stott 1966); however, they are likely to be present in those children who appear motorically slow and clumsy.

Other tests include the Yale Children's Inventory, used in the USA for history evaluation (Shaywitz *et al.* 1986); the Peabody Picture Vocabulary Test, a standardized test of receptive language; the Ayres' test for sensorimotor integration (Ayres 1972); the Bruininks-Oseretsky Motor Proficiency Scale (Bruininks 1978); the Frostig Developmental Test of Visual Perception (Frostig 1963); tests for kinaesthesis (Laszlo and Bairstow 1985); the Basic Motor Ability Test–Revised (Arnheim and Sinclair 1979); and the Stott, Moyes and Henderson (1984) Test of Motor Impairment.

It is possible that testing at-risk infants in their first year may reveal transient neurological signs or neuromaturational signs indicative of the development in childhood of the signs of MBD. Drillien in 1972 made a study of 300 infants of low birth weight (less than 2000 g) in an attempt to identify at an early age the infants who might present with minor impairment at school age. He described a syndrome he called transient abnormal neurological signs in the first year of life and suggested that this syndrome may be indicative of the MBD evident at a later age.

It is possible, therefore, that tests will eventually be able to anticipate with some reliability those infants whose failure to become suitably competent in various areas of function will become obvious as they grow older. The

Brazelton Neonatal Behavioral Assessment Scale (Brazelton 1975; Tronick and Brazelton 1975) may be one such test; Prechtl's (1977) another. These authors stress the importance of very early infant evaluation because of the tendency for early abnormal signs or behaviour to disappear, sometimes to reappear months or years later. These assessments can be combined with an evaluation of the infant's maturity at birth and of intrauterine conditions of nutrition and/or depletion (the dysmaturity scale of Dubowitz *et al.* 1970). It should then follow that programmes can be developed for these infants which will enable them to develop their potential – that is, to become more competent than they would without special guidance.

Description

Learning disability

The term learning disability (LD) includes difficulty with language and reading (dyslexia) with arithmetic (dyscalculia), with writing (dysgraphia) and with spelling. This group of children is generally held to be very heterogeneous (Satz *et al.* 1985). Studies have identified cognitive processing deficits which include deficits in linguistic processing, visual perception and attention. Some children with LD have memory deficits and may have difficulty holding one thing in mind while doing another (Levine 1987). Children in this group are typically slow in performing school-based tasks. It is generally accepted that LD can be associated with all levels of intelligence performance, including the gifted. However, children with LD frequently have feelings of poor self-esteem, may be motivated by fear of failure and consequently are often anxious individuals (Bryan *et al.* 1983). Some children with LD have problems with motor control, seen principally in hand use and balancing activities. Some studies suggest that children with LD more frequently demonstrate motor performance deficits than their peers (Das 1986). Taylor (1982) found significantly poorer performance in children with reading disability on 11 of 15 common childhood games such as catch-and-throw and balancing on one leg. She identified several problems, including an inability to follow a pattern and to recognize errors; deficiencies in specific skills and inability to use advice on what strategies to attempt. The relationship between cognitive function and action is stressed by many authors (Neisser 1976; Whiting 1982). This is not a difficult concept to accept given the necessity for paying attention, for planning and for decision-making in acquiring competence in motor performance (Das 1986).

Dyslexia is the term used for difficulty with language, specifically with the significance of words and spelling. Affected children are poor readers and have an increased incidence of delayed speech (Frith 1981). This disorder is thought to be familial (DeFries 1978) and possibly genetic. Children with this problem may have no other identifiable dysfunction.

Motor control deficit (clumsiness)

Although movement dysfunction is usually clearly evident in this group of children, the nature of the motor deficit and the distinction between the primary deficit and the secondary (adaptive) dyscontrol are not at all clear. The motor problems are often generally described as involving poor balance and poor interlimb and/or total body coordination (Baker 1986).

Motor dyscontrol may be due to primary defects of sensory integration, seen in agnosia or dyspraxia, or to disorders of motor control, seen in athetosis, ataxia, hyperreflexia or immature motor behaviour. Specific examples of clumsiness may include poor manual skills or poor balance. A child may appear to have muscle weakness or hypotonus and lack of physical energy. Different kinds of movement, for example, swinging, spinning, motor car or boat movement, may not be tolerated.

There is no universally accepted set of characteristics of the movement disorders. It is generally assumed that there is no cognitive or marked motor, sensory or neurological impairment (Gubbay 1978; Smyth and Glencross 1986). However, speech defects and auditory imperception have been described as coexisting with clumsiness (Paine *et al.* 1968). Motor dyscontrol is typically evident in such actions as jumping and hopping and in bimanual activities.

On observation, it appears that many motor-impaired children demonstrate motor control deficits similar to those found in individuals with cerebellar lesions. These deficits may include dysmetria, seen on pointing, at heel strike in walking, and when standing on one leg. The problems commonly seen in jumping are also similar to those seen in ataxic children. The timing deficits and difficulty coordinating the flexion counter-movement with the subsequent propulsive extension phase appear to illustrate dyssynergia. Another problem with jumping and hopping seems to be the inability to absorb forces through the lower-limb joints on landing (Larkin and Hoare 1991). This phase of the action is normally accomplished by an eccentric (lengthening) muscle contraction of the lower-limb extensor muscles. Difficulty with eccentric muscle activity (to brake a movement) is typical of the dysfunction seen in individuals with cerebellar dysfunction, and is seen also in difficulty braking the ballistic phase of reaching. Difficulty in eliminating unwanted muscle activity is frequently seen in these children and probably illustrates their motor immaturity. They may persist in such immature associated movements as moving the fingers of both hands when one hand picks up an object. This problem is seen, for example, in the excessive force generated in throwing, the extraneous arm movements in jumping and hopping.

Interestingly, there appear to be no reports showing results of neurological tests typically used to identify dysmetria and dyssynergia (see Chapter 4). When the motor performance of these children is more commonly investigated using techniques to test for motor control during specific tasks, it can be expected that the underlying control deficits will become clarified. A few studies have recently reported such findings.

For example, children have been shown to have difficulty controlling movements of the distal extremities (Williams 1983). In one study (Williams *et al.* 1992), 13 normal and 12 clumsy children aged 6–7 years and 9–10 years, within a normal range of intellectual and academic achievement, were investigated. The clumsy children were significantly more variable than the normal children in a test which required them to time repetitive motor responses with the index finger. The authors considered that the timing difficulties were due to deficits in a central timing mechanism.

Forsstrom and von Hofsten (1982) reported findings from a study of 4–11-year-old children with MBD reaching to catch a moving target. These children made more devious approach paths than normal controls. By aiming at a point further ahead from the target, the children seemed to take account of their decreased efficiency and by this strategy managed to catch the ball on most attempts.

These findings, as the authors point out, suggest cerebellar dysfunction, since the cerebellum is generally considered to be involved in the control and regulation of timed movements (e.g. Arshansky *et al.* 1983; Brooks 1984; Dichgans and Diener 1984; Ivry and Keele 1989).

Specific sensory and motor problems

These vary greatly from child to child, but there are some particularly common problems which should be considered.

Hand function may be poor in some children and can be seen in the following problems:

1   Inability to adapt to the load force required to lift different objects under different conditions and to the slippage afforded by the object. That is, the child may have difficulty generating the amount of force in the finger muscles to prevent a glass from slipping through the fingers. The child may be unable to control grasp appropriately for the particular characteristics of an object. Some children have difficulty maintaining the necessary grip force as they move about (as they do two things at once).
2   Difficulty maintaining the thumb in the abducted position required to oppose forefinger to thumb for holding small objects, a pencil or cutlery. The difficulty seems to be in stabilizing the thumb at the carpometacarpal joint.
3   Related to this is poor pincer grasp. The child may be able to pick up a pen but not a pin, because a pin requires precise opposition of the tips of the thumb and forefinger.
4   Inaccurate reaching with dysmetric under- or overshooting.
5   Difficulty with rapid repetitive movements such as writing and tapping with the fingers.
6   Difficulty catching and throwing a ball.

Balance, that is, the ability to make postural adjustments that are specific to an action and to the context in which it is performed, is typically a problem for this group of children. Balance dysfunction is seen in the following problems:

1   Inability to stand on one leg without excessive movement of the body mass about the fixed foot and without excessive arm movements.
2   Difficulty walking under conditions which require more control, for example, across an elevated beam. The child may be able to walk across quickly but not slowly, since fast movement requires less postural control.
3   Loss of balance when visual inputs are eliminated. This condition forces the child to depend on somatosensory (proprioceptive, tactile) and vestibular information. If this is deficient, balancing will be impaired.
4   Difficulty reaching to the limits of stability, in sitting and/or standing. The perimeter within which the body mass can move without balance being lost appears smaller than usual.

These difficulties may be seen in combination with what appears to be poor attention to relevant sensory input.

Inadequate sensory discrimination may be seen in poor tactile localization, problems in stereognosis, in joint position sense and in two-point discrimination.

Visuospatial orientation (VSO) Infants are thought to become aware of spatial relationships by integrating vision with somaesthetic inputs from tactile, kinaesthetic and proprioceptive senses. VSO is the recognition and discrimination amongst patterns and their spatial relationships. It enables one to do such actions as doing up buttons and tying shoelaces. Visual perceptual problems are considered to contribute to motor deficits (Lord and Hulme 1987). Problems in VSO may be illustrated by lack of coordination between eye and hand in throwing, catching and batting.

Oculomotor deficits Some children have difficulty with the control of eye movements. This will be demonstrated by difficulty dissociating eye and head movements, poor control of saccadic eye movements and visual pursuit (Bala *et al.* 1981).

Sensory integrative dysfunction Ayres (1972) has proposed that disorders of sensory integrative function are common in these children. Following her studies of children with cognitive, perceptual and/or motor dysfunction, she suggested that perceptual-motor dysfunction may be classified into a number of syndromes:

1 Vestibular and bilateral integration dysfunction, which she considered is a dysfunction in brainstem processing.
2 Developmental apraxia, with either a vestibular or a somatosensory basis.
3 Generalized dysfunction.

For historical interest, the reader should refer to Ayres (1972) for this author's description of the problems associated with sensory integrative dysfunction and her approach to treatment.

Dominance In the absence of normative data, undue emphasis should probably not be placed on tests for dominance. Mixed dominance may be as common in the normal population as in the population with dysfunction.

Vestibular dysfunction Problems in vestibular function have been attributed to brain-damaged children (Bobath and Bobath 1972) as well as to children with MBD (Ayres 1972). Abnormal responses to vestibular stimulation have been reported also in autistic children (Ritvo *et al.* 1969) and in Down's syndrome children (Kantner *et al.* 1976).

Stimulation of the semicircular canals normally produces nystagmus, although it can be inhibited in states of dreaminess (reverie), where the reticular activating system is unstimulated, and by fixation of the eyes. Responses to stimulation of the semicircular canals in children with MBD are reported to be either hypo- or hyperactive, and may vary in quality. In addition to changes in nystagmus, some children demonstrate considerable fear during or following the post-rotatory nystagmus tests; others become dizzy and vomit. Fear may be a sign of postural insecurity; the other signs appear to indicate an adversive reaction to movement.

The vestibular system is thought to affect the excitatory state of spinal cord motoneurones through the connections between the labyrinths and the facilitatory reticular formation of the brainstem (Ayres 1972; O'Connell and Gardner 1972; Pompeiano 1972). The vestibular system together with the proprioceptive, tactile and visual systems is also involved in the control of postural adjustments and balance.

Steinberg and Rendle-Short (1977) found significant differences in post-rotatory nystagmus and head-righting between a group of children with normal intelligence referred with minimal problems and a control group of randomly selected children without known problems. All the children were aged between 3 and 6 years. The authors tested head-righting in the horizontal and vertical positions. Poor head-righting was greatest in the horizontal position with vision eliminated. In all, 88% of the children showed complete lack of head correction. Even with vision, head-righting remained inefficient. Some of these children also demonstrated loss of postural tone when held in the horizontal and vertical positions.

The relevance of these abnormal responses is not clear. Nor is it clear whether the deficits reported reflect only vestibular dysfunction. Understanding the relationship between sensation as tested and functional motor performance is fraught with problems, not the least of which is the apparent specificity with which sensory inputs are utilized by the control system. That is, the system appears to pay attention only to those inputs (out of many) that are relevant to the task being attempted and the relevant inputs would be interactive.

Attention deficit disorder

Symptoms include inattention, hyperactivity or poor impulse control. It is principally evidenced by its behavioural manifestations. ADD is seen in children who have had a head injury as well as children with no history of trauma. A large percentage of children with ADD have learning difficulties (Safer and Allen 1976).

Selective attention is often a problem with these children. It is illustrated by an inability to focus purposefully for appropriate lengths of time on incoming information. The child may show impersistence, difficulty in delaying gratification, inconsistent performance, and a low tolerance for frustration. Parents sometimes report that, as an infant, the child appeared insatiable, irritable and unpredictable.

Hyperactive behaviour is difficult to define. To some extent it is relative. A child may appear hyperactive in a family where all the other children are quiet. Nevertheless, hyperactive children demonstrate behaviour which differs markedly in both extent and quality from the behaviour seen in normal high-spirited children at certain ages.

Hyperactivity is characterized by excessive restlessness and inattentiveness. The child's activities and reactions are excessive. Toys may be hurled instead of thrown. The child may appear unable to eliminate irrelevant stimuli, and, in paying attention to everything, may run from one toy to the next, taking heed of all sounds without discriminating between the most important. The child appears a 'naughty' child but the behaviour is largely a manifestation of an inability to control impulses. Sitting still or listening to stories for any length of time is often difficult for such children. In both speech and action, some tend to perseverate and be compulsive. The behaviour of the hyperactive child tends to be immature, with impulsivity and temper tantrums.

In addition, the hyperactive child may demonstrate other problems seen in children with MBD. Perceptual–motor and cognitive disorders may be present, and particularly evident when school starts. Problems of motor coordination may result in clumsiness and inability to catch a ball or hold a pencil. Problems in balance may make it difficult to stand on one leg or walk along a raised beam. Visual motor coordination is often poor, with difficulty in gaining eye–hand control, which will affect the acquisition of skill in reading and writing, for example.

Assessment

Overall assessment may involve the skills of paediatrician, psychologist, audiologist, speech pathologist, paediatric neurologist and physical educator, as well as occupational and physical therapist. Some tests typically performed are listed earlier in the chapter.

A careful history from the parents, supplemented by a history from the school teacher, together with observation of the child during various activities, will indicate to the therapist what areas of function are difficult. As the therapist gets to know the child and family better, other problems may become obvious or previously recognized problems clarified.

In general, assessment may be performed in the areas of motor ability (including prehension and postural adjustments), significant neurological signs, tactile, proprioceptive, vestibular and spatial functioning, visual and auditory function.

Assessment in general should also be directed at the coping mechanisms present within the family. Strengths and weaknesses of the child and parents should be evaluated and should include behaviour as well as function.

Hoare and Larkin (1991) have identified five distinct patterns of motor dysfunction in a group of 80 children with motor impairment. They used tests of kinaesthetic acuity, visual perception, visual–motor integration, peg assembly, static balance and running. They identified three tasks as reliable determinators of motor dysfunction: hopping on the spot on one leg; balancing on one leg; and a 50-metre sprint. Testing of these tasks may help in the identification of children with motor dysfunction associated with MBD.

Further testing by the physiotherapist should be directed towards the assessment of any action with which the child is having difficulty, including everyday actions (see Chapter 3). In addition, analysis of other actions can be evaluated against the increasing account of normative data gradually accumulating on jumping (e.g. Clark and Phillips 1985), hopping (Halverson and Williams 1981); throwing (Roberton 1978) and kicking (Elliott *et al.* 1980).

Intervention

Many children with MBD are not seen by a physiotherapist until they are at least 3 or 4 years old, and often not until they have been at school for 2 or 3 years. The child may then be referred with a combination of clumsiness, hyperactivity, educational underachievement and behaviour disorders.

Not all children with motor control deficits or delayed motor development require physiotherapy. Some children will benefit from structured exercise classes and sporting activities designed to develop skill in, for example, ball-handling, which can be organized and run by physical education teachers at school. Group activities may also be organized and run by a physiotherapist or occupational therapist where specific problems requiring the input of a therapist are needed. Some children will benefit from dance lessons.

Those children who also have behaviour and/or learning difficulties will require remedial teaching, psychiatric or psychological counselling and behaviour control. Children with specific hearing and speech problems will receive treatment from the appropriate source.

There is evidence that improvement in motor skills and in schoolwork will affect behaviour when behavioural problems stem from these causes. Hence it seems reasonable to suggest that children with problems in motor function, learning and behaviour should have a trial period of physical education or physical therapy and remedial teaching before being referred for specific behaviour therapy.

The physiotherapist should be prepared to assess and deal with the child's problems away from a medical setting, preferably in child-care centres, in school or gymnasium. The child should not see movement training as treatment, because that suggests sickness, but should see it as good fun, and an opportunity to acquire skill.

Group activity performs a useful social function. Some children will improve in social skills even if they remain relatively unskilled in motor function. As Abbie and colleagues (1978) point out, a person can lead a fulfilled happy life without being particularly skilled in a motoric sense. None the less, these children should still be given the chance to develop skills which would not develop without guidance. Group activity is described by Abbie *et al.* (1978).

Motor training must be specific to each child's problems, which requires that assessment of motor performance be as detailed as possible (see Chapter 3). It is not sufficient to determine, for example, that a child has poor balance. Balance needs to be analysed and training will be specific to the areas in which the child has difficulty. Larkin and Hoare (1991) describe methods of training specific actions in this group of children and the reader should consult this text.

A child who has an aversive reaction to movements which stimulate the vestibular system may be helped by therapy to improve the tolerance to externally imposed movement. This therapy may need to be combined with anti-motion sickness medication (Frank and Levinson 1973).

Parents may require advice on child-rearing and on how to decrease the level of tension at home. They may need to appreciate how to anticipate routine restlessness and channel it into meaningful activity. They and the school teacher should know how to aim at the child's strengths so the child can experience success.

Methods of treating hyperactivity are very controversial and include drug therapy, diet and behaviour control. Treatment which quietens the child may be good or bad, depending upon whether the child's newly found control can be used to improve learning and socializing. There is also a considerable difference between treatment which controls the child and treatment which enables the child to control him- or herself.

Behavioural management may consist of biofeedback to increase self-control and desensitization as well as other forms of behaviour therapy. Hampstead (1979) reported on the effects of electromyogram (EMG)-assisted relaxation training of 6 hyperactive children aged 6–9 years. EMG electrodes were placed on the forehead and the children received auditory feedback about the level of muscle activation. All the children decreased EMG activity and 5 of the 6 made behavioural improvements at home and school. Stewart and Olds (1973) give suggestions for parents on raising a hyperactive child.

Safer and Allen (1976) describe the medical (drug) and behavioural management of hyperactive children. Their studies and others (Ottenbacher and Cooper 1983) have shown that a group of children on stimulant medication (such as methylphenidate or dextroamphetamine) demonstrated a statistically significant improvement in their hyperactive behaviour, with less classroom restlessness, increased attention span, increased academic output and improved emotional and social behaviour. These children became happier, more motivated, more successful and were, therefore, better accepted into society.

Summary

In this chapter the author has set out to introduce the reader to the variety of problems found in children who do not fit easily into family and school life and whose lives are adversely affected by their social, behavioural and motor deficits. The most effective means of evaluating and training children with MBD is not yet established, primarily due to the paucity of studies describing the motor deficits and the lack of knowledge related to the pathophysiological mechanisms. Intervention typically comprises remedial education, behaviour therapy, pharmacology, activities to improve sensorimotor integration, the training of motor control and the promotion of physical fitness.

Testing and intervention are, where possible, in a non-medical setting, and both child and parents should receive help and encouragement in optimizing the child's performance and behaviour.

References

Abbie, M., Douglas, M.H. and Ross, K.E. (1978) The clumsy child: observations in cases referred to the gymnasium of Adelaide Children's Hospital over a three year period. *Med. J. Aust.*, **1**, 65.

Arnheim, D.D. and Sinclair, W.A. (1979) *The Clumsy Child: A Program of Motor Therapy*, 2nd edn. St Louis, MO: C.V. Mosby.

Arshansky, Y., Gelfand, I. and Orlovsky, G. (1983) The cerebellum and control of rhythmical movements. *Trends Neurosci.*, **6**, 417–422.

Ayres, A.J. (1972) *Sensory Integration and Learning Disorders*. Los Angeles, CA: Western Psychological Services.

Baker, J. (1986) A psycho-motor approach to the assessment and treatment of clumsy children. *Physiotherapy*, **67**, 356–363.

Bala, S.P., Cohen, B., Morris, A.G. *et al.* (1981) Saccades of hyperactive and normal boys during ocular pursuit. *Dev. Med. Child Neurol.*, **23**, 323–336.

Bobath, K. and Bobath, B. (1972) Cerebral palsy. In: *Therapy Services in Developmental Disabilities*, edited by P.H. Pearson and C.E. Williams. Springfield IL: Charles C. Thomas.

Brazelton, T.B. (1975) *The Brazelton Neonatal Behavioral Assessment Scale*. London: Heinemann.

Brooks, V. (1984) Cerebellar functions in motor control. *Hum. Neurobiol.*, **2**, 251–260.

Bruininks, R.H. (1978) *Bruininks-Oseretzky Test of Motor Proficiency. Examiner's Manual*. Circle Pines, MN: American Guidance Service.

Bryan, J.H., Sonnefeld, L.J. and Grabowski, B. (1983) The relationship between fear of failure and learning disabilities. *Learn. Disabil. Q.*, **6**, 217.

Carr, J.H. and Shepherd, R.B. (eds) (1987) *Movement Science: Foundations for Physical Therapy in Rehabilitation*. Rockville, MD: Aspen Publishers.

Clark, J.E. and Phillips, S.J. (1985) A developmental sequence of the standing long jump. In: *Motor Development: Current Selected Research*, edited by J.E. Clark and J.H. Humphrey. Princeton, NJ: Princeton Books.

Clements, S.D. (1966) *Minimal Brain Dysfunction in Children: Terminology and Identification*. NINDB Monograph 3. Washington: N.I.H.

Critchley, M. (1981) Dyslexia: an overview. In: *Dyslexia Research and its Application to Education*, edited by G.T. Pavlidis and T.R. Miles. Chichester: John Wiley.

Das, J.P. (1986) Information processing and motivation as determinants of performance in children with learning disabilities. In: *Themes in Motor Development*, edited by H.T.A. Whiting and M.G. Wade. Dordrecht: Martinus Nijhoff.

DeFries, J.C. (1978) Familial nature of reading disability. *Br. J. Psychiatry*, **132**, 361.

Dichgans, J. and Diener, H. (1984) Clinical evidence for functional compartmentalization of the cerebellum. In: *Cerebellum Function*, edited by J. Bloedel, J. Dichgans and W. Precht. Berlin: Springer-Verlag.

Drillien, C.M. (1972) Abnormal neurologic signs in the first year of life in low-birthweight infants: possible prognostic significance. *Dev. Med. Child Neurol.*, **14**, 575.

Dubowitz, L.M., Dubowitz, V. and Goldberg, C. (1970) Clinical assessment of gestational age in the newborn infants. *Pediatrics*, **77**, 1.

Elliott, B.C., Bloomfield, J. and Davies, C.M. (1980) Development of the punt kick: a cinematographic analysis. *J. Hum. Movement Stud.*, **6**, 142–150.

Forsstrom, A. and von Hofsten, C. (1982) Visually directed reaching of children with motor impairments. *Dev. Med. Child Neurol.*, **24**, 653–661.

Frith, U. (1981) Experimental approaches to developmental dyslexia. *Psychol. Res.*, **43**, 97.

Frank, J. and Levinson, H. (1973) Dysmetric dyslexia and dyspraxia. Hypothesis and study. *J. Child Psychol.*, 690–701.

Frostig, M. (1963) *Development Test for Visual Perception*. Los Angeles, CA: Consulting Psychologists' Press.

Galaburda, A.M., Sherman, G.F., Rosen, G.B., Aboitiz, F. and Geschwind, N. (1985) Developmental dyslexia: four consecutive patients with cortical anomalies. *Ann. Neurol.*, **18**, 222–223.

Gubbay, S.A. (1975) *The Clumsy Child: A Study of Developmental Apraxia and Agnostic Ataxia*. London: Saunders.

Gubbay, S.A. (1978) The management of developmental apraxia. *Dev. Med. Child Neurol.*, **20**, 643–646.

Halverson, L. and Williams, K. (1981) Developmental sequence for hopping over distance: a prelongitudinal screening. *Res. Q. Ex. Sport.*, **56**, 37–44.

Hampstead, W.J. (1979) The effects of EMG-assisted relaxation training with hyperkinetic children. A behavioral alternative. *Biofeedback Self-Regulation*, **4**, 2, 113–181.

Henderson, S.E. (1987) The assessment of 'clumsy' children: old and new approaches. *J. Child Psychol. Psychiatry*, **28**, 4, 511–527.

Hier, D., Le May, M., Rosenberger, P.B. and Perlo, V.P. (1979) Developmental dyslexia: evidence for a subgroup with reversal of cerebral asymmetry. *Arch. Neurol.*, **35**, 90.

Hoare, D. and Larkin, D. (1991) Coordination problems in children. In: *State of the Art Review 18*. Australian Sports Commission: National Sports Research Centre.

Illingworth, R.S. (1968) Delayed motor development. *Pediatr. Clin. North Am.*, **15**, 569.

Ivry, R.B. and Keele, S.W. (1989) Timing functions of the cerebellum. *J. Cognitive Neurosci.*, **6**, 136–152.

Kantner, R.M., Clark, D.L., Allen, L.C. and Chase, M.F. (1976) Effects of vestibular stimulation on nystagmus response and motor performance in the developmentally delayed infant. *Phys. Ther.*, **56**, 414.

Knuckey, N.W. and Gubbay, S.S. (1983) Clumsy children: a prognostic study. *Aust. Paediatr. J.*, **19**, 9–13.

Knuckey, N.W., Apsimon, T.T. and Gubbay, S.S. (1983) Computerised axial tomography in clumsy children with developmental apraxia and agnosia. *Brain Dev.*, **5**, 14–19.

Larkin, D. and Hoare, D. (1991) *Out of Step: Coordinating Kids' Movements*. Nedlands, Western Australia: Active Life Foundation, Dept of Human Movement and Recreation Studies, University of West Australia.

Larkin, D. and Hoare, D. (1992) The movement approach: a window to understanding the clumsy child. In: *Approaches to the Study of Motor Control and Learning*, edited by J.J. Summers. Amsterdam: Elsevier Science Publishers.

Laszlo, J.I. and Bairstow, P.J. (1985) *Perceptual-Motor Behavior. Developmental Assessment and Therapy.* London: Holt, Rinehart and Winston.

Levine, M. (1987) Developmental dysfunction – school age children. In: *Nelson Textbook of Pediatrics*, 13th edn, edited by R.E. Behrman and V.C. Vaughan. Philadelphia, PA: W.B. Saunders.

Lockwood, R.J., Larkin, D. and Wann, J.P. (1987) Specific motor disabilities. In: *Physical Education and Disability*, edited by R.J. Lockwood. Parkside, SA: ACHPER, pp. 80–86.

Lord, R. and Hulme, C. (1987) Kinaesthetic sensitivity of normal and clumsy children. *Dev. Med. Child Neurol.*, **29**, 720–725.

Losse, A., Henderson, S., Elliman, D., Hall, D.B., Knight, E. and Jongmans, M. (1990) Clumsiness in children – do they grow out of it? *Dev. Med. Child Neurol.*, **32**, 1099–1122.

Lou, H.C., Henriksen, L. and Bruhn, P. (1984) Focal cerebral hypoperfusion in children with dysphasia and/or attention deficit disorder. *Arch. Neurol.*, **42**, 825.

Neisser, U. (1976) *Cognition and Reality*. San Francisco, CA: W.H. Freeman.

O'Connell, A.L. and Gardner, E.B. (1972) *Understanding the Scientific Bases of Human Movement*. Baltimore, MD: Williams & Wilkins.

Ottenbacher, K.J. and Cooper, M.M. (1983) Drug treatment for hyperactivity in children. *Dev. Med. Child Neurol.*, **25**, 358.

Paine, R.S., Werry, J.C. and Quay, H.C. (1968) A study of minimal cerebral dysfunction. *Dev. Med. Child Neurol.*, **10**, 505.

Pompeiano, O. (1972) Vestibulo-spinal relations: vestibular influences on gamma motoneurons and primary afferents. *Prog. Brain Res.*, **37**, 197.

Prechtl, H. (1977) *The Neurological Examination of the Full-term Newborn Infant*, 2nd edn. London: Heinemann.

Prechtl, H. and Dijkstra, J. (1960) Neurological diagnoses of cerebral injury in the newborn. In: *Prenatal Care*, edited by B. tenBerge. Groningen: Noordhoff.

Ritvo, E.R., Ornitz, E., Eviatar, A., Markham, C.H., Brown, M.B. and Mason, A. (1969) Decreased post-rotatory nystagmus in early infantile autism. *Neurology*, **19**, 653.

Roberton, M.A. (1978) Stages in movement development. In: *Motor Development: Issues and Applications*, edited by M. Ridenour. Princeton, NJ: Princeton Book Company.

Safer, D.J. and Allen, R.P. (1976) *Hyperactive Children. Diagnosis and Management.* Baltimore, MD: University Park Press.

Satz, P., Morris, R. and Fletcher, J.M. (1985) Hypotheses, subtypes, and individual differences in dyslexia: some reflections. In: *Biobehavioral Measures of Dyslexia*, edited by D.B. Gray and J.F. Kavanagh. Baltimore, MD: York Press.

Shaywitz, B.A. and Shaywitz, S.E. (1989) Learning disabilities. In: *Pediatric Neurology, vol. 1.* edited by K.F. Swaiman. St Louis, MO: C.V. Mosby, pp. 857–894.

Shaywitz, S.E., Shaywitz, B.A., McGraw, K. and Groll, S. (1984) Current status of the neuromaturational examination as an index of learning disability. *J. Pediatr.*, **104**, 819–825.

Shaywitz, S.E. *et al.* (1986) Yale Children's Inventory (YCI): an instrument to assess children with attentional deficits and learning disabilities. 1. Scale development and psychometric properties. *J. Abnorm. Child Psychol.*, **14**, 347.

Smyth, T.R. and Glencross, D. (1986) Information processing deficits in clumsy children. *Aust. J. Psychol.*, **38**, 13–22.

Steinberg, M. and Rendle-Short, J. (1977) Vestibular dysfunction in young children with minor neurological impairment. *Dev. Med. Child Neurol.*, **19**, 639.

Stewart, M. and Olds, S. (1973) *Raising a Hyperactive Child.* New York: Harper & Row.

Stott, D.H. (1966) A general test of motor impairment for children. *Dev. Med. Child Neurol.*, **8**, 705.

Stott, D.H., Moyes, F. and Henderson, S. (1984) *Test of Motor Impairment.* Ontario: Brook Education Publishing.

Taylor, K.J. (1982) Physical awkwardness of reading disability: a descriptive study. Cited in Larkin, D. and Hoare, D. (1991) *Out of Step: Coordinating Kid's Movements.* Amsterdam: Elsevier Science Publishers.

Tronick, E. and Brazelton, T.B. (1975) Clinical uses of the Brazelton neonatal behavioral assessment scale. In: *Exceptional Infant, vol. 3*, edited by B.Z. Friedlander *et al.* New York: Brunner-Mazel.

Wender, P.H. (1971) *Minimal Brain Dysfunction in Children.* New York: Wiley.

Whiting, H.T.A. (1982) Image of the act. In: *Theory and Research in Learning Disabilities*, edited by J.P. Das, R.F. Mulcahy and A.E. Wall. New York: Plenum Press.

Williams, H.G. (1983) *Perceptual-Motor Development in Young Children.* Englewood Cliffs. NJ: Prentice-Hall.

Williams, H.G., Woollacott, M.H. and Ivry, R. (1992) Timing and motor control in clumsy children. *J. Motor Behav.*, **24**, 2, 165–172.

Further reading

Connolly, K. and Stratton, P. (1968) Developmental changes in associated movements. *Dev. Med. Child Neurol.*, **10**, 49.

Denkla, M.B. (1984) Developmental apraxia: the clumsy child. In: *Middle Childhood: Development and Dysfunction*, edited by M.D. Levine and P. Satz. Baltimore, MD: University Park Press, pp. 245–260.

Gordon, N. and McKinlay, I. (1980) *Helping Clumsy Children*. New York: Churchill Livingstone.

Kalverbroer, A.F. (1975) *A Neurobehavioral Study in Pre-School Children*. Oxford: Butterworth-Heinemann.

Kephart, N. (1971) *The Slow Learner in the Classroom*. Columbus, OH: Merrill.

8

Mental retardation: cognitive impairment and developmental delay

The term mental retardation is commonly used to categorize children with impaired intelligence and inadequate learning abilities (Swaiman 1989). The term cognitive impairment is used in this chapter in order to highlight the relationship between cognition and action (Neisser 1976). In this group of children, motor performance may be impaired either as a result of the causative brain dysfunction or because of an impaired ability to pay attention, develop abstract concepts, match intention to action, learn motor skills, as well as lack of curiosity about the surroundings and lack of motivation to explore. Children with cognitive impairment have difficulty with everyday life because of a poor ability to link intention with action.

Mental retardation is an intellectual deficit which is present from birth (Walton 1971). Children are typically classified as severely or profoundly retarded (IQ below 35), moderately (trainable) retarded (IQ between 36 and 51), mildly retarded (IQ between 52 and 67) and borderline retarded (IQ between 70 and 79).

Generally speaking, the profoundly retarded are incapable of protecting or caring for themselves, often being looked after in institutions, while the mildly retarded approach the lower limits of normal intelligence and manage to live and work in society. Illingworth (1974) has suggested that a child with an IQ over 50 will probably be able to earn a living in some capacity. Whether the child will be educable or not will depend on the presence and the degree of physical handicap. A very hyperactive child with an IQ in the borderline normal group may, for example, be ineducable because of hyperactivity.

Aetiology

There is no wholly satisfactory aetiological classification of mentally retarded infants. However, any classification will include the following groups (see also Swaiman 1989):

1　Metabolic and endocrine disorders (e.g. congenital hypothyroidism or cretinism, phenylketonuria, Wilson's disease).
2　Genetic or chromosomal abnormalities (e.g. Down's syndrome, Klinefelter's syndrome).
3　Malformations of the central nervous system (microcephaly, hydrocephaly, encephalocele).

In addition, many syndromes have been described, including Noonan's, Möbius, Laurence–Moon, and Apert's syndromes (Holmes *et al.* 1972). Mental retardation occurs in some children with cerebral palsy, in some who are born dysmature or premature, or whose mothers were infected by rubella or herpes virus during pregnancy. Certain toxins are known to affect fetal development (tobacco, alcohol and other drugs). Mental retardation may also develop in children with epilepsy or following encephalitis, meningitis or head injury, and as a result of child abuse.

A degree of mental retardation has been found to be associated with muscular dystrophy (Dubowitz 1965) and spina bifida cystica (Soare and Raimondi 1977). Deprived children are frequently found to have motor and cognitive impairment which may resolve when their social situation improves. In severe cases of malnutrition, however, the full development of cognitive abilities may never occur even when nutrition becomes adequate. This must be a subject of great concern given the extent of famine and poverty in many countries. If the child is in an institution, stimulation may be lacking, and because many institutions are overcrowded and short-staffed, children may be left to their own devices all day with no opportunity for developing whatever their potential abilities might have been.

It is also possible for a child with a severe motor handicap from earliest infancy to suffer cognitive impairment which is secondary to the motor disability. This should, however, be preventable to some extent, with early treatment designed to overcome the motor handicap and provide environmental stimulation.

Many mentally retarded infants have ophthalmological problems including primary optic atrophy, cortical blindness, strabismus, congenital ocular anomalies and refractive errors (Ghose and Chandra Sekhar 1986). Visual impairment may further impair the child's ability to learn, to acquire motor control and become skilled in motor tasks.

The importance of accurate diagnosis and assessment of children with developmental disorders in order to plan appropriate intervention strategies cannot be too greatly stressed. Infants and children with developmental delay which is secondary to sensorimotor disability (e.g. cerebral palsy), to deprivation, or to specific learning difficulties (e.g. dyslexia, dysgraphia) must be distinguished from those whose developmental delay is due to primary cognitive impairment.

Developmental assessment typically includes the use of objective scales such as the Denver Developmental Screening Test (Frankenburg and Dodds 1967) and Bayley Scales of Infant Development (Bayley 1969). Assessment may also include an examination of developmental reflexes and milestones as an indication of maturation of physiological processes and anatomical structures (Illingworth 1974; Swaiman 1989).

Electroencephalography and sensory-evoked potentials aid in recognition of seizures, integrity of visual pathways (visual-evoked potentials) and auditory system (brainstem auditory-evoked potentials). Computed tomography and magnetic resonance imaging are the common means of assessing brain structure. It is now recognized that individuals with Down's syndrome (DS) should be tested for atlantoaxial instability before participation in vigorous exercise placing strain on the neck (Cooke 1991).

Specific clinical tests aid the identification of syndromes and diseases. Chromosomal analysis is critical to the diagnosis of genetically transmitted conditions (Lemieux 1989). Neuropsychological and intelligence testing (Swaiman 1989) is particularly important when the child reaches school age. Commonly used measures of intelligence are the Stanford Binet Intelligence Scale and the Wechsler Intelligence Test for Children. The level of social functioning and adaptive behaviour may be assessed using the Vineland Adaptive Behavior Scale (Gould 1977) and the Minnesota Child Development Inventory (Ireton and Thwing 1972). There are many problems in assessing the intelligence of severely motorically handicapped children and the tests may be of doubtful value as they require verbal or manual skills for their performance.

Cognitive impairment, motor development and performance

Infants with brain dysfunction may show the clinical sign called *hypotonia* for the first few months of life. This is particularly characteristic of infants with DS. Hypotonus in these infants has been defined as a lack of descending excitation to the spinal cord motoneuron pool (Gilman *et al.* 1981). Davis and Kelso (1982) have suggested that individuals with DS have a deficit in the specification of stiffness and damping parameters and that this may explain the clinical features associated with hypotonus, including hyperextensibility of joints. Recent work casts doubt on this hypothesis (Shumway-Cooke and Woollacott 1985), since motoneuron pool excitability appears within normal limits for the first few months of life. Cowie (1970) has suggested that hypotonia may be due to delayed maturation of the cerebellum and cortical pathways. Other deficits reported in DS individuals, which are possibly relevant to hypotonia, include smaller brain weight, particularly of cerebellum and brainstem (Crome *et al.* 1966). Lower levels of the amino acid 5-hydroxytryptophan (Coleman 1975; Koch and de la Cruz 1975), thought to play an important role in neural transmission and muscle contraction (Ahlman *et al.* 1971), have been reported. Signs suggestive of cerebellar dysfunction have been reported in individuals with DS. Davis and Kelso's results (1982) show an increased oscillation about final end-position, a tendency to overshoot targets and lack of smoothness in movement, which may be the result of delayed cerebellar maturation. Few studies, however, have explored the specific motor control deficits associated with DS.

The earliest signs of mental retardation may be *feeding* problems, with the infant unable to suck or swallow effectively, and apparently uninterested in feeding; delay in *social responses* such as smiling and recognition of a parent's face; an excessive number of hours spent *sleeping*; a weak *cry*; *apathy* and little *spontaneous activity*. The infant may be slow to *vocalize*, and then lack the repertoire of sounds which a normal infant demonstrates. *Speech* may be very slow to develop, and in the severely retarded may not develop at all. Persistent *hand regard* may develop. *Mouthing* of toys and hands typically continues beyond the normal limit of 12 months of age. The baby may also develop *perseverant* or *stereotyped actions*, repetitive pointless movements such as hand-flapping, head-rolling, or rocking, which seem to occur at the stage when the infant is 'stuck' in a particular position (MacLean and Baumeister 1981), lacking the movement organization and incentive which would enable movement out of that position (Fig. 8.1). In playing, the child may not go after toys if they are dropped, appearing to forget about them, and there may be no attempt to get a toy which is out of reach.

The extent to which movement develops in a mentally retarded child depends to some extent on the severity of the mental handicap. The lack of incentive, of a desire to move from one place to another, to reach a particular toy, to explored the possibilities of the environment, are critical causative factors in the cognitively impaired child's motor impairment. Also critical must be the lack of interest in exploring the dynamic possibilities of the

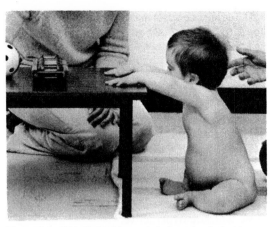

Figure 8.1 This little girl can sit independently but her wide base of support limits the actions she can perform and prevents her from getting out of the position.

linked body segments in interacting with objects.

Generally in the mildly handicapped child motor development proceeds as in a normal child but at a slower rate with, in the case of DS, plateaux (Carr 1975). Movements may be relatively normal, although many children do not achieve a fully extended posture when upright, maintaining some flexion of the hips, knees and trunk in standing. Whole-body movements, such as walking and sit-to-stand, may appear to be less involved than speech, manipulation and social behaviour. However, as more studies of the biomechanics and motor control of children with mental retardation are being published, it is becoming evident that the control of so-called gross movements may also be impaired.

The achievement of motor milestones is usually delayed to some extent. For example, where on average normal infants sit independently at 6 months, stand at 11 months and walk at 12 months, infants with DS have been reported to achieve these milestones at 9, 18 and 19 months (Henderson 1985). Interestingly, it has been shown that infants with DS aged between 7 and 11 months were able to take alternating steps on a treadmill on average 8–19 months before they began to walk independently (Ulrich *et al.* 1992). The results showed that these infants were responding to the treadmill in a similar manner to younger normal infants. The results further support the view expressed by Thelen (1986) that the pattern of walking is innate in normal infants, extending this to include infants with DS. It is very likely that two major reasons for delay in independent walking in mentally retarded children are deficits in motor control and muscle strength in the linking of postural control to action and lack of practice.

Mentally retarded children are generally considered to have poor *muscular strength*. Asmussen and Heeboll-Neilsen (1956) suggested that low intelligence is associated with less muscular strength and endurance. In addition, movements often appear to be performed more slowly by these children, although not by those who are hyperactive.

Motor development may come to a halt at any stage. In the severely retarded child this may occur at an early age. In assessment, the difference between, for example, a child with cerebral palsy and one who has an intellectual impairment may show itself by the difference in the progress of development. The cerebral palsied child's development may be patchy, with particular milestones left out, while others may have developed. On the other hand, the development of a mentally retarded child usually shows a generalized arrest. It is as if the child has become fixed at this point and can go no further with a particular action. The child may learn how to pull to standing, but may not go on to cruise around the furniture and walk alone for some time.

This arrested development once a low level of attainment has been achieved typically illustrates the relationship between cognition and action. Cognitively intact infants and children are continually practising new actions so as to gain increased skill and master their environment. Once in sitting or standing, the normal infant strives to become independent, falling over many times in the process of experimenting and in the process of learning and achieving. Piaget (1960) identified action as a basis for early learning. It has been demonstrated that an infant's opportunity for learning and socializing increases as more control is gained over the body (Campos *et al.* 1982; Gustafson 1984; Berthenthal and Campos 1987).

Control of the head is usually slow to develop, particularly in the floppy child. This may be partly due in some cases to the reluctance of parents to handle the infant, and play. An unresponsive baby gives parents little reward for their efforts at communicating

and the infant may as a consequence be relatively unstimulated. Similarly, an infant who cries little and does not demand attention may also suffer such unintentional neglect. It is often this infant, appearing to parents as good, docile and such little trouble, who spends the day lying in supine, a position which will accentuate a lack of interest in the surroundings and a general apathy. If the infant is picked up only rarely, this stimulus to gaining head and trunk control will be absent also. Lack of experience and slowness in learning to hold the head vertical may impair the infant's ability to develop visuomotor function. Lack of the experience of seeing the limbs move actively may also, as has been shown in kittens, impair the development of neural control of the limbs.

Balance is typically slow to develop, particularly if the child is lying down all day, or is propped securely in sitting, a position from which there is no stimulus to regain or maintain a balanced position. Head, trunk and arm movements in response to tilting in supine and sitting have been shown to be very delayed in mentally retarded infants in findings reported by Molnar (1974), suggesting that the dysfunction or anomaly causing the cognitive impairment may also affect sensorimotor areas of the brain.

For postural adjustments to develop in a particular position (e.g. sitting or standing), it is probably necessary for goal-directed actions to be practised in that position. Postural adjustments are muscle activation patterns that form part of the muscular synergy involved in particular actions. They have been shown to be specific to the task and to the context in which it is being performed (see Chapter 2). Infants with DS have been reported as having delayed postural adjustments (Butterworth and Cicchetti 1978). Shumway-Cooke and Woollacott (1985) have shown that DS children can make directionally specific muscle responses to platform (support surface) perturbations just as normal children. The children with DS, however, showed poor adaptation to changing task conditions in comparison to normal peers. The responses of the DS children showed that monosynaptic reflexes were present, suggesting that the balance deficits are not associated with the hypotonus as such (as is frequently proposed) but result from defects in higher-level postural mechanisms.

Infants with developmental delay typically develop *adaptive motor behaviours* in compensation for their inability to make the necessary adjustments to movements of the body mass over the base of support (see Chapter 3). These adaptive behaviours usually involve widening the base of support (e.g. sitting or standing with the hips relatively abducted) and using the hands for support, a behaviour which further enlarges the base of support and allows postural adjustments to occur using a different pattern of muscle activation. It has been suggested (Lydic and Steele 1979) that wide-based sitting reflects an inability to rotate about the body axis. This observation, however, illustrates the difficulty in the clinic of distinguishing between primary and secondary problems. In this case, the primary problem is an inability to make the necessary preparatory and ongoing postural adjustments as the infant moves about in that position. Failure to turn around in sitting is very likely to be secondary, a device to avoid disturbing body alignment, thereby decreasing the need to control the muscle activations necessary for postural adjustment. In addition, wide-based floor-sitting imposes a physical restriction on trunk rotation. The infants with DS in Figures 8.1 and 8.7 typify the strategy of infants with poor movement control when placed in sitting: legs apart, and using the hands for support. These figures also illustrate how the infant can adapt the context of an action in order to fit in with the adaptive behaviour.

Adaptive behaviours are probably reinforced by the persistence in therapy and at home of sitting on the floor, since the size of the possible support surface enables a wide base of support. Sitting on a stool does not allow this behaviour. Figure 8.6a illustrates how habituation of a posture in one position (in this case, sitting) carries over into another. The little boy in this picture had had little practice of standing and at this point it was not possible to get him to bear weight through the feet.

Orofacial dysfunction, specifically early feeding difficulty and the development of persistent tongue protrusion in children with DS, may be related to abnormalities of skeletal development which are reported to lead to a decrease in the volume of the oral cavity (Cohen and Winer 1965; Gullickson 1973). Malocclusion has been noted and attributed to underdevelopment of the maxilla and/or protrusion of the

mandible. Underdevelopment of the sinuses may lead to mouth-breathing. An abnormally large tongue has also been reported in these children (Lemperle and Radu 1980).

Impoverished *manipulation* is particularly evident, even in quite young infants. Persistent and perseverant sucking on objects replaces the exploratory manipulation which normally develops. Infants with DS have been reported as developing normal prehensile patterns (Hogg and Moss 1983). However, other studies have demonstrated inaccuracy on tasks such as finger-tapping (Seyfort and Spreen 1979) and slowness of movement with overshooting and oscillation around a target (Davis and Kelso 1982). It has been suggested that deficits in manual tracking may be due to an inability to use sensory information to generate properly timed movements (Henderson, *et al.* 1981), just as balance difficulties appear to result from deficent integration of visual, vestibular and somatosensory inputs as well as difficulty adapting to changing environmental conditions (Shumway-Cooke and Woollacott 1985). Cole *et al.* (1988) investigated the ability of 8 adults with DS to make adaptive grip force adjustments. The authors report aberrations in control of grasping force and in adapting grasp to changing environmental conditions. The subjects tended at all times to use excessive force. Normally the level of grip force is slightly greater than that needed to prevent the object from slipping and we match increases in the load or slipperiness of an object with an appropriate increase in grip force (Johansson and Westling 1984). The use of excessive force by individuals with DS may have been a learned adaptation by which always producing large forces would ensure a large range of objects would not be dropped. This strategy has been observed in individuals with impaired sensation in the hand (Johansson and Westling 1984). However, sensory abnormalities have not been reported in individuals with DS.

As with able-bodied children, there seem to be important periods in the child's progress at which the impetus towards a particular stage of development is strong. If this opportunity is missed in the retarded child it may be difficult to recreate. For example, if the child is not stood on the feet at an early age, an aversion to having the feet on the ground may develop and the child will flex the legs and refuse to stand. The relationship between vision, reaching and manipulation may be slow to develop and, although this may be due to a visual defect or to poor control of the head, trunk and limb muscles, it may also be due primarily to an attention deficit. Paying attention to what one is doing or to what others are doing is a critical aspect of learning, both motor and scholastic.

For most children, the ultimate level of achievement and the rate at which the child reaches it will depend upon the severity of cognitive impairment. However, for some children, developmental progress will depend on improved nutrition and nurturing, and on the provision of special training. Eventual motor development seems to be influenced by the amount of help, training and guidance the child receives from birth onwards. If the child is referred for treatment for the first time when already 2 years old, some benefit may be derived but it may be less likely that the child will achieve the potential that might have been reached had training to acquire 'good' habits of learning taken place in infancy.

Physiotherapy intervention

Infants with cognitive impairment typically have problems or are slow in developing motor control and acquiring skill in motor actions, including those of everyday life. Problems in developing postural adjustments are particularly common and result in infants being rather slow to sit and stand independently and to be able to use their hands when unsupported. Independent walking may be slow to develop and manual dexterity and skill may never develop.

The *major emphasis in physiotherapy* should be on the training of actions such as standing up and sitting down, walking (or, in the case of severely handicapped children, some form of ambulation), independent sitting and standing, and reaching and manipulation – actions which are critical for the child to be able to contribute to and learn from everyday life. Physiotherapy also involves the prevention of soft tissue adaptations to immobility and deformities in the severely impaired infant, and, for older children, developing exercise programmes to promote fitness.

In addition, the role of the physiotherapist and other health professionals (occupational therapist, speech therapist, psychologist,

orthoptist) involves providing guidance to parents and caregivers about training eating and drinking and encouraging vocalization, ensuring appropriate adaptive devices (e.g. seating) are available, preventing respiratory complications and developing behaviour modification strategies for improving motivation or for extinguishing unwanted behaviours. Parents are trained to organize the infant's and child's environment to encourage competence (Hunt 1976) and minimize the effects of the intellectual impairment.

Typical motor control problems in the performance of everyday actions and some training methods are described in Chapter 3. In this present chapter, some specific problems in training infants with mental retardation are described, with emphasis on infants with DS. This group of children are particularly able to benefit from motor training and exercise programmes.

Commonly used therapeutic approaches to the movement problems associated with intellectual impairment include the so-called neurophysiological approaches (for discussion, see Gordon 1987), particularly the facilitation approach of Bobath. It has been suggested that a facilitation approach is particularly relevant for children with cognitive impairment (Bobath 1963; Lunnen 1991) since such an approach is directed at gaining an automatic response to a perturbation or to handling provided by a person or a piece of equipment. A motor control approach (Gordon 1987; Ostrovsky 1990), on the other hand, requires cognitive participation by the patient (Lunnen 1991).

With small infants, there may be some value in facilitating head, body and limb adjustment to externally imposed displacements of body mass. It is possible that in normal infants such righting movements may well develop naturally as a result of parental handling as the infant is carried around and played with, whereas infants with mental retardation, particularly if they are hypotonic and relatively unresponsive, may be moved about less vigorously.

Nevertheless, the first stage in acquiring skill in movement is said to be cognitive (Fitts 1964). Given the link between cognition and action, a motor learning approach may be preferable for infants and children with mental retardation. In other words, movement that is not linked to intention, that is, to a goal, and is merely automatic or responsive, may be irrelevant to function. Furthermore, such a training programme could be expected to optimize cognitive function. For effective self-initiated motor actions (e.g. reaching to grasp an object) to be acquired, it is probably critical that the child learns to control such actions and receives feedback about the result of the action. There is no evidence that facilitation of automatic responses to outside-induced body displacements will carry over into improved performance of self-initiated movements. The evidence from experiments which illustrate the task- and context-specificity of motor control mechanisms, for example, is that it may not be so (see Chapter 2). In addition, since the infant must learn to initiate movement and control the interactions between body segments, it is very likely that the most direct way for effective motor actions to be learned is for them to be specifically practised.

Understanding the nature of the problems underlying movement deficits helps clarify the nature of the intervention process. For example, children with profound cognitive impairment may be unable to learn how to link intention with action and intervention consists of methods of preventing contracture and deformity and techniques for modifying aberrant – including self-abusive – behaviour.

Measures of effectiveness There is general acceptance now of the need for early stimulation or training of mentally retarded infants. Several studies indicate the benefits for this group of children (Connolly and Russell 1976; Montgomery and Richter 1977; Wolpert *et al.* 1978). The issue is, however, controversial and evidence of the effectiveness of early intervention programmes on developmentally delayed children is variable (Simeonsson *et al.* 1982). Vohr and colleagues (1979) found that 90% of low birth-weight infants considered at risk for poor outcome who were enrolled in a 3-year 'enrichment' programme approached normality at 2 years. In another study (Sloper *et al.* 1986), 24 infants with DS showed a significantly improved attention span following an intensive programme of intervention.

Conductive education over a 22-month period was found in one study to be no more effective in a group of children over the age of 4 years with profound intellectual retardation than traditional classroom teaching (Cottam and Sutton 1985). Montgomery and Richter

(1977) describe the effects of a sensory integrative therapy programme on a group of mentally retarded children from age 5 to 12 years. They quote Ayres's (1972) hypothesis that improvement in sensorimotor integration will result in improvement in motor skills, academic achievement and language ability. The authors do not give details of their programme. In a study on the effects of vestibular stimulation on infants with DS aged between 6 and 24 months, Kantner and colleagues (1976) reported improved motor performance. There are also reports of vestibular stimulation causing a decrease in self-stimulating behaviours (Whitman *et al.* 1983). However, it is not certain that the positive effects are maintained once the vestibular stimulation ceases.

When therapeutic objectives are not directed at improving the performance of functional activities, intervention cannot really be expected to be effective if functional actions are tested. In one study of children with DS who received either neurodevelopmental therapy (NDT) or were on a learning programme (Harris 1981), the therapeutic objectives of the NDT programme were achieved. However, there was a non-significant outcome in terms of the motor development tests used (Bayley Motor Scales and Peabody Gross Motor Scales). The authors suggested that the disparity between the results of the different tests was due to the inappropriateness of the items in the developmental scales. It may also have been, however, that the therapeutic goals were not particularly relevant to the acquisition of skill in performance of the actions tested in the developmental scales. A goal for one infant (the ages of the infants in the study ranged from 2.7 to 21.5 months), for example, was to sit propped with weight on hands for 10 seconds. Infants with DS, once placed in sitting, quickly become habituated (see Fig. 8.7), becoming 'stuck' in the position whether or not they receive physiotherapy. Postural adjustments are typically very poorly developed in this position. It can be difficult, therefore, to teach the child to progress on from this point. That is, to have this type of sitting as a therapeutic goal may be to ensure an adaptive behaviour from which it is difficult for the infant to progress.

The effectiveness of intervention programmes must depend to a large extent both on the type of intervention given and on the severity of the intellectual handicap. Effective intervention needs to incorporate methods of training attention and visuomotor control; behaviour modification techniques; exercises for strengthening specific .muscle groups as well as training of critical functional tasks. Effective measurement needs to test the effects of particular methods on the acquisition of particular attributes. For example, the effectiveness of training standing up needs to be measured by a test of standing up ability, such as movement duration and paths of body parts. Many investigations have instead examined the overall effects of a generalized programme so that it is difficult to know not only what the programme comprised but also whether or not motor performance on functional actions changed. In one study (Kirby and Holborn 1986), the effects of gross motor skill training were found not to generalize into fine motor or social behaviour or even into gross motor skill in different settings. Given the large body of research findings showing the specificity effects of training and exercising, it would be surprising if there were generalization from one action into another, dissimilar, action, particularly in this group of children, who have difficulty developing flexible behaviour.

Without stimulation the mentally retarded infant demonstrates certain predictable delays, all of which have an effect upon the relationship of the infant with adults and peers, the ability to go from one place to another and the ability to develop his or her potential learning capacity, no matter at what level that may be. Training of effective motor performance and the necessary modifications to the environment need to be planned so they can be carried out at home and at school, since this is where the most effective training will occur. The therapist's role involves helping the parents understand the infant's needs, and the ways of bringing out the best in the child, for example, to improve the child's ability to attend to the necessary environmental cues. Parents needs to understand not only what actions have to be trained but also what problems to anticipate and strategies for avoiding them.

For the child to begin to learn even simple concepts, the ability to concentrate and pay attention is critical. Several programmes have been developed with the objective of *improving the learning capacity* of infants with DS. Williams (1978) suggested that mentally retarded children may be more handicapped by their overt behaviour than by lack of development of internal concepts. He stresses that the child must be assisted to develop skills which will enable independence. The gradual development of object permanence in infants with DS is described by Morss (1983), who illustrated the use of structured practice to aid acquisition of the skill. Langley (1990) stresses the importance of the child gaining a sense of control over the environment. She discusses the use of microswitches and computers in making activities meaningful and functional in order to promote practice and skill acquisition. Automated learning devices can be utilized to encourage desired behaviour following the principles of behaviour modification.

Behaviour modification is a critical part of a training programme for the cognitively impaired. A target behaviour is selected and the obstacles to that behaviour defined. Correctly completed behaviour is reinforced. Lunnen (1990, p. 280) describes the steps as:

1 Specify the target behaviour, if necessary breaking the behaviour into component parts.
2 Determine the method of measuring change.
3 Choose appropriate reinforcers.
4 Specify the contingencies under which the desired behaviour will be rewarded.
5 Establish a plan providing for consistent reinforcement and ensuring frequent success.
6 Monitor the effectiveness of the contingencies.
7 Modify as necessary.

The use of a concrete action reinforced immediately by a pleasant consequence has been shown to be effective in training mentally retarded children (Frielander *et al.* 1974; Ball and McGrady 1975; Maloney and Kurtz 1982).

Other studies have also reported positive outcomes following behaviour modification (Chandler and Adams 1972; Westervelt and Luiselli 1975). When a child has developed a habitual response that is maladaptive, training may not be able to proceed until the adaptive behaviour can be controlled. For example, a severely retarded little girl aged 6 years would only stand and walk when she could lean backwards for support and the support had to be provided by a person standing behind her. Training designed to achieve independent standing and walking could not be attempted until a period of behaviour modification had been completed. Not only the child's leaning-backward behaviour but also the behaviour of the adults in the institution who cared for her had to be modified, since it was the adults' acquiescence in the leaning behaviour that was working to reinforce the behaviour.

Training movement control

A critical feature in training control over movement is the use of environmental manipulation – the setting up of an environment that will elicit muscle activity and optimize the development of coordination and the ability to interact with objects and people.

The mentally retarded infant is better sitting in a chair rather than lying supine during the day. Hughes (1971) suggested that head-rolling, a fairly common occupation of cognitively impaired infants and children, may be prevented from developing if the supine position is avoided. Repetitive perseverant movement can occur in any position in which the infant becomes 'stuck', unable to move about, and seems to be related to the infant's inability to perform any more meaningful action.

The erect position encourages the development of control of head position and visual abilities. Sitting in an inclined seat, the young infant may be encouraged to play with graspable toys that elicit both looking and arm movement and that invite interaction; these toys can be hung from a frame within reach. Toys need to be particularly bright and attractive in order to attract attention and to provide feedback and positive reinforcement.

Extension exercises for the trunk, head and lower limbs in prone, abdominal exercises and push-ups are used to encourage the development of control and muscle strength. In Figure 8.2, the 10-month-old boy tended to use his tongue repetitively and rake with his hands (a). Extension exercises and push-ups in prone apparently gave him some idea of the possibilities of action in prone (b and c). With practice, he was able to take weight through his hands (d), and within a few days to reach out for a toy without falling over.

The little girl in Figure 8.3 had a similar problem in four-foot kneeling. In this position, she could not hold her legs in adduction and therefore could not move (a). Supported in this position, however, (b), she could reach out and grasp toys and play games (c). As she played, her leg muscles were being exercised specifically for moving about in four-foot kneeling. If necessary, the legs can be prevented from abducting by a light harness (for a suggested design, see Sellers and Capi 1989).

Repetitive practice of actions such as standing up from the floor using the hands for support may be necessary. Once the little girl in Figure 8.1 was taken through the action (Fig. 8.4) she soon learned to do it herself and to get back down to the floor. She got the idea of the means by which she could reach the objects on the table (which she could not reach unless she stood up), and although she devised a number

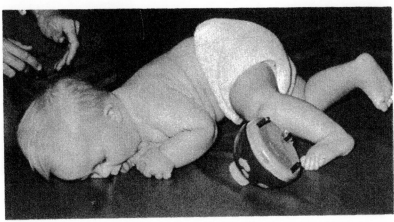

a

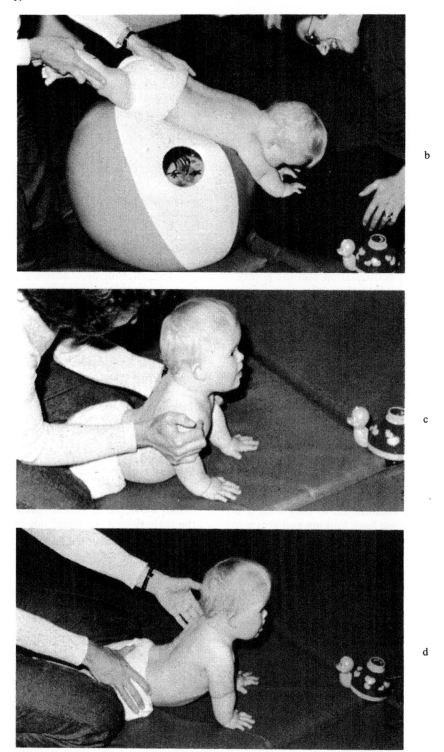

b

c

d

Figure 8.2   (a) Limited motor behaviour in prone. (b) Extension exercises over a ball. (c) Practice of "push-ups" to strengthen his upper body and lower-limb extensor muscles. (d) Now he has the idea of some possibilities offered by the prone position.

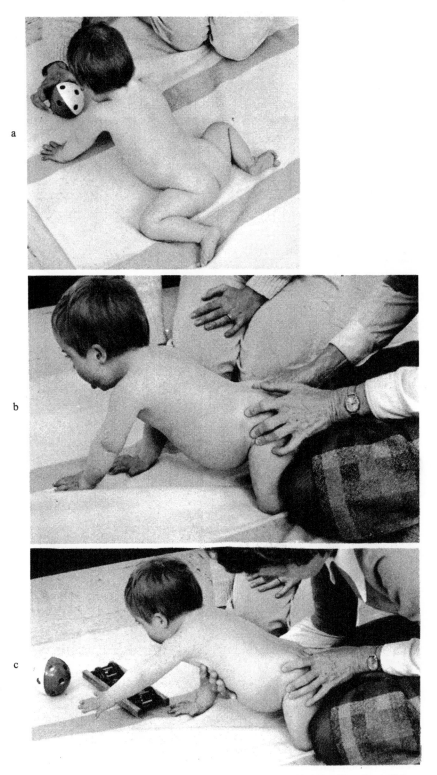

Figure 8.3   (a) She is 'stuck' in this position and cannot adduct her hips. (b, c) If her legs are held adducted, she is able to reach out for a toy.

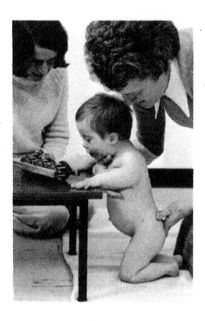
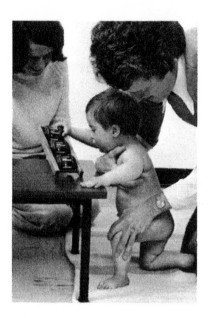
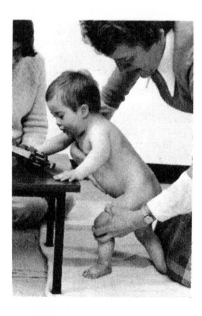
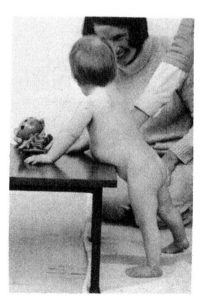

Figure 8.4   This little girl is shown how to get from kneeling to standing. She will need repetitive practice with guidance until she can do it independently as a means to a desired end.

of variations in her initial independent attempts, she was learning how to problem-solve, that is, how to relate her body to the environment as a means of achieving her intentions.

The infant needs early experience of standing. Parents normally stand their infants (in some cultures a great deal of practice in standing is given), so infants typically experience supported standing long before they are able to balance and stand independently. The infant with DS, for example, is unlikely to be stood early because hypotonia makes it difficult for the infant to be held upright without the legs collapsing. At this stage, the provision of wraparounds (Fig. 8.5) makes it possible for the infant to practise standing. There are several reasons for the early institution of standing and these are discussed in Chapter 3. For the cognitively impaired infant, however, it is particularly necessary to experience and become accustomed to weight-bearing through the feet, as some children appear to develop an aversion to tactile and pressure sensation

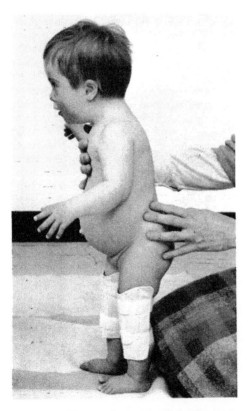

Figure 8.5 The use of wraparounds is often necessary to enable standing to be practised.

through the soles of the feet and will draw the legs into flexion when placed in standing.

If the infant is not given the opportunity to stand, the ability to support and balance the body mass through the lower limbs may not develop even when the lower limb extensor muscles are able to generate sufficient force. The little boy in Figure 8.6a, at the age of 10 months, seemed to have no idea how to support himself on his feet and could not be held in standing. After a few minutes supported in standing at a table, with wraparounds preventing his knees from collapsing, he was able to stand with support (Fig. 8.6b). The wraparounds, together with the opportunity to play at a table, seemed to give him the idea of what to do. The next step was to teach him to move around in standing, for example, walk sideways around the table and reach out for toys, so that he would eventually be able to stand independently, without using his hands for support.

Some cognitively impaired children also develop aversive reactions to taking weight through the hands and holding objects in the hands. These children hold their hands fisted and resist any attempt to have them use their hands. This aversive response seems to arise when infants are not given the opportunity to use their hands for support and for manipulation and, therefore, it should be possible to avoid. Once an aversion to sensory inputs to the hands or feet has developed, however, some method of desensitization may be needed. A mechanical vibrator placed on the limb proximal to the foot or hand, then moved distally as the child's tolerance increases, may have the necessary effect. As soon as the child can tolerate vibration to the plantar or palmar surface, standing can be attempted. Behaviour modification techniques may need to be used in conjunction.

As the child gets older, activities are encouraged to increase endurance and promote physical fitness. Poor motor skills with an inactive lifestyle in children with DS have been proposed to contribute to the excess body fat noted in many of these children (Pueschal 1987).

Swimming instruction is important for safety as well as enjoyment and mobility. The child is taught how to float, encouraged to put the face in the water without inhaling, and how to swim. Two points in teaching body control in the water are the control of respiration, which

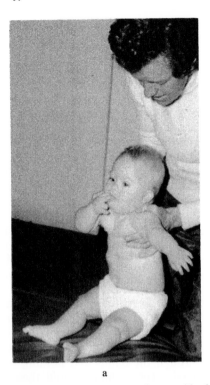 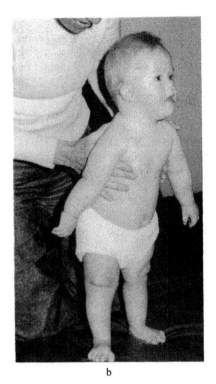

a   b

Figure 8.6   (a) He appears to have no idea how to use his legs for support. (b) After some
practice standing in wraparounds he has the idea. Now he needs to learn how to move
about (balance) in standing and to take steps.

involves relaxation, plus the instinctive knowledge that movement of the head influences the
position of the trunk and legs. That is, extension of the head in prone and flexion in supine
cause the legs to sink down, while flexion of the
head in prone and extension in supine cause the
legs to float on the surface (Reid Campion
1991).

Training postural adjustments

It has been suggested (Shumway-Cook and
Woollacott 1985) that focus in establishing
more effective balance in DS infants should be
on enhancing motor coordination by improving
spatiotemporal   coupling   between   muscle
groups and on improving the organizational
processes for adapting postural adjustments to
changing task conditions. Chapter 3 contains a
description of some task- and context-specific
training strategies which have been developed
in an attempt to meet these criteria. This present section contains some examples specifically
directed at the problems of motor behaviour
associated with mental retardation.

In sitting, the infant typically acquires the
ability to reach forwards but cannot reach sideways or turn the body to look behind. Allowing
floor-sitting for such children appears to encourage this behaviour since there may be few
demands on the postural system. Figure 8.7
shows the typical sitting position of an infant
with DS who would only reach for an object if it
were held directly in front (a). She would only
look up after she had moved the body mass
forwards and supported herself on her hands
(b). Normally, looking up displaces the body
mass backwards and anticipatory postural
adjustments would ensure that balance would
not be lost. This little girl has learned to manipulate the environment and the individual with
whom she is playing to ensure that she need
make only limited postural adjustment.

The girl in Figure 8.8 could reach further in a
lateral direction when sitting on a seat with feet
on floor (b), compared to when she sat on the
floor with legs abducted and flexed (a). When
she was first placed on a seat, it was wide
enough to allow her to sit with legs flexed and
abducted in the same posture as on the floor,

and she strongly resisted any attempt to put her feet on the floor. This meant that she was having no practice at using her legs for assisting balance. However, when the environment was modified to ensure her favourite posture was impossible (when she was sat on a narrow seat), she was able to sit and reach out for a toy. Sitting at a table to play, learning to stand up and sit down, and to reach down to pick up toys from the floor forwards and laterally were the next objectives.

Since these adaptive behaviours (see Figs 8.7 and 8.8) are common in sitting in infants with cognitive impairment and tend to persist once developed, it is probably good practice to encourage the development of postural adjustments and independent sitting on a seat with feet on the floor rather than on the floor. Avoiding floor-sitting may seem to be depriving the child of a place to play. However, with many of these children, the development of independent sitting with effective postural adjustments can be very slow, and floor-sitting can effectively immobilize the child. The major aims of intervention in sitting are to train the child to reach out for objects to manipulate, which requires the ability to move the upper body about over the base of support which comprises the thighs and the feet. The critical muscle activations in sitting are those which link the upper body to the thighs and the lower limbs to the feet.

The little girl in Figure 8.9 could only stand with her feet wide apart (a). When her legs were held together she flexed them. She needed to wear wraparounds while she was encouraged to play in standing (Figs 8.5 and 8.10) and until her habitual wide-based stance was eliminated. Playing was designed to encourage postural adjustments to self-initiated movements of the body mass with the aim of independent standing.

Training eating and drinking

The infant with DS may have a thick, hypotonic tongue which, together with poor motor control, may be a reason for difficulty suckling and swallowing. Perhaps because of their low expectations of the child and the lack of help they so often receive with feeding, many parents tend to keep the infant on the bottle and on sloppy food for much longer than normal (Carr 1979). Lateral vibration to the tongue, done vigorously with the finger, with downwards pressure on the tongue (Mueller 1977; Carr 1979) is considered to be effective in stimulating the tongue. When combined with

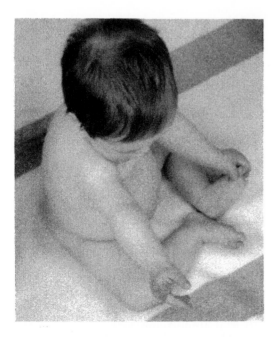
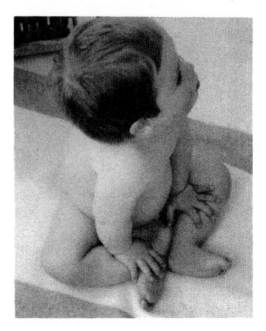

Figure 8.7 Typical adaptive behaviours in sitting.

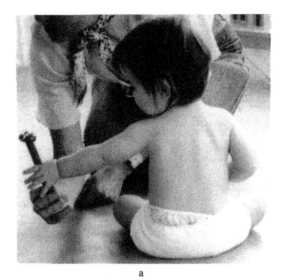
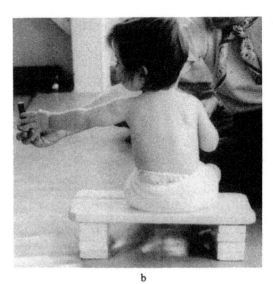

a   b

Figure 8.8   (a) This was the extent of lateral reaching in floor-sitting. (b) Sitting on a seat, training was given to develop postural adjustments with the feet and thighs forming the base of support.

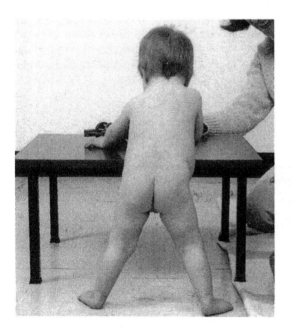

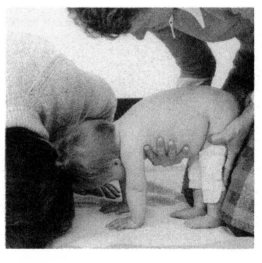

Figure 8.10   Learning to stand with legs adducted on a narrow base of support.

Figure 8.9   Typical posture in standing.

treatment to desensitize the oral area if it is hypersensitive and to train control of lip and jaw closure and swallowing, the process of feeding the infant may become much simpler.

The infant should start on solid food at the normal time and should gradually be introduced to food which needs chewing. One way to stimulate chewing is to place a strip of under-

cooked meat between the infant's gums or teeth (Mueller 1977), which is followed by stimulation of lip and jaw closure (Chapter 5). Parents should introduce the infant to foods of different flavours and textures early so as to avoid the development of an aversion to different foods. Finger-feeding should also be introduced as soon as possible, both as an early step towards independence and to enable the child to gain pleasure from eating.

Behaviour therapy can be used to modify unwanted behaviour, such as food spillage when eating (Cipani 1981) and to encourage more appropriate behaviour. Both behaviour modification and oromotor training appear to be effective in reducing tongue protrusion in young children with DS (Purdy *et al.* 1987).

Aspiration of food can cause pneumonia or death (Chaney 1978). Mentally retarded infants and children frequently have poor respiratory function which may be due to a combination of factors, such as poor positioning (supine), muscle weakness and incoordination (affecting coughing), poor coordination between oromotor and respiratory movements and increase in volume of saliva with poor clearance. These factors increase the likelihood of aspiration of food and saliva.

Social and psychological factors

The trend in management in many countries is away from institutionalization and towards keeping the child at home with support services provided. Foster home placement provides an alternative when parents cannot cope with the stress imposed on the family. Where possible, cognitively impaired youngsters are brought up and educated in the 'normal' environment of the able-bodied. It is believed that a home or similar environment encourages the development of social skills and interpersonal relationships. The severely cognitively impaired, however, probably require to live in institutions which have the necessary staff and facilities.

The birth of a mentally retarded infant brings a sense of loss and grief to the parents. Many authors have discussed these effects and the stresses facing parents of a mentally retarded infant. If parents have a negative view of the infant's future capabilities, this may have an effect upon their developing relationship with the infant and upon the infant's immediate environment. There is a reciprocal relationship between infant responses to handling and parental behaviour. It is probable that young infants, by their patterns of behaviour, influence well-established child-rearing practices (Hopkins and Westra 1988). It has been suggested that specific parental handling procedures may positively affect infant behaviour which in turn leads to a more positive attitude on the part of the parent (Solkoff *et al.* 1969). It is important that parents realize the help they

and the infant can receive from therapists and teachers and can understand the need for specific training in motor and other skills. This point can be discussed with parents without giving them unrealistic hopes for the infant's future. Discussions with the parents of older children with DS are usually helpful in giving new parents insight into the pleasures and difficulties involved in rearing a child who has DS.

Parents are helped to understand that the child will need extra stimulus to explore the environment and to develop the motor and other skills that other children will achieve with minimum help. They are taught strategies to avoid and, when necessary, to deal with aberrant behaviour, which can be more of an obstacle to the success of an intervention programme and to child-rearing itself than the cognitive impairment (Hutt and Gibby 1979).

Summary

Motor development and the acquisition of skill is delayed in the mentally retarded child, who may be floppy with poor motor control, lacking the ability to move about, with poor balance, and a tendency to develop habitual responses which further hinder progress. Movement is an integral part of the development of social, emotional and cognitive functions, since it enables the infant to interact with objects and people in the environment. Training should begin in early infancy in order to assist the infant to develop his or her potential, and to guide the parents in establishing a bond with the infant. It requires patience and affection to assist these children to acquire motor skill, and also the conviction that something can be done to help them. It does seem certain that many mentally retarded infants will gain considerably from training designed to improve motor function, and from parents trained to understand their infant's special needs.

References

Ahlman, H., Grillner, S. and Udo, M. (1971) The effect of 5-HTP on the static fusimotor and the tonic stretch reflexes of an extensor muscle. *Brain Res.*, 27, 393–396.

Asmussen, E. and Heeboll-Neilsen, K. (1956) Physical performance and growth in children. Influence of sex, age and intelligence. *J. Appl. Physiol.*, **8**, 4, 371.

Ayres, A.J. (1972) *Sensory Integration and Learning Disorders.* Los Angeles, CA: Western Psychological Services.

Ball, T.S. and McGrady, R.E. (1975) Automated finger praxis training with a cerebral palsied retarded adolescent. *Ment. Retard.*, **13**, 41.

Bayley, N. (1969) *Bayley Scales in Infant Development.* New York: The Psychological Corporation.

Berthenthal, B. and Campos, J. (1987) New directions in the study of early experience. *Child Dev.*, **58**, 560–567.

Butterworth, G. and Cicchetti, D. (1978) Visual calibration of posture in normal and motor retarded Down syndrome infants. *Perception*, **7**, 513–525.

Campos, J., Svejda, M., Campos, R. *et al.* (1982) The emergence of self-produced locomotion: its importance for psychological development in infancy. In: *Intervention with At-Risk and Handicapped Infants*, edited by D. Bricker. Baltimore, MD: University Park Press.

Carr, J. (1975) *Young Children with Down's Syndrome.* IRMMH monograph 4. London: Butterworths.

Carr, J.H. (1979) *Oral Function in Infancy – Its Importance for Future Development.* Aust. J. Physiother. Paediatric Monograph. Melbourne: Australian Physiotherapy Association.

Chandler, L.S. and Adams, M.A. (1972) Multiply handicapped child motivated for ambulation through behaviour modification. Case report. *Phys. Ther.*, **52**, 399.

Chaney, R.H. (1978) Respiratory complications in the profoundly retarded compared to those less retarded. In: *The Profoundly Mentally Retarded IX*, edited by J.D. Schwartz, P.C. Eyman, C.C. Cleland *et al.* Austin, TX: Western Research Conference.

Cipani, E. (1981) Modifying food spillage behavior in an institutionalized retarded client. *J. Behav. Ther. Exp. Psychiatry*, **12**, 3, 261–265.

Cohen, M.M. and Winer, R.A. (1965) Dental and facial characteristics in Down's syndrome. *J. Dent. Res.*, **44** (suppl.), 197–298.

Cole, K.J., Abbs, J.H. and Turner, G.S. (1988) Deficits in the production of grip forces in Down syndrome. *Dev. Med. Child Neurol.*, **30**, 752–758.

Coleman, M. (1975) The use of 5-hydroxytryptophan in patients with Down's syndrome. In: *Down's Syndrome (Mongolism): Research, Prevention, and Management*, edited by R. Koch and F.F. de la Cruz. New York: Brunner-Mazel.

Connolly, B. and Russell, F. (1976) Interdisciplinary early intervention programme. *Phys. Ther.*, **56**, 2, 155.

Cooke, R. (1991) Atlantoaxial instability in individuals with Down syndrome. *Bulletin of Aust. Physiother. Assoc. (NSW)*, **Oct**, 4,7.

Cottam, P.J. and Sutton, A. (eds) (1985) *Conductive Education a System for Overcoming Motor Disorder.* London: Croom Helm.

Cowie, V.A. (1970) *A Study of Early Development of Mongols.* London: Pergamon.

Crome, I., Cowie, V. and Slater, E. (1966) Statistical note on cerebellar and brain stem weight in mongolism. *J. Ment. Defic. Res.*, **10**, 69–72.

Davis, W.E. and Kelso, J.A.S. (1982) Analysis of 'invariant characteristics' in the motor control of Down's syndrome and normal subjects. *J. Motor Behav.*, **14**, 3, 194–212.

Dubowitz, V. (1965) Intellectual impairment in muscular dystrophy. *Arch. Dis. Child.*, **40**, 296–301.

Frankenburg, W.K. and Dodds, J.B. (1967) Denver developmental screening test. *J. Pediatr.*, **71**, 181.

Frielander, B.Z., Kamin, P. and Hesse, G.W. (1974) Operant therapy for prehension disabilities in moderately and severely retarded young children. *Train. Sch. Bull. (Vincl)*, **71**, 101.

Ghose, S. and Chandra Sekhar, G. (1986) The eye in idiopathic mental retardation. *Jpn. J. Ophthalmol.*, **30**, 431.

Gilman, S., Bloedel, J.R. and Lechtenberg, R. (eds) (1981) *Disorders of the Cerebellum.* Philadelphia, PA: F.A. Davis.

Gordon, J. (1987) Assumptions underlying physical therapy intervention: theoretical and historical perspectives. In: *Movement Science. Foundations for Physical Therapy in Rehabilitation*, edited by J.H. Carr and R.B. Shepherd. Rockville, MD: Aspen Publications.

Gould, J. (1977) The use of the Vineland social maturity scale, the Merrill-Palmer scale of mental tests (non verbal items) and the Reynell developmental language scales with children in contact with the services for severe mental retardation. *J. Ment. Defic. Res.*, **21**, 213.

Gullickson, J.S. (1973) Oral findings in children with Down's syndrome. *J. Dent. Child.*, **40**, 293–297.

Gustafson, G.E. (1984) Effects of the ability to locomote on infants' social and exploratory behaviours: an experimental study. *Dev. Psychol.*, **20**, 397–405.

Harris, S.R. (1981) Effects of neurodevelopmental therapy on motor performance of infants with Down's syndrome. *Dev. Med. Child Neurol.*, **23**, 477.

Henderson, S.E. (1985) Some aspects of the development of motor control in Down's syndrome. In: *Themes in Motor Development*, edited by H.T.A. Whiting and M.G. Wade. Dordrecht: Martinus Nijhoff.

Henderson, S.E., Morris, J. and Frith, U. (1981) The motor deficit in Down's syndrome children: a problem of timing? *J. Child Psychol. Psychiatry*, **22**, 233–245.

Hogg, J. and Moss, S.C. (1983) Prehensile development in Down's syndrome and non-handicapped pre-school children. *Br. J. Dev. Psychol.*, **1**, 189–204.

Holmes, L.B., Moser, H.W., Halldorsson, S., Mack, C., Pant, S.S. and Matzilevich, B. (1972) *Mental Retardation. An Atlas of Diseases with Associated Physical Abnormalities.* New York: Macmillan.

Hopkins, B. and Westra, T. (1988) Maternal handling and motor development: an intracultural study. *Genet. Soc. Gen. Psych. Mongr.*, **114**, 379–408.

Hughes, N.A.S. (1971) Developmental physiotherapy for mentally handicapped babies. *Physiotherapy*, **57**, 9, 399.

Hunt, J.M. (1976) Environmental programming to foster competence and prevent mental retardation in infancy. In: *Environments as Therapy for Brain Dysfunction*, edited by R.N. Walsh and W.T. Greenough. New York: Plenum Press.

Hutt, M.L. and Gibby, R.G. (1979) *The Mentally Retarded Child: Development, Training and Education*, 4th edn. Boston, MA: Allyn and Bacon.

Illingworth, R.S. (1974) *The Development of the Infant and Young Child*, 5th edn. London: Churchill Livingstone.

Ireton, H.R. and Thwing, E.J. (1972) *Manual for the Minnesota Child Development Inventory. Interpretive Scoring System*.

Johansson, R.S. and Westling, G. (1984) Roles of glabrous skin receptors and sensorimotor memory in automatic control of precision grip when lifting rougher or more slippery objects. *Exp. Brain Res.*, **56**, 550–564.

Kantner, R.M., Clark, D.L., Allen, L.C. and Chase, M.P. (1976) Effects of vestibular stimulation on nystagmus response and motor performance in the developmentally delayed infant. *Phys. Ther.*, **56**, 4, 414.

Kirby, K.C. and Holborn, S.W. (1986) Trained, generalized and collateral behavior changes of preschool children receiving gross-motor skills training. *J. Appl. Behav. Anal.*, **19**, 283–288.

Koch, R. and de la Cruz, F.F. (1975) *Down's Syndrome (Mongolism): Research, Prevention, and Management*. New York: Brunner-Mazel.

Langley, M.B. (1990) A developmental approach to the use of toys for facilitation of environmental control. *Phys. Occup. Ther. Pediatr.*, **10**, 2, 83.

Lemieux, B.G. (1989) Chromosomal-linked diseases. In: *Pediatric Neurology. Principles and Practice*, edited by K.F. Swaiman. St Louis, MO: C.V. Mosby.

Lemperle, G. and Radu, D. (1980) Facial plastic surgery in children with Down's syndrome. *Plast. Reconstructr. Surg.*, **66**, 337–342.

Lunnen, K.Y. (1991) Children with severe and profound retardation. In: *Pediatric Neurologic Physical Therapy*, 2nd edn, edited by S.K. Campbell. New York: Churchill Livingstone.

Lydic, J.S. and Steele, C. (1979) Assessment of the quality of sitting and gait patterns in children with Down's syndrome. *Phys. Ther.*, **59**, 12, 1489–1494.

MacLean, W. and Baumeister, A. (1981) Observational analysis of the stereotyped mannerisms of a developmentally delayed infant. *Appl. Res. Ment. Retard.*, **2**, 257.

Maloney, F.P. and Kurtz, P.A. (1982) The use of a mercury switch head control device in profoundly retarded, multiply handicapped children. *Phys. Occup. Ther. Pediatr.*, **2**, 4, 11.

Molnar, G.E. (1974) Motor deficit of retarded infants and young children. *Arch. Phys. Med. Rehabil.*, **55**, 393.

Montgomery, P. and Richter, E. (1977) Effect of sensory integrative therapy on the neuromotor development of retarded children. *Phys. Ther.*, **57**, 7, 799.

Morss, J.R. (1983) Cognitive development in the Down's syndrome infant; slow or difficult? *Br. J. Educ. Psychol.*, **53**, 40–47.

Mueller, H. (1977) Personal communication.

Neisser, U. (1976) *Cognition and Reality*. San Francisco, CA: W.H. Freeman.

Ostrovsky, K.M. (1990) Facilitation vs motor control. *Clin. Management*, **10**, 34.

Piaget, J. (1960) The general problems of the psychobiological development of the child. In: *Discussions on Child Development*, vol. 4, edited by J.M. Tanner and B. Inhelder. New York: International Universities Press.

Pueschal, S.M. (1987) Health concerns in persons with Down syndrome. In: *New Perspectives on Down Syndrome*, edited by S. Pueschal, C. Tingey, J. Rynders *et al.* Baltimore, MD: P.H. Brooks.

Purdy, A.H., Deitz, J.C. and Harris, S.R. (1987) Efficacy of two treatment approaches to reduce tongue protrusion of children with Down syndrome. *Dev. Med. Child Neurol.*, **29**, 469–478.

Reid Campion, M. (1991) *Hydrotherapy in Paediatrics*, 2nd edn. Oxford: Butterworth-Heinemann.

Sellers, J.S. and Capi, B. (1989) Use of abduction restraint in facilitating selected motor patterns in a child with Down syndrome: a case report. *Phys. Occup. Ther. Pediatr.*, **9**, 4, 63–68.

Seyfort, B. and Spreen, O. (1979) Two-plated tapping performance by Down's syndrome and non-Down's syndrome retardates. *J. Child Psychol. Psychiatry*, **20**, 351–355.

Shumway-Cooke, A. and Woollacott, M.H. (1985) Dynamics of postural control in the child with Down syndrome. *Phys. Ther.*, **65**, 9, 1315–1322.

Simeonsson, R.J., Cooper, D.H. and Scheiner, A.P. (1982) A review and analysis of the effectiveness of early intervention with Down's syndrome infants. *Pediatrics*, **69**, 635–641.

Sloper, P., Glenn, S.M. and Cunningham, C.C. (1986) The effect of intensity of training on sensori-motor development in infants with Down's syndrome. *J. Ment. Defic. Res.*, **30**, 149–162.

Soare, P.L. and Raimondi, A.J. (1977) Interactional and perceptual-motor characteristics of treated myelomeningocele children. *Am. J. Dis. Child.*, **131**, 199–204.

Solkoff, N., Yafte, S., Weintraub, D. and Blase, B. (1969) Effects of handling on subsequent development of premature infants. *Dev. Psychol.*, **1**, 765–768.

Swaiman, K.F. (1989) Mental retardation. In: *Pediatric Neurology. Principles and Practice*, edited by K.F. Swaiman. St Louis, MO: C.V. Mosby.

Thelen, E. (1986) Treadmill-elicited stepping in seven-month-old infants. *Child Dev.*, **57**, 1498–1506.

Ulrich, B., Ulrich, D. and Collier, D.H. (1992) Alternating stepping patterns: hidden abilities of 11-month old infants with Down syndrome. *Dev. Med. Child Neurol.*, **34**, 233–239.

Vohr, B.R., Oh, W., Rosenfield, A.G. *et al.* (1979) The preterm small for gestational age infant: a two year follow-up study. *Am. J. Obstet. Gynecol.*, **133**, 425.

Walton, J. (1971) *The Essentials of Neurology*. London: Pitman.

Westervelt, V.D. and Luiselli, J.K. (1975) Establishing standing and walking behaviour in a physically handicapped, retarded child. *Phys. Ther.*, **55**, 76.

Whitman, T.L., Scibak, J.W. and Reid, D.H. (1983) *Behaviour Modification with the Severely and Profoundly Retarded: Research and Application.* San Diego, CA: Academic Press.

Williams, C. (1978) An introduction to behavioural principles in teaching the profoundly handicapped. *Child*, **4**, 21.

Wolpert, R., Gouse-Sheese, J., Leuchter, S.L. and Sandmann, M. (1978) Stimulating developmentally delayed infants: evaluation of a short term project. *Physiother. Can.*, **30**, 2, 78.

Further reading

Alberto, P.A. and Troutman, A.C. (1987) *Applied Behavioural Analysis for Teachers – Influencing Student Performance*, 2nd edn. Columbia, OH: Charles E. Merrill.

Holt, K.S. (1958) The home care of severely retarded children. *Pediatrics*, **22**, 744.

La Frenais, M. (1971) *Language Stimulus with Retarded Children*. London: National Society for Mentally Handicapped Children.

Levy, J. (1973) *The Baby Exercise Book* New York: Pantheon.

National Society for Mentally Handicapped Children (1967) *Stress in Families with a Mentally Handicapped Child. Report of a Working Party*. London: NSMHC.

9

Infections of the nervous system

Encephalitis, encephalomyelitis and meningitis

Inflammation of the central nervous system (CNS) may result from many causative factors, and the clinical features will depend upon the severity of the infection and the specific area of the nervous system involved. The majority of infants and children who suffer from encephalitis, encephalomyelitis and meningitis recover without any apparent sequelae. However, some are left with permanent evidence of neurological damage – mental retardation, behavioural abnormalities, speech disturbances, epilepsy and motor disability.

Neurological syndromes may complicate certain common childhood illnesses such as mumps, measles, chickenpox or pertussis, or may be the result of vaccination. Infants may be born with congenital rubella encephalopathy due to maternal rubella, and may demonstrate cardiac defects, mental retardation, cataracts, deafness and skeletal deformities. Bacterial meningitis may be caused by Haemophilus influenzae, Escherichia coli, meningococcus or pneumococcus. The young infant may be particularly susceptible to bacterial meningeal infection during the period between passively gained immunity and the development of active immunity. An encephalopathy may be caused by lead intoxication in children who chew on toys or furniture coated with paint containing lead. It is the accumulation of lead which causes damage to the brain and peripheral nerves as well as to other organs.

The neurological complications of encephalopathy are due to subdural effusion, hydrocephalus, brain abscess, to necrosis or to haemorrhage. The signs evident during the acute stage include pyrexia, headache, vomiting, coma and convulsions, opisthotonus and irritability, and the cry may be high-pitched.

Management of these children in the early stages is supportive. Treatment of the unconscious child is described briefly in Chapter 27.

Physiotherapy in the stage of recovery from encephalopathy is directed towards the particular functional problems demonstrated by each child, and is as described in Chapter 4.

Viral encephalomyelitis may be caused by the poliomyelitis virus, and Guillain–Barré syndrome is an encephalomyelitis of unknown origin. Management of children suffering from these diseases and their aftermath is described below.

Anterior poliomyelitis

This is an infectious disease caused by one of three strains of polioenterovirus. Transmission is human to human, principally through secretions of the upper respiratory tract and by faecal contamination. The virus travels from the pharynx or lower alimentary tract via the circulatory system to the CNS, causing meningitic symptoms and, in a small percentage of individuals, destroying the motor cells of the anterior horn of the spinal cord and brain-stem, causing a flaccid lower motor neuron-type of paralysis. Physical effort or localized trauma during the initial stage of infection apparently predisposes those particular cells to destruction (Sharrard 1971; Walton 1971). If the muscles of respiration are paralysed and adequate ventilation cannot be maintained, or if respiratory tract infection cannot be prevented or controlled, death may ensue.

The effects of the viral invasion can be prevented or inactivated by oral vaccines, and consequently the disease is no longer common in countries in which large-scale inoculation programmes are practised. However, infrequent outbursts provide evidence of the potential of poliomyelitis occurring in poorly immunized populations. In tropical and subtropical developing countries, it is estimated that an average of 400 000 new cases occur each year (Raymond 1986). Outbreaks occur even in countries with immunization programmes (Hovi *et al.* 1986).

Pathology

The neuronal lesions occur in the anterior horn cells of the spinal cord, the medullary and pontine reticular formation, the cranial nerve cells of the medulla, the cerebellum, midbrain (grey matter, substantia nigra), thalamus and hypothalamus, pallidum and cerebral cortex (motor areas only). Polioencephalitic changes have been found in post-mortem studies even in cases without spinal motoneuron damage (Bruno *et al.* 1991). Extraneural pathology, such as bronchopulmonary changes, is usually secondary owing, for example, to impairment of cough and decreased thoracic movement.

The nerve cells are either destroyed, in which case no recovery of function will occur, or temporarily disabled. This disability is due either to inflammatory oedema occurring around the cells or to relatively minor damage being done to the cells. The pathological reactions include chromatolysis, neurolysis and eventually neuronophagia (Swaiman 1989). There is an inflammatory reaction in the region of the cells involved, characterized by diffuse oedema and cellular exudation. The axons of the damaged cells demonstrate Wallerian degeneration throughout the entire length of the nerve fibre. Cells concerned with the innervation of the abdominal organs including the bladder may

be affected where there are areas of severe destruction. As a result of the inflammatory reaction and the destruction of the cells, the cerebrospinal fluid, when tested, shows an increase in cells which returns to normal 10–14 days after onset of the disease, as well as an increase in protein. The virus can be isolated in the stools and the child is said to be infectious while this situation continues.

Recovery processes

Functional recovery is generally attributed to reinnervation of muscles by collateral axonal sprouting from surviving lower motoneurons (Wohlfart 1958). Axonal sprouting enables uninvolved or recovered motoneurons to make connections with up to five additional muscle fibres. The effectiveness of this process is probably responsible for muscles testing normal, even when a large percentage of the original motoneurons have been damaged (Halstead 1988). In muscle biopsies, fibre-type grouping has shown that there are fewer but larger motor units (Drachman *et al.* 1967) in recovered individuals.

Clinical features

Approximately 90% of those infected will be asymptomatic. Others suffer a transient minor illness. A small percentage of those infected develop paralysis (Mandell *et al.* 1985).

The clinical features may be described as occurring in three stages – preparalytic and paralytic stages, followed by the recovery stage. In the *preparalytic stage* the features are those of a febrile illness, with fever, malaise, vomiting and, if there is meningeal involvement, pain in the neck, trunk and limbs. Symptoms may mimic a mild attack of influenza. Many children have a short symptom-free period before the onset of a second phase which may or may not result in paralysis.

In a small percentage of those affected the disease progresses to a *paralytic stage* in which there is gradually developing weakness and paralysis with muscle tenderness. Reflexes are absent or diminished. The nerve cell involvement is haphazard in distribution and may cause paralysis of single muscles or almost total paralysis of trunk and limb muscles and the muscles of swallowing. In the spinal form, there is weakness of muscles of the neck, trunk and limbs. In the bulbar form, there is weakness of muscles supplied by cranial nerves. In the encephalitic form, there may be irritability, drowsiness or disorientation.

Certain muscles have been found to be more susceptible to paralysis than others. Sharrard (1955, 1957) lists the following: tibialis anterior, tibialis posterior, the long toe flexors and extensors, the peronei, the calf muscles and, in the upper limbs, the intrinsic muscles of the hand, the deltoid and tricep brachii.

The degree of muscle weakness depends on the percentage of nerve cells destroyed. More than 60% of motor cells supplying a muscle have to be destroyed before weakness becomes clinically detectable (Sharrard 1953), suggesting that muscles which are apparently spared may have undergone subclinical lesions (Klingman *et al.* 1988).

Respiratory problems may arise in the presence of one or more factors: paralysis of the diaphragm due to involvement of the phrenic nerve, paralysis of the intercostal muscles, paralysis of the abdominal muscles resulting in poor expiratory power and difficulty in clearing airways, involvement of cranial nerves resulting in paralysis or weakness of the muscles of swallowing and the danger of aspiration of saliva, food, fluid or vomitus.

Pain and tenderness cause protective muscle spasm. The child resents handling while the disease is acute and may lie with the part protectively flexed. Apart from the pain and tenderness there are no other sensory changes. The child will be irritable and restless while the disease is in the acute stage.

The *stage of recovery* begins when the acute symptoms subside, leaving the child with weakness and paralysis of movement. Muscle length changes occur as a result of unbalanced muscle activity and immobility. Muscular atrophy occurs due to denervation and disuse.

The main period of recovery is in the few weeks following the acute phase of the disease, and this recovery is probably due to the resolution of inflammatory oedema which compresses but does not necessarily destroy the nerve cells. Further improvement takes place in the next 12 months. Damaged cells will not regenerate so the residual paralysis will be permanent. Any further recovery is probably due to adaptive changes in the nervous system, as well as to muscle hypertrophy through exercise of those muscle fibres still innervated and the learning of trick or substitution movements.

Post-polio syndrome

Poliomyelitis has been considered a stable chronic disease following recovery from the acute phase. However, a significant number of adults who had poliomyelitis as children are being found to experience new and debilitating symptoms of fatigue, muscle weakness and atrophy, pain and respiratory problems many years later (Dalakas *et al.* 1984; *Polio Network News* 1992; Westbrook 1992). In a US survey done in 1985 of 676 individuals who had survived polio, 91% reported new or increased fatigue (Bruno and Frick 1987).

The pathogenesis is unknown but hypotheses include neuromuscular overuse, muscle cell breakdown, normal and/or premature ageing, an immune response and hormonal imbalance deficit (Klingman *et al.* 1988; Bruno *et al.* 1991; Dean 1991; *Polio Network News* 1992). It has been suggested that the enlarged motor units may carry an increased susceptibility for dysfunction and/or degeneration (Klingman *et al.* 1988). The maintenance of these larger motor units would impose large metabolic demands on both motoneuron and sarcomere and could predispose to such dysfunction.

Management

Preparalytic stage

During this stage the child must have complete bed rest. Analgesics may be prescribed to relieve pain, and hot packs may provide relief. During the initial stages, attention is paid to ensuring adequate fluid and electrolyte balance, providing respiratory support and treating bladder and bowel dysfunction where necessary.

Paralytic stage

This regime is continued during the active paralytic stage, and the child is disturbed as little as possible. Handling will increase discomfort, and the muscles are often tender to touch. Management here consists largely of measures of prevention.

Respiratory condition must be assessed at frequent intervals day and night in case paralysis of the respiratory muscles or of the muscles of swallowing should suddenly develop. Should paralysis of the swallowing muscles occur, the child may aspirate food or mucus and develop serious respiratory difficulty. In this case, the child is nursed from side to side or in prone with the foot of the bed elevated in order to minimize the risk of aspiration.

If paralysis or severe weakness of the respiratory muscles occurs, the child may be nursed in a tank respirator which exerts a negative pressure upon the thorax. As air is pumped into the tank in which the child lies, the lungs deflate and air is expelled. As the air is removed from the tank, the lungs expand under the influence of the negative atmospheric pressure within the tank and air is drawn into the lungs. The advantage of this method of ventilation over intermittent positive pressure ventilation lies in the relative freedom from infection, compared to the risk of infection present in positive pressure ventilation unless it is administered under scrupulously sterile conditions. The child is easily nursed in the tank respirator and can be given passive movements and warm packs through the portholes.

However, if the child also has paralysis of the swallowing muscles there is a definite risk of aspiration of mucus and food during the negative pressure phase of the cycle, as the negative pressure exerted by the machine will suck mucus and food from the oral cavity into the lungs. For this reason the child will be tracheostomized and ventilated on an intermittent positive pressure machine with a humidifier attached. Physical therapy under these conditions is briefly described in Chapter 27.

Where paralysis results in unopposed muscle action, and where it allows part of a limb to lose its ability to withstand the force of gravity, adaptive muscle length changes will occur if steps are not taken to prevent this early. If positioning of the child is poor, certain muscles are pre-disposed to length-associated changes. A pillow placed under the knees will allow hip and knee flexor contractures to occur if the child cannot move the legs. A soft mattress may have a similar effect. Pain and protective muscle spasm may result in prolonged maintenance of a flexed position. The child should be nursed on a firm mattress, with a bed cradle to prevent the bedclothes from pressing the feet into plantarflexion. If there is a need to prevent the knees from resting in a hyperextended position, it is better to apply a posterior splint with

the knee in 2 or 3° of flexion, than run the risk of hip and knee flexor contractures by placing a pillow under the knee. Warm packs will effectively relieve pain and spasm in most cases, and will make it easier for the child to tolerate movements in the maximum painfree range. The child may also gain relief by lying on a sheepskin mattress.

Active and passive movements are done gently but in the fullest possible painfree range, and with as little handling of the tender muscle bellies as possible. To avoid distressing the child these may be done at intervals during the day for short periods only. Passive movements, provided they are frequently and effectively done, are probably more effective than splinting for the prevention of soft contractures in these early stages, as splinting may cause pain and further spasm. However, it may be necessary to apply a posterior splint to the lower limb to prevent contractures of the triceps surae and the long toe flexors. Similarly, for the forearm and hand, a splint will help prevent contracture of the wrist and finger flexors. A long sandbag placed down the lateral side of the leg will prevent contracture of the hip external rotators while the child is lying in supine. Where splints are used they should not become substitutes for full-range movements done several times a day to preserve the extensibility of the soft tissues in this early stage.

Stage of recovery

This stage usually begins some 3 weeks after the onset of the disease. While the disease is active the child is encouraged to lie as quietly as possible, since there is some evidence that activity increases the possibility of damage within the CNS. However, once the active stage is over, signalled by a loss of the clinical features associated with the viral illness, the child may begin gentle active exercise.

If there is bulbar involvement or paralysis of the respiratory muscles, recovery will depend very largely on the recovery of respiratory function. Artificial ventilation will continue until the muscular function is sufficiently improved. The child will gradually be weaned from the respirator, spending increasingly longer periods of time without it. The child may progress to the stage where all day can be spent out of the respirator, going back into it at night, or doing without its assistance completely. An older child may be able to use glossopharyngeal breathing in order to spend periods of the day independent of the respirator. At this stage physical treatment may be done during the periods when the child is out of the respirator with the physiotherapist keeping a check on respiratory rate. The child is always at risk of developing a respiratory tract infection and this should be prevented if possible and, if it occurs, treated by antibiotics and postural drainage.

Investigation of coping strategies used by individuals with paralysis following poliomyelitis infection many years after the illness has revealed the ways in which they coped with their disabilities. Bozarth (1987) found, for example, that denial of feelings and minimization of loss were common. Such individuals frequently became 'super-independent achievers' in order to prove they were equal to the able-bodied. The extraordinary performance of many poliomyelitis survivors has been referred to in several recent publications (Bruno and Frick 1987, 1991). Westbrook (1992) speculates that the 'nature of the disease and the philosophy associated with polio rehabilitation encouraged high levels of determination and persistence' (p. 90).

Assessment

As soon as possible the extent of the child's disability is assessed. A detailed assessment will not be done until the active stage is over, in order to avoid unnecessary disturbance to the child.

Muscle strength testing

A complete muscle chart may be done in order to establish the range and extent of weakness and paralysis. The methods of testing the individual muscles are described by Kendall and McCreary (1983).

Unfortunately this method of assessment is very subjective. Above grade 3, it is not possible to quantify the amount of resistive force applied by the physiotherapist, which is a major problem inherent in manual muscle testing. However, test–retest reliability can be optimized if the same therapist does subsequent reassessments.

Manual muscle testing does not give an accurate picture of, for example, spinal muscle involvement, as the small muscles of the spine cannot be charted. The chart may also be inaccurate because of the difficulty the therapist, particularly if inexperienced, has in discriminating between a trick movement which is effective and a movement in which the normal coordination of muscles is present.

The strength of a particular muscle and, therefore, the grade it is given will also depend on the degree of weakness of the muscles with a synergic or fixator action when the child performs a movement or holds a joint steady against resistance. The grade given will also depend on the experience and skill of the therapist in assessing the relative strength of muscles. For example, if the hip abductors, adductors and rotators, and the abdominal muscles are weak, the hip flexors will test as weak because of the poor movement which results. These muscles may potentially be capable of generating more force if the segments to which they are attached were stabilized. No group of muscles can perform a movement without the aid of synergist and fixator muscles, therefore, in the absence of normal function in these groups, it is very difficult to assess the real strength of the prime mover. The therapist is really assessing the strength of the movement rather than of the muscle.

Despite the difficulties and inaccuracies it is hard to think of a more suitable clinical method of establishing either the extent of paralysis or improvement in strength of muscles. There are certain positive features of muscle charting to keep in mind. It enables the therapist to estimate potential deformities which may arise as a result of muscle imbalance, and to take steps to prevent these by suitable splinting and exercise.

When an infant or small child is too young to obey instructions, the evaluation procedure is difficult and time-consuming. Testing involves watching for spontaneous movement and eliciting reactions to stimulation where possible. The therapist may stimulate reflex movements in the infant. Flexion of the toes, for example, may be tested by stimulating the tonic reaction of the toe flexors.

The clinical usefulness of muscle charting may be explained by a look at the mechanism of nerve cell recovery. Singer and Rose-Innes (1963) have suggested that recovery occurs in some anterior horn cells during the stage of recovery in two ways. Those cells which have suffered a neurapraxia, probably due to inflammatory oedema, but which have suffered no actual histological change, will recover quickly. Those which have undergone some histological changes which stop short of complete chromotolysis will return to normal within a few months. The function of charting individual muscle does, therefore, give an indication of the rate of improvement in nerve cells, as well as of the degree of hypertrophy of those muscle fibres which are still innervated. EMG and nerve conduction tests provide methods of quantifying motor output. As soon as the child can be more active, measures of functional activities such as sit-to-stand, walking, stair-climbing, reaching to pick up an object (see Chapter 3) are carried out. This will serve as a guide for further management, for splinting, surgery or self-help apparatus.

Muscle length testing

The muscles which will be affected by length changes can be predicted with a degree of certainty from knowledge of weak or paralysed muscles and the effects of gravity and positioning. Muscle length can be estimated by passive movement of the joint over which the muscle passes. This method is not reliable as a repetitive measure, however, since the joint angle achieved by a passive stretch is a reflection of the amount of force applied by the therapist as much as real muscle length. In addition, if a muscle is tender, a reflex contraction will prevent angular displacement going beyond a certain point. Muscle length may be better estimated during active exercise, when any discrepancy in length should be obvious to an observant therapist as the child practises functional activities or does exercises.

Muscle length is measured at intervals using a standardized test (e.g., Ada and Canning 1990; Moseley and Adams 1991; see also Chapter 5). Where there is respiratory involvement, function is tested regularly by the measurement of vital capacity and forced expiratory volume (see Chapter 27).

Physical treatment

As soon as the acute stage has passed, active movements are started within the limits of the child's comfort. Exercises must be begun gently. For the first few weeks any resistance given to a movement, whether by the therapist or the child's own body weight, should be minimal to avoid strain to the soft tissues, and should progress slowly to maximal effort.

Exercises are given to encourage both isolated movements, that is, those movements performed by using the weak muscle as prime mover, as synergist or as fixator, and actions in which the weak muscle is encouraged to work in conjunction with other muscles in performing a specific function. For example, if the quadriceps femoris is weak, it can be strengthened by exercises involving knee extension and by stepping up and down, stair-climbing and descent, and standing up and sitting down. These actions may need to be modified to avoid over-exerting weak muscles and straining soft tissues around relatively unprotected joints.

Some techniques for strengthening muscles and improving motor control are described below, demonstrating the methods used at various stages of the muscle's recovery.

When a muscle appears paralysed, various methods may be employed to elicit a minimum contraction, if this is a possibility. For example, if tibialis anterior is charted as grade 1, a contraction may be elicited in whichever muscle fibres are still innervated in one of the following ways:

1 Sitting up from supine or semireclined with the feet held (modified if abdominal muscles are weak).
2 Manual or electrical stimulation to the belly of the muscle plus pressure on the dorsum of the foot while the child attempts to dorsiflex the foot.
3 Sitting on a stool with the feet on the floor, manual stimulation under the toes will facilitate any potential ability of the dorsiflexor muscles and toe extensors to contract.
4 Supine lying with the plantar surface of the heel in the therapist's hand, pushing the heel down into the hand as though to elongate the leg.
5 Supine lying, resisting hip and knee flexion with resistance given at the thigh, and the other hand at the dorsum of the foot.
6 Standing up and sitting down, modifying to a high seat if necessary (see Chapter 3).

Electromyographic (EMG) feedback as the child attempts any of the above exercises will provide information to the child about muscle activity even if no joint movement can be observed and is, therefore, reinforcing and motivating. In addition, EMG provides information for the physiotherapist about recovery in muscle activation.

When muscles recover to the stage where they are able to perform a movement, and as they become progressively stronger, so they can be trained progressively by practice of a variety of actions.

Assistance to a movement is gained manually, or by using springs and pulleys. Resistance to a movement can be applied by slings, springs, weights and body weight. Exercise machines which give feedback about the level of effort being applied are motivating and are interesting and fun for the child. Actions are practised which include isometric and isotonic, concentric and eccentric, muscle activity.

Muscles are not only re-educated by specific exercises directed mainly at the particular muscle group involved, but also by more general activities involving the maintenance and regaining of balance, and the movement of the whole body (see Chapter 3). Games are structured to facilitate the best response from the muscles to be re-educated. For example, a child with weak elbow extensors will use these muscles when playing pat-ball with a balloon, and later with a light rubber ball. The elbow will be extended in different parts of its range if the ball is returned at different heights. Walking while pushing a weighted pram will strengthen weak lower limb extensors. Trunk and head extensors will be strengthened by wriggling in prone through a cardboard tunnel.

Activities should be planned that increase endurance and agility. Responding to the unexpected perturbations of a balance board or electronic balance platform while standing on it will train muscle control in the lower limbs and trunk by requiring them to adjust quickly to changes in direction. Increasing the number of times the child steps up on a stool will increase the endurance of knee and hip extensors. Throwing and catching a ball while lying in prone with a pillow under the chest will increase the endurance of trunk and head extensors, if the time spent in this activity is increased each day. Riding a prone scooter (see Fig. 15.4) will have a similar effect.

If a child is too young to cooperate or follow simple instructions, movements are trained by placing the child in an environment that 'forces' the desired action.

The child may be treated in a warm pool. If nervous when first allowed out of bed, it may be easier to move about in a pool than on dry land. If the disability is severe the ability to move in the water with so little effort will be encouraging. Exercises in the water can again be divided into those which are specifically for the muscles involved, and those which are more general, in which the muscles work in conjunction with others in swimming and games. The water is used both for assistance, in which case it is buoyancy which gives assistance, and for resistance, when it is the weight of the water which resists. Walking is practised, first in deeper water using its buoyancy to hold the child upright. Respiratory function is improved by techniques which encourage the child to breathe deeply, hold the breath and breathe out effectively. Activities such as blowing a sailing boat across the surface of the pool, swimming with the face in the water, picking up toys from the bottom of the pool are all useful activities as well as being good fun (Reid-Campion 1991). The water temperature should be neither too warm, which will be enervating, nor too cold, which will inhibit muscle action. The best temperature is said to be between 32 and 34°C. The child should not remain in a heated pool too long as it is enervating.

Once the child is discharged home, the parents will take over responsibility for supervising exercises, returning to the physiotherapist periodically to learn how to progress exercises and activities. The parents (and the child, if old enough) are taught how to care for the limbs. A flail limb has poor circulation and this will inhibit growth if the child is young. The limb will also be subject to trophic changes, including osteoporosis, with the danger of fracture on minimal strain. Skin ulceration will occur if the skin is not carefully protected, and these lesions are slow to heal. In cold weather chilblains are common and the child should be kept as warm as possible in winter, wearing woollen socks or stockings, and gloves.

Splinting

Splinting is designed for the child as soon as it is found to be necessary. In the early stages this applies particularly to the lower limbs and trunk. The child will not be allowed to stand or walk unsplinted if there is severe instability in the lower limbs. Weakness of the trunk muscles which may lead to a paralytic scoliosis if the child is allowed to remain upright without support. The instability which results from weakness or paralysis of muscles surrounding a joint results in trauma to the surrounding soft tissues and eventually to permanent deformity if the child is allowed to bear weight without adequate support.

If weakness of the abdominal muscles or spinal musculature is present, a spinal support may be necessary; a specially designed brace is particularly necessary in the prevention and treatment of paralytic scoliosis.

Splinting for the limbs is similarly designed according to the distribution of the paralysis, to prevent the deforming effects of muscle imbalance and gravity, to give stability, to allow activity where paralysis or weakness prevents it, and to prevent strain being thrown on other parts of the body.

Paralysis of the quadriceps makes it impossible for the child to take weight on that leg without fully extending the knee, which will result eventually in a genu recurvatum deformity. Paralysis of the hamstrings and anterior tibial muscles also causes this deformity. A caliper with a posterior knee piece as well as a knee pad gives stability in either case. If the muscles remain paralysed, a knee-locking mechanism is added to the caliper to allow knee flexion when the child sits down.

Paralysis of the anterior tibial muscles prevents a heel–toe gait and causes the child to step high with that leg to clear the toes from the ground. Paralysis of the tibialis anterior allows the foot to roll into pronation on weight-bearing. An ankle–foot orthosis may be necessary to provide stability for the ankle.

Paralysis of the hip extensors causes the child to jack-knife forwards from the hips, and a reciprocating gait orthosis may be necessary (see Fig. 15.12). Eventually the child develops, or is taught, compensatory or substitution movements if there is no recovery in hip extensors. These allow walking and standing without a pelvic support, by thrusting the pelvis forwards, gaining stability for the hips anteriorly.

Upper-limb splints are designed to allow maximum hand function by holding the wrist extended or the thumb abducted to allow better grasp. It should be remembered that these splints will be useless and soon discarded if they do not give the child improved hand function. It will be of more use to encourage and teach substitution movements if these prove more effective for function.

The problem of deciding which is the most suitable splinting for the child is difficult. It is necessary to prevent deformity developing if possible, but splinting to fulfil this aim may conflict with the aim of allowing the child to function with maximum effectiveness.

The progressive deformities following as a result of paralysis may be formidable. Their full extent in children is only seen several years after the illness. They result probably from several factors, the most important probably being the effect of growth and of stereotyped movement. The child continues to grow, but a flail limb, or a limb severely affected by muscle paralysis, does not grow at the same rate as the normal one, and by the time the child's growth is completed the flail limb will be shorter, sometimes by several centimetres, than the other. Another factor in the progression of deformity is the increasing mechanical advantage of stronger muscles over their paralysed or weakened antagonists. These weakened antagonists may eventually be unable to contract at all, so great may the mechanical disadvantage become. This occurs because of the gradual lengthening of the paralysed muscles and their adjacent soft tissues as the pull of gravity and the abnormal posture of the joint gradually force the part further into the deformed position. One 12-year-old boy known to the author, severely paralysed since the age of 18 months, demonstrated the effect of walking for several years in a long caliper with the hip held in full external rotation. The soft tissues on the medial side of the knee gradually lengthened and bone growth was influenced by the effect of the boy's weight being borne laterally at the knee. This resulted in a gross genu valgum deformity which the caliper was unable to prevent. However, it was only by maintaining this position that the boy had taught himself to walk.

Exercises and splints cannot hope to prevent the development of such deformities against these mechanical factors. It may be possible to slow their development by treatment and splinting designed to minimize the effects of gravity and posture, and splinting is continued for as long as recovery is occurring. Once improvement has ceased, the orthopaedic surgeon considers what reconstructive or stabilizing surgery may be necessary either to gain more effective function or to prevent future deformities. Where the child's bone growth is still immature, splinting is continued until the child is old enough for surgery, and longer if it increases functional independence.

Gait dysfunction, use of orthoses and walking aids are associated with considerable energy cost (Waters *et al.* 1978; Patterson and Fisher 1981) and would contribute to fatigue and decreased endurance. The severely disabled child, when old enough to make the decision, may prefer to use a wheelchair rather than endure the effort of being ambulant in splints.

The recognition of post-poliomyelitis sequelae has resulted in histories of poliomyelitis survivors being studied. Such information may be of value in determining rehabilitation strategies for children who develop poliomyelitis today. Reviewing their past rehabilitation, poliomyelitis survivors report having found that their vigorous rehabilitation regimes enabled them to gain a significant degree of functional ability (Scheer and Luborsky 1991). However, many describe learning to ignore pain and fatigue in their attempts to achieve normal levels of performance. It is apparent that encouraging polio survivors to achieve in all spheres of living despite their disabilities, although it probably had considerable benefits in the early period of disability, may also have had some negative effects particularly evident as survivors grew older. In rehabilitation, it may be that encouraging 'high levels of determination and persistence' (Westbrook 1992, p. 90) needs to be tempered with assistance in dealing with loss and encouragement to develop a realistic view of impairment rather than minimizing any limitations, with real needs being acknowledged rather than denied.

Polyneuropathy

Peripheral neuropathy may arise from one of many different causative factors. The cause may be infectious (e.g. herpes zoster), toxic (e.g. post-immunization, heavy metal poisoning), traumatic, metabolic (e.g. diabetes, vitamin

B_1 deficiency), vascular (e.g. dermatomyositis, lupus erythematosus), or neoplastic (e.g. leukaemia, neurofibromatosis). It may also be idiopathic, as in Guillain–Barré syndrome.

Symptoms are muscle weakness and sensory impairment, and depend upon whether the site of involvement is the anterior or posterior nerve root or a mixed peripheral nerve.

Guillain–Barré syndrome

Guillain–Barré syndrome is a polyneuropathy of unknown origin, although it has been suggested that the cause may indicate a hypersensitivity phenomenon, as it frequently follows an acute viral infection (Beghi *et al.* 1985).

In countries where poliomyelitis also occurs, Guillain–Barré syndrome must be distinguished from poliomyelitis, which it closely resembles symptomatically. A feverish illness with vomiting and pyrexia precedes the sudden development of paralysis. However, the polyneuritis is symmetrical in distribution and usually affects all the muscles in a limb, often spreading gradually from lower limbs to upper. There is usually sensory involvement, the child complaining of pain, numbness and paraesthesiae, and suffering loss of proprioception. The peripheral nerves with their roots are involved and in some cases the cranial nerves, particularly the facial nerve (Markland and Riley 1967). There is muscle tenderness, absence or diminution of tendon reflexes and a varying degree of weakness or paralysis of muscle. Autonomic involvement may include postural hypotension and bladder and bowel dysfunction. The disease tends to resolve slowly. Most children make a good recovery, but some suffer remissions and exacerbations of symptoms. Due to paralysis of respiratory muscles and uncontrolled respiratory infection, a few may die.

Pathology

Changes found in peripheral nerves and their roots include axonal degeneration. Oedema, endoneurial lymphocyte cell infiltration and segmental demyelination occur. Proximal roots of nerves are commonly more affected than distal. Eventually, in most cases, regeneration of the nerve structure occurs, but recovery is seldom complete.

Management

Treatment is symptomatic. The value of drug therapy is uncertain. Plasmaphoresis appears effective in adults if started within 7 days of onset (Swaiman 1989).

Physical treatment is as described for poliomyelitis. However, due to the involvement of the sensory fibres of the peripheral nerves and the anaesthesia which may result, appropriate care must be taken to avoid damage to the skin from pressure of bedclothes and ill-fitting splints. Tracheostomy or a negative-pressure cuirass respirator may be needed in some cases (Gracey *et al.* 1982; Lands and Zinman 1986).

Transverse myelitis

Transverse myelitis is the term given to an inflammation involving several spinal cord segments. The inflammation may progress upwards (ascending myelitis) or remain stationary. Transverse myelitis may be associated with childhood viral diseases such as mumps and rubella or with certain vaccinations.

Clinical manifestations depend upon the part of the cord involved. For example, anterior horn cell damage causes muscle paralysis or weakness. Involvement of sensory pathways results in sensory loss up to the level of the cord lesion. Involvement of autonomic pathways causes autonomic dysfunction, such as lack of sweating. Hyperreflexia will be present if central control over intact anterior horn cells is interrupted. Prognosis is usually poor in terms of full recovery of function.

Physical treatment depends upon the problems with which the child presents. Emphasis must be on stimulating growth and development, which requires that soft tissue contractures must be prevented, mobility must be ensured and social and educational isolation avoided.

Summary

The main infections of the brain, spinal cord and peripheral nerves seen in children are described, with anterior poliomyelitis described in detail. Physical treatment is symptomatic and preventive, aiming at maintaining the child in a condition which will allow maximum recovery of function to occur, by ensuring efficient ventilation, and by preventing soft tissue contractions. Motor training encourages weakened muscles to develop their optimal strength, endurance and coordination. The management of the residual paralysis is the province of the orthopaedic surgeon and those skilled in designing apparatus for self-help.

References

Ada, L. and Canning, C. (1990) Anticipating and avoiding muscle shortening. In: *Key Issues in Neurological Physiotherapy*, edited by L. Ada and C. Canning. Oxford: Butterworth-Heinemann, pp. 219–236.

Beghi, E., Kurland, L.T., Mulder, D.W. *et al.* (1985) Guillain–Barré syndrome. Clinicoepidemiologic features and effect of influenza vaccine. *Arch. Neurol.*, **42**, 1053.

Bozarth, C.H. (1987) *Unfinished Business: Some Feelings Surrounding the Late Effects of Polio*. Michigan: Polio Survivors Group of Lansing.

Bruno, R.L. and Frick, N.M. (1987) Stress and 'type A' behavior as precipitants of post-polio sequelae. In: *Research and Clinical Aspects of the Late Effects of Poliomyelitis*, edited by L.S. Halstead and D.O. Wiechers. White Plains, NY: March of Dimes.

Bruno, R.L. and Frick, N.M. (1991) The psychology of polio as prelude to post-polio sequelae: behavior modification and psychotherapy. *Orthopedics*, **14**, 1185–1193.

Bruno, R.L., Frick, N.M. and Cohen, J. (1991) Poliomyelitis, stress, and the etiology of post-polio sequelae. *Orthopedics*, **14**, 11, 1269–1276.

Dalakas, M.C., Sever, J.L., Madden, D.L. *et al.* (1984) Late poliomyelitis muscular atrophy: clinical, virologic, and immunologic studies. *Rev. Infect. Dis.*, **6** (suppl. 2), 562–567.

Dean, E. (1991) Post-poliomyelitis sequelae: a pathophysiologic basis for management. *Aust. J. Physiother.*, **37**, 2, 79–86.

Drachman, D.B., Murphy, S.R., Nigam, M.P. *et al.* (1967) Myopathic changes in chronically denervated muscle. *Arch. Neurol.*, **16**, 14–24.

Gracey, D.R., McMichan, J.C. and Divertie, M.B. (1982) Respiratory failure in Guillain–Barré syndrome. *Mayo Clin. Proc.*, **57**, 742.

Halstead, L.S. (1988) The residual of polio in the aged. *Topics Geriatr. Rehabil.*, **3**, 4, 9–26.

Hovi, T., Cantell, K., Huovilainen, A. *et al.* (1986) Outbreak of paralytic poliomyelitis in Finland: widespread circulation of antigenically altered poliovirus type 3 in a vaccinated population. *Lancet*, **1**, 1427–1432.

Kendall, F.P. and McCreary, E.K. (1983) *Muscles Testing and Function*, 3rd edn. Baltimore, MD: Williams & Wilkins.

Klingman, J., Chui, H., Corgiat, M. and Perry, J. (1988) Functional recovery. A major risk factor for the development of postpoliomyelitis muscular atrophy. *Arch. Neurol.*, **45**, 645–647.

Lands, L. and Zinman, R. (1986) Maximal static pressure and lung volumes in a child with Guillain–Barré syndrome ventilated by a cuirass respiratory. *Chest*, **89**, 757.

Mandell, G.L., Douglas, G. and Bennett, J.E. (1985) *Principles and Practices of Infectious Diseases*. New York: John Wiley.

Markland, L.D. and Riley, H.D. (1967) The Guillain–Barré syndrome in childhood. *Clin. Pediatr.*, **6**, 3, 162.

Moseley, A. and Adams, R. (1991) Measurement of passive ankle dorsiflexion: procedure and reliability. *Aust. J. Physiotherapy*, **37**, 3, 175–181.

Patterson, R. and Fisher, S.V. (1981) Cardiovascular stress of crutch walking. *Arch. Phys. Med. Rehabil.*, **62**, 257–260.

Polio Network News (1992), **8**, 3.

Raymond, C.A. (1986) Worldwide assault on poliomyelitis gathering support, garnering results. *Med. News Perspect.*, **255**, 12, 1541–1546.

Reid-Campion, M. (1991) *Hydrotherapy in Paediatrics*, 2nd edn. Oxford: Butterworth-Heinemann.

Scheer, J. and Luborsky, M.L. (1991) Post-polio sequelae. The cultural context of polio biographies. *Orthopedics*, **14**, 11, 1173–1181.

Sharrard, W.J.W. (1953) Correlation between changes in spinal cord and muscle paralysis in poliomyelitis. *Proc. R. Soc. Med.*, **40**, 364.

Sharrard, W.J.W. (1955) The distribution of permanent paralysis in the lower limb in poliomyelitis. *J. Bone Joint Surg.*, **37B**, 540.

Sharrard, W.J.W. (1957) Muscle paralysis in poliomyelitis. *Br. J. Surg.*, **44**, 471.

Sharrard, W.J.W. (1971) *Paediatric Orthopaedics and Fractures*. Oxford and Edinburgh: Blackwell.

Singer, M. and Rose-Innes, T. (1963) *The Recovery from Poliomyelitis. A Study of the Convalescent Phase*. Edinburgh: Livingstone.

Swaiman, K.F. (ed) (1989) *Pediatric Neurology. Principles and Practice*. St Louis, MO: C.V. Mosby.

Walton, J.N. (1971) *Essentials of Neurology*. London: Pitman.

Waters, R.L., Hislop, H.J., Perry, J. and Antonelli, D. (1978) Energetics: application to the study and management of locomotor disorders. *Orthoped. Clin. North Am.*, **9**, 351–362.

Westbrook, M.T. (1992) A survey of post-poliomyelitis sequelae: manifestations, effects on people's lives and responses to treatment. *Aust. J. Physiother.*, **37**, 2, 89–102.

Wohlfart, G. (1958) Collateral regeneration in partially denervated muscles. *Neurology*, **8**, 175–180.

Further reading

Barr, J.S. (1949) The management of poliomyelitis. In: *Poliomyelitis: Papers and Discussions, Presented at First International Poliomyelitis Conference*. London: Lippincott.

Block, H.S. and Wilbourn, A.J. (1986) Progressive post-polio atrophy: the EMG findings. *Neurology*, **36**, (suppl. 1), 137.

Edds, M.V. (1950) Hypertrophy of nerve fibres to functionally overloaded muscles. *J. Comp. Anat.*, **93**, 259.

Feldman, R.M. (1985) The use of strengthening exercises in post-polio sequelae. *Orthopedics*, **8**, 889.

Halstead, L.S. and Wiechers, D.O. (1987) (eds) *Research and Clinical Aspects of the Late Effects of Poliomyelitis*. NY: March of Dimes Birth Defects Foundation.

McFarland, H.R. and Heller, G.L. (1966) Guillain–Barré disease complex. *Arch. Neurol.*, **14**, 196.

Seddon, H.G. (1954) Poliomyelitis. In: *British Surgical Practice*. London: Butterworth.

10

Brachial plexus lesions in infancy

The brachial plexus of an infant may be injured during a difficult birth (Sjoberg *et al.* 1988), for example, when a traction force is applied to the head during delivery of the shoulder. Babies involved are frequently of high birth weight, and breech presentations with an after-coming head. The traction on the plexus may cause injury to the upper roots (C5 and 6), resulting in the upper plexus type known as Erb's palsy, or to the lower roots (C7, 8, T1), resulting in paralysis of the muscles of the hand, known as Klumpke's paralysis. Rarely, all the nerve roots may be injured and the infant will have a completely flail arm, an Erb–Klumpke-type paralysis. Exact localization of the anatomical lesion is often difficult (Wickstrom 1962; Adler and Patterson 1967). Many infants demonstrate a mixed upper and lower type.

The type of lesion varies from oedema affecting one or two nerve roots to total avulsion of the plexus. The facial nerve may also be involved in the trauma, resulting in a mild facial paralysis (Eng 1971). In addition, clavicular or humeral fractures, traction to the cervical spinal cord, subluxation of the shoulder and torticollis may be additional complications.

As Adler and Patterson (1967) pointed out, recognition by obstetricians of disproportion between the infant's head and the mother's pelvis and improved means of managing this complication dramatically decreased the incidence of so-called obstetrical paralysis of the upper limb. However, the incidence of brachial plexus injury is still not negligible (Eng 1971;

Davis *et al.* 1978; Jackson *et al.* 1988) and the resultant handicap can be very severe.

Pathology

Figure 10.1 shows a diagrammatic representation of the brachial plexus. Any force which alters the anatomical relationship of neck, shoulder girdle and humerus may potentially injure the plexus, which is attached to the first rib and to the coracoid process of the scapula. Lateral movement of the head with depression

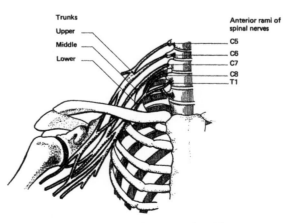

Figure 10.1 The brachial plexus. Reprinted from Campbell, S.K. (ed.) (1991), *Pediatric Neurologic Physical Therapy*, 2nd edn. New York: Churchill Livingstone, with permission.

of the shoulder girdle stretches the nerves, compressing them against the first ribs. This may cause injury to the upper plexus, whereas the lower plexus can be injured by hyperabduction of the shoulder with traction on the arm, this action stretching and compressing the nerves under the coracoid process (Shepherd 1992).

A forceful stretch of the nerve roots or trunk of the plexus may result in injuries varying from swelling of the neural sheath with blocking of nerve conduction, to haemorrhage and scar formation, to complete axonal rupture (Eng *et al.* 1978). Somatosensory cortical-evoked potentials may be used to aid in the diagnosis of dorsal root avulsion (Zverina and Kredba 1977; Landi *et al.* 1980).

Serial electromyographic (EMG) studies help track the recovery process. Initially there is decreased voluntary motor unit activity and denervation potentials. Regeneration is signalled by the appearance of small polyphasic motor units. As recovery proceeds, the number of recorded motor units increases, denervation potentials decrease and eventually there is a return of excitability of the nerves to electrical stimuli. Degenerative changes in muscles are indicated by an absence of motor unit activity, few denervation potentials and non-conduction (Eng 1971). Studies of infants suggest that denervation changes at birth can result in impairment of the normal developmental changes which occur postnatally in muscle contractile properties (Stefanova-Uzanova *et al.* 1981).

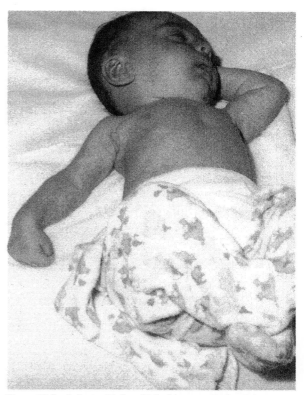

Figure 10.2 Infant with brachial plexus paralysis of the right arm. Note the pronated forearm and flexed wrist and fingers. Reprinted from Campbell, S.K. (ed.) (1991) *Pediatric Neurologic Physical Therapy*, 2nd edn. New York: Churchill Livingstone, with permission.

Description

The baby, immediately after birth, is noticed to lie asymmetrically, with the affected arm limply at the side instead of maintained in the predominantly flexed posture of the neonate. In the upper-arm-type of paralysis, the following muscles may be affected: rhomboids, levator scapulae, serratus anterior, deltoid, supraspinatus, infraspinatus, biceps brachii, brachioradialis, brachialis, supinator and long extensors of the wrist, fingers and thumb (Fig. 10.2). In the lower-arm-type, these muscles may be affected: the extensors of wrist and fingers, and intrinsic muscles of the hand.

Muscle weakness or paralysis results in the substitution of intact muscles to produce adaptive motor performance, soft tissue contracture

and the possibility of learned non-use. The performance of such actions as balancing in sitting and bimanual activities is affected, as well as actions involving the affected arm.

Motor dysfunction occurs as a result of the combination of muscle weakness or paralysis, the unopposed activity of muscles with intact innervation and the functional imbalance which stems from these factors. As the infant attempts to reach out for a toy, adaptive motor behaviour will be evident, the action being performed in the best possible way given the dynamics of the musculo-skeletal linkage and the state of the muscular system (Fig. 10.3).

Soft tissue contracture results from the immobility of joints and the resting position of the limb. The muscles linking the humerus to the scapula (subscapularis, teres minor, latis-

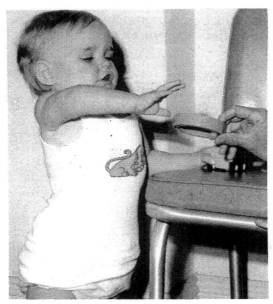

Figure 10.3 Note the adaptive movement as the child reaches for a toy. She has weak shoulder flexor, external rotator and supinator muscles. Abduction at the shoulder enables her to reach forwards with the arm in internal rotation and pronation. Reprinted from Campbell, S.K. (ed.) (1991) *Pediatric Neurologic Physical Therapy*, 2nd edn. New York: Churchill Livingstone, with permission.

simus dorsi) are those most at risk of shortening in the upper-arm-type of lesion.

Sensory loss may occur over the lateral aspect of the arm but this is usually less than the corresponding motor loss. Where there is complete sensory loss in a severe whole-arm paralysis, there will be absence of all sensation – pain, temperature, touch and proprioception.

Prognosis

Prognosis depends on the extent of injury to the plexus. Times for maximum recovery vary from 1 to 18 months. Regeneration is unlikely after complete axonal rupture. Most injuries are, however, less severe and, following a neuropraxis with no damage to the neurilemmal sheath, axis cylinder or neurofibrils, resolution of oedema and haemorrhage will result in spontaneous recovery of function in a month. If the lesion is an axonotmesis in which the axis cylinder is disrupted but the nerve fibres remain

intact, regrowth will occur at approximately 1 mm/day. In the upper-arm-type, therefore, regeneration may be complete in 4–5 months, while in the lower-arm-type it will take from 7 to 9 months.

If there is complete division of the axon, muscle wasting will be noticeable after the first few weeks. If recovery does not occur, normal growth will not take place in the limb, which will be noticeably smaller than the normal limb as the child grows. The child with a complete paralysis is left with a flail insensible arm which may dislocate at the shoulder and is totally useless. In the case of an upper-arm paralysis which fails to recover, it is remarkable how well the child can adapt the use of the shoulder girdle and arm to compensate for the disability if it is not severe. Many of these children require surgery when they are older in order to improve function. Relevant surgery is described by Sharrard (1971) and Zancolli (1981).

Assessment

The infant is sent for physiotherapy treatment as soon as the injury is recognized and diagnosed. Assessment is carried out with the infant undressed and in a warm room.

Movement is tested by observation of spontaneous movement as the infant lies in supine and prone, is moved around, cuddled and talked to, and by observation of motor behaviour during the testing of reflexes and reactions (e.g. Moro reflex, placing reaction of the hand, Galant reflex, neck-righting reaction, grasp reflex). Observation will provide some indication of muscle activity which can be recorded, as for example:

0 = absent
1 = present but lacking full range
2 = present throughout available range
    (Shepherd 1992).

The Moro reflex may be asymmetrical, with insufficient arm abduction, although the elbow and fingers may extend. The grasp reflex will be present in the upper-arm-type but not in the lower-arm-type. The finger flexion is normally accompanied by elbow flexion, hence absence of elbow flexor muscle activity will cause the grasp to be weaker on the affected side.

Testing of the neck-righting reflex will indicate whether or not the infant has any ability to abduct and flex the shoulder.

EMG is considered a useful method of determining the extent and severity of the injury and providing information related to potential outcome (Eng 1971). EMG is also a useful tool for the physiotherapist, since signs of recovery on EMG usually precede clinical signs of function by several weeks. The appearance of these signs could be followed by intensified training to stimulate activity in the recovering muscles. It is likely that specific training of arm movements at this point in recovery may be critical to the infant's ability to maximize neural and functional recovery. EMG should, therefore, be used more extensively than at present for guiding the motor-training programme.

It is better for the physiotherapist to carry out an assessment about 1 hour after feeding, when the infant will be alert and active.

Joint range is tested by moving the whole arm through abduction, elevation, flexion, extension and rotation, and each joint separately through its range of motion. Care should be exercised in moving the limb passively in order not to impose an excessive stretch to the relatively unprotected soft tissues around the glenohumeral joint. When checking joint range, movement of the scapula should be noted, since shortening of muscles which link the scapula to the humerus (e.g. subscapularis) will cause the scapula to be pulled further around the thorax than normal when the arm is flexed or abducted.

Treatment

The baby's arm is rested for 1–2 weeks after birth to allow haemorrhage and oedema to resolve.

The major goals of physiotherapy are to ensure the optimal conditions for recovery of motor function, to provide the environmental conditions necessary for muscles to resume function as soon as neural regeneration has taken place and to train motor control by the practice of actions such as reaching to grasp (Shepherd 1992).

Ensuring optimal conditions for functional recovery includes preventing soft tissue contracture and skeletal deformity; adaptive motor behaviour; and neglect of the limb.

Ensuring that the maximum potential functional recovery will follow neural regeneration, motor training of specific actions must be aggressively pursued by therapist and parents as soon as muscles are reinnervated and capable of contraction. Should recovery not occur, the goal of physiotherapy becomes one of training optimal function after microsurgery to repair nerves (Boome and Kaye 1988) or orthopaedic surgery to transplant muscles or arthrodese joints.

Passive movements are commonly recommended as a means of preventing soft tissue contracture, particularly scapulohumeral adhesion (Fig. 10.4). Parents should be warned to be careful not to overstretch soft tissues around the shoulder joint in particular and, in the case of whole-arm paralysis, care must be taken not to move the shoulder beyond a conservative estimate of normal range due to the risk of glenohumeral dislocation. Forceful manipulation of the arm is said to be one of the factors contributing to alteration in the anatomy of the glenohumeral joint following brachial plexus injury (Zancolli 1981). The scapula should not be manually restrained after the humerus has moved through the first 30°, as humeral movement without scapular rotation will cause the humerus to impact on the acromion process.

Splinting to prevent soft tissue shortening is controversial, although the evidence strongly suggests that splinting in abduction leads to

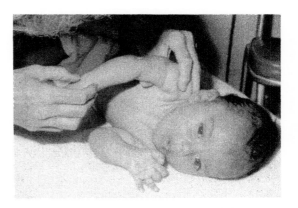

Figure 10.4 In side lying, gentle stretching of the shoulder adductors and extensors is done to maintain extensibility of these muscles. Reprinted from Campbell, S.K. (ed.) (1991) *Pediatric Neurologic Physical Therapy*, 2nd edn. New York: Churchill Livingstone, with permission.

excessive mobility of the glenohumeral joint and may lead to joint injury and dislocation (Eng *et al.* 1978). Sever, in 1925, following observation of 1100 children, reported that splinting appeared to delay recovery. External rotation/abduction contractures have been found to occur in infants splinted without access to physiotherapy.

Motor training follows along the lines described in Chapter 3 and in Shepherd (1992), and should start within the first month of life. Although there will be no activity in denervated muscles at this stage, early training probably serves to elicit activity in muscles which are only temporarily denervated and to minimize soft tissue contracture and neglect. In addition, early training sets up a regular pattern of behaviour in the parents, which ensures that muscles will be stimulated to contract for appropriate motor actions as soon as nerve regeneration has occurred.

Motor training should be specifically directed to relevant age-related actions with particular emphasis on reaching to touch and eventually to grasping and manipulating different objects. The infant's actions are monitored, using manual guidance (Fig. 10.5) and verbal feedback to ensure the infant activates the appropriate muscles for the action required. Emphasis should be placed on activating abductors, flexors and external rotators of the shoulder, which are

prime movers for reaching sideways or forwards; the supinators of the forearm; wrist extensors; and thumb palmar abductor. These muscles are not trained in isolation but are encouraged to function as part of the necessary synergy for a specific action. Tasks and objects are chosen that by their nature force the action required (Fig. 10.6).

Training should be carried out under optimal conditions for the weak muscles, that is, taking account of leverage, alignment of segments and weight of arm to be lifted, trying to elicit eccentric activity if concentric activity is difficult. The task may have to be modified to be achievable. For example, the deltoid may not be strong enough to lift the arm through range to the horizontal position but may be able to hold the arm and lower it a few degrees if the arm is held horizontal (Fig. 10.7).

Specific games can be played with the older infant with the purpose of improving sensory awareness of the affected limb. Games such as

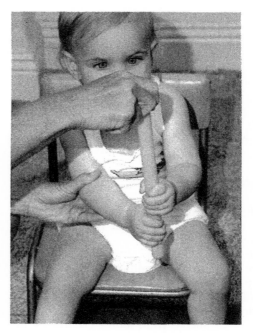

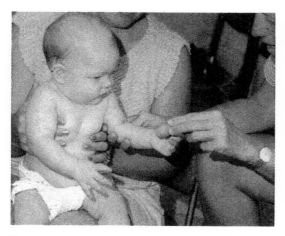

Figure 10.5 Objects are presented to encourage supination. Reprinted from Campbell, S.K. (ed.) (1991) *Pediatric Neurologic Physical Therapy*, 2nd edn. New York: Churchill Livingstone, with permission.

Figure 10.6 Bimanual activities train coordination between the two limbs and, if carefully planned, optimize activation of the weak muscles. Reprinted from Campbell, S.K. (ed.) (1991) *Pediatric Neurologic Physical Therapy*, 2nd edn. New York: Churchill Livingstone, with permission.

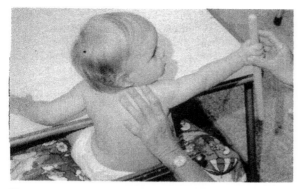

Figure 10.7 The rod is used to give feedback about supination and pronation. The child is encouraged to reach out in this position. Reprinted from Campbell, S.K. (ed.) (1991) *Pediatric Neurologic Physical Therapy*, 2nd edn. New York: Churchill Livingstone, with permission.

finding particular objects in the sand, localizing touch, recognizing and naming common objects while blindfolded are some examples.

Training should continue for as long as recovery is still occurring. Gatcheva (1979) has reported EMG evidence of reinnervation and return of nerve conduction for 6–8 years after brachial plexus injury and has suggested that it is essential to continue rehabilitation for several years. It is probably advisable to monitor recovery using EMG, using this as a guide as to whether or not training should continue.

Neglect of the affected limb may contribute to a failure of recovery of muscle function when nerve regeneration has occurred. There have been several reports of infants with good return of muscle function who nevertheless did not use the arm (Eng 1971; Rose 1979). This neglect has been attributed to the lack of development of 'functional patterns of coordination' (Wickstrom 1962) and to the failure of normal patterns of movement to develop (Zalis *et al.* 1965). Taub (1980) described a behaviour he called 'learned non-use' seen in monkeys following deafferentation involving the upper limb, which he considered was primarily due to a learning phenomenon. The monkeys learned *not* to use their affected limb as they could carry out the actions they wanted with the remaining limbs with little incentive to use the affected one. Of relevance to brachial plexus injury is that the monkeys' habitual non-use of the limb persisted so that even when the limb became potentially useful the animal did

not seem to be aware of it. Similar findings have been reported elsewhere (Yu 1976). Interestingly, in this study, the combination of restraint of the intact upper limb and specific training of the affected limb was found to result in improved function of that limb. A study of 2 children with hemiplegia (Schwartzman 1974) utilized restraint of the intact arm during early training sessions for short periods during the day. After 6 months of training both children could use their previously paretic limb.

Since the phenomenon of learned non-use could also occur in infants with brachial plexus injury, it is probable that the motor training programme should incorporate periods of restraint of the intact upper limb. Restraint can be imposed by keeping the intact arm inside the infant's clothing, or by lightly binding it to the side, or by organizing the environment so the infant can only reach a desired object by using the affected arm (Fig. 10.8; see also Fig. 3.26a). It is important that the restraint should be accompanied by training of the affected limb, and subsequent training of

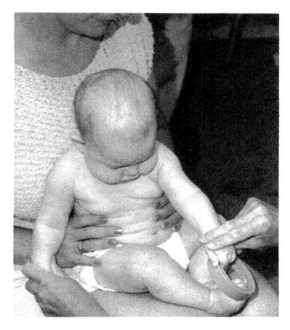

Figure 10.8 The intact arm can be restrained while the infant practises reaching with the affected left arm. Reprinted from Campbell, S.K. (ed.) (1991) *Pediatric Neurologic Physical Therapy*, 2nd edn. New York: Churchill Livingstone, with permission.

bimanual actions once there is some movement possible in the affected limb.

Biofeedback therapy, although not commonly used in children, is potentially a means of training and reinforcing the required motor behaviour. Devices have yet to be developed which can be used to train upper limb motor control by providing irresistible entertainment for an infant and young child. Such devices could be turned on or off at the movement of a joint or a twitch of a muscle.

Electrical stimulation is controversial and its effectiveness has not been adequately tested. It has been suggested that stimulation of denervated muscles prevents muscle atrophy (Eng 1971; Liberson and Terzis 1987). It is probable that electrical stimulation should be given for longer periods and with different equipment than is typical in clinical practice, and that it should be functionally oriented and associated with active training of the limb.

Orthoses

Splinting or strapping can be used to prevent excessive use of unopposed muscles, and may also force weak muscles to contract (Perry *et al.* 1974; Draznin *et al.* 1984). A small light splint may be worn for part of the day. For example, a moulded plastic splint may be used to hold the thumb in some abduction, or a wrist splint to encourage activity in the wrist extensors at the usual length for grasping. Dynamic splinting may also be useful (Eng 1971).

Summary

Brachial plexus injury at birth causes paralysis or weakness of muscles of the upper limb and loss of sensation, followed subsequently by sympathetic changes, soft tissue contracture and limb deformity. The infant, therefore, has a considerable loss of function, with difficulty reaching out and using the affected hand, and impaired bimanual function. Prognosis depends principally on the extent of the injury, and is very poor with severe lesions. However, the potential for recovery is also influenced by the development of learned non-use of the limb and soft tissue contracture, and the nature and intensity of rehabilitation. The role of the physiotherapist is in developing a programme for the parents involving methods of eliciting mus-

cle activity, preventing soft tissue contractures, preventing learned non-use and training reaching and functional use of the hand where reinnervation occurs.

References

Adler, J.B. and Patterson, R.L. (1967) Erb's palsy. *J. Bone Joint Surg.*, **49A**, 6, 1052–1064.

Boome, R.S. and Kaye, J.C. (1988) Obstetric traction injuries of the brachial plexus. *J. Bone Joint Surg.*, **70-B**, 4, 571–576.

Davis, D.H., Onofrio, B.M. and MacCarty, C.S. (1978) Brachial plexus injuries. *Mayo Clin. Proc.*, **53**, 12, 799.

Draznin, E., Maloney, F.P. and Brammell, C. (1984) Functional strapping for incomplete Erb palsy: a case report. *Arch. Phys. Med. Rehabil.*, **65**, 731–732.

Eng, G.D. (1971) Brachial plexus palsy in newborn infants. *Pediatrics*, **48**, 18–28.

Eng, G.D., Kroch, B. and Smokvina, M.D. (1978) Brachial plexus palsy in neonates and children. *Arch. Phys. Med. Rehabil.*, **59**, 458–464.

Gatcheva, J. (1979) Early diagnosis and long-term management of obstetric paralysis. *Int. Rehabil. Med.*, **3**, 1, 126.

Jackson, S.T., Hoffer, M.M. and Parrish, N. (1988) Brachial plexus palsy in the newborn. *J. Bone Joint Surg.*, **70-A**, 8, 1217–1220.

Landi, A., Copeland, S.A., Wynn-Parry C.B. *et al.* (1980) The role of somatosensory evoked potentials and nerve conduction studies in the surgical management of brachial plexus injuries. *J. Bone Joint Surg.*, **62-B**, 4, 492.

Liberson, W.T. and Terzis, J.K. (1987) Some novel techniques of clinical electrophysiology applied to the management of brachial plexus palsy. *Electromyogr. Clin. Neurophysiol.*, **27**, 371–383.

Perry, J., Hsu, J., Barber, L. *et al.* (1974) Orthoses in patients with brachial plexus injuries. *Arch. Phys. Med. Rehabil.*, **55**, 134–137.

Rose, F.C. (1979) *Paediatric Neurology*. Oxford: Blackwell.

Schwartzman, R.J. (1974) Rehabilitation of infantile hemiplegia. *Am. J. Phys. Med.*, **53**, 75–81.

Sever, J.W. (1925) Obstetric paralysis: report of 1100 cases. *J.A.M.A.*, **85**, 1862–1865.

Sharrard, W.J.W. (1971) *Paediatric Orthopaedics and Fractures*. Oxford: Blackwell.

Shepherd, R.B. (1992) Brachial plexus injury. In: *Pediatric Neurologic Physical Therapy*, 2nd edn. edited by S.K. Campbell. New York: Churchill Livingstone.

Sjoberg, I., Erichs, K. and Bjerre, I. (1988) Cause and effect of obstetric (neonatal) brachial plexus palsy. *Acta Paediatr. Scand.*, **77**, 357–364.

Stefanova-Uzanova, M., Stamatova, L. and Gatev, V. (1981) Dynamic properties of partially denervated muscle in children with brachial plexus birth palsy. *J. Neurol. Neurosurg. Psychiatry*, **44**, 497.

Taub, E. (1980) Somato-sensory deafferentation research with monkeys: implications for rehabilitation medicine.

In: *Behavioral Psychology in Rehabilitation Medicine: Clinical Applications*, edited by L.P. Ince. Baltimore, MD: Williams & Wilkins, pp. 371–401.

Wickstrom, J. (1962) Birth injuries of the brachial plexus: treatment of defects of the shoulder. *Clin. Orthop.*, **23**, 187–195.

Yu, J. (1976) Functional recovery with and without training following brain damage in experimental animals: a review. *Arch. Phys. Med. Rehabil.*, **57**, 38.

Zalis, O.S., Zalis, A.W., Barron, K.D. *et al.* (1965) Motor patterning following transitory sensory-motor deprivation. *Arch. Neurol.*, **13**, 487–494.

Zancolli, E.A. (1981) Classification and management of the shoulder in birth palsy. *Orthop. Clin. North Am.*, **12**, 433.

Zverina, E. and Kredba, J. (1977) Somatosensory cerebral evoked potentials in diagnosing brachial plexus injuries. *Scand. J. Rehabil. Med.*, **19**, 47.

Further reading

Jeannerod, M. (1984) The timing of natural prehension movements. *J. Motor Behav.*, **16**, 3, 235–254.

von Hofsten, C. (1979) Development of visually directed reaching: the approach phase. *J. Hum. Movement Stud.*, **5**, 160–178.

von Hofsten, C. (1982) Eye–hand coordination in the newborn. *Dev. Psychol.*, **18**, 450.

Section III

Congenital abnormalities

11   Talipes equinovarus
12   Talipes calcaneovalgus
13   Congenital dislocation of the hip
14   Arthrogryposis multiplex congenita
15   Spina bifida
16   Congenital limb deficiencies

Talipes equinovarus

Talipes equinovarus (TEV) is said to be the commonest congenital abnormality of the foot (Sharrard 1971), with an incidence of 1–2 per 1000 live births. The foot is plantarflexed at the ankle, inverted and adducted at the subtaloid (talocalcaneal) and mid tarsal joints. In severe cases the deformities may be fixed and the foot almost immobile. In milder postural cases the foot may be relatively mobile but the infant has difficulty in actively everting and dorsiflexing it.

This deformity may occur in an otherwise normal infant, but it is also seen in association with other congenital deformities such as dislocation of the hip, or as one of the deformities associated with arthrogryposis multiplex congenita or myelomeningocele. It also occurs in infants with congenital absence of the tibia. The deformity is often bilateral, in which case one foot is always more deformed than the other, but it may also be unilateral.

The cause of the defect is usually unknown, although causes are generally considered to be developmental, environmental and/or genetic (Wynne-Davies 1964; Beals 1978; Cowell and Wein 1980). Browne (1936) suggested increased intrauterine pressure as an environmental cause.

Other environmental causes cited are a decrease in the capacity of the uterine cavity secondary to loss of amniotic fluid and drugs ingested by the mother (Cowell and Wein 1980). Early germplasm defect (Irani and Sherman 1963) and neuromuscular abnormality (Isaacs *et al.* 1977) have been suggested as causative.

Developmental arrest has also been suggested since an equinovarus foot posture is normally found in 5-week-old embryos (Diaz 1979). An acquired equinovarus deformity will result from muscle imbalance in poliomyelitis or in muscular dystrophy, caused by paralysis of the anterior tibial and peroneal muscles.

Types

The deformity may be classified into one of two groups – those which are 'postural', in which there is at first no bony or arthrotic abnormality; and those in which there are abnormalities of the bones themselves, with malpositioning of the joints, and soft tissue abnormality. Where the deformity is severe (Figs 11.1–11.3), the affected foot is smaller in appearance than the other. The heel is usually small and underdeveloped, the calf thin with poor development of the gastrocnemius. The talus is prominent on the dorsum of the foot. The skin on the medial side is wrinkled and on the lateral side stretched. The great toe may be abducted away from the other toes. The foot may be so displaced that its medial border is in contact with the medial side of the leg. If the foot is viewed from behind, the extreme degree of plantarflexion with shortening of the tendo Achilles is clearly seen (Fig. 11.2). The degree of inversion and adduction is noticed from the plantar aspect when the foot is seen to be curved in

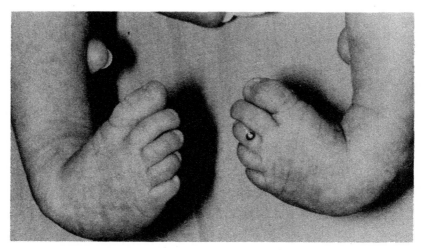

Figure 11.1 A severe degree of talipes equinovarus. Note the extreme degree of inversion and metatarsus varus.

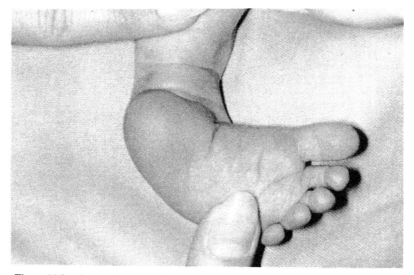

Figure 11.2 A posterior view demonstrates the degree of plantarflexion and inversion. The contracted tendo Achilles is clearly visible.

a banana shape. The foot with a postural equinovarus deformity may be of relatively normal size and shape, but held in an equinus and varus position (Fig. 11.4).

Pathological anatomy

The underlying pathological mechanism is still unknown. There have been several anatomical studies of club foot. In 1963, Schlicht reported a study he made of TEV in stillborn babies and babies who died soon after birth. He performed dissections on the feet, all of which showed a severe degree of deformity. He did not, unfortunately, state whether the deformities were associated with myelomeningocele or arthrogryposis. He noted that the bones themselves showed distortion, particularly the talus, calcaneus, navicular, cuboid and metatarsals, the

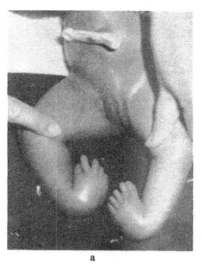 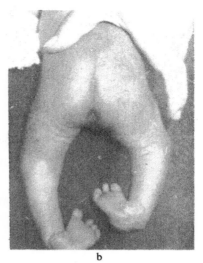

a   b

Figure 11.3 A severe degree of talipes in an infant with arthrogryposis. In (b) note the poor muscular development of the lower limbs.

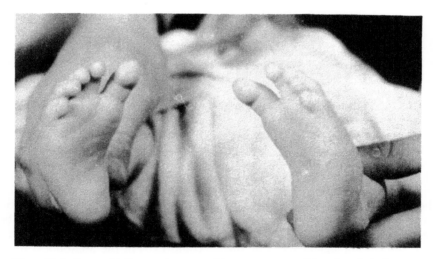

Figure 11.4 Postural talipes equinovarus with metarsus varus. Note the relatively normal shape of the foot compared to Figures 11.1 and 11.3.

talus being the most affected. Not only were the bones themselves malformed, but their relationships with each other were also distorted (Fig. 11.5). In all the feet he dissected, the talus showed distortion of the facets on the superior surface and therefore the bone could not fit properly into the tibiofibular mortice. He suggested that this bony block was an important cause of the persistence of the equinus deformity.

The talus and calcaneus in severely deformed feet are often smaller than normal, this factor contributing to the smallness of the affected foot in relation to the unaffected one. The convex shape of the outer border of the foot is due not only to the pull of the contracted muscles on the inner side of the foot and leg, but also to the subluxation of the calcaneocuboid joint, the ligaments and capsule of which are stretched.

SKELETON OF FOOT

viewed from above

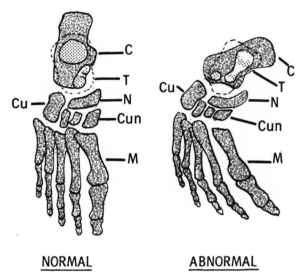

NORMAL   ABNORMAL

Figure 11.5 Normal and abnormal skeletal structure. Note the distortion of the bones as well as their abnormal relationships to each other. C = Calcaneum; T = Talus; N = Navicular; Cu = Cuboid; Cun = Cuneiform; M = Metatarsal. (From Schlicht, D. (1963) The pathological anatomy of talipes equinovarus. *Aust. N.Z. J. Surg.*, **33**, 1.)

Schlicht found that the soft tissues were affected in all the feet he dissected and he considered the equinus and varus deformities to be maintained by tension in these tissues. Certainly contracture of gastrocnemius, soleus, tibialis posterior, flexor hallucis longus and flexor digitorum longus all appear to contribute to the equinus element, while contracture of tibialis anterior and posterior, flexor hallucis longus and flexor digitorum longus, of the deltoid and spring ligaments, and the small muscles along the inner side of the foot contribute to the varus element. Surgeons have noticed the preponderance of fibres of the tendo Achilles inserted into the medial half of the posterior surface of the calcaneus, and this is probably also an important factor in the varus deformity.

In another anatomical study (Waisbrod 1973), the feet of 8 fetuses were dissected. This study is interesting since it provides an anatomical reason for the difference between so-called postural and structural TEV described clinically and also explains the resistance of the structural type to treatment which

has been reported (Lloyd-Roberts 1964). In each of the 5 cases which could not forcibly be manipulated into the plantigrade position, the talus bone was found to be deformed, as Schlicht had reported. The tali were smaller and misshapen. The vascular channels of the feet were abnormal and the ossification centres small. The tendon and insertion of tibialis posterior were also found to be abnormal. The author considered that the talar abnormality could explain the anatomical deformity of the whole foot. In the 3 cases in which the feet could be manipulated into a plantigrade position, the tali were normal.

The proposal that the principal deformity is in the talus has been confirmed by several studies (Settle 1963; Irani and Sherman 1963). More recent studies have shown that the anterior aspect of the calcaneus is rotated medially and the posterior aspect laterally (McKay 1982; Simons and Sarrafian 1983). Smith in 1983 noted a contracture of the deltoid and calcaneofibular ligaments in 7 feet with a decreased size of head and attenuated neck of talus. The essential lesion was considered to be a dislocation of the talocalcaneona-vicular joint. The movements of the calcaneus under the talus are very complex and under-standing the normal relationship between the two bones and the altered anatomy and mechanics associated with TEV is critical if treatment is to be effective and further defor-mity is to be avoided (Campos da Paz and de Souza 1978). Three-dimensional computer modelling has added to the understanding of the bony relationships (Herzenberg *et al.* 1988).

Wasting of the calf muscles, found in the fetus as well as at term, is characteristic of TEV (Irani and Sherman 1963; Laaveg and Ponseti 1980), and several studies have investi-gated the reason for this. Structure of calf mus-cles appears normal, with wasting apparently due to a reduction in number of fibres rather than in fibre size (Gray and Katz 1981). However, a higher proportion of type 1 fibres has been found in the soleus muscle compared to normal (Gray and Katz 1981; Handelsman and Badalamente 1981), although maturation of other calf muscles appears to proceed nor-mally. An increase in type 1 could be due to immobility. However, according to Gray and Katz (1981), since the maturation of slow mus-cles such as soleus is dependent upon the integ-rity of the spinal cord, the findings of changes in the soleus muscle only suggest a neurogenic basis for structural TEV.

Prognosis

Most postural cases of TEV correct with con-servative treatment in an uncomplicated man-ner. It should be remembered that in the case of postural TEV, although according to anatomi-cal studies the bones are not initially deformed, deformity will occur over time as growth takes place if the foot posture is not corrected and if the muscles which should control the foot are not trained to do so. Many structural cases show a tendency to relapse despite treatment, although Sharrard (1971) suggests that this may not be a relapse in the sense of a loss of correction, but rather an indication that the deformities have not been completely cor-rected. If the foot does not yield where it should (at the ankle and subtalar joints) when force is directed towards making the plantarflexed and inverted foot plantigrade (e.g. during both treatment and walking), pseudocorrection can occur in both the verti-cal and horizontal planes. The vertical breach occurs at the mid tarsal joints, causing a rocker-bottom foot. The horizontal breach occurs at the ankle, causing a bean-shaped foot. The mechanism is described in detail by Lloyd-Roberts and Fixsen (1990).

If the deformity is either untreated or inade-quately treated, secondary bony deformities will develop as the child grows. The relationship between the articular surfaces will alter, the

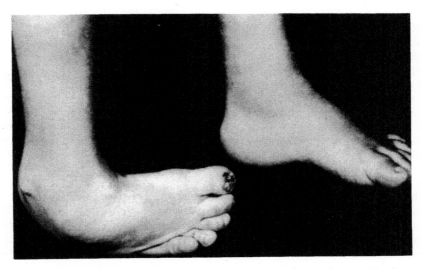

Figure 11.6 Untreated talipes equinovarus with weight-bearing on the lateral border of the foot.

subtaloid and calcaneocuboid joints in particular being altered in alignment (Lloyd-Roberts and Fixsen 1990). Eventually the child may weight-bear on the lateral border of the feet, with painful callosities forming under the cuboid and cuneiform bones (Fig. 11.6).

Management

It is generally considered that the mild postural TEV will be corrected by mobilization and strapping, that the moderately severe structural deformity will require mobilization and plaster casting, and that the severe deformity will require surgical correction, which is usually delayed until the infant is 4–6 months of age (Cummings and Lovell 1988). In the case of structural TEV, the earlier the deformity begins in intrauterine life the more difficult it is considered reduction will be, due to the extent of the anatomical changes (Campos da Paz and de Souza 1978).

When the anatomical evidence of structural abnormalities of the talus in severe cases is considered, it is difficult to see how mobilizing and splinting could be expected to correct the hindfoot part of the deformity, although the forefoot could be corrected by these methods. It may be that the hindfoot deformity can only be compensated for by surgical reconstruction of the talocalcaneal area. Treatment of this deformity has long been the subject of controversy.

The methods of manipulating or mobilizing the joints of the foot into a corrected position, and the types of splinting used, vary from hospital to hospital. The author describes below one method of mobilizing the foot, and several methods of splinting. These methods of splinting have been reported to be successful in the short term. Long-term results have not been adequately assessed. Until clinical trials on the various methods in use in different hospitals have been set up and their results made known, the student must expect to be confronted with a confusing number of alternatives of treatment. There is a disappointing tendency for many treated structural deformities to relapse. The only effective methods of treatment will be those which prevent this tendency. This is an area of therapeutics in which the physiotherapist should institute clinical

trials in collaboration with an orthopaedic surgeon.

Assessment

Details of family history and the infant's birth history are recorded by the physiotherapist. It is sometimes found that similar deformities, TEV or a short tendo Achilles, have been present in other members of the family. Note is made of any other congenital abnormalities which are also present, such as spina bifida occulta, dislocated hips, or the deformities associated with arthrogryposis.

The feet are examined and details of their shape, the extent of the deformity and the degree of mobility are noted, together with the degree of passive and active correction which can be obtained. This can be measured using a goniometric device incorporating a dynamometer to record a known force. The effectiveness of the evertors and dorsiflexors in a young infant is tested by stroking the lateral border of the foot. The normal infant will respond immediately and strongly. In the infant with severe deformity, the response will indicate the deficiencies of the peroneal and anterior tibial muscles, or the degree to which they are inhibited by their contracted antagonists.

Photographs of the infant's feet are taken before treatment commences, and at frequent intervals until eventual discharge. Periodic radiographs as the child grows are useful in showing the true position of the joints (Lloyd-Roberts and Fixsen 1990).

Physical and orthopaedic treatment

There have been a few recent investigations into the relative effectiveness of various forms of treatment (Ryoppy and Sairanen 1983; Green and Lloyd-Roberts 1985). Conservative treatment consisting of mobilizing and splinting begins as early as possible after the infant's birth in order to take advantage of the pliability of ligaments conferred by maternal hormones (Bates and Chung 1989). It should be remembered that the deformity is present in an infant who will be subject to the mechanics of growth and development. Mechanical structures (bone and soft tissue) develop according to the stresses put upon them. If the equinovarus foot is left untreated, the bony structure of the foot and lower leg will be subject to unnatural stresses, the soft tissues will undergo further adaptive changes, and the actual deformity will be increased. The older the child is before treatment is commenced, the poorer the end-result will probably be.

Mobilization

Passive correction is a gradual closed reduction of the malaligned joints and should be frequent, repetitive and gentle (Bates and Chung 1989). This technique takes into account the need to mobilize the foot as well as to correct the deformity, and in this way is probably more effective than the rigid forms of splinting sometimes used.

Traditionally there has been controversy as to the order in which correction should be gained, with two conflicting views. In the first, emphasis is placed on the early correction of the hindfoot equinus (Lloyd-Roberts and Fixsen 1990). Attenborough (1966), however, made the observation that the infant's heel cannot be put in a valgus position – that is, everted – while the foot is in equinus. In the second view, the emphasis is on early correction of the mid tarsal and subtaloid adduction and inversion before attempting correction of the equinus element (Browne 1936; Sharrard 1971; Bates and Chung 1989). The technique described below allows for attempting correction of the subtalar malalignment (inversion and adduction) followed by the plantarflexion element.

The mobilization of these feet should be attempted only by an experienced physiotherapist with detailed knowledge of the normal and pathological anatomy of the foot, plus an awareness of the plasticity of the infant foot. The foot should always be mobilized with due regard to the damage which may be caused to the undeveloped bones, to the epiphyseal areas of the tibia and fibula, and to the soft tissues around the foot by forcible manipulation (Sharrard 1971).

Technique

One hand holds the lower ends of the tibia and fibula and the calcaneus. This enables the therapist to protect the tibial and fibular epiphyses

from a shearing strain, and to hold the hindfoot steady while the other hand mobilizes the forefoot away from its adducted position in relation to the hindfoot (Fig. 11.7a). When this part of the foot (tarsometatarsal and mid tarsal joints) has been mobilized, the therapist changes the grip slightly, holding the foot with the thumb over the talus, giving gentle pressure downwards and backwards on the prominent talus, in an attempt to guide its articular facet back into the ankle joint mortice and gain as much dorsiflexion and eversion as possible. When some correction has been gained, the tendo Achilles may be more effectively stretched by the method shown in Figure 11.7b. The foot is held in one hand, the heel pulled down to stretch the plantarflexors, and into eversion. Care is taken that it is the hindfoot that is corrected, and not the forefoot. If the foot is immobile, emphasis is on mobilization of the various joints rather than on maintenance of a passive stretch.

Precautions

The knee must be held flexed while the foot is being mobilized in order to avoid strain on the medial ligament of the knee. If the foot is everted on an extended leg it is possible to exert such strain on the medial ligament of the knee that a valgus deformity results. The risk in attempting to correct the plantarflexion element too early and vigorously lies in the tendency of the foot to 'break' at the mid tarsal joints, giving the foot a rocker-shaped appearance. This pseudocorrection can be avoided if the therapist corrects the subtalar malalignment first and proceeds slowly with the correction of the hindfoot, gently increasing the mobility gained rather than attempting too great a degree of correction.

This mobilization is done by the therapist several times a day while the infant and mother are in the maternity hospital, and the mother is taught the procedure, and does it herself under the therapist's supervision. When they return home the infant is seen by the therapist regularly, and emphasis at this point is on ensuring that the parents understand the mobilizing techniques well enough to do them several times a day. If the parent mobilizes the foot with excessive zeal with the risk of injuring it, the mobilizing may be better left to the therapist.

Mobilization is usually followed by the application of some form of splinting.

Splinting

There are several methods of splinting in current use. Some are designed to allow active correction by the child while kicking the legs; others are more rigid, holding the foot immobile in a position of some correction. Rigid splinting is avoided by some surgeons (Sharrard 1971) as it may result in a stiff immobile foot. Many prefer to correct the foot in an adjustable or removable splint or strapping, which allows the joints to be mobilized regularly. However, following surgery a full cast may need to be worn for several weeks. The applications of three types of splinting are described below.

Strapping

This method of strapping holds the foot in a corrected position, the degree of correction being altered by adjusting the pull from the buckle (Fig. 11.8). Once the foot can be held in some eversion the infant will facilitate active contraction of the evertor and dorsiflexor muscles each time the leg is extended. In some centres, the single strap is replaced by two, one to pull the foot into dorsiflexion, the other to pull it into eversion. Lloyd-Roberts and Fixsen (1990) describe in detail the alternative Robert-Jones strapping.

Materials

Non-allergenic strapping 8 cm wide.
Tincture benzoin compound.
Buckle.

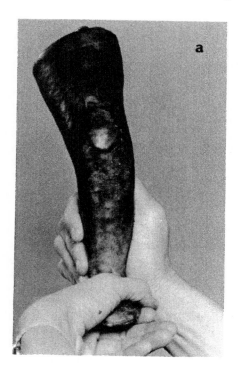

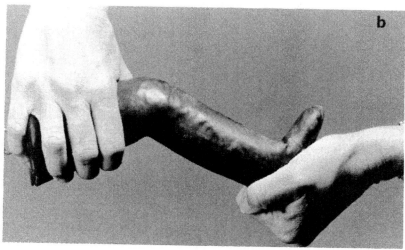

Figure 11.7   Left talipes equinovarus: mobilizing technique. (a) Mobilizing the forefoot in relation to the hindfoot. (b) Stretching the tendo Achilles.

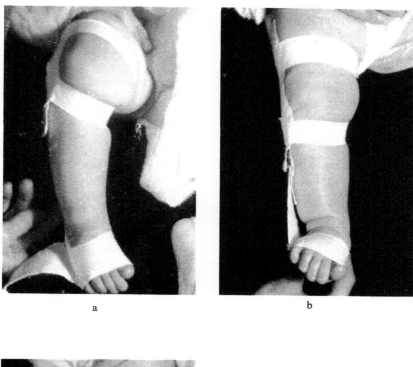

a

b

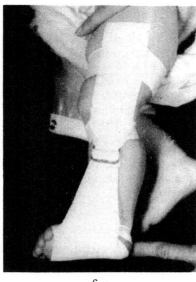

c

Figure 11.8 Talipes equinovarus: strap and buckle splinting. (a) Before being buckled up. (b) Anterior view of strap and buckle maintaining correction. (c) Lateral view.

Method (Fig. 11.9)

The strapping is cut into pieces, the buckle is attached, and the strapping is sewn. Alternatively, Velcro can be used. The therapist mobilizes the foot before applying the strapping. Tincture benzoin compound is applied to the skin with cotton wool and allowed to dry before the strapping is applied. This will give some protection to the skin, but if the infant is allergic to strapping it should not be used.

Step 1: Piece A is applied to the foot. It should be wide enough to extend from the back of the heel to the web of the toes. The cut-out piece is deep enough to avoid cutting into the front of the ankle when the foot is dorsiflexed. The entire piece is long enough to extend from the lateral side of the dorsum of the foot, around the medial side, under the plantar aspect and up to the knee.

Step 2: Piece B is applied to the dorsum of the foot, extending from the medial side across the dorsum to join piece A laterally. This piece is the lining for piece A, to which it is joined as near to the plantar surface as possible in order to pull the foot into dorsiflexion and eversion.

Step 3: Piece C is now applied. The point at which the two pieces of strapping are sewn is placed at the medial side of the calcaneum with the horizontal piece passing from the great toe around the heel to the base of the fifth toe. The broader vertical strip is then taken under the heel and is attached to the combined pieces A and B. This piece reinforces the pull into dorsiflexion and eversion.

Step 4: With the foot pieces in place, piece D is applied to the lateral side of the thigh with the buckle just below the knee. Its exact position depends on the angle of pull required to correct the foot.

Step 5: Pieces E and F are applied around the top of the thigh and top of the leg in order to hold piece D in position. They are placed carefully, without tension, in order to avoid occlusion of the circulation. Piece F should not be placed over the popliteal fossa.

Step 6: The strapping is now too wide to pass through the buckle, so it is made narrower, being cut away anteriorly as far as necessary. As the pull is required particularly from the hindfoot, the strapping is not cut posteriorly.

Step 7: The combined pieces A, B and C are attached to the buckle after the foot has been pulled into the position of correction.

It has been suggested above that the foot be mobilized gently in order to avoid trauma to bones, joints and soft tissues, and this applies also to the splinting, which should not be applied too rigorously. A rocker-bottom foot may result if the strapping pulls the forefoot into dorsiflexion by 'breaking' the foot at the mid tarsal joints instead of pulling the foot into dorsiflexion at the ankle joint.

If the foot is flexed at the mid tarsal joints and the strapping does not correct this, a flat thin piece of aluminium shaped to the foot may be strapped to the plantar surface after the strapping has been applied. Similarly, if the strapping does not correct a severe degree of metatarsus varus, a small metal splint is attached to the medial side of the foot from the calcaneus to the great toe.

The circulation of the foot is carefully checked by observing the capillary response to pressure on the toes. If the toes become dusky in colour, normal circulation can usually be restored by loosening the strapping at the buckle. Instructions are given to the baby's parents about caring for the strapping and the skin, and the purpose of the strapping is explained. The strapping should be kept dry when the baby is bathed, and the nappy put on firmly and changed regularly in order to avoid soiling and soaking. The buckle is undone in order to mobilize the foot during the day. The strapping is replaced each week. If the infant's skin suffers an allergic reaction to the strapping, other forms of splinting may have to be considered.

Anteromedial plaster splint

This splint is useful when a foot is so severely deformed and so immobile that strapping cannot be put on effectively or safely, that is, when other splinting cannot be applied without a force which would damage the infant's foot. It is used for the first few days of treatment until some correction of the adduction and inversion element is obtained, and is followed as soon as possible by strapping which encourages some active correction on the part of the child.

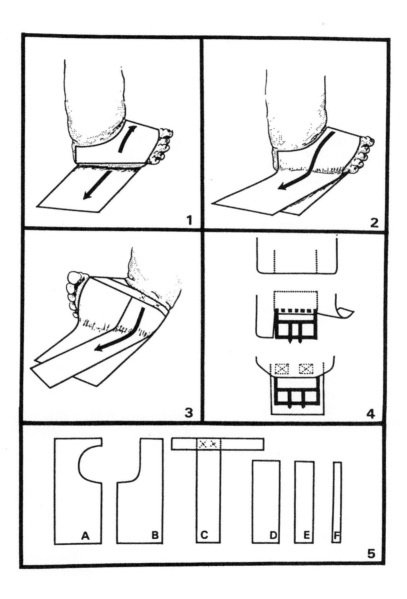

Figure 11.9 Method of applying strap and buckle splinting to the right foot.

Materials

Plaster bandage 10 cm wide.
Piece of foam padding 1.25 cm thick.
Elastoplast strapping 5 cm wide.

Method

A piece of plastic foam and a plaster slab of six thicknesses are cut to fit the anterior, medial and posterior surfaces of the foot and leg, from below the tibial tubercle to the tips of the toes. A narrow strip down the lateral side is left free. The foot is mobilized before the application of the plaster. The plaster slab is wet and is placed on the padding with any wrinkles smoothed out. This combined slab is applied (padding against the skin) to the leg and foot. The adduction and inversion element is corrected gently as in the mobilizing technique and held there until the plaster sets (Fig. 11.10). Indentations from finger pressure must be avoided. The Elastoplast strapping is bandaged around the splint and foot, leaving the toes free.

The capillary response is checked in the toes immediately after the plaster is applied, and at intervals for the next 10 minutes. If the toes become dusky in colour, the splint is removed and reapplied.

This splint is removed three to four times a day for passive mobilizing and stretching. A new splint may be applied daily until sufficient correction has been gained and either strapping or a plaster cast can be applied. The parent is advised to check the circulation of the foot each day, and to remove the splint if the capillary response is not normal.

The combination of mobilization by the physiotherapist and parent and strapping may continue for up to 12 weeks. If at that time the hindfoot remains in equinus, posterior and posterior-medial release surgery may be performed. This is followed by a plaster cast and then strapping and mobilization are resumed. Treatment continues until the foot can be actively everted and dorsiflexed beyond the neutral position.

Denis Browne metal splints

This form of splinting is not often used. It consists of two pieces of aluminium moulded into footplates with extensions for the lateral side of the leg (Fig. 11.11). It is important that the foot pieces are the same size as the baby's feet. If they are too wide, the strapping will not be able to control the adduction element. The lateral extension should extend well up the leg. If it is too short it will eliminate the leverage required to hold the foot everted. In the case of a unilateral deformity the normal foot must be splinted as well. The splints are joined together by a removable crossbar which attaches by butterfly nuts to the footplates. The crossbar may be bent downwards to a small degree, and if the footplates are attached with the legs in some external rotation, the position of the legs and feet probably helps facilitate eversion and dorsiflexion as the infant kicks into extension.

The effectiveness of this splint is questioned by some surgeons (Fripp and Shaw 1967) on the grounds that the feet are stiff and immobile after the splint is removed.

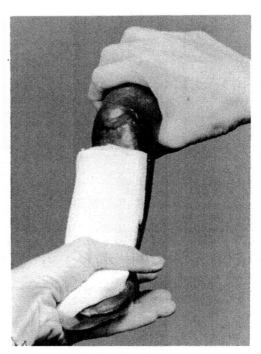

Figure 11.10 Method of applying an anteromedial plaster splint to the left foot. The foot and leg are held in the splint by elastoplast strapping.

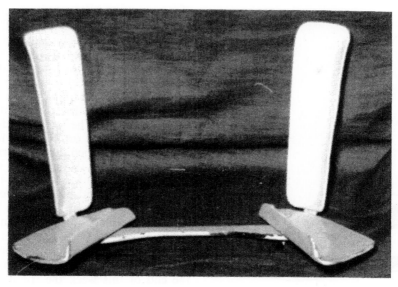

Figure 11.11   Denis Browne splints.

Materials

Denis Browne metal splints made to measure.
Adhesive felt 0.5 cm thick.
Strapping 3 cm wide.

Method

The splints are covered with felt which overlaps the edges a little. Small wedges of felt are cut out to pass from under the cuboid along the lateral border of the plantar surface of the foot. The number of pieces of felt in each wedge, that is, the height of the wedge, depends on the degree of correction obtainable (Fig. 11.12).

A narrow strip of felt is cut out which is long enough to pass along the medial side of the foot from the great toe to the calcaneus. It is difficult to apply this splint without help, so assistance is needed. One therapist, or the baby's parent, holds the foot firmly on the splint in order to gain the best correction; the other straps the foot on to the splint. At no time should force be used. The therapist, holding the foot, holds with one hand at the toes and the other at the knee. The knee is flexed and gentle pressure downwards will keep the ankle in as much dorsiflexion as is obtainable. Tincture benzoin compound is applied to the skin from the web of the toes to the knee, making sure to cover the skin thoroughly.

The wedges are applied either to the splint or to the foot, extending laterally from the cuboid to the toes. These will hold the foot everted. The strapping is wound in circular fashion, leaving no gaps and starting from the web of the toes. Emphasis is placed on holding the ankle in as much dorsiflexion as possible by several turns around the ankle and under the heel, and the strapping is continued up the leg to the top of the splint. A narrow piece of felt is strapped on medially from the heel to the great toe to prevent the foot adducting from the splint. Alternatively, a small piece of padded aluminium may be applied in the same way.

The screws underneath the footplates must be free from strapping. The crossbar is attached (if it is curved, the curve must be convex downwards) to the screws with the legs in as much external rotation as required. The butterfly nuts are then done up tightly (Fig. 11.13).

It is easy to occlude the circulation during the application of the strapping, so the colour of the toes is checked carefully over a period of 10 minutes, and the baby's parent is advised to continue these checks periodically for at least the next few hours. If the circulation does appear to be occluded and the obstruction cannot be relieved, the splint must be removed and reapplied.

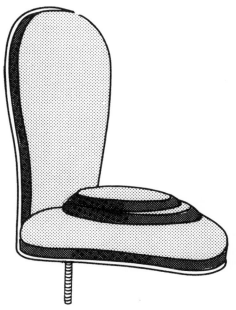

Figure 11.12   Denis Browne splint for the left foot with felt and wedges attached.

Care must be taken when applying this splint that the dorsiflexion obtained is at the ankle joint and not at the mid tarsal joints.

The normal foot is placed flat on the footplate with a piece of felt under the medial longitudinal arch, and is strapped on as described above.

If it is difficult to gain sufficient eversion by the above method, a strip of felt may be applied, with the sticky side against the skin, to pass from the medial side of the calcaneum and under the heel. At this point tension on the felt will pull the heel into some eversion. The felt is then attached to the lateral side of the leg, and acts as lining for the splint as well as a corrective force. The lateral wedges of felt are attached as before or on to the foot itself, and the splint is strapped on as described above.

Some advice to the parents is necessary, and they are told how to look after the splint, and how to remove and reapply the crossbar which will have to be done when the baby is being dressed. The splint remains in place for 1 week. Ferguson (1968) suggests that the feet be suspended at times by a cord attached to the bar so the baby can kick more freely. At the end of this week the splint is removed by cutting the strapping along the lateral side. The baby may now be bathed and allowed to kick free for a few hours before the splint is reapplied.

Posterior plaster splint

A padded plaster splint is made to hold the foot either in the mid-position or in eversion and dorsiflexion. It is of no value in severe TEV with its tendency to relapse, as even with firm

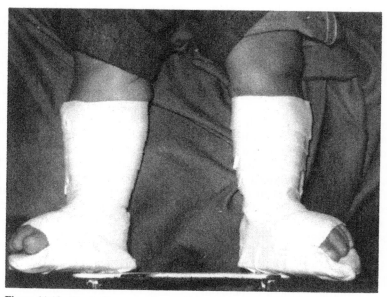

Figure 11.13   Denis Browne splints, with strapping applied.

bandaging it cannot control the tendency to return to an equinovarus position. However, the splint is useful in mild postural deformities to maintain correction until the infant can do so actively, in infants with myelomeningocele where the leg is flaccid, and when correction must be maintained until stabilizing surgery can be performed.

Denis Browne bootee splints

This splint is sometimes prescribed as a means of maintaining correction gained by strapping. It consists of a pair of boots attached to metal plates on a crossbar (Fig. 11.14). The principle is similar to that of the metal splint described above. The legs are held in external rotation and the feet are everted and dorsiflexed. The splint is worn at night.

During the day, a child old enough to stand and walk may wear a pair of boots without heels, with 3 mm outer sole and heel raises.

Active correction

This is an important aspect of treatment. Mobilization of the infant's foot is followed by an attempt at stimulating active eversion and dorsiflexion by stroking the lateral border of the foot firmly with the tip of the finger in the direction of the heel.

With postural TEV, as soon as the foot can be passively moved to plantigrade, the infant should be given practice of standing. The parents are shown how to stand the infant with the affected foot in the optimal position, and how to encourage standing up from crouch with the heels on the floor (see Fig. 3.1), sit-to-stand (see Fig. 3.9) and stepping up (see Fig. 3.18). The depth of the crouch position is increased gradually as the degree of ankle plantarflexion is increased. The parents need to understand why no force should be used to keep the heel on the ground, and this understanding can probably best be acquired when they have some knowledge of the anatomy of the foot, of the fragility of the structures of the infant's foot and the ease with which a false plantarflexion can be achieved if force is used.

At 5 months of age the normal infant in the supine position reaches up to grasp the toes and to play with them, and this should be encouraged by the parents as another way of gaining active correction. The baby should be encouraged to hold the lateral toes in order to stimulate eversion. Similarly, when sitting at 6 or 7 months the baby can be encouraged to play with the feet. Mechanical vibration over the muscles required to contract has also been suggested (Bishop 1975). Stimulation of the foot-placing reaction (Appendix 1) will also facilitate active dorsiflexion in infants. There are other methods of stimulating movement and these should be explored by the therapist.

Surgical management

Surgical intervention for severe club feet can be divided into three groups according to Cummings and Lovell (1988), involving soft

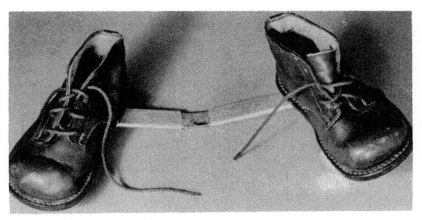

Figure 11.14 Denis Browne bootee splint.

tissues, bone or a combination of these. *Soft tissue procedures* include release or lengthening of soft tissues (ligaments, joint capsules, tendons) and tendon transfers to remove a deforming force or correct muscle imbalance. *Bony procedures* include metatarsal or calcaneus osteotomy and triple arthrodesis. An example of a *combined procedure* is a wedge osteotomy of the calcaneus together with soft tissue release. Aronson and Puskarich (1990), in their retrospective study of 29 children, found that operative intervention demonstrated three significant effects:

1 Subtalar release increased the talocrural index and eventual foot length.
2 Capsulotomy of the ankle joint decreased ankle motion.
3 Multiple tendo Achilles lengthenings decreased muscle strength and calf circumference.

Summary

Talipes equinovarus is the commonest congenital deformity of the foot. The severe, structural type is difficult to treat successfully and shows a tendency to relapse despite treatment. Methods of conservative treatment are still controversial. To some extent this is due to the lack of clinical trials on the various methods available. Mobilization of the joints of the foot is used to correct the deformity, and the physiotherapist must do this mobilizing with a thorough understanding of the anatomy of the foot, as well as with an awareness of the potential damage that may be caused by careless or forcible techniques. The promotion of active correction is a significant part of physiotherapy. When the foot is plantigrade, the infant is helped to practise actions in which the body mass is moved over the feet (e.g., crouch-to-stand). These actions assist in the maintenance of correction by actively increasing soft tissue extensibility and providing the opportunity to strengthen the leg muscles as the infant grows.

References

Aronson, J. and Puskarich, C.L. (1990) Deformity and disability from treated clubfoot. *J. Pediatr. Orthop.*, **10**, 109–119.

Attenborough, C.G. (1966) Severe congenital talipes equinovarus. *J. Bone Joint Surg.*, **48B**, 1, 31

Bates, E.H. and Chung, W.K. (1989) Congenital talipes equinovarus. In *The Foot. Its Disorders and their Management*, edited by Helal and Wilson. London: Churchill Livingstone.

Beals, R.K. (1978) The snapping knee of infancy. *J. Bone Joint Surg.*, **60**, 679–680.

Bishop, B. (1975) Vibratory stimulation 3. *Phys. Ther.*, **55**, 2, 139–143.

Browne, D. (1936) Congenital deformities of mechanical origin. *Proc. R. Soc. Med.*, **29**, 1, 409.

Campos da Paz, A. and de Souza, V. (1978) Talipes equinovarus: pathomechanical basis of treatment. *Orthop. Clin. North Am.*, **9**, 1, 171–185.

Cowell, H.R. and Wein, B.K. (1980) Current concepts review. Genetic aspects of club foot. *J. Bone Joint Surg.*, **62A**, 8, 1381–1384.

Cummings, R.J. and Lovell, W.W. (1988) Current concepts review. Operative treatment of congenital idiopathic club foot. *J. Bone Joint Surg.*, **70-A**, 7, 1108–1112.

Diaz, A.V. (1979) Embryological contribution to the aetiopathology of idiopathic clubfoot. *J. Bone Joint Surg.*, **61-B**, 127.

Ferguson, A. (1968) *Orthopaedic Surgery in Infancy and Childhood*. Baltimore, MD: Williams & Wilkins.

Fripp, A.T. and Shaw, N.R. (1967) *Clubfoot*. Edinburgh: Livingstone.

Gray, D.H. and Katz, J.M. (1981) A histochemical study of muscles in club foot. *J. Bone Joint Surg.*, **63-B**, 3, 417–423.

Green, A.D. and Lloyd-Roberts, G.C. (1985) The results of early posterior release in resistant club feet. A long term review. *J. Bone Joint Surg.*, **67**, 588–593.

Handelsman, J.E. and Badalamente, M.A. (1981) Neuromuscular studies in clubfoot. *J. Pediatr. Orthop.*, **1**, 23–32.

Herzenberg, J.E., Carroll, N.C., Christofersen, M.R., Lee, E.H., White, S. and Munroe, R. (1988) Club foot analysis with three-dimensional computer modelling. *J. Pediatr. Orthop.*, **8**, 257–262.

Irani, R.N. and Sherman, M.S. (1963) The pathological anatomy of club foot. *J. Bone Joint Surg.*, **45-A**, 45–52.

Isaacs, H., Handelsman, J.E., Badenhorst, M. and Pickering, A. (1977) The muscles in clubfoot – a histological, histochemical and electron microscopic study. *J. Bone Joint Surg.*, **59-B**, 465–477.

Laaveg, S.J. and Ponseti, I.V. (1980) Long-term results of treatment of congenital club foot. *J. Bone Joint Surg.*, **62-A**, 23–31.

Lloyds-Roberts, G.C. (1964) Congenital club foot. *J. Bone Joint Surg.*, **46B**, 369–371.

Lloyd-Roberts, G.C. and Fixsen, J.A. (1990) *Orthopaedics in Infancy and Childhood*, 2nd edn. Oxford: Butterworth-Heinemann.

McKay, D.W. (1982) New concept of and approach to clubfoot treatment. Section 1. Principles and morbid anatomy. *J. Pediatr. Orthop.*, **2**, 347–356.

Ponseti, I.V., El-Khoury, G.Y., Ippolito, E. *et al.* (1980) A radiographic study of skeletal deformities in treated club-feet. *Clin. Orthop. Rel. Res.*, **160**, 30–42.

Ryoppy, S. and Sairanen, H. (1983) Neonatal operative treatment of club foot. *J. Bone Joint Surg.*, **65-B**, 320–325.

Schlicht, D. (1963) The pathological anatomy of talipes equinovarus. *Aust. N.Z. J. Surg.*, **33**, 1, 2–10.

Settle, G.W. (1963) The anatomy of congenital talipes equinovarus. Sixteen dissected specimens. *J. Bone Joint Surg.*, **45-A**, 1341–1354.

Sharrard, W.J.W. (1971) *Paediatric Orthopaedics and Fractures*. Oxford: Blackwell.

Simons, G.W. and Sarrafian, S. (1983) The microsurgical dissection of a stillborn fetal clubfoot. *Clin. Orthop.*, **173**, 275–283.

Smith, R.B. (1983) Dysplasia and the effects of soft tissue release in congenital talipes equinovarus. *Clin. Orthop.*, **174**, 303–309.

Waisbrod, H. (1973) Congenital club foot. *J. Bone Joint Surg.*, **55B**, 4, 796–801.

Wynne-Davies, R. (1964) Family studies and the cause of congenital clubfoot. *J. Bone Joint Surg.*, **46B**, 445–463.

Further reading

Böhm, M. (1929) The embryological origin of clubfoot. *J. Bone Joint Surg.*, **11**, 229–259.

Brockman, E.P. (1930) *Congenital Clubfoot*. Bristol: Wright.

Browne, D. (1956) Splinting for controlled movement. *Clin. Orthop.*, **8**, 91.

Coleman, S.S. (1983) *Complex Foot Deformities in Children*. Philadelphia, PA: Lea & Febiger.

Fixsen, J.A. and Lloyd-Roberts, G.C. (1988) *The Foot in Childhood*. New York: Churchill Livingstone.

Kite, J.H. (1964) *The Clubfoot*. New York: Grune & Stratton.

Lehman, W.B. (1980) *The Clubfoot*. Philadelphia, PA: J.B. Lippincott.

Tachdjian, M.O. (1985) *The Child's Foot*. Philadelphia, PA: W.B. Saunders.

12

Talipes calcaneovalgus

In this congenital deformity (Fig. 12.1), the foot is held in dorsiflexion at the ankle joint and eversion at the subtaloid joint, and it cannot be moved passively into full inversion or plantarflexion. The soft tissues on the anterior surface of the ankle are contracted. The deformity is thought to be a postural one if unaccompanied by spina bifida or bony abnormality of the foot. In children with spina bifida cystica, the deformity, although present at birth, is probably be the result of muscle imbalance.

The aetiology is unknown, although Jolly (1968) noted that it is seen in post-mature infants. The hips of the neonate with talipes calcaneovalgus (TCV) should be carefully examined to exclude congenital hip dislocation since there is an increased incidence of hip instability associated with TCV and other foot deformities (Lloyd-Roberts and Fixsen 1990). Prognosis is good in the otherwise normal child and, with passive movements done daily by the parents and encouragement to move the foot actively into plantarflexion, full-range movement should be gained within a few weeks. However, in the child with muscle imbalance, although passive correction may be achieved, its maintenance is very difficult, and the effects of gravity and positioning frequently result in a secondary deformity involving plantarflexion of the mid tarsal joints with the ankle remaining in dorsiflexion.

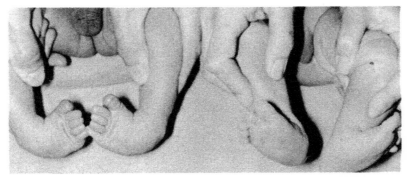

Figure 12.1 Compare the postures of the feet with talipes equinovarus on the left with those on the right with talipes calcaneovalgus. (Courtesy of W. Cumming.)

Congenital vertical talus

This uncommon disorder must be differentiated from TCV which, at first sight, it resembles (Fig. 12.2). Subtaloid rigidity and an equinus heel distinguish vertical talus from TCV. The foot is convex on the medial side, the head of the talus protrudes in the sole and there is rigidity of the subtaloid joint. Radiographs, with the foot at 90° to the shank, show the calcaneus to be in equinus with the talus continuing in a vertical line from the tibia (Fig. 12.3). The talonavicular joint is dislocated.

This condition is treated conservatively in infancy by the application of a serial plaster cast applied with the foot in full plantarflexion (Fig. 12.4) followed by a posterior release to restore the plantigrade position. If the child is not seen in early infancy, surgery, including posterior release, dorsal capsulotomies and muscle transplantation (Lloyd-Roberts and Fixsen 1990) may be necessary.

Management

Physical treatment of TCV aims at mobilizing the foot by stretching the short anterior structures and by stimulating the calf and posterior tibial muscles to plantarflex and invert the foot. The mobilization is done by the parents at home with supervision by the physiotherapist. Serial plaster splinting is useful for maintaining the correction gained. Surgery may be necessary eventually for the infant whose deformity is due to muscle imbalance

Assessment

The physiotherapist takes note of the appearance of the foot, and tests the range of movement at the ankle and subtaloid joints. Photographs of the foot are a useful guide to progress.

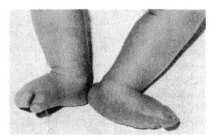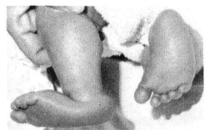

Figure 12.2 The left foot has a vertical talus. (Courtesy of the Royal Alexandra Hospital for Children, Sydney, Australia.)

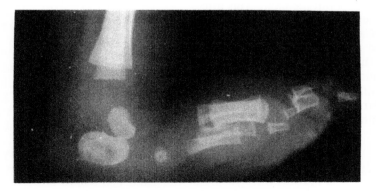

Figure 12.3 A radiograph of the same foot showing abnormal bony relationships. (Courtesy of the Royal Alexandra Hospital for Children, Sydney, Australia.)

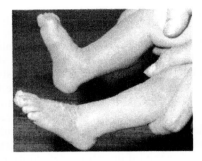

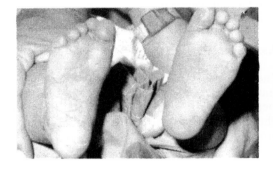

Figure 12.4   These photographs show the altered position of the left foot after several applications of moulded plaster casts. (Courtesy of the Royal Alexandra Hospital for Children, Sydney, Australia.)

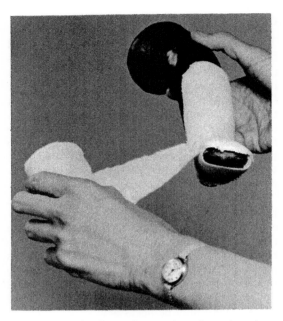

Figure 12.5   Left talipes calcaneovalgus. Anterolateral plaster slab seen from the medial side. The heel must be bandaged up into the splint to gain as much plantarflexion as possible.

Physical treatment

Mobilization

The foot is held in a handshake grasp with the lateral border of the foot in the palm. This grip enables the calcaneus to be inverted as the foot is plantarflexed. Care is taken to hold the foot near the ankle so plantarflexion will occur at this joint rather than at the mid tarsal joints, otherwise a pseudocorrection will occur, with the ankle remaining in dorsiflexion while the forefoot is plantarflexed. This mobilization is done for a few minutes several times a day.

Splinting

A plaster slab is made to fit the anterolateral aspect of the foot and leg. It is padded with plastic foam, which is particularly necessary in

the case of the myelomeningocele infant with absent or abnormal sensation. The splint extends from below the knee to cover the toes. Laterally it covers the calcaneus in order to obtain maximum correction of the eversion element. The wet plaster slab is applied using the same grip as in the mobilization technique, and the foot is gently corrected as much as possible, making sure it is true plantarflexion that is being gained. The splint is bandaged on with a 5 cm crêpe bandage (Fig. 12.5).

When the splint is being bandaged on, care is taken to hold the heel firmly enough to allow the anterior aspect of the ankle to fit well into the splint. If the splint is bandaged on with the heel sagging there will again be a tendency towards pseudocorrection. This must be carefully explained to the infant's parents. The circulation of the toes is checked after the splint is bandaged on.

A new splint is made every few days as the position of the foot improves. It may be worn day and night until correction is gained, with periods of the day spent in kicking freely without it, and eventually only at night until the baby can maintain active correction.

Active correction

In infants with intact neural control of muscles, weight-bearing on a flat surface and practice of crouch-to-stand and sit-to-stand will stimulate plantarflexor activation, as will pressure upwards against the sole of the foot.

Summary

In an otherwise normal baby, TCV poses no problems in management; the affected foot regains full-range movement and a normal posture within a few weeks of treatment commencing. Where the deformity is the result of muscle imbalance, as may occur in a baby with myelomeningocele, maintenance of correction is difficult, and the infant may require surgery to correct the effects of the muscular imbalance.

References

Jolly, H. (1968) *Diseases of Children*. London: Blackwell.

Lloyd-Roberts, G.C. and Fixsen, J.A. (1990) *Orthopaedics in Infancy and Childhood*, 2nd edn. Oxford: Butterworth-Heinemann.

Further reading

Coleman, S.S. (1983) *Complex Foot Deformities in Children*. Philadelphia, PA: Lea & Febiger.

Fixsen, J.A. and Lloyd-Roberts, G.C. (1988) *The Foot in Childhood*. New York: Churchill Livingstone.

Helal, B. and Wilson, D.W. (1989). *The Foot. Its Disorders and their Management*. London: Churchill Livingstone.

Lehman, W.B. (1980) *The Clubfoot*. Philadelphia, PA: J.B. Lippincott.

Tachdjian, M.O. (1985) *The Child's Foot*. Philadelphia, PA: W.B. Saunders.

13

Congenital dislocation of the hip

Congenital dislocation (or dysplasia) of the hip (CDH) results from abnormal development of one or more of the components of the hip joint – the femoral head, the acetabulum or the soft tissues, including the capsule, surrounding the joint. Dislocation may, however, also be associated with hypermobility of joints (Rose 1986). The treatment of unstable hips in infants and of dislocated and subluxated hips in infants and older children is the province of the orthopaedic surgeon. The physiotherapist plays a role in the detection of hip dislocation and in assisting parents to understand and apply splinting. Following any period of immobilization associated with either splinting or surgery, the physiotherapist's primary role involves exercise and motor training to ensure flexibility of the lower-limb joints and soft tissues, and efficient movement control in locomotion and other actions. In many paediatric departments the physiotherapist is responsible for the application of splinting, and a description of the methods of application of the most commonly used forms of splinting is given below.

Description

A hip is said to be *dislocated* when the head of the femur is completely outside the acetabulum (Fig. 13.1); it is *subluxed* when the femoral head lies partially beneath the roof of the acetabulum; it is *dislocatable* when the femoral head can be dislocated from the acetabulum and

relocated either spontaneously or by manipulation and positioning. If a hip remains dislocated, the psoas, adductor and hamstring muscles shorten and eventually the head of the femur changes shape, becoming flattened in appearance.

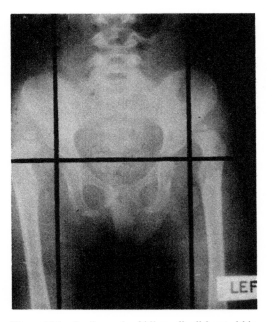

Figure 13.1 Radiograph of bilaterally dislocated hips. Note the position of the head of the femur in relation to the acetabulum.

Aetiology

The reported incidence of CDH is variable (Catford *et al.* 1982). It is more common in girls than in boys, and occurs more often unilaterally than bilaterally.

The aetiology is multifactorial (Sharrard 1971; Behrman and Vaughan 1987; Lloyd-Roberts and Fixsen 1990). There appear to be genetic factors. Since it is sometimes associated with a breech delivery, uterine position or birth trauma is implicated. Congenital dysplasia is also found associated with other congenital abnormalities such as arthrogryposis or talipes equinovarus.

Diagnosis

Catford and colleagues (1982) stress the importance of the screening of infants and children under 1 year of age for hip dysplasia, suggesting that all health professionals who come into contact with children in the first year of life should examine the hip as part of normal practice (p. 1529). Screening is performed initially soon after birth. The aim of screening is to detect hip instability early enough to prevent frank dislocation, and to commence treatment of babies with actual dislocation as early as possible. Earlier treatment appears more effective than treatment commenced later. It is therefore critical that the physiotherapist who suspects or, on examination, detects hip dysplasia or dislocation refers the infant immediately to the medical practitioner.

Tests for hip instability in infants

There are two tests for detecting hip instability in common use – Barlow's test and Ortolani's manoeuvre.

Barlow's test and Ortolani's manoeuvre

With the baby in supine on an examination table, the hips and knees are flexed to 90°, and the hips abducted. In the neonate, the hip should abduct to approximately 90°. With the hip in mid-rotation (Fig. 13.2), pressure is applied longitudinally down towards the table (Barlow's test). If a click or jerk is felt, it indicates that the head of the femur has slipped posteriorly over the rim of the acetabulum and out of the socket. Pressure by the fingers through the greater trochanter as the hip is gently abducted will push the head of the femur back into the acetabulum (Ortolani's manoeuvre).

Other signs to look for which may indicate *unilateral dislocation* in an infant may be:

1 Decreased abduction in one hip (Fig. 13.3).
2 Asymmetrical skin creases.
3 Apparent shortness of one leg (Fig. 13.4).
4 On palpation, one greater trochanter is felt to be higher than the other.

In the case of *bilateral dislocation* the signs may include:

1 Wide perineum.
2 Wide pelvis.
3 Increased lumbar lordosis.

Once the child begins to bear weight and walk the following signs will be evident:

1 Trendelenburg sign demonstrating lateral hip instability.
2 Abnormal gait:
   (a) Unilateral: limp due to apparent shortness of the limb and lateral hip instability.
   (b) Bilateral: waddling gait due to lateral hip instability.

Management

Orthopaedic treatment is usually conservative. If this is unsuccessful surgery may be necessary. In both cases, the objective is to reduce the dislocation and maintain its reduction with minimum trauma to the head of the femur and the soft tissues around the hip joint. Treatment varies from one paediatric centre to another, and is described in detail by Lloyd-Roberts and Fixsen (1990). It may consist of one or more of the following modalities: manipulation under anaesthesia, manipulation followed by a period in traction, plaster of Paris in a modified Lorenz position, splints, harnesses and surgery.

In a neonate with subluxation (that is, normal hip with lax capsule), the legs are held in abduction by a splint such as a von Rosen

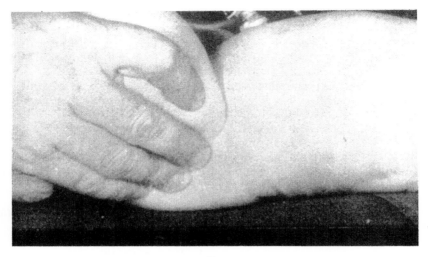

a

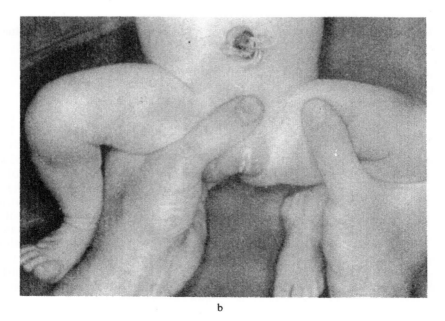

b

Figure 13.2   (a) Barlow's test for dislocation of the hips. (b) Ortolani's manoeuvre.
(Courtesy of W. Cumming.)

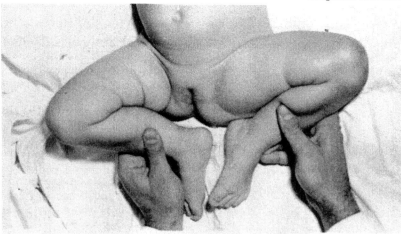

Figure 13.3   Dislocation of the right hip. Note the limited abduction of this hip compared with the left.

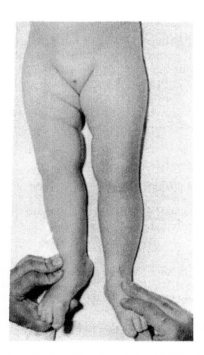

Figure 13.4   Dislocation of the right hip. Note the apparent shortness of the right leg and the asymmetrical skin creases.

splint, a Frejka pillow or Pavlik or Denis Browne hip harness. The objective is to encourage the capsule to tighten. For the infant with a dislocatable hip, a Pavlik harness or von Rosen splint are usually prescribed, since these do not have to be removed with each nappy change.

Frejka pillow (Fig. 13.5)

This consists of a moulded piece of firm rubber or felt, covered with waterproof material. The pillow is enclosed in a jacket into which the child is fitted, the pillow fitting between the legs, holding them in abduction and flexion to 90°. The pillow itself extends from the lumbar spine posteriorly to the umbilicus anteriorly. This splint is an alternative to double nappies and may be prescribed for a small infant with unstable or subluxated hips.

Von Rosen splint (Fig. 13.6)

This splint also holds the baby's legs in flexion and abduction to 90°, and is used particularly for the young infant with either dislocation or instability of the hip. It allows movement in a small range at the hip, with the joint always returning to the required position. The parents are taught to care for the baby's skin under the splint, making sure there are no pressure areas.

Abduction splints (including plaster splints in the Lorenz position of 90° abduction) have been associated with a small incidence of damage to the capital femoral epiphysis leading to avascular necrosis. Severe forms of avascular necrosis can cause permanent damage to the hip.

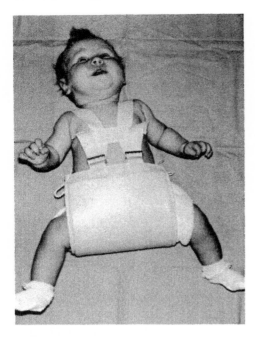

Figure 13.5 Frejka pillow. (Courtesy of W. Cumming.)

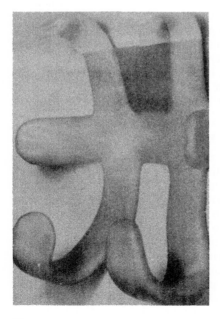

Figure 13.6 Von Rosen splint. (Courtesy of W. Cumming.)

Denis Browne hip harness

This splint also holds the hips in flexion and abduction, and permits a small amount of movement at the hips. The splint permits full rotation but limits limb flexion and extension, abduction and adduction to a range of approximately 30° in each direction from the modified Lorenz position (50° abduction and more than 90° flexion). The splint cannot be removed without the surgeon's knowledge. The harness allows crawling and walking. Both the Denis Browne and the Pavlek harnesses, by allowing movement, encourage the development of the articular cartilage and muscle.

Pavlek harness (Fig. 13.7)

This webbing harness also holds the hips in flexion and abduction, and allows the child to crawl about.

If the infant is older than 6–9 months, traction, closed reduction and sometimes tenotomy of adductor muscles may be the treatment of choice. Closed reduction under general anaesthesia is usually followed by the application of a hip spica with the hips abducted 40–50° and flexed above 90°.

Plaster hip spica

This is usually applied under anaesthesia and may be preceded by 2–3 weeks in traction in order that shortened soft tissues around the hip may be stretched, and to enable the hip to be replaced within the acetabulum by a closed reduction.

Parents are taught correct lifting techniques for their own protection, as the weight of child plus plaster may be considerable. The child may also move about with the aid of a trolley on castors. Carpenter (1970) describes some suitable equipment.

Precautions

The child is put on a plaster chart in the ward and circulation is checked at regular intervals for the first 24 hours and then rechecked at 24-hour intervals. If the plaster inhibits respiration by being too tight or too high around the thorax, it must be cut down a little to relieve the pressure.

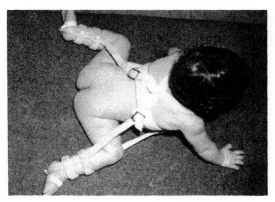

Figure 13.7 Pavlek harness. (Courtesy of W. Cumming.)

Plaster splinting may be followed by a period in a Denis Browne hip harness, for example. If conservative measures such as those outlined above are unsuccessful, surgery may be necessary to realign the angle of weight-bearing or to reconstruct the superior aspect of the acetabulum. Surgery is described by Lloyd-Roberts and Fixsen (1990).

Physical treatment

Infants and children will usually need physiotherapy following a period of immobilization. Small children do not, however, suffer the stiffness and lack of function that follow long periods of splinting in adults. Motor problems to be addressed usually include diminished range of motion in lower-limb joints due to soft tissue shortening, and decreased muscle strength due to disuse. As splinting involves both legs, motor problems will not just involve the affected leg. During splinting and casting, muscles will become weak at lengths other than those at which they were immobilized (for example, the hip and knee extensors could be expected to be weak at their shorter lengths, that is in the inner range of hip or knee extension). Muscles will also be weaker in performing actions which involve supporting, moving and balancing the body mass with the feet as the fixed base of support (for example, stair-climbing, walking, standing up). A child may, in addition, be fearful of moving following a period spent in a hip spica cast. In this latter case, exercises can be given in a warm pool, involving weight-bearing through the feet (walking, jump-

ing), kicking on a body board and swimming. Exercises out of the pool should be specific to the particular muscle activation patterns to be trained. The knee extensors, for example, will need to be strengthened in the mid to inner range of knee extension, preferably with the foot on the floor and as part of practice of functional actions. Indeed, most exercises should emphasize weight-bearing through the feet as it is the muscle activation patterns associated with this type of activity which will not have been practised for some time, if they ever have. Care should be taken that exercise is not so vigorous that a strain is put on the reduced hip.

Gait training can be commenced when the child can stand with the lower limbs in relatively normal alignment. If assistance is needed at first, crutches are probably preferable to walking frames as they allow a more normal extent of hip extension. A slow-moving treadmill can be an interesting way of practising walking for an older child and has the advantage of promoting hip extension and improving endurance.

Summary

The physiotherapist should be able to test for hip dislocation whenever suspicious signs are noted, such as apparent shortening in one leg or limited abduction at the hip, in babies being treated for other conditions. The place of physical treatment in the management of subluxation or dislocation lies in the application of splinting, in the explanation of care to the baby's parents, and in the provision of a specific exercise and motor training programme.

References

Behrman, R.E. and Vaughan, V.C. (1987) *Nelson Textbook of Pediatrics*, 13th edn. Philadelphia, PA: W.B. Saunders.
Carpenter, E.M. (1970) Equipment for children in plaster. *Occup. Ther.*, **35**, 10.
Catford, J.C., Bennet, G.C. and Wilkinson, J.A. (1982) Congenital hip dislocation: an increasing and still uncontrolled disability? *Br. Med. J.*, **285**, 1527–1530.
Lloyd-Roberts, G.C. and Fixsen, J.A. (1990) *Orthopaedics in Infancy and Childhood*, 2nd edn. Oxford: Butterworth-Heinemann.
Rose, G.K. (1986) *Orthotics: Principles and Practice*. Oxford: Butterworth-Heinemann.
Sharrard, W.J.W. (1971) *Paediatric Orthopaedics and Fractures*. Oxford: Blackwell.

Further reading

Somerville, E.W. (1982) *Displacement of the Hip in Childhood*. New York: Springer-Verlag.

Tachdjian, M.O. (1982) *Congenital Dislocation of the Hip*. New York: Churchill Livingstone.

Wilkinson, J.A. (1985) *Congenital Displacement of the Hip Joint*. New York: Springer-Verlag.

14

Arthrogryposis multiplex congenita

Description

Arthrogryposis is a heterogeneous group of congenital disorders. It is non-progressive. The infant is born with multiple deformities, joint stiffness and soft tissue contractures. The pattern will vary from child to child, but all four extremities may be involved with talipes equinovarus, flexed or extended knees, dislocated hips, flexed hips either abducted or adducted, clubbed and clawed hands, flexed or extended elbows and adducted shoulders. The joints are held rigidly in these positions. This is a non-progressive disorder, but the degree of deformity is frequently very severe. The affected limbs appear cylindrical and featureless, with loss of normal contours. There may be dimpling near the joints. The joints appear at first sight to be involved; however, there is no bony ankylosis. The joint rigidity is extra-articular, resulting from short muscles and capsular contracture. There are thickened inelastic joint capsules (Walton 1969). Atrophic muscle fibres with fibrosis and fatty infiltration have been noted at autopsy (Behrman and Vaughan 1987). The deformities appear to be due to the poor development of muscles, to their replacement by fibrous tissue, or to muscle imbalance *in utero*.

Aetiology

This is a relatively uncommon disorder. Its aetiology is unknown. Muscle biopsy is usually the most important diagnostic procedure as it allows a distinction to be made between neurogenic and myopathic processes. X-ray investigation is useful in determining the nature of deformities such as scoliosis, but there may be multiple causes. Children with congenital hypotonia and severe but non-progressive muscle weakness with histology typical of muscular dystrophy have been found to have associated arthrogryposis (Pearson and Fowler 1963). Other cases have been found at autopsy to lack anterior horn cells in spinal cord segments which correspond to the paralysed muscles. This has led to a classification in which these children with their congenital deformities are grouped under the two headings of neuropathic and myopathic arthrogryposis (Adams *et al.* 1962).

Management

Clinical management of these children is very complex due to the combination of movement disability, deformity, genetic implications, psychological problems and self-care considerations. The health care team typically involves physician, surgeon, physiotherapist, occupational therapist, social worker and psychologist. An orthotist and rehabilitation engineer may also be involved in designing seating and upper-limb adaptive equipment.

The deformities with which these children are born are extremely difficult to correct as they tend to be rigid, and maintenance of correction is difficult because of lack of muscle strength. However, if they are treated early enough with passive mobilizing and splinting, and if this is followed by mobilizing or reconstructive surgery, many children will make surprisingly good progress. Although the deformities can seem irremediably severe, it is very worthwhile for the physiotherapist to spend time in mobilizing these infants. Many of these children are intelligent and have good personalities, and with help and encouragement may accomplish far more as they grow older than would have seemed possible when they were infants.

Physical treatment

A major part of physiotherapy comprises stretching the tightened soft tissues, gentle mobilizing of joints, encouragement of active limb and trunk movements and assistance with the attaining of skill in functional actions. Progressive splinting is applied to maintain the correction gained. This regime should be pursued as intensively as possible, especially during the child's first year, but it is likely that treatment and support will be needed at least until adult life, then assistance when necessary.

The parents' help is enlisted in carrying out treatment at home. The mobilizing techniques and stretching should be done for short periods several times a day, although this should not be made too demanding of the parents' time. Care should be taken to teach them how to be gentle and effective in their treatment, and they will need encouragement to be patient, for results are slow to be gained.

Severe talipes equinovarus may be splinted with serial plaster splints applied medially, progressing as soon as possible to strapping which allows the physiotherapist and parents to mobilize the foot. Rigid splinting is avoided where possible, the emphasis being on mobility. Prone lying is encouraged as soon as practicable, to stretch the structures anterior to the hip, or to maintain hip extension after surgery to correct hip flexion deformity.

All splints and calipers should be as light and unencumbering as possible, so the child will be less likely to reject them, and will have as little extra weight to lift as possible without limiting effectiveness.

Where deformity makes it difficult to play and to explore the environment, the child may need assistance, and this part of management could be taken over by the occupational therapist. Toys may have to be altered or specially designed, self-feeding may be taught using adjusted tools, and time spent by both therapists in encouraging the child in explorative activities.

These children have a reputation for adaptability and intelligence, being capable of making the most of whatever is available to them. Despite the severity of the deformities, these attributes make it very worthwhile concentrating considerable efforts in planning and implementing interventions.

Surgical treatment

Reconstructive surgery will eventually be needed in the majority of cases, but probably not until as much movement as possible has been gained by conservative means. Capsulotomy of the structures posterior to the knee and elongation of the tendo Achilles are commonly done to release soft tissue tightness, while reconstructive surgery is often necessary to correct resistant talipes equinovarus and other limb deformities. Dislocated hips are treated by traction, adduction tenotomy, release of a tight psoas muscle and splinting, or if necessary, open reduction of the hips with iliopsoas transplant if hip extensors are non-functioning. Surgery for the upper limbs is usually not attempted until the child's future needs can be in some measure assessed, although self-feeding remains a major target, and the child with extended arms will need surgery to provide sufficient flexion to enable the hands to be taken to the mouth.

Summary

The infant with arthrogryposis demonstrates a picture of congenital abnormalities consistent with intrauterine neurological or muscular pathology. The role of the physiotherapist lies in the correction of the deformities by physical methods, frequently in conjunction with surgical correction, and in encouraging and training optimal skills in everyday actions.

References

Adams, R.D., Denny Brown, D. and Pearson, C.M. (1962) *Diseases of Muscle: A Study in Pathology*. New York: Hoeber.

Behrman, R.E. and Vaughan, V.C. (1987) *Nelson Textbook of Pediatrics*, 13th edn. Philadelphia, PA: W.B. Saunders.

Pearson, C.M. and Fowler, W.G. (1963) Hereditary non-progressive muscular dystrophy including arthrogryposis syndrome. *Brain*, **86**, 75.

Walton, J.N. (1969) *Disorders of Voluntary Muscles*. Baltimore, MD: Williams & Wilkins.

Further reading

Brown, L.M. and Sharrard, W.J.W. (1980) The pathophysiology of arthrogryposis multiplex congenita neurologica. *J. Bone Joint Surg.*, **62-B**, 291.

Drachman, D.B. and Banker, B.Q. (1961) Arthrogryposis multiplex congenita. *Arch. Neurol.*, **5**, 77.

Dubowitz, V. (1970) The myopathies. *Physiotherapy*, **56**, 4, 384.

Friedlander, H.L., Westin, G.W. and Wood, W.L. (1968) Arthrogryposis multiplex congenita. *J. Bone Joint Surg.*, **50A**, 89.

Lloyds-Roberts, G.C. and Lettin, A.W.F. (1970) Arthrogryposis multiplex congenita. *J. Bone Joint Surg.*, **52B**, 494.

Mead, N.G., Lithgow, W.C. and Sweeney, H.J. (1958) Arthrogryposis multiplex congenita. *J. Bone Joint Surg.*, **40A**, 1285.

Swinyard, R.A. (1982) Concepts of multiple congenital contracture (arthrogryposis) in man and animals. *Teratology*, **25**, 247.

Thompson, G. and Bilenker, R. (1985) Comprehensive management of arthrogryposis multiplex congenita. *Clin. Orthop. Rel. Res.*, **194**, 6–14.

15

Spina bifida

Description

Spina bifida or myelodysplasia is a congenital abnormality in which there is a developmental defect in the spinal column with incomplete closure of the vertebral canal due to a failure of fusion of the vertebral arches. There may or may not be protrusion and dysplasia of the spinal cord or its membranes.

The primary developmental defect is thought to arise in the first few weeks of gestation, due to a failure of the neural tube to close (Patten 1953; Swaiman 1989). In the third week of gestation, the neural plate normally differentiates into the neural tube which will eventually become the brain and spinal cord (Table 4.1).

Spina bifida is the commonest of the major congenital abnormalities, with a variable incidence from country to country and decade to decade, typically ranging from 1 to 4:1000 live births (Lorber 1968a; Elwood and Elwood 1980; Windham and Edmonds 1982; Swaiman 1989). Spina bifida affects the neuromusculoskeletal and genitourinary systems. Early closure of the defect together with improved methods of controlling hydrocephalus have resulted in increased survival rates. However, some children who now survive do so with severe impairments.

The aetiology is unknown but is generally considered to be multifactorial. Myelodysplasia may be caused by teratogenic agents (Janzer 1986) acting prior to the fourth gesta-tional week, when closure of the neural tube normally occurs. There appears an increased risk with subsequent births once one infant has been born with spina bifida (McKusick 1983). The presence of abnormally high levels of alpha-fetoprotein in the amniotic fluid is strong evidence of myelomeningocele and ultrasonography can detect the extent of neural tube defect (Chamberlain, 1978; Hood and Robinson, 1978; Milunsky et al. 1989).

Classification

A number of varieties of myelodysplasia have been described, from spina bifida occulta, the subtlest defect, to the complex and symptomatic myelomeningocele. It is the child with myelomeningocele who most concerns the physiotherapist. However, occasionally a child with neurological signs arising from spina bifida occulta may be referred for treatment.

Spina bifida occulta

In this defect, the vertebral arches are unfused; however, there is no herniation or displacement of neural tissue. Skin changes over the defect, pathological changes in the spinal cord, and therefore neurological signs, may or may not be present. This form is usually asymptomatic and is most common in the lower lumbar spine, involving the laminae of L5 and S1.

Table 4.1 The development of the central nervous system

	Structure	Function
Week 2	*Blastocyst* (future embryo and placenta), embedded in the uterine mucosa, begins its specific development	
Week 3	Ectoderm thickens to form *neural plate*	
	Neural plate develops *neural groove*	
	Neural crest cells form	
	Neural groove deepens → formation of *neural folds*	
Week 4	Fusion of neural folds → *neural tube*	Heart beats
	Neural tube dilates → *forebrain vesicle*	
	midbrain vesicle	
	hindbrain vesicle	
	Remainder of tube elongates → *spinal cord*	
	Neural crest cells differentiate into various sensory and autonomic ganglia	
Week 5	Forebrain and hindbrain vesicles divide	
	Their cavities form lateral, third and fourth *ventricles* and *aqueduct of Sylvius*	
	Cerebral hemispheres begin to expand	
Week 6	*Thalamus* indicated	
	Cerebellum appears	
	Cerebral commissures appear	
	Motor and sensory nuclei of *cranial nerves* IX–XII originate in medulla oblongata	
	Capillary system formed (*cerebral vascular system*)	
Week 8	*Corpus striatum* differentiates into *caudate nucleus* and *lentiform nucleus*	First reflex arc functional
	Lentiform nucleus divides into *putamen* and *globus pallidus*	Reflex responses to tactile
	Expansion of cerebral hemisphere → overlapping of mid- and hindbrain	stimulation
	Formation of *frontal, temporal* and *occipital* lobes	Irritation of upper lip →
	Spinal cord same length as vertebral column	withdrawal of head
	Development of *sense organs* progressing	Neck and trunk movement
	Meninges (pia, arachnoid, dura mater) are distinct	
	Brain has a human appearance	
Week 10	*Corpus callosum* appears and connects right and left cerebral hemispheres	Spontaneous movements
	Epithalamus, thalamus and *hypothalamus* developing from forebrain	observable and stereotyped
		Tactile stimulation of lips →
		swallowing movement
Week 12	*Vermis* and *cerebellar hemisphere* recognizable	Less stereotyped movements
	Anterior commissure develops and connects right and left cerebral hemispheres	becoming more individuated
		Movements increase in force
	Taste buds appear	Mouth opening and closing
	inner ear developing adult configuration	Chest muscles contract
Week 14	*General sense organs* (pain, temperature, deep pressure and tactile endings, chemical endings, neuromuscular spindles and neurotendinous end organs) begin to differentiate	Tactile stimulation of face → head turning, contraction of contralateral trunk muscles, trunk extension, rotation of pelvis to other side
Week 16	Characteristic folia of adult *cerebellum* gradually develop	Tongue movements
	Three small apertures (f. of *Luschka* and f. of *Magendie*) appear → *free passage* of CSF between ventricles and subarachnoid space	Abdominal muscles contract
	Cervical *spinal cord* developing *myelin*	
	Cervical and *lumbar enlargements* form	
Week 20	Main components of middle and external *ear* have assumed adult form	Effective but weak grasp
	Pacinian corpuscles appear	Protrusion and pursing of lips
	Muscle spindles in almost all muscles	Contraction of diaphragm
	Golgi endings and rudimentary *joint endings* present	Sucking
Week 24	*Myelination* in brain begins in *basal ganglia, pons, medulla, midbrain*	Temporary respirations if born
	Spinal cord extends to S1 vertebra	
	Posterior columns *myelinated*	
	Vestibulospinal, reticulospinal tracts *myelinated*	
Week 28	*Cerebral* and *cerebellar connections* myelinated	Permanent respiratory movements established on birth
	Spinocerebellar, spinothalamic tracts myelinated	Eye sensitive to light
		Maintained grasp
		Olfactory perception
Final 12 weeks	Differentiation of some *sense organs* completed	Reflex mechanisms for sucking, swallowing well-established
	Taste buds reach functional maturity	

From Carr, J.H. and Shepherd, R.B. (1980) *Physiotherapy in Disorders of the Brain*. London: Heinemann.

With *occult spinal dysraphism*, there may be spinal cord or nerve root distortion due to fibrous bands or adhesions and in these cases it is quite common for the spinal cord to be tethered. The severity of symptoms depends on the degree and extent of neural involvement. Slowly progressing weakness or sensory loss in the lower limbs, disturbances of walking, bowel or bladder dysfunction may be evident. Common associated findings include decreased Achilles tendon reflexes, shortened calf muscles, talipes equinovarus and unequal leg length (Swaiman 1989). Diagnosis is usually by magnetic resonance imaging and ultrasonography and surgical treatment may be necessary.

Spina bifida cystica

Meningocele

The vertebral arches are unfused and there is herniation of the meninges, producing a protrusion containing cerebrospinal fluid. The sac is covered by skin or membrane (Fig. 15.1). Neither myelodysplasia of the spinal cord nor neurological signs are present. Part of the cord or nerve roots may be present in the sac, but if so they conduct impulses normally.

Myelomeningocele

Myelomeningocele involves spinal cord, nerve roots and meninges, all of which may protrude through the vertebral defect. Neural tissue, itself abnormal, may be attached to the inner surface of a covering membrane or exposed on the surface (Fig. 15.2) because of complete failure of neural closure or myeloschisis. The defect can occur at any level of the neuraxis but is most common in the lumbosacral area. Durham Smith noted in 1965 that 'with the declining incidence of poliomyelitis and tuberculous bone and joint diseases, myelomeningocele now stands second only in importance to cerebral palsy as a cause of chronic locomotor disability in childhood.' The situation is probably similar today.

Pathology of myelomeningocele

Spinal cord and nerve roots

Some anterior and posterior horn cells may be recognizable histologically in the protruding neural tissue and may have connections with muscles, which can be shown by electrical stimulation. Nerve roots and posterior root ganglia are often well-formed. The spinal cord may be tethered low in the vertebral canal and the

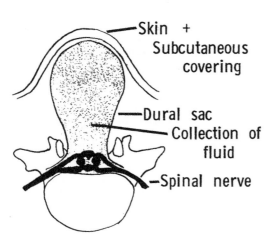

Figure 15.1 Diagram of the defect in meningocele.

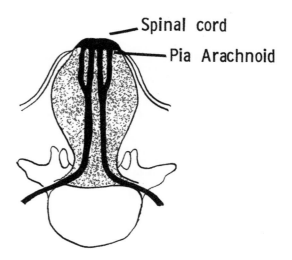

Figure 15.2 Diagram of the defect in myelomeningocele.

nerve roots will then pass laterally to their for-
amina instead of caudally.

Tethering of the cord may cause progressive
neurological deficits (e.g. hyperreflexia, muscle
weakness, decreased sensation) caused by traction on the conus medullaris and cauda equina.
Onset of clinical signs seems to be related to the
level of the lesion, age and height (Petersen
1992).

The spinal cord is abnormal in every case.
The dysplastic changes usually extend below
the level of the main myelomeningocele mass,
which means that if the mass is in the lumbar
or sacral region, the dysplasia may extend
down to the conus medullaris. If the cord is
dysplastic below the level of the main mass
there will be no anterior horn cells intact. As
the final common pathway is interrupted, there
will be no stretch reflex reaction, and hence the
lower motoneuron flaccidity usually found in
these children. However, if part of the cord is
intact below the level of the lesion there may
be some anterior horn cells intact, and the
child will show some signs of hyperreflexia.
This manifestation of an upper motoneuron
lesion will be due to the interruption of descending inhibitory and facilitatory pathways.
Hyperreflexia in these cases is usually isolated
to particular muscle groups, such as the hip
and knee flexors.

Vertebrae

Lamina growth is apparently arrested at various stages of development; some vertebrae
show a failure of laminae and spines to fuse
posteriorly, while others show a failure of the
laminae to develop at all.

Skin

The skin is rarely intact over the lesion. The
myelomeningocele mass shows itself as a raised
mass on the back, covered laterally and at its
base by normal skin, the summit of the mass
being devoid of skin (Fig. 15.3). The surface
may appear ulcerated and granulated. The
dura mater is usually fused with the edges of
the skin defect, the sac being covered by ara-
chnoid membrane only.

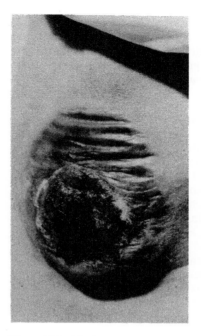

Figure 15.3 Myelomeningocele mass in newborn baby.
Note the central area devoid of skin.

Brain

Over 80% of infants born with myelomeningocele are said to have an associated hydrocephalus (Behrman and Vaughan 1987). A common
cause is the Arnold–Chiari malformation.
There are several types of malformation. In
the most common, there is displacement caudally of a tongue of cerebellar tissue comprising
the inferior part of the cerebellar vermis and
an elongated medulla oblongata, into the cervical part of the spinal canal via the foramen
magnum. The hydrocephalus may be caused
by aqueductal stenosis or by an obstruction
of the flow of cerebrospinal fluid from the
fourth ventricle into the cerebral subarachnoid space, so interfering with its absorption.
The exact cause is unknown (Gilbert *et al.*
1986). Distension of the cerebral ventricles
occurs. If the hydrocephalus is left untreated,
the ventricular distension will eventually lead
to pressure on the bones of the skull, which
become thin. The cranial sutures separate, the
anterior fontanelle enlarges and there is
marked congestion of the veins of the scalp.
However, signs of increased intracranial pressure are usually minor due to the expansibility

of the skull in infancy. In uncontrolled hydrocephalus, neurological signs become evident as the child develops, and there will almost certainly be a degree of mental as well as motor retardation as a result.

Clinical features

The type and degree of neurological and functional impairment are determined by the location and extent of the defect. The commonest site of myelomeningocele is the lumbosacral region. The clinical features evident in the infant and young child with a lumbosacral myelomeningocele are:

1 Flaccid paralysis.
2 Muscle weakness.
3 Muscle wasting.
4 Decreased or absent tendon reflexes.
5 Decreased or absent exteroceptive and proprioceptive sensation.
6 Rectal and bladder incontinence.
7 Paralytic and congenital deformities.
8 Hydrocephalus.

As well as the above features, children with lumbar or thoracic lesions may demonstrate muscle activity in isolated muscle groups due to the influence of isolated intact reflex arcs.

Eventually secondary clinical features will almost certainly develop:

1 Pressure ulceration of the skin due to absent sensation and poor skin nutrition.
2 Severe vasomotor changes.
3 Osteoporosis with probability of fractures.
4 Retarded mental, physical and emotional development due to the child's inability to move about and explore the environment, to play normally and to interrelate with other children.
5 Soft tissue contractures and eventual skeletal deformity, due to unopposed muscle action, gravity and posture.

Associated with the congenital malformation of the spine and spinal cord there may be other congenital abnormalities such as dislocated hips, talipes equinovarus, hemivertebrae with resultant scoliosis, local kyphosis due to the vertebral anomaly, hare lip, cleft palate, cardiac and urinary tract abnormalities.

The problems involved and their management

The problems involved in this complex congenital disorder are extremely wide-ranging and cannot be considered in isolation. Their management requires the cooperation of a large team of people: the child and parents, a neurosurgeon, urologist, psychologist, physiotherapist, social worker and orthopaedic surgeon. Significant progress has been made in the medical and surgical management of children with myelomeningocele and hydrocephalus.

The problems are described under the following headings:

1 The myelomeningocele mass.
2 Hydrocephalus.
3 Social and psychological factors.
4 Incontinence of bladder and bowel.
5 Deformity.
6 Absence of sensation.
7 Movement dysfunction.

The myelomeningocele mass

Surgery to repair the defect is usually performed within the first few hours of birth, usually within the first 24–48 hours. Microsurgical techniques are used that allow some anatomical reconstruction of the spinal cord and improved preservation of functional neural tissue (McLone 1980). Surgical repair is thought (Sharrard *et al.* 1967) to minimize the risk of ascending meningitis and of further damage to the spinal cord with resultant paralysis. During the surgery, as much of the neurological tissue as possible is conserved and the defect is covered with dura mater and sound skin.

Early surgical repair is considered to be appropriate for the majority of newborns with myelodysplasia (McLaughlin *et al.* 1985). Infants with high cord lesions and hydrocephalus, because of poor prognosis and poor results of treatment, may not be included in this group (Lorber 1973).

Hydrocephalus

If the hydrocephalus is uncontrolled the infant will suffer brain dysfunction and will not survive. Survival may be accompanied by severe intellectual and physical disability. Infants with Arnold–Chiari malformation are monitored carefully (Venes *et al.* 1986). Closure of the back lesion will, in infants with this malformation, result in an increase in pressure of cerebrospinal fluid within the cranium.

Treatment of hydrocephalus usually requires surgical insertion of a ventriculoperitoneal shunt which drains the cerebrospinal fluid from the lateral ventricle on a route passing down the neck, behind the clavicle and down the chest wall to the peritoneum, where the fluid is absorbed.

As the child grows, the tube is periodically replaced by a longer one. Surgery may also be necessary to revise the shunt should the tube become blocked by growing brain tissue. This blockage will cause the pressure within the cranium to rise. The clinical signs of a blocked shunt and consequent raised intracranial pressure include a high-pitched cry, irritability, seizures, downward deviation of the eyes ('sunset' eyes), bulging fontanelle, vomiting, lethargy and headache. However, by using modern radiological techniques, such as computed tomography scans, it is now known that an absence of clinical signs does not necessarily mean that hydrocephalus is arrested. Such children have been found to have dilated ventricles or compensating hydromyelia and these brain changes are thought to be the cause of the gradual loss of function in both upper and lower limbs, scoliosis and decrease in cognitive function that are noted in some children (Hall *et al.* 1979).

Even when the hydrocephalus is controlled, in some infants the weight of the enlarged head will make head control slow to develop and the child's general motor development will be correspondingly slowed. The child may sit later than usual and balance may be slower to develop. Many children show some degree of cognitive impairment despite control of their hydrocephalus. It has been reported that a major factor in influencing the intelligence of children with spina bifida is the development of hydrocephalus (Hunt and Holmes 1975; Soare and Raimondi 1977; Tew 1978). Tew and Laurence (1975) found that visuoperceptual functioning (tested using the Frostig test of visual perception) closely correlated with defects in intelligence. McLone and colleagues (1982), following a study of 167 children with myelomeningocele, found that cognitive impair-

ment appeared to be primarily related to the presence of infection (ventriculitis and/or meningitis) associated with the presence of a shunt. They pointed out the difficulty of predicting intellectual function from simple hydrocephalus and the need for early detection and treatment of infection in children with hydrocephalus.

Social and psychological factors

The parents

After the child is born the immediate problem for the parents is one of acceptance of the child, who is often the first-born. There may be feelings of resentment or guilt, or a sense of inadequacy with regard to the problems ahead. There will be an atmosphere of sorrow around the birth of the child, where the parents had expected only joy. At this time the parents are seen by the social worker and by the physician in charge of treatment, who will be able to give them some idea of what lies ahead, of the treatment required, and any other counselling that may be necessary in order to allay fear and anxiety.

Practical problems for the parents include the expense of medical and hospital care, with apparatus by no means a small consideration. There is the problem of schooling and eventual habilitation. There is the fear of having further affected children. The other children in the family may feel neglected by parents who feel the need to spend extra time with the disabled child. Parents will need advice on nutrition, since a relatively inactive child may become obese.

There is a profound stress on all those who come in contact with this child, and it is one of the responsibilities of the physiotherapist to watch for signs of mounting anxiety in the family and to refer them where they will find help. The physiotherapist, who spends so much time in the company of the child and parents, has the opportunity of developing a close relationship with them, and may allay some of the parents' anxiety, especially at the time when the child is learning to walk, by counselling patience, and by giving encouragement. An atmosphere of hopefulness should prevail at all times. Parents who have a positive attitude towards their child are more willing to develop and adopt apparatus and toys, and realize the importance of the stimulus to development which they can give the child.

Parents' associations have been formed in many countries where the abnormality is prevalent. These associations provide help, both social and economic, to their members, and most of them issue booklets or news-sheets which explain the child's problems in non-medical language, and contain helpful, practical hints (Lorber 1968b).

The child

Bowlby (1953) and others have shown that long periods of hospitalization result in deprivation of the infant and young child. This may be manifested by extreme apathy in the infant, and disturbances of behaviour in the child and adolescent (Douglas 1975; Quintern and Rutter 1976). As soon as the general condition allows, the infant should be picked up, nursed and talked to. Particular care should be taken when carrying a baby with hydrocephalus to support the head and neck, because of the enlarged head and lack of head control. The infant should not be left lying in a cot all day, with no stimulus of any kind. Colourful mobiles can be hung over the bed, close enough to be seen and reached. Even the young infant will respond to shapes made from tin foil as these move about and reflect the light. Where possible, the infant's parent is able to stay in or close to the hospital.

Those who come in contact with the young child in hospital should try to maintain links with home and parents, by talking about them, by asking questions, and by finding out from parents about favourite toys, games and pets.

When the child is discharged home it is suggested that outpatient physiotherapy is required only as often as is necessary for parents to be taught a home programme, which will change from month to month as the infant develops. As much treatment and training as possible is carried out at home. The child will need intensive physiotherapy only when starting to stand and walk, after orthopaedic surgery, or if there is severe deformity.

The child's ability to learn about the world and to develop as an individual may be impaired by difficulty in achieving actively upright (sitting, standing) positions and in the ability to move about. One has only to watch a normal child of 12 months exploring the environment to realize how deprived of experience of the world the disabled child may be if positive steps are not taken to prevent this occurring. Whether or not the child is cognitively impaired, there is probably a degree of secondary impairment due to the inability to learn in an uninhibited manner. Keeping up with other children, both mentally and physically, is one of the greatest problems. The child needs great perseverance and boldness in order to do things which come naturally to other children. Learning may be further impaired by the failure of parents to encourage independence.

Physically and mentally the child may be neglected by parents who are unable to cope with the situation, because it is after all a situation which demands a great deal from them. The child may develop pressure areas, or may be deprived of contact with other children. These problems can sometimes be anticipated by the physiotherapist and talked over with the parents and with the social worker or psychologist. In some cases the parents cannot cope with the strain of caring for their child and prefer to enrol the child in a special residential school.

During growth and development, the child has to learn to understand and to come to terms with disability, according to his or her gradually broadening horizons, and there will be certain times when encouragement and support are more particularly needed. The physician, or another individual with a similar disability, or some other suitable person from the team, should set aside time for talking to the child at different stages, particularly approaching adolescence. The child will know that there is someone of whom questions can be asked about the future, about sexual function, the possibility of marriage and family life, and other questions about which there may be a need to talk.

These children often have what Durham Smith (1965) called a brittle mental capacity, tending to be less adaptable to stresses and strains than other children. They often lack confidence, tend to be emotionally immature and to become dependent. A study comparing 20 adolescents with myelodysplasia with a control group (Hayden *et al.* 1979) found that the areas of most concern were self-esteem and social/sexual adjustment. They suggested that decreased opportunity for interaction and competition with peers, unreliable bowel and bladder function and a tendency for the disabled children to be given fewer household responsibilities may be obstacles to emotional growth.

From early infancy parents are encouraged to handle the infant as they would a normal child. It has been found to be easier to teach a child to walk at 18 months than to wait until the child is 4 or 5 years old and has lost the urge to walk which is so strong in the baby's second year. With children who are incapable of moving around by themselves, curiosity should be aroused, and games played which teach simple spatial concepts such as being 'under' a table or 'in' a box. A padded board fitted with castors (Fig. 15.4) enables the child to propel himself along the floor using the arms. The Chailey chariot (Fig. 15.5), or the Shasbah trolley which was adapted from it, were designed to enable children to move about by themselves in the sitting position.

Although the chariot is a useful way of enabling the child to get about, it has one serious disadvantage. The child who spends a large part of the day in the sitting position, with knees extended, quickly develops contracture of iliopsoas, rectus femoris and hip adductor muscles. Some degree of hip flexor contracture may be impossible to prevent. Nevertheless, the child who uses a chariot should have the day carefully planned to include activities to counteract this tendency.

The child should be given the experience of moving through space and of falling, all with as little fear as possible. The child can be placed, for example, on top of a large ball, in sitting or in lying, with movement of the ball to stimulate the need to respond to support surface perturbations and provide the pleasure of rough-and-tumble activity. Confidence-building activities like ball games, swimming, horse-riding and camping expeditions (Bodzioch *et al.* 1986) should be encouraged so that the child develops confidence, self-esteem and learns to deal with competition, uncertainty and fear.

If fear is to be avoided, great care must be taken during these and similar activities, because if the child is seriously frightened, it will take much time and patience to restore confidence.

Incontinence of bladder and bowel

The bladder is normally innervated from the sacral segments of the cord, therefore it is commonly paralysed in children with spina bifida, particularly if the lesion is lumbosacral. These children suffer from overflow incontinence,

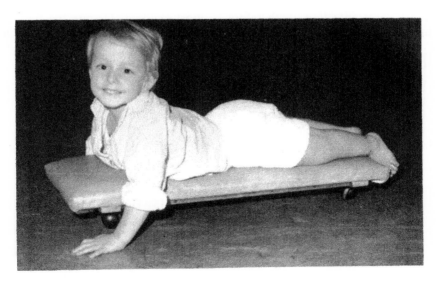

Figure 15.4 Using a prone scooter can encourage active head, trunk and hip extension and enables a non-ambulant child to be mobile.

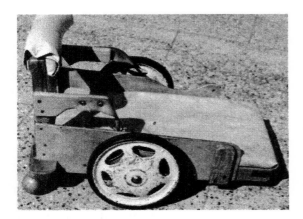

Figure 15.5 The Chailey chariot. Another means of gaining mobility for the non-ambulant child. (Courtesy of Chailey Heritage, Sussex, England.)

which means that the bladder never completely empties; urine dribbles from it as it becomes full. The child does not have any sensation of fullness as there is no sensory feedback from the denervated bladder.

Although boys may be fitted with external collecting devices, many children now have an ileocutaneous ureterostomy or ileal loop diversion operation, afterwards wearing a bag in which urine is collected. This surgery (Fig. 15.6) involves the diversion of urine direct from the ureters, via a piece of ileum, to the skin, thereby bypassing the bladder. A primary cause of urinary tract infection is therefore avoided as urine can no longer be retained in

the flaccid bladder, leading to infection which may track back to the kidneys. Retention of urine in a paralysed bladder contributes to urinary tract infection and this is considered to be the greatest threat to the child's life after hydrocephalus has been controlled.

Surgical urinary diversion procedures are only carried out where conservative methods have failed. There are several conservative measures used. *External manual pressure* to the lower abdomen may be applied in a downwards and backwards direction to assist bladder drainage. This is done by a parent whenever the nappy is changed. Older children can be taught to do the drainage themselves. This method reduces residual urine. *Intermittent catheterization* involves the insertion of a catheter through the urethra into the bladder. Complete emptying of the bladder can in this way be achieved at regular intervals (every 2–4 hours).

If the child has had a urinary diversion operation the collecting bag is held in place by a belt. Unfortunately this belt is sometimes a cause of pressure areas around the waist, especially in hot climates, but these may be prevented by lining the belt with lambswool. The child is taught to care for and empty the urinary apparatus when old enough. Once the apparatus is fitting correctly or a routine of intermittent catheterization or manual expression is established, there is no reason why the child should not be allowed to go swimming.

Bowel-training presents few problems with most children. Despite the flaccid bowel, with perseverance on the part of parents, the child

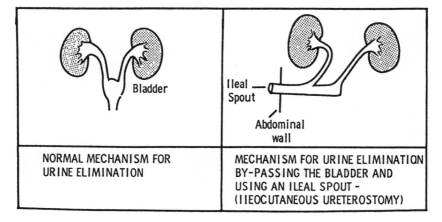

Figure 15.6 Diagram of an ileocutaneous ureterostomy showing the means by which urine is diverted directly from the kidneys via an ileal conduit, thus bypassing the bladder.

will usually manage a regular bowel evacuation. Diet may need to be regulated to prevent either constipation or loose stools, and many children need to take an aperient regularly. A few children are difficult to train. A child may appear to have loose stools, but this may be caused by chronic constipation, and should therefore be corrected by an aperient rather than by an anti-dysenteric. Sometimes the failure in bowel-training can be due to the rush of the early morning, as the parent tries to get the family fed and off to work and school, as well as trying to find time to toilet-train the disabled child. In these cases it can be suggested that there is no reason why the child's bowel action should take place in the morning, and the child should be trained in the evening instead, when there may be more time.

Some follow-up studies of children having intermittent catheterization, bowel-training and dietary planning have shown a pattern of delayed independence that suggests that psychosocial factors may be more significant limiting factors to independence than physical disability (Okamoto *et al.* 1984; Shurtleff and Mayo 1986).

Deformity

Deformities in these children are common, difficult to treat and may be so severe as to hold back the child's developmental progress. Secondary deformities, arising from prolonged positioning or muscle imbalances may not be as severe as congenital deformities unless they are left untreated for a long period of time. Once a deformity has become established, it may progress, eventually becoming fixed as the child grows. One of the most severe deformities in a large number of infants is the kyphosis noticed from birth in the region of the spina bifida. It is progressive as the child grows, with a compensatory lordosis developing above the kyphosis. The erector spinae, because of their relatively anterior position, act as flexors and add a further deforming force.

A true congenital dislocation of the hip may be seen in these children as in otherwise normal children. An arthrogrypotic type of fixed talipes equinovarus deformity is also seen in some children with myelomeningocele and is very resistant to conservative treatment. Figure 15.7 shows a list of acquired deformities and their possible causative factors.

It seems that a number of the deformities mentioned could be prevented by intensive care from the child's birth onwards. The infant may be born with certain deformities due to muscle imbalance, such as talipes equinovarus, but there is no need for these to become worse, and indeed they should begin to improve from the day treatment starts. Deformities due to unopposed muscle action and posture which will develop as the child develops and moves about can very often be prevented by conservative means in infancy, followed by surgery to correct the imbalance when the child is old enough.

A modified muscle chart is done soon after the baby's birth (for e.g., see Fig. 15.8; see also McDonald *et al.* 1986; Umphred 1985; Garber 1991) from which can be established any potential deformities which may occur due to the baby's particular distribution of paralysis. From then on, prevention is a matter of foresight and care.

Parents are taught how to give the baby daily treatment, consisting of passive muscle lengthening (see Chapter 11), stimulation of active corrective movements and the application and care of light plaster splints where these are necessary to prevent deformity due to unopposed muscle action. A small cradle or a pillow at the end of the bed will prevent the bedclothes pushing a flail or calcaneus foot into equinus. When the baby's parent is taught how to do passive movements, care must be taken to teach the normal range of movement in order that enthusiastic stretching does not damage the soft tissues around a joint.

Where there is already established deformity, treatment is instituted as soon after birth as the baby's general condition allows. In the case of talipes equinovarus and calcaneovalgus, treatment is as described in Chapters 11 and 12, although extra care will need to be exercised because of the poorly nourished skin and the lack of sensation. All plaster splints must be lined with orthopaedic felt or plastic foam, and particular attention is paid to skin under strapping should this be applied for an equinovarus deformity.

Where there is unopposed toe flexor activity, the toes will develop flexion deformities if they are not moved through a full range passively each day. All babies in the first few weeks

Feet.	
Weakness or paralysis of gastrocnemius and soleus with active anterior tibial muscles.	→ Calcaneo-valgus or calcaneo-varus deformity.
Weakness or paralysis of anterior tibial muscles and evertors.	→ Equinovarus deformity.
Unopposed lumbrical action.	→ Flexion deformity of metatarso-phalangeal joints.
Total lower limb paralysis + pressure of bedclothes + gravity.	→ Equinus deformity with flexion at the metatarso-phalangeal joints and tarso-metatarsal joints.
Uncorrected calcaneus deformity + pressure of bedclothes + gravity.	→ Flexion deformity of fore-foot.

Knees.	
Unopposed sartorius action leading to a lower limb posture of flexion, abduction and external rotation.	→ Flexion deformity.
Unopposed hip flexion and adduction.	→ Flexion deformity.
Unopposed quadriceps action.	→ Hyperextension deformity.

Hips.	
Total lower limb paralysis + lower limb posture of flexion, abduction and external rotation.	→ Flexion, abduction, external rotation deformity.
Unopposed flexion and adduction.	→ Dislocation of hip and flexion/adduction deformity

Spine.	
Hip flexor contracture.	→ Lordosis.
Imbalance of spinal muscul-ature.	→ Scoliosis

Figure 15.7   The deformities which may occur and their possible causes.

ASSESSMENT CHART FOR SPINA BIFIDA CYSTICA

Date: ....

Name: ....   Date of Birth:..............

Address: ....

Approximate level of lesion: ....

Muscle Power:

Left		Right
	Abdominals	
	Erector Spinae	
	Hip flexors	
	Hip extensors	
	Hip adductors	
	Hip abductors	
	Hamstrings	
	Quadriceps	
	Foot dorsiflexors	
	Foot plantarflexors	
	Foot invertors	
	Foot evertors	
	Toe extensors	
	Toe flexors	

Sensation:
(Tested by pinprick)

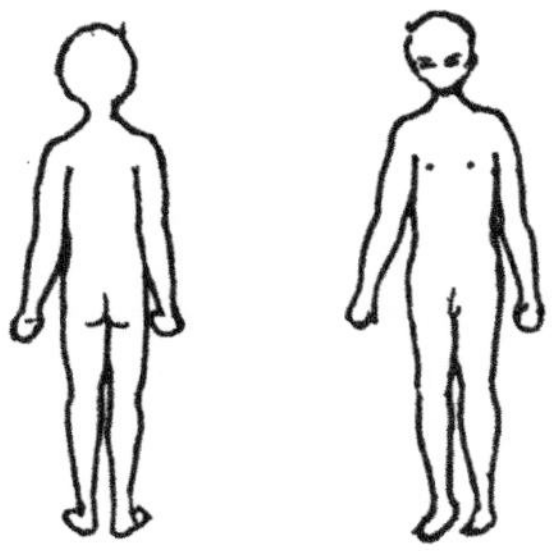

Contractures
and
Deformities: ....
....

Figure 15.8 Assessment chart for spina bifida cystica.

after birth hold their hips in flexion, and it is not until they are several weeks old that their hips can be fully extended. Perhaps because of this, in the child with inactive hip extensors, it can escape notice that the hips are becoming more flexed. Particular attention is paid to the hip flexors and adductors in the early stages to prevent, as far as possible, contracture of these muscles, and to encourage as much hip mobility as possible. The prone position is useful for encouraging more extension in the hip, and the baby can be placed in this position for periods during the day.

Dislocation of the hip may be a congenital deformity or occur as a secondary deformity due to unopposed hip flexor and adductor activity. Where the treatment regime is conservative, the child is subjected, often unsuccessfully, to long periods of recumbency and splinting, with possible effects of pressure ulceration, maternal deprivation, and slowed physical and mental development. Dislocated hips in these children may be reduced successfully, but maintenance of reduction is difficult and frequently impossible because of the continuing threat to hip stability posed by unopposed flexion and adduction, and by total paralysis of the lower limbs. The alternative is operative intervention, and an iliopsoas transplant operation, such as the one devised by Sharrard (1969) may be performed. This surgery involves the transplanting of the iliopsoas muscle through the ilium to the greater trochanter, resulting in greater hip stability. The period of fixation in a plaster hip spica is followed by physiotherapy to mobilize the lower limbs, to encourage balance in standing and to develop the child's ability to walk. Follow-up studies indicate that iliopsoas transfer surgery is likely to be more effective if done to children with relatively normal quadriceps activation and a good potential for ambulation (Menelaus 1980b). In other children, soft tissue release (including iliopsoas and adductor muscles) or femoral osteotomy is used when there is hip flexion deformity. Unfortunately it is difficult for some children to recover mobility after the immobilization that frequently follows surgery (Findley *et al.* 1987).

If the hips are not reduced and if they remain unstable, walking is difficult, the child may develop further flexion contractures at the hips and a marked lumbar lordosis. Strain is transmitted to the lumbar spine, and even if the child does learn to walk, the effort may prove too much, and he or she may prefer a wheelchair.

Scoliosis may require surgical correction and stabilization with anterior and/or posterior spinal fusion with instrumentation (Ward *et al.* 1989). Such surgery also requires a period of immobilization.

Plaster or thermoplastic splints

Light padded splints are worn at night by a baby who may be expected to develop contractures due either to unopposed muscle action or to complete paralysis of muscles around a joint combined with the effect of gravity. They are also worn by a baby who has already acquired contractures, in order to stretch the soft tissues. They may be applied anterolaterally to correct a calcaneovalgus foot, or posteriorly to hold a foot in a plantigrade position. In this latter splint, the sole of the splint must be flat and straight to prevent the foot developing a rocker shape, and the medial border should also be straight to prevent the great toe from abducting away from the midline of the foot. The feet and legs are left free for a part of the day to allow as much movement as possible to occur.

Sharrard (1979) suggests that night splinting is of little use in correcting or preventing deformity where unopposed muscle action is present. However, if splinting is worn also during part of the day, and if it is combined with passive movements, it is the experience of some clinicians that acquired deformities of the feet occur with less severity than if the foot were left free. Similarly, although splinting will not necessarily gain full correction of a congenital foot deformity, nor will it indefinitely maintain correction where muscle imbalance exists, it will bring about improvement in the position of the foot and maintain this improvement until surgery can be performed. It is probably critical that infants and small children wear the appropriate orthoses whenever they are supported in   standing. Details of the surgery performed for correction of deformity may be found in Menelaus (1980a) and Sharrard (1979).

Absence of sensation

Sensory loss does not always correspond with motor loss and is difficult to assess accurately. Absence of sensation, both exteroceptive and somatosensory, results in two major problems:

1 Risk of injury to soft tissues through the inability to feel pain, pressure and temperature.
2 Loss of information and feedback normally gained through the various sense organs.

The skin is prone to pressure areas and ulceration due to anaesthesia, excessive pressure from orthoses or support surfaces, and faecal and urinary soiling, and is a source of considerable morbidity (Menelaus 1980a; Okamoto *et al.* 1983). The areas most affected are the bony prominences of the feet and spine. An early sign of prolonged pressure is redness of the skin.

Once the child starts to move about on the floor, the malleoli and the dorsum of the feet and toes become prone to friction burns and ulceration. Ill-fitting plaster splints, boots or calipers may cause pressure areas. Careless fitting of a boot may result in a great toe being flexed within the boot, and the child may walk around for some time without complaining of pain. Soft tissues of the lower limbs and the bones themselves may be injured or broken because the child is unaware of the position of the limbs. Warmth and swelling of a leg may be the only indication of a fracture.

Splints are lined with orthopaedic felt or plastic foam material. When the child is ready to stand, a pair of lambswool-lined boots which open and lace up from the toes are fitted. Ordinary boots are too difficult to fit correctly on an anaesthetic foot.

The child's poor or absent somato-sensation makes learning to move about in sitting and standing difficult. The child may not know where the lower limbs are in space without looking, and will have to be taught to note the position of the feet when learning to stand and walk.

Normally an infant will investigate and discover the various parts of the body by exploration. By 5 months the infant will play with the feet when in supine. The myelomeningocele infant will have to be helped to play with the feet when there is no somatosensory feedback from the lower limbs.

Problems resulting from lack of sensation are added to by the poor circulation found in paraplegic children. The normal pumping action of the muscles being poor or non-existent, circulation in the lower limbs may be very deficient. Should ulceration occur, the skin will heal slowly and may need a graft to restore its integrity. In some cases infection occurs and in extreme cases may necessitate amputation (Sharrard 1979). In the cold weather these children suffer chilblains and trophic changes in the skin because of the sluggish circulation, and again ulceration may result.

Parents are warned of the difficulties involved in skin healing and advised to check the skin carefully as a routine each day. When the child is able, he or she will take over this task, which is probably not possible until at least the age of 7 years. In the winter the child is dressed in warm clothes of wool or cotton; many synthetic materials are unsuitable as they may cause friction on the skin. Leggings, trousers or warm stockings may be worn, and when the weather becomes very cold, leggings may be made of quilted material. The child must be kept clear of hot water bottles, radiators and fires because of the lack of temperature sensation.

Movement dysfunction

Lloyd-Roberts and Fixsen (1990) have suggested the following system of grading of the paralysis:

Group 1: Flaccid paralysis of the lower limbs. The level of the lesion is from T12 to L1 downwards. There are typically no active deforming forces in the lower limbs.
Group 2: Hip flexion and adduction are present, and knee extension to some extent. All other muscles in the lower limbs are paralysed. The level of the lesion extends from L4 downwards. Hip deformity and dislocation are likely to occur.
Group 3: The paralysis is principally below the knee. The level of the lesion extends from S1 downwards.

The Denver Developmental Screening Test (Frankenburg *et al.* 1970) can be used until the age of 6 and the Bayley Scale of Infant Development Mental Scale (Bayley 1969) is also suggested. However, of future value will be the use of biomechanical tests that measure, for example, postural adjustments in sitting and standing (in terms of both stability and ability to move about), reaching and grasping, aided gait, and the use of physiological tests that provide information about the physical work involved in various aided gaits. Standardized videotapes allow a record to be kept of a child's performance on critical motor actions (e.g. sit-to-stand, walking, wheelchair activities). A checklist of critical biomechanical features derived from studies of normal subjects (see Chapter 3; Carr and Shepherd 1987) can provide guidance in motor training.

There are as yet few biomechanical studies which have investigated adaptive motor performance in children or adults with different levels of spinal cord lesion. Such studies would provide information which could lead to the development of training methods designed to optimize performance in children with spina bifida. In one study of adults with paraplegia resulting from a complete lesion below T3 (Seelen and Vuurman 1991), it was found that when subjects reached out in the sitting position, latissimus dorsi and trapezius muscles appeared to be active in stabilizing the sitting position. This muscle activity can be taken to signify compensatory (adaptive) muscle activity since it occurred when body movement was registered by seat force transducers. As would be expected, given the difficulty with making preparatory postural adjustments, reaction time was slower in these individuals than normal. Further investigations of effective adaptive motor behaviours in paraplegic children will provide information of value in promoting the learning of effective functional compensations.

As has been noted, the child's development is hindered by the time that may be spent in hospital undergoing surgery for the myelomeningocele mass, hydrocephalus, urinary tract incontinence and dislocated hips. In the first few months of life, the child may spend several periods in hospital, and even with care on the part of staff, there will be times when there will be little freedom to move about. All these factors may result in a degree of motor retardation, quite apart from the motor disability which results from muscle paralysis and imbalance. Soare and Raimondi (1977), following their study of 173 children with spina bifida, pointed out that all the children scored lower than their siblings on perceptuomotor functions. The authors suggested that this may be due to the decreased stimulation associated with prolonged hospital stay, decreased opportunity for exploration or primary brain damage.

However, upper limb and cognitive–perceptual deficits may also be due to central nervous system dysfunction (Tew and Laurence 1975; Anderson and Plewis 1977; Brunt 1980; Mazur et al. 1986). Visuomotor dysfunction, including visual tracking disturbances (Lennerstrand and Gallo 1990; Lennerstrand et al. 1990) also affect the attainment of manual motor skills, reading, writing, and may also affect the development of balance.

The child may be slow to develop head and upper body control, particularly if there is hydrocephalus. However, control will develop more quickly if the infant is picked up, carried about and nursed, than if left lying in a cot. It is interesting to note that African babies whose mothers carry them about all day on their backs seem to develop head control more quickly than western babies who are wheeled about in prams (see Chapter 2). The myelomeningocele baby, partly because of long stays in hospital, partly because of being more awkward to handle, may lack the stimulus of being picked up and carried.

The child will be slow to develop balance in sitting if head control is poor and if a neck collar to assist head support is not provided. The child will also be slow to develop task- and context-specific postural adjustments because the paralysis of lower-limb muscles limits the effectiveness of postural adjustments in sitting which require support from feet and/or thighs. The child will have to learn to use arms and trunk as well as the active leg muscles in order to balance.

Children normally pull themselves to standing independently at around 9 months, although parents assist and support standing much earlier than this, and walking begins at approximately 13 months. At this stage of development the urge to stand and walk is very strong. Many disabled children, however, lack not only the physical ability to initiate these functions themselves but also lack the incentive or the drive to do so. It is probably essential that the child is helped to practise sitting, standing and walking as early as possible. If standing and walking are left until later, the child may have become accustomed to being mobile with relative ease in a chariot or mobile chair and will have developed fears and anxieties which make it difficult to encourage standing and walking. It is also important for standing to be instituted early in order to minimize muscle and bone atrophy (Curtis 1972).

In the infant, muscle activity is encouraged in several ways, by putting the infant in positions which encourage movement. Exercises are given to strengthen the innervated lower limb muscles, particularly the extensors, and the muscles of the upper limb. Upper-limb extensor muscles need to be strong enough to provide weight-bearing pressure while walking with aids. In the absence of muscle power, extension at the hips and knees and a plantigrade foot position must be obtained and maintained by passive movement, surgery and splinting. In training the development of postural adjustments, it may be necessary to teach the child to use the upper body and arms for making adjustments to movements of the body mass if leg muscles cannot be activated.

Lying in prone over a foam wedge (Fig. 5.15) or over the therapist's knee (Fig. 5.11) will develop strength and control of the head, trunk and, if active, hip extensors. In addition, the child will learn to weight-bear on the hands while reaching out to play with toys. Crawling or the maintenance of four-point kneeling is encouraged by the use of a crawler or with a towel held under the baby's abdomen for support. The legs must be well-protected by long pants and socks in order to avoid friction burns. It may be preferable to replace training of crawling with additional training in standing and sitting, where there is little likelihood of the infant being able to crawl independently.

As soon as possible, emphasis is placed on strengthening the arms in preparation for walking with apparatus. The child may be wheel-barrowed when old enough and strong enough to take body weight through the arms, but the physiotherapist must hold the thighs rather than the lower legs or feet in order not to put unnecessary strain on possibly osteoporotic bones. In sitting, the child learns to push down on the hands in order to lift up from the floor, but small wooden blocks may be needed under the hands if arms are too short to afford much movement.

Supine lying should be avoided for any longer than necessary. In sitting, the infant will be able to develop an interest in surroundings, which is not possible when lying looking up at a ceiling or at a blank wall. As soon as possible, the infant is sat up against pillows in a corner of the sofa or an inclined chair. When old enough, the child can move around sitting in a Chailey chariot. Periods of sitting are alternated with periods spent supported in standing, with short periods in prone or on a prone scooter, as prolonged sitting will increase the tendency towards flexion contractures at the hips and knees.

When the child is ready to stand independently, and this should be some time before 12 months of age, apparatus may need to be provided which will give support and confidence and allow play. A standing table will be useful at home. By shifting the body mass about during play, some balancing ability will be developed. Some form of splinting for the legs to correct deformity will probable be necessary for many infants before they will be able to stand.

Orthoses

The type of orthosis prescribed is influenced by the child's level of motor function. The stage at which an orthosis for promoting standing is prescribed should probably be as early as possible. It has been suggested that this should be correlated with the time at which children normally stand and walk (Drennan 1976) and when the child demonstrates interest in being upright (Carroll 1974). However, infants normally experience supported standing earlier than 9 months and interest in standing may be best aroused by giving early experience of standing. Fitting expensive orthoses to infants may be unrealistic. However, experience of supported standing with wraparounds to support the knees (see Fig. 8.5) and with the infant wearing the appropriate foot orthoses to ensure an appropriate weight-bearing surface, may be critical factors in optimizing the infant's visual and motor development.

Several types of orthosis are in common use. *Moulded foot orthoses* are aimed to prevent pronation of the foot by holding the calcaneus in an optimal position. *Anterior floor-reaction ankle–foot orthoses* (AFO) are recommended for children who stand with knees flexed, this position being attributed to elongated Achilles tendon. This type of AFO consists of an anterior shell, in contrast to the posterior shell typical of the usual AFO. In addition, knee–ankle–foot orthoses and various types of parapodium with either one lock for both hip and knee (Toronto parapodium) or separate hip and knee locks (Rochester parapodium; Motlock 1971; Kinnen *et al.* 1984) are commonly prescribed.

Orthotic use can be evaluated in terms of walking speed, heart rate and oxygen consumption, and these measures can be used to give an indication of the best orthosis for a particular child at a particular stage (Yngve *et al.* 1984; Flandry *et al.* 1986). In addition, the child's apparatus is checked for fit and length periodically, as ill-fitting apparatus can cause deformity and pressure ulceration. Effectiveness of apparatus is also checked, since 'braces should be used to enlarge not limit a child's horizon' (Ferguson 1968).

Deciding on the apparatus necessary for a particular child at this stage is very difficult and cannot be decided merely upon knowledge of the grade of paralysis. It is to some extent a matter of trial and error, although Spiers (1972) suggested that it may be preferable to start with too much apparatus and gradually discard unnecessary parts as the effects of the child's disability on function become clarified. Ambulatory ability appears to be closely related to the strength of the quadriceps muscles (Schopler and Menelaus 1987) and early emphasis should be placed on exercises designed to strengthen the lower-limb extensors with supportive force through the feet. A child with some paralysis or weakness localized below the knee may manage to stand in AFOs or may be better able to manage in the beginning with knee–ankle–foot orthoses until balancing ability improves. A child with extensive paralysis may require support in a swivel walker such as a Shrewsbury splint (Fig. 15.9) or a parapodium (Fig. 15.10). This can be changed to a pelvic band jointed on to calipers

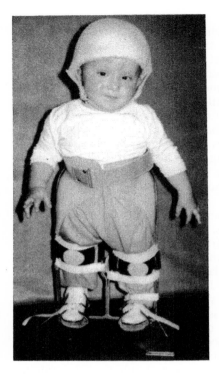

Figure 15.9 The Shrewsbury splint.

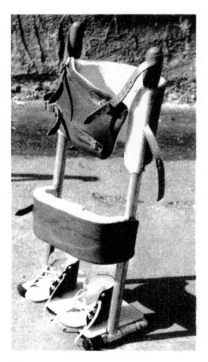

Figure 15.10 Canadian parapodium. (Courtesy of Chailey Heritage, Sussex, England.)

(Fig. 15.11) or calipers alone, or to a reciprocating gait orthosis (Fig. 15.12).

In standing the child must learn to balance by transferring weight with the upper body if there is extensive lower-limb paralysis, and the stimulus to any adjustment of balance will have to come from sensory feedback from the muscles and joints of the upper body rather than the lower limbs, as well as from visual receptors and the vestibular system. There are many activities which the physiotherapist can use for training balance and gaining confidence in standing. These may include standing with hands on the wall, moving one hand, then both hands on to differently coloured marks; pushing against the physiotherapist; standing with hands on a large ball while the physiotherapist moves the ball backwards, and forwards, from side to side; reaching in different directions for objects, both uni- and bimanually. These and other activities should emphasize the need for the paraplegic child to keep the body mass forwards, and stress the fact that falling should be forward on to the hands.

Walking should be expected of most children, even if only for part of the day. Provided deformities are corrected, and the child has suitable intelligence, and provided attempts to encourage walking are made early enough, most children with lesions below L4 should be capable of independent walking (Samuelsson and Skoog 1988). For some, those with higher lesions and many of those with scoliosis and/or

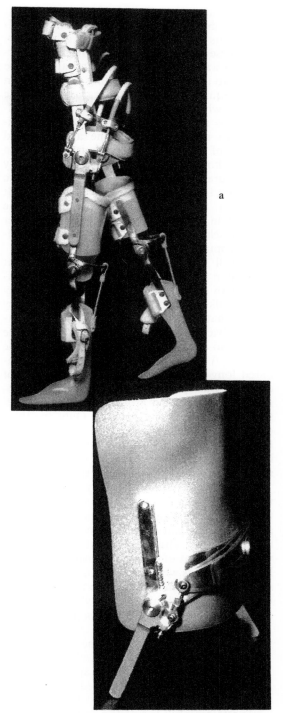

a

b

Figure 15.12 (a) Reciprocating gait orthosis. (b) Recent modification to the hip mechanism. (Courtesy of the Orthotics Department, Prince of Wales Hospital, Sydney, Australia.)

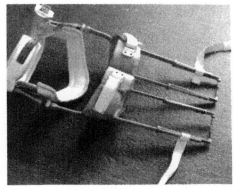

Figure 15.11 Pelvic band and calipers. (Courtesy of Chailey Heritage, Sussex, England.)

hydrocephalus, the effort may prove too great and they may eventually decide that a wheelchair offers the greatest possibility of mobility. All of these children should be given the opportunity to walk if they want to, and all must be enabled to maintain the standing position, even if this requires extensive apparatus. For those children who prefer to ambulate in a wheelchair, it is necessary to provide a chair of suitable size and type, given the age, size and abilities of the child. Wheelchair mobility in adults is known to involve considerable energy expenditure (Glaser *et al.* 1981a). It is therefore important for the child's fitness level to be built up by a task-oriented training programme directed in particular to strengthening upper limb muscles (Glaser *et al.* 1981b) and wheelchair propulsion activities.

Stillwell and Menelaus (1983) found that more than two-thirds of a group of 50 individuals with spina bifida (aged 15+) were functional walkers at the time of the review. They suggest that a combination of hip flexion deformity, pelvic obliquity and scoliosis, or any one of these to a severe degree, is likely to preclude walking. A study by Mazur *et al.* (1989) compared long-term walking ability in a group of children who participated in a walking programme with another group who had been prescribed a wheelchair early in life. Only one-third of the early walkers were still walking at ages from 12 to 20 years. However, the early walkers had experienced fewer pressure sores and were more independent than the wheelchair users.

A child with severe disability may learn to walk pushing a weighted pram, a large wooden toy on wheels, using a reverse-facing walker, in a reciprocating gait orthosis, a swivel walker or a parapodium. The child may learn better by walking in front of an adult, pushing down on his or her hands while taking a step. There is no stick or crutch which is suitable for every child with this type of disability and while some children manage well with quadripod sticks (Fig. 15.13), others may do better with crutches with a small ski tip instead of the usual ferrule.

Other children will learn to walk in a swivel walker. The advantage of this apparatus is in the ability of a severely disabled and perhaps cognitively-impaired child to be ambulant while retaining full use of the hands. The child walks by transferring weight to one plate, rotating the trunk towards that side, then transfer-

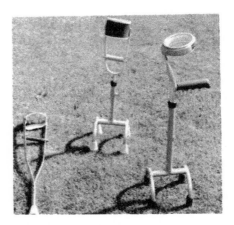

Figure 15.13 A selection of walking aids. (Courtesy of Chailey Heritage, Sussex, England.)

ring weight to the opposite plate. The plates are returned to their starting position by springs. Most children need to wear crash helmets while in their walkers, although the splint is stable under normal circumstances. This apparatus should not be considered as any but a temporary means of getting a child to stand and walk. As soon as possible the child should progress to apparatus which allows greater mobility and a more normal gait.

Most children with orthoses and crutches will learn to walk using a four-point and a swing-through gait, the latter being preferred by children who have developed the confidence to use it because of the extra speed it allows. The child should not be hurried at this stage and care must be taken to maintain confidence. The child cannot be made to walk before there is the desire to do so, but once this stage is reached, the child will need all the help and patience parents can give.

Hand function has been considered to be relatively normal in children with thoracic or lower-level lesion (Sharrard 1979), probably in comparison to the severity of the lower-limb disability. A recent study of 33 individuals aged from 4 to 17 years showed, however, that, according to the criteria used, only 2 subjects had 'normal' upper-limb function and 85% of the group had signs of cerebellar ataxia, sometimes combined with upper motoneuron lesion signs. Abnormal hand function has also been described by others (MacKenzie and Emery 1971; Grimm 1976). Problems described include difficulty with bimanual coordination, fine finger movement, manipulation of small objects requiring eye–hand coordination, 'clumsiness' and tremor.

As a result of these studies and given the particular importance of hand function to paraplegic children, the physiotherapist should specifically train reaching and manipulation, with bimanual as well as unimanual tasks, and evaluate hand function as part of the motor assessment of the child (Stott *et al.* 1972). Kinematic analysis of reaching would be an effective means of comparing performance with a normal model, since several studies have reported details of normal performance (see Chapter 3).

Sport

Swimming is a good sport for children once their incontinence has been overcome. They are taught to float, to swim, and to get in and out of the water, and as they develop proficiency can participate in races against each other. It takes some children a while to overcome their fear of the water. With paralysed lower limbs, children with myelomeningocele are quickly out of their depth in a pool. Dowrick and Dove (1980) report the successful use of self-modelling, using videotape replay, in 3 children with spina bifida learning to swim. Self-modelling is defined by the authors as a behavioural change resulting from repeated observation of oneself performing only desirable behaviours. The children viewed themselves frequently on short (usually 2-minute) videotapes. Evidence of distress and of physical support given to the child were edited out so the child saw in essence a behaviour slightly exceed-ing their own ability. Archery, wheelchair basketball, sprinting and ball games provide other outlets for their sporting aspirations.

Children with high lesions frequently lack normal respiratory movement due to spinal and thoracic deformity, weak abdominals and poor sitting posture, and may require daily breathing exercises or exercises that promote deep breathing. If the child is prone to respiratory tract infection, parents will give postural drainage at home when necessary

Summary

The overall goal of the physiotherapist for the child with spina bifida, as it is of the other members of the team, is the promotion of functional independence. For this to be a reality, the physiotherapist has several specific aims: *prevention* of adaptive deformity, of pressure ulceration, of secondary cognitive impairment, and *correction* of deformity already present at birth, *promotion of the learning of critical motor skills*, including effective postural adjustments as part of actions performed in sitting and standing, and a method of independent ambulation, *strengthening* of arm, trunk and relevant lower limb muscles, and, where necessary, *training wheelchair activities*.

Motor performance in paraplegic children can be viewed as compensatory (adaptive) and residual rather than as impaired and disabled. Taking this view should lead to a promising avenue of research, in which the most effective adaptations are determined given certain residual muscle activations. From this information, training would then be directed at promoting the learning of effective adaptive motor behaviours.

References

Anderson, E.M. and Plewis, I. (1977) Impairment of a motor skill in children with spina bifida cystica and hydrocephalus. *Br. J. Psychol.*, **68**, 61.

Bayley, N. (1969) *Manual for the Bayley Scales of Infant Development*. New York: The Psychological Corporation.

Behrman, R.E. and Vaughan, V.C. (1987) *Nelson Textbook of Pediatrics*, 13th edn. Philadelphia, PA: W.B. Saunders.

Bodzioch, J., Roach, J.W. and Schkade, J. (1986) Promoting independence in adolescent paraplegics: a 2-week 'camping' experience. *J. Pediatr. Orthop.*, **6**, 198–201.

Bowlby, J. (1953) *Child Care and the Growth of Love*. London: Penguin.

Brunt, D. (1980) Characteristics of upper limb movements in a sample of meningomyelocele children. *Percept. Motor Skills*, **51**, 431.

Carr, J.H. and Shepherd, R.B. (1987) *A Motor Relearning Programme for Stroke*, 2nd edn. Oxford: Butterworth-Heinemann.

Carroll, N. (1974) The orthotic management of the spina bifida child. *Clin. Orthop.*, **102**, 108–114.

Chamberlain, J. (1978) Human benefits and costs of a national screening programme for neural tube defects. *Lancet*, **2**, 1293.

Curtis, B.H. (1972) Principles of orthopaedic management in myelomeningocele. In: *Symposium on myelomeningocoele*. American Academy of Orthopedic Surgeons. St Louis, MO: Mosby.

Douglas, J. (1975) Early hospital admissions and later disturbances of behaviour and learning. *Dev. Med. Child Neurol.*, **17**, 426.

Dowrick, P.W. and Dove, C. (1980) The use of self-modelling to improve the swimming performance of spina bifida children. *J. Appl. Behav. Anal.*, **13**, 51–56.

Drennan, J.C. (1976) Orthotic management of the myelomeningocele spine. *Dev. Med. Child Neurol.*, **37** (suppl. 18), 97–103.

Durham Smith, E. (1965) *Spina Bifida and the Total Care of Myelomeningocele*. Illinois: Thomas.

Elwood, J.M. and Elwood, J.H. (1980) *Epidemiology of Anencephalus and Spina Bifida*. Oxford: Oxford University Press.

Ferguson, A.B. (1968) *Orthopaedic Surgery in Infancy and Childhood*. Baltimore, MD: Williams & Wilkins.

Findley, T.W., Agre, J.C., Habeck, R.V. *et al.* (1987) Ambulation in adolescents with myelomeningocele: 1. Early childhood predictors. *Arch. Phys. Med. Rehabil.*, **68**, 518–522.

Flandry, F., Burke, S., Roberts, J.M., Hall, S., Drouilhet, A., Davis, G. and Cook, S. (1986) Functional ambulation in myelodysplasia: the effect of orthotic selection on physical and physiologic performance. *J. Pediatr. Orthop.*, **6**, 661–665.

Frankenburg, W.K., Dobbs, J.B. and Fandel, A. (1970) *The Revised Denver Developmental Screening Test Manual*. Denver, CO: University of Colorado Press.

Garber, J.B. (1991) Myelodysplasia. In: *Pediatric Neurologic Physical Therapy*, edited by S.K. Campbell, 2nd edn. New York: Churchill Livingstone, pp. 169–212.

Gilbert, J.N., Jones, K.L., Rorke, L.B. *et al.* (1986) Central nervous system anomalies associated with myelomeningocele, hydrocephalus, and the Arnold-Chiari malformation: reappraisal of theories regarding the pathogenesis of posterior neural tube closure defects. *Neurosurgery*, **18**, 559.

Glaser, R.M., Sawka, M.N., Wilde, S. *et al.* (1981a) Energy cost and cardiopulmonary responses for wheelchair locomotion and walking on tile and on carpet. *Paraplegia*, **19**, 220.

Glaser, R.M., Sawka, M.N., Durbin, R.J. *et al.* (1981b) Exercise program for wheelchair activity. *Am. J. Phys. Med.*, **60**, 67.

Grimm, R.A. (1976) Hand function and tactile perception in a sample of children with myelomeningocele. *Am. J. Occup. Ther.*, **30**, 234–240.

Hall, P., Lindseth, R., Campbell, R. *et al.* (1979) Scoliosis and hydrocephalus in myelomeningocele patients: the effects of ventricular shunting. *J. Neurosurg.*, **50**, 174–178.

Hayden, P.W., Davenport, S.L.H. and Campbell, M.M. (1979) Adolescents with myelodysplasia: impact of physical disability on emotional maturation. *Pediatrics*, **64**, 1, 53–59.

Hood, V.D. and Robinson, H.P. (1978) Diagnosis of closed neural tube defects by ultrasound in second trimester of pregnancy. *Br. Med. J.*, **417**, 931.

Hunt, G.M. and Holmes, A.E. (1975) Some factors relating to intelligence in treated children with spina bifida cystica. *Dev. Med. Child Neurol.*, **17** (suppl. 35), 65.

Janzer, R.C. (1986) Neural tube defects: experimental findings and concepts of pathogenesis. In: *Spina Bifida– Neural Tube Defects*, edited by D. Voth and P. Glees. New York: Walter de Gruyte, p. 21.

Kinnen, E., Gram, M., Jackman, K.V. *et al.* (1984) Rochester parapodium. *Clin. Prosthet. Orthot.*, **8**, 4, 24–25.

Lennerstrand, G. and Gallo, J.E. (1990) Neuro-ophthalmological evaluation of patients with myelomeningocele and Chiari malformations. *Dev. Med. Child Neurol.*, **32**, 415.

Lennerstrand, G., Gallo, J.E. and Samuelsson, L. (1990) Neuro-ophthalmological findings in relation to CNS lesions in patients with myelomeningocele. *Dev. Med. Child Neurol.*, **32**, 423.

Lloyd-Roberts, G.C. and Fixsen, J.A. (1990) *Orthopaedics in Infancy and Childhood*, 2nd edn. Oxford: Butterworth-Heinemann.

Lorber, J. (1968a) The child with spina bifida. *Physiotherapy*, **54**, 11, 390.

Lorber, J. (1968b) *Your Child with Spina Bifida*. London: Association for Spina Bifida and Hydrocephalus.

Lorber, J. (1973) Early results of selective treatment of spina bifida cystica. *Br. Med. J.*, **4**, 201.

McDonald, C., Jaffe, K. and Shurtleff, D.B. (1986) Assessment of muscle strength in children with meningomyelocele: accuracy and stability of measurements over time. *Arch. Phys. Med. Rehabil.*, **67**, 855–861.

MacKenzie, N.G. and Emery, J.L. (1971) Deformities of the cervical cord in children with neurospinal dysraphism. *Dev. Med. Child Neurol.*, **13** (suppl. 25), 58–67.

McKusick, V.A. (1983) *Mendelian Inheritance in Man: Catalogs of Autosomal Dominant, Autosomal Recessive, and X-linked Phenotypes*, 6th edn. Baltimore, MD: Johns Hopkins University Press.

McLaughlin, J.F., Shurtleff, D.B., Lamers, J.Y. *et al.* (1985) Influence of prognosis on decisions regarding the care of newborns with myelodysplasia. *N. Engl. J. Med.*, **312**, 1589.

McLone, D.G. (1980) Technique for closure of myelomeningocele. *Child Brain*, **6**, 65.

McLone, D.G., Czyzewski, D., Raimondi, A.J. and Sommers, R.C. (1982) Central nervous system infections as a limiting factor in the intelligence of children with myelomeningocele. *Pediatrics*, **70**, 3, 338–342.

Mazur, J.M., Menelaus, M.B., Hudson, I. and Stillwell, A. (1986) Hand function in patients with spina bifida cystica. *J. Pediatr. Orthop.*, **6**, 442–447.

Mazur, J.M., Shurtleff, D., Menelaus, M.B. and Colliver, J. (1989) Orthopaedic management of high-level spina bifida. *J. Bone Joint Surg.*, **71-A**, 1, 56–61.

Menelaus, M.B. (1980a) *The Orthopaedic Management of Spina Bifida Cystica*, 2nd edn. Edinburgh: Livingstone.

Menelaus, M.B. (1980b) Progress in the management of the paralytic hip in myelomeningocele. *Orthop. Clin. North Am.*, **11**, 17.

Milunsky, A., Jick, S.S., Bruell, C.L. *et al.* (1989) Predictive values, relative risks, and overall benefits of high and low maternal serum alpha-fetoprotein screening in singleton pregnancies: new epidemiological data. *Am. J. Obstet. Gynecol.*, **161**, 291.

Motlock, W.M. (1971) The parapodium: an orthotic device for neuromuscular disorders. *Artificial Limbs*, **15**, 36–47.

Okamoto, G.A., Lamers, J.V. and Shurtleff, D.B. (1983) Skin breakdown in patients with myelomeningocele. *Arch. Phys. Med. Rehabil.*, **64**, 20–23.

Okamoto, G.A., Sousa, J., Telzrow, R.W. *et al.* (1984) Toileting skills in children with meningomyelocele: rates of learning. *Arch. Phys. Med. Rehabil.*, **65**, 182.

Patten, B.M. (1953) Embryological stages in the establishing of myeloschisis with spina bifida. *Am. J. Anat.*, **93**, 365.

Petersen, M.C. (1992) Tethered cord syndrome in myelodysplasia: correlation between level of lesion and height at time of presentation. *Dev. Med. Child Neurol.*, **34**, 604–610.

Quintern, D. and Rutter, M. (1976) Early hospital admissions and later disturbances of behaviour. *Dev. Med. Child Neurol.*, **18**, 447.

Samuelsson, L. and Skoog, M. (1988) Ambulation of patients with myelomeningocele: a multivariate statistical analysis. *J. Pediatr. Orthop.*, **8**, 569–575.

Schopler, S.A. and Menelaus, M.B. (1987) Significance of the strength of the quadriceps muscles in children with myelomeningocele, *J. Pediatr. Orthop.*, **7**, 507–512.

Seelen, H.A.M. and Vuurman, E.F.P.M. (1991) Compensatory muscle activity for sitting posture during upper extremity task performance in paraplegic persons. *Scand. J. Rehabil. Med.*, **23**, 89–96.

Sharrard, W.J.W. (1969) Posterior ilio-psoas transplantation. In: *Operative Surgery*, vol 8. London: Butterworth.

Sharrard, W.J.W. (1979) *Paediatric Orthopaedics and Fractures*, 2nd edn. Oxford: Blackwell Scientific Publications.

Sharrard, W.J.W., Zachary, R.B. and Lorber, J. (1967) Survival and paralysis in open myelomeningocele with special reference to the time of repair of the spinal lesion. *Dev. Med. Child Neurol. Suppl.*, **13**, 35.

Shurtleff, D. and Mayo, M. (1986) Toilet training: the Seattle experience and conclusions. In: *Myelodysplasia and Exstrophies: Significance, Prevention and Treatment*, edited by D.B. Shurtleff. Orlando, FL: Grune & Stratton, p. 267.

Soare, P.L. and Raimondi, A.J. (1977) Intellectual and perceptual-motor characteristics of treated myelomeningocele children. *Arch. Dis. Child*, **131**, 199–204.

Spiers, B.W. (1972) Personal communication.

Stillwell, A. and Menelaus, M.B. (1983) Walking ability in mature patients with spina bifida. *J. Pediatr. Orthop.*, **3**, 184–190.

Stott, D.H., Moyes, F.A. and Henderson, S.E. (1972) *Test of Motor Impairment*. Guelph: Brook International.

Swaiman, K.F. (ed) (1989) *Pediatric Neurology. Principles and Practice*. St Louis, MO: C.V. Mosby.

Tew, B. (1978) The psychological and educational consequences of spina bifida and its complications. *Dev. Med. Child Neurol.*, **20**, 240.

Tew, B. and Laurence, K.M. (1975) The effects of hydrocephalus on intelligence, visual perception and school attainment. *Dev. Med. Child Neurol.*, **17**, (suppl. 35), 129–134.

Umphred, D.A. (ed) (1985) *Neurological Rehabilitation*. St Louis, MO: C.V. Mosby.

Venes, J.L., Black, K.L. and Latack, J.T. (1986) Preoperative evaluation and surgical management of the Arnold-Chiari II malformation. *J. Neurosurg.*, **64**, 363.

Ward, W.T., Wenger, D.R. and Roach, S.W. (1989) Surgical correction of myelomeningocele scoliosis: a critical appraisal of various spinal intrumentation systems. *J. Pediatr. Orthop.*, **9**, 3, 262.

Windham, G.C. and Edmonds, L.D. (1982) Current trends in the incidence of neural tube defects. *Pediatrics*, **70**, 3, 333–337.

Yngve, D., Douglas, R. and Roberts, J.M. (1984) The reciprocating gait orthosis in myelomeningocele. *J. Pediatr. Orthop.*, **4**, 304–310.

Further reading

Buvisson, J.S. and Hamblen, D.L. (1972) Electromyographic assessment of the transplanted ilio-psoas muscle in spina bifida cystica. *Dev. Med. Child Neurol.*, **4**, 1, suppl. 27.

Hare, E.H., Lawrence, K.M., Payne, H. and Rawnsley, K. (1966) Spina bifida cystica and family stress. *Br. Med. J.*, **2**, 757.

James, C.C.M. (1970) Fractures of the lower limbs in spina bifida children. *Dev. Med. Child Neurol.*, **12**, suppl. 22.

Knutson, L.M. and Clark, D.E. (1991) Orthotic devices for ambulation in children with cerebral palsy and myelomeningocele. *Phys. Ther.*, **71**, 12, 947–960.

Lorber, J. (1970) *Your Child with Hydrocephalus*. London: Association for Spina Bifida and Hydrocephalus.

Ryan, K.D., Ploski, C. and Emaus, T.B. (1991) Myelodysplasia – the musculo-skeletal problems: habilitation from infancy to childhood. *Phys. Ther.*, **71**, 12, 935–946.

Sand, P. *et al.* (1973) Performance of children with spina bifida manifesta on the Frostig developmental test of visual perception. *Percept. Motor Skills*, **37**, 539–546.

Scobie, W.G., Eckstein, H.B. and Long, W.J. (1970) Bowel function in myelomeningocele. *Dev. Med. Child Neurol.*, **12**, suppl. 22.

Turner, A. (1985) Hand function in children with myelomeningocele. *J. Bone Joint Surg.*, **67-B**, 2, 268–272.

Williamson, G.G. (1987) *Children with Spina Bifida. Early Intervention and Preschool Programming*. Baltimore, MD: Paul H. Brookes.

16

Congenital limb deficiencies

Although the commonest type of limb reduction or amputation in children is congenital in origin, trauma, tumour and other diseases are additional causes of amputation seen in paediatric practice (Krebs and Fishman 1984). There has been some difficulty in finding a classification system which will include all the varieties of limb deficiency or *dysmelia*, and amputation. Frantz and O'Rahilly (1961), Henkel and Willert (1969) and others have attempted classifications depending upon morphology or clinical observation.

Two terms in common usage are phocomelia and amelia. Rubin (1967) described *phocomelia* (Figs 16.1 and 16.2) as an incomplete development of the limbs. *Amelia* (Fig. 16.3) infers complete absence of a limb. The varieties seen range from amelia of one limb to complete amelia of all four limbs.

Congenital anomalies are currently classified as *transverse* if all skeletal elements distal to the level of loss are absent, or *longitudinal* if some distal elements remain (Day 1988). Transverse limb deficiencies are similar in appearance to surgical amputations, while longitudinal ones are more variable. In the lower limb, the fibula and the fourth and fifth rays of the foot may be missing; in the upper limb the ulna may be missing. In proximal femoral focal deficiency, the femur is shortened and the tibia, fibula and foot are relatively normal. In phocomelia the foot may be in close proximity to the pelvis. The commonest site of congenital deficiency is the upper limb, and below-elbow deficiencies are the most frequently seen anomalies (Krebs and Fishman 1984).

The causes of developmental failure are usually unknown, although it has been shown to be the result of certain drugs taken by the mother in the first weeks of pregnancy. The developmental breakdown probably occurs

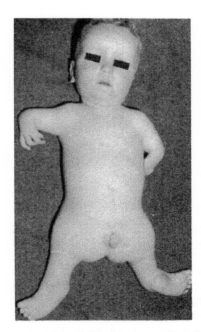

Figure 16.1 Child with phocomelic limbs (thalidomide syndrome).

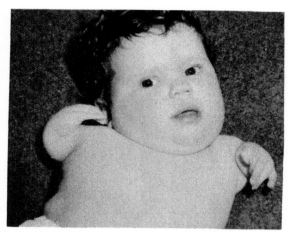

Figure 16.2 Child with phocomelic upper limbs (thalidomide syndrome).

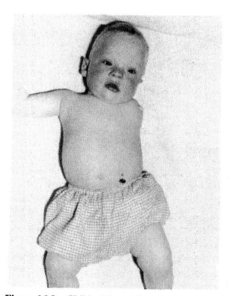

Figure 16.3 Child with amelia of the left upper limb.

during the fourth to the eighth gestational week, at the time when the limb buds are forming.

The effects of the drug thalidomide are now well-known. The affected children suffered a variety of congenital abnormalities including complete or partial absence of limbs, disorders of other systems, amongst them cardiac and intestinal abnormalities, and facial anomalies.

The thalidomide tragedy focused attention on all children with limb deficiencies and stimulated research into prosthetic design and management. The problems described below are particularly applicable to those families in which a severely limb-deficient child has been born, although they will be present to a varying degree in all similarly affected families.

The parents of a child born with severe limb deficiencies suffer profound shock. They need to make considerable adjustment in order to cope with their grief and disappointment, and their feelings of guilt and shame. The parents' inability to come to terms with their child's problems may lead them to reject the child, either unconsciously or overtly, and consequently to overprotection. Unconscious rejection may lead the parents to seek help in the form of artificial aids for the child which he or she will never use, and practical suggestions which will never be put into practice. It is not enough just to teach a child to be independent, as those responsible for the management of these children have found out, but it will be the parents' attitudes which will in the end determine how independent the child will be.

It is said to be fear and anxiety which lead to rejection, and parents need expert counselling to help them see the child's problems in a realistic light, to gain some knowledge of the assistance they will receive, and to be reassured that they need feel no guilt about their child's deficiencies. Whether or not they will be able to lose their negative feelings probably depends to a large extent on how the infant is accepted by relatives, friends and the community. Shame is sometimes connected with the disappointment all parents must feel if their newborn baby is not all they had hoped for, if they are not able to experience the pride of showing the infant off to their relatives and friends.

The child should be encouraged from as early an age as possible to have a positive attitude towards life, so new challenges can be overcome. From an early age the child has to accept being considered different. Independence and a creative approach to solving problems posed by the environment need to be encouraged in even the youngest child, and exercise and play need to be designed to promote confidence, self-esteem and boldness.

Fear of falling is often considerable in children whose balance is severely affected due to lack of arms or to an inability to feel connected with the ground while wearing a lower-limb prosthesis. Children with lower-limb deficiencies plus hip instability suffer considerable balance difficulty initially. However, it is lack of mobility which appears to be the greatest handicap in these children, and it is the lower-limb-deficient children who suffer most in this respect.

Clinical features

Motor deficits

Children with limb deficiency usually suffer some delay in motor development, which may be localized, as in the child with absent fingers, or more general in the case of a child with one or more limbs involved. The most handicapped is the child with total amelia.

Normal motor development demands amongst other things intact skeletal and muscular systems, and, in the presence of defects in these systems, development will be both delayed and abnormal unless treatment is directed at overcoming the difficulties.

A child who has no legs will not be able to sit or to develop skills in sitting or standing unless provided with an external aid which enables erect sitting and standing positions to be maintained.

A child with no arms will be slow to develop the ability to get into sitting from prone or supine as well as to balance while moving about (e.g. reaching) in sitting and standing. Although lack of hands may seem a severe deterrent to the sensitive exploration of the world around the child, the feet can develop remarkable dexterity and sensitivity if the child is encouraged to use them. If there is an absence of both hands and feet, the child is taught to use lips and tongue as vehicles for sensory and motor exploration. The use of the mouth or the feet as substitutes for hands is essential for the development of these children. There may be increased sensitivity at the tips of phocomelic limbs and the child will consequently prefer the use of these tiny limbs to any prosthesis which has so far been designed. No prosthesis, however sophisticated, can provide the knowledge that comes from somatosensory inputs.

Problems arising from the delayed development of balance in phocomelic and amelic children cannot be overemphasized. Special balance training is required for the child with bilateral upper-extremity amelia or phocomelia as arms are essential for balance, especially in early standing and walking. A child with severe bilateral lower-extremity deficiency will also develop balance slowly, partly because of a lack of sensory inputs from the feet. Special apparatus is needed to enable the child to develop balance in the upright position, and emphasis in treatment is on training head and trunk movements in response to both self-initiated and externally imposed alterations to segmental alignment.

In normal children, increasing height caused by both growth and the ability to achieve the sitting and standing positions enables the visualization of the environment from different levels – chair legs, the seat, a table top and so on. Prostheses are lengthened gradually to keep pace with chronological progression in order to optimize cognitive and perceptual development. As the child gets older, prostheses may need lengthening in response to the child's concern about the height of peers or siblings. Adjustments for growth are also made in order to ensure that a deficient limb is maintained at a length equal to the sound limb. This is done as often as every 1 or 2 years in infants and small children.

The development of a normal child proceeds, if unimpeded, in an effortless manner, one step leading on to the next, the child driven on to achieve the next skill, repeating each new action until it is effective. It is assumed, therefore, that it is easier to teach a handicapped child how to walk, for example, when at a stage of development at which the urge to walk and explore is strong, than to wait until the child is older when the urge may be less strong. The older child having adapted to a more sedentary existence. With this in mind it is important to try, with the aid of prosthetic devices, to help the child achieve milestones when the natural drive to do so is present.

Deformities

As in the case of any infant born with a congenital defect there is always the possibility of other defects, and many children born with limb deficiencies have deformities associated with the deficiency. These deformities may include talipes equinovarus, talipes calcaneus, dislocated hips or spina bifida. Deformities may be very severe. If an existing foreshortened limb is also grossly deformed, further problems of management arise, especially when it is necessary to make decisions about the fitting of prostheses.

Surgical conversion of a congenital anomaly is only undertaken after consultation between members of the health team and the family. It is necessary to consider present and future prosthetic options and cosmetic and functional expectations (Krebs *et al.* 1991).

There is also a risk of contractures, particularly in children with foreshortened limbs. A child with a phocomelic upper limb may develop contracture of the anterior shoulder muscles through the repeated action of taking the limb to the mouth. Acquired soft tissue contractures must be prevented so the child will have maximum range of movement and be able to take full advantage of whatever limb remnants are present and of any prosthesis which may be designed in the future.

Loss of surface area

Some children have such an extensive loss of surface area that marked interference with the body cooling system occurs. Such children sweat heavily, and in warm weather and during exercise care must be taken to dress them lightly to allow maximum circulation of air to take place.

Management

A large team of people is involved in the care of these children: an orthopaedic surgeon, specialist prosthetist, social worker, physiotherapist and occupational therapist. The child's parents and school teacher also have important roles to play in the child's habilitation.

The infant's family is seen by the social worker as soon as practicable after birth, and this support is continuous from then on, offering practical advice about financial assistance, schooling and to some extent acting as coordinator between the various people responsible for the child's management.

The physiotherapist sees the infant as soon as possible to assess what functional training is

necessary, and what exercises must be done to prepare the child for a prosthesis.

Parental instruction in the strengthening and coordination exercises and games of a home programme is essential in preparing the child for independent function. Parents are also instructed in the care, maintenance and operation of prostheses.

Prosthetic options

Most authorities agree that a limb-deficient child be fitted with a prosthesis to coincide with the appropriate stage of development. In this way a lower-limb-deficient child will begin wearing a prosthesis when ready to stand, usually between 10 and 18 months, and an upper-limb-deficient child when sitting balance is gained at 6-8 months. The early fitting of a prosthesis will, it is hoped, make more likely its incorporation into the child's body image, and there is some evidence that apparatus is more readily acceptable at an early age even if it is rejected by the child when older.

The complexity of the apparatus depends in part on the maturation of the child's central nervous system. As the child matures, a prosthesis of increasing complexity can be used. This applies particularly to upper-limb prostheses, but it is difficult at the moment to realize this aim as there are many problems of design to be overcome and complex electronic devices are very expensive. Unfortunately, at this stage of technological development, the more complex the equipment the heavier it is. However, there are many centres throughout the world where research is directed at refinements in design.

Limb prostheses for children are similar in general to those used by adults; however, prosthetic design for children is complex because of the child's small size and physical, cognitive and emotional immaturity.

Prosthetic options for infants and children are chosen on the basis of function (present and future), comfort and appearance. Present psychological and physiological needs are weighed up against eventual functional requirements (Turgay and Sonuvar 1983). The options are discussed with the parents and if possible with the child.

Basically, prostheses can be divided into two categories, the cosmetic and the functional, and frequently the cosmetic apparatus is provided for the parents' sake as much as for the child's. The fitting of a cosmetic limb, especially an upper limb, is often necessary to give the parents the confidence to take the child out into the community. The child usually prefers the functional prosthesis, but many children prefer to use their upper-limb remnants and remaining limbs, as these give more speed of movement and more dexterity due in part to the presence of sensory inputs. Functional upper-limb prostheses remain an ideal to be achieved in the future. While lower-limb prostheses present fewer problems, many children find their activities too restricted, and remove the prosthesis in order to be more mobile. The child with bilateral hip instability may prefer to be mobile in a wheelchair rather than struggle to maintain balance in a prosthesis (Robertson 1971).

Children with four limbs affected, who are aged 10–24 months, are usually fitted with a bucket-shaped device on castors, a swivel walker or an electric cart for mobility (Lineberger 1962; Sauter 1972; Aitken 1972; Zazula and Foulds 1983).

It is important to keep in mind that whatever device the child uses for the upper limb, any limb remnants, no matter how small, are left free and are not enclosed within the apparatus, as these remnants may be used to operate the apparatus (Fig. 16.4).

Upper-limb prostheses

Upper-limb prostheses include a terminal device or hand, a wrist unit, a forearm section, an elbow unit and a socket. The prosthesis typically involves a harness and cable system (Fig. 16.4). The terminal device may be a passive, cosmetic hand or a hook device which allows grasp and release with cables which may be powered by air and/or body movement. Pinch force may be controlled by rubber bands. Recreational devices are also manufactured, enabling various pieces of sporting equipment to be manipulated.

Recent developments in technology have led to the development of myoelectric prostheses for children with congenital below-elbow limb amputations. Although these prostheses have been used largely for teenagers, they have recently been shown to be effective also for preschool children as young as 18 months of age (Sorbye 1977; Hubbard *et al.* 1985; Sauter

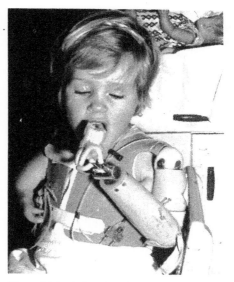

Figure 16.4 A functional prosthesis powered from a carbon dioxide cylinder and operated by the child using the right phocomelic limb.

1988). These units tend to be both heavy and fragile compared to the cable-operated devices. Children are trained in muscle control before they are fitted with the prosthesis (see Hubbard *et al.* 1985 for details). The child practises flexing and extending the wrist of the normal arm, with visual electromyogram feedback from the appropriate muscles. The same procedure is then carried out on the stump side in order to achieve a muscle response from the residual soft tissue at the end of the stump. Once the prosthesis is fitted, the child is given functional training, learning to use the prosthetic extremity as assistive or stabilizing while objects are manipulated with the natural hand. Such training is typically given by the physiotherapist. However, it has been shown that parents can train the child at home just as effectively once the therapist has given the necessary explanations and instructions (Hubbard *et al.* 1985).

Lower-limb prostheses

Prostheses for toddlers are designed to allow for a wide walking base with some hip external rotation typical of the age group. Children with below-knee deficiencies require a prosthesis with a foot–ankle assembly, a shank, a socket and a suspension. Infants are given a simple SACH (solid-ankle cushion heel) foot which gives a stable standing base of support. By the age of 2 years, toddlers can often manage a basic prosthetic foot. Older children may be provided with energy storing and releasing feet which have flexible soles which store energy in early stance and release it in late stance. Modern prostheses have the capacity to give the wearer more flexibility in the type of ground over which they walk. However, their provision depends on the financial resources of the parents and the health service. In developing countries, where many of the children with traumatic lower-limb amputations live, lower-limb prostheses are usually much simpler, providing the wearer with support and equal leg length.

Children with above-knee amputations require foot and shank components as above plus extra components which vary according to the child's age and special requirements. An infant may need an ischial-bearing socket or a bucket-shaped arrangement in which the pelvis sits (see Fig. 16.12). Knee components for older children may be hydraulic or pneumatic, in which the frictional control adjusts to changes in walking velocity. Total suction suspension can be used even by children as young as 5 years (Fishman *et al.* 1987). When older, children with phocomelia or a very short stump will need a hip disarticulation prosthesis or, if bilateral, a modified reciprocating gait orthosis. Children with bilateral phocomelia may opt eventually for a wheelchair as the energy cost of ambulation is so great.

Physiotherapy

Assessment

The child's stage of development is assessed at regular intervals as this will be one of the major factors in treatment and training. Specific measurements of joint range and muscle strength are done at regular intervals and particularly before the prescription of a prosthesis is made. Once fitted with a prosthesis, measurements and evaluation of function to determine how the child and parents are managing are made in the child's home, where strengths and weaknesses may be more clearly seen than in the hospital (Robertson 1971).

Exploration

This is encouraged from infancy, with the child using mouth, feet or hands in order to explore the body and its surroundings. The infant is put in positions from which it is easy to see the events of the household. A child with no arms, for example, may lie in prone, with a pillow under the chest encouraging head and trunk extension for looking around and to strengthen the trunk extensor muscles.

Early sitting should be organized for infants with upper-limb deficiencies and colourful objects arranged to encourage the use of feet in play.

Prehension

The hands are normally necessary for prehension, but the feet, lips or tongue may be effectively used in the absence of hands. The feet should be left free of socks and shoes except where these are necessary. It may be difficult for the parents to accept this unconventional use of the feet for prehension and they may have to be persuaded to allow the child to use them in an unembarrassed manner. Toys are selected or adapted to be held in the mouth, the upper-limb remnants or the toes. The child is encouraged to be creative, for example, learning to transfer a toy from one limb remnant to the other via the chin.

The attachments of an upper-limb prosthesis are no substitute for upper-limb remnants or toes, but the child may learn to use an artificial limb effectively for limited activities. The earliest apparatus, fitted when the child has good sitting balance, may allow bimanual grasp activated by shoulder girdle movement. An active terminal device such as a split hook on a conventional upper-limb prosthesis cannot usually be operated by a child of less than $2\frac{1}{2}$ years. Most of the prostheses in use for amelic and phocomelic children are activated by on–off switches. These allow a variety of movements including elbow flexion and extension, forearm supination and pronation, and opening and closing of the split hook. The child may operate the switches with limb remnants, chin or by shoulder movement. Some surveys, including a report by Robertson (1971), have suggested that some children are unenthusiastic about upper-limb prostheses if bilateral. The exceptions seem to be children with severe bilateral upper and lower deficiencies who must depend on prostheses for any function at all.

The occupational therapist works with the physiotherapist in training the child to perform everyday functional activities and to play, by using unaffected limbs and limb remnants. The child with amelia is taught to hold a toy between chin and shoulder, in the toes (Fig. 16.5), or in the remnants of upper limbs.

The child learns to be independent in dressing, eating, drinking and playing, by using whatever method is most effective. Krebs and colleagues (1991) list some of the normal developmental skills which also need to be acquired by the child, although very often using adaptive (substitution) movements.

The occupational therapist helps parents to make alterations to clothing and designs equipment such as toothbrush and cutlery suitable to the child's needs. When fitted with a prosthesis for upper limbs, the occupational therapist and physiotherapist teach its use. Both therapists work closely with parents, who carry out much of the child's training at home under guidance.

Mobility of limbs and trunk

An essential part of early treatment is concerned with preparing the child for maximum functional independence both with and without prostheses. Important for this maximum independence is the gaining of a range of movement in joints which exceeds the range typically found for the everyday activities of a child or adult. This is achieved by encouraging activities that ensure the length of soft tissues essential for the activities to be performed by the child. To this end, training begins in infancy to maintain and where necessary increase the mobility of limbs and trunk. The upper-limb amelic child needs to use the feet for dressing (Fig. 16.6), feeding (Figs 16.7–16.9), writing and toileting. The last function, which requires that the child reach the perineal area with a foot, requires a wide range of hip, knee and foot movement, greater than is typically required by the individual with limbs intact. The child with phocomelic upper limbs needs sufficient movement at the shoulder girdle in order to bring the small limb remnants as near to the mouth as possible (Fig. 16.10).

General mobility is required as well as mobility of specific limbs. It is difficult for a limbless child to move around, and this is partly a mechanical problem and partly the result of fear. General mobility is encouraged by teaching the infant to roll over, and this can be pro-

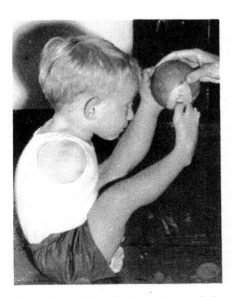

Figure 16.5 Child with bilateral upper-limb amelia training to improve balance and lower-limb dexterity.

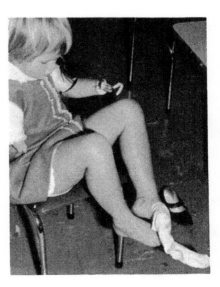

Figure 16.6 Practising dressing.

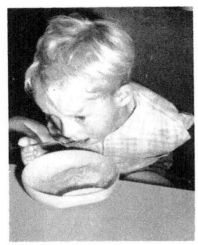

Figure 16.7 Developing dexterity with the feet.

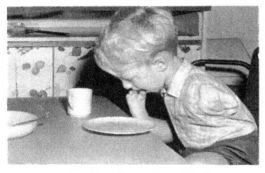

Figure 16.8 Developing dexterity with the feet.

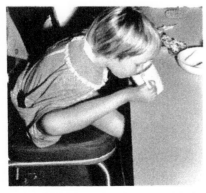

Figure 16.9 Developing dexterity with the feet.

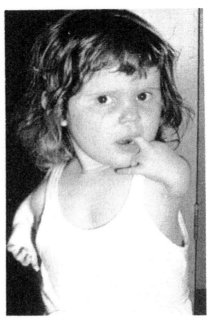

Figure 16.10 Child with bilateral upper-limb phocomelia has sufficient upper-limb dexterity to enable her to take her fingers to her mouth.

gressed to rolling down a sloping board. The upper-limb amelic child can use rolling to help gain the sitting position. In a small pool or in the bath, well-supported by the physiotherapist or by floats, the child can play using the remaining limbs, trunk and head in order to move about. Moving from place to place around the house or garden is facilitated by the provision of a cart, a prone scooter (Fig. 15.4) or a Chailey Chariot (Fig. 15.5). The upper-limb-deficient child needs to be taught such movements as standing up (Fig. 16.11) through half-kneeling and squatting, as well as from a chair, making sure the movement can be done in reverse.

As soon as the child with lower-limb deficiency shows a desire to pull to standing, apparatus is provided which will enable a form of ambulation to be learned. This may be in the form of a simple lower-limb prosthesis or pylon, or, in the case of a bilaterally deficient child, a pair of rigid legs on rockers which he or she will eventually be able to use for walking by using weight transference and trunk rotation (Figs 16.12 and 16.13).

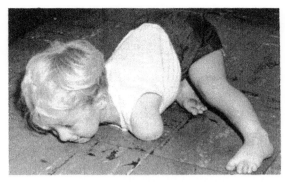

Figure 16.11 The same child as in Figure 16.5 practising rising from supine to sitting.

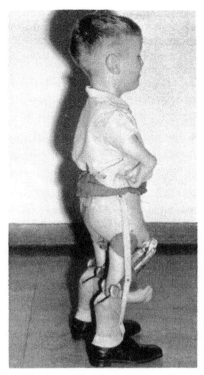

Figure 16.13 He then walked in this apparatus, which enabled hip and knee movement.

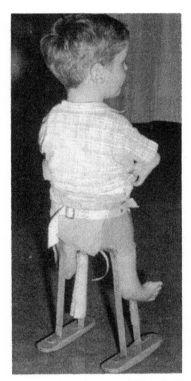

Figure 16.12 The same child as in Figure 16.1 in his first walking apparatus which was operated by shifting weight laterally and rotating the upper body.

Muscle strength and endurance

If the child is to move about in a balanced manner despite limb deficiencies, muscle power and coordination need to be developed specifically for the action to be carried out. The therapist, child and parents need to be creative in working on the best (in terms of energy expenditure and effectiveness) way for a goal to be achieved, then in developing an exercise programme to strengthen the necessary muscles and develop the motor skill required. Similarly, strength and endurance need to be trained to ensure the best possible use is made of the prosthesis.

Deformities

If maximum function is to be gained from dysmelic limbs it is sometimes necessary to correct existing deformities such as talipes equinovarus. An equinovarus deformity is not usually corrected, however, if the foot position makes prehension with the limb easier. Correction of deformities by splinting is frequently disappointing and surgical correction may eventually be necessary. Deformities of the upper limb are thought to be best left untouched until the child is older, when the usefulness of the limbs can be more accurately assessed, the child's own opinion being sought at this stage.

The skeletal and muscular structure of phocomelic limbs is so relatively undifferentiated that accurate assessment of their potential is very difficult. Even a small limb remnant may be indispensable to the child's function.

Postural adjustments

Most children, unless they have only minor deficiencies, need help to develop balance. Postural adjustments are normally made by muscles linking fixed segments (thighs and feet in sitting; feet in standing) to segments above (see Chapter 3). Children with lower-limb deficiencies may need to learn to make these adjustments higher up the segmental linkage and with no sensory information from the base of support (the prosthesis). Such children need considerable opportunity to practise balancing in simple prosthetic devices, as they learn to pay attention to and utilize the sensory information they have available. Children with severe upper-limb deficiencies will also need practice in making postural adjustments in sitting and standing without their arms for either support or balance.

Body movements in response to a changing relationship to gravity and to support surface perturbations may be trained in lying and sitting by using a large ball or a balance board, or with the child held by the therapist in such a way that a response is necessary. However, the acquisition of postural adjustments associated with intentional movement is the major focus of training, since the child must learn to make preparatory as well as ongoing adjustments to voluntary self-initiated movements and not just to respond to support surface perturbations.

The lower-limb amelic or phocomelic child who cannot otherwise sit is placed in a 'flower-pot' apparatus in which postural adjustments are trained using head, trunk and arms. It is difficult for children with upper-limb deficiencies to stand up from the floor and balance training is given in kneeling and half-kneeling in addition to practice of standing up from a seat. The child may be fearful of standing on the first few attempts. There is no protective extension of the arms to brake a fall, and all protective adjustments must be made with head, trunk and legs. The child is taught how to fall, beginning in upright kneeling, falling against the wall or against the therapist, learning to fall sideways on to the shoulder, thereby protecting the head.

A crash helmet may be necessary until the child can walk without falling over.

The reader is referred to Chapter 3 for some detailed suggestions for training postural adjustments.

Summary

The child with a limb deficiency may have problems of emotional, intellectual and motor development stemming from the movement limitations imposed by the absence or abnormality of the limbs. These problems will be principally in the areas of locomotion, balance and manipulation, but will extend much further into the development of the family unit and the child's ability to learn.

Physical treatment consists principally in training the most effective adaptive movements possible for the child, teaching prosthetics use where this is necessary. Those responsible for the training of the child must be sufficiently adaptable and imaginative to be able to encourage unorthodox development of activities where this will enable the child to function more effectively.

References

Aitken, G.T. (1972) Child amputee: overview. *Orthop. Clin. North Am.*, **3**, 447–472.

Day, H.J.B. (1988) Nomenclature and classification of congenital limb deficiency. In: *Amputation Surgery and Lower Limb Prosthetics*, edited by G. Murdoch and R.G. Donovan. Oxford: Blackwell Scientific Publications, pp. 271–278.

Fishman, S., Edelstein, J.E. and Krebs, D.E. (1987) Icelandic-Swedish-New York above-knee prosthetic sockets: pediatric experience. *J. Pediatr. Orthop.*, **7**, 557–562.

Frantz, C.H. and O'Rahilly, R. (1961) Congenital skeletal limb deficiencies. *J. Bone Joint Surg.*, **43A**, 1202.

Henkel, L. and Willert, H. (1969) Dysmelia. *J. Bone Joint Surg.*, **51B**, 3, 399.

Hubbard, S., Galway, H.R. and Milner, M. (1985) Myoelectric training methods for the preschool child with congenital below-elbow amputation. *J. Bone Joint Surg.*, **67-B**, 2, 273–277.

Krebs, D.E. and Fishman, S. (1984) Characteristics of a child amputee population. *J. Pediatr. Orthop.*, **4**, 89–95.

Krebs, D.E., Edelstein, J.E. and Thornby, M.A. (1991) Prosthetic management of children with limb deficiencies. *Phys. Ther.*, **71**, 12, 920–934.

Lineberger, M.I. (1962) Habilitation of child amputees. *J. Am. Phys. Ther. Assoc.*, **42**, 397–401.

Robertson, E.S. (1971) *Follow-up Study into the Functional Abilities at Home and at School of Multiple Limb Deficient Children*. London: Queen Mary's Hospital.

Rubin, A. (1967) *Handbook of Congenital Malformations*. Philadelphia, PA: Saunders.

Sauter, W.F. (1972) Prostheses for child amputee. *Orthop. Clin. North Am.*, **3**, 483–494.

Sauter, W.F. (1988) Electric pediatric and adult prosthetic components. In: *Comprehensive Management of the Upper-Limb Amputee*, edited by D.J. Atkins and R.H. Meier. New York: Springer-Verlag.

Sorbye, R. (1977) Myoelectric controlled hand prostheses in children. *Int. J. Rehabil. Res.*, **1**, 15–25.

Turgay, A. and Sonuvar, B. (1983) Emotional aspects of arm or leg amputation in children. *Can. J. Psychiatry*, **28**, 294–297.

Zazula, J.L. and Foulds, R.A. (1983) Mobility device for a child with phocomelia. *Arch. Phys. Med. Rehabil.*, **64**, 137–139.

Further reading

American Academy of Orthopaedic Surgeons (1981) *Atlas of Limb Prosthetics: Surgical and Prosthetic Principles*. St Louis, MO: C.V. Mosby.

Atkins, D.J. and Meier, R.H. (eds) (1988) *Comprehensive Mangement of the Upper-Limb Amputee*. New York: Springer-Verlag.

Blakeslee, B. (1973) *The Limb Deficient Child*. Los Angeles, CA: University of California Press.

Hoy, M.G., Whiting, W.C. and Zernicke, R.F. (1982) Stride kinematics and knee joint kinetics of child amputee gait. *Arch. Phys. Med. Rehabil.*, **63**, 74–82.

Krebs, D. (ed) (1987) *Prehension Assessment: Prosthetic Therapy for the Upper-Limb Child Amputee*. Thorofare, NJ: Slack.

Lamb, D.W. and Law, H.T. (1987) *Upper-limb Deficiencies in Children: Prosthetic, Orthotic, and Surgical Management*. Boston, MA: Little, Brown.

Lee, K.S. and Thomas, D.J. (1990) *Control of Computer-based Technology for People with Physical Disabilities: An Assessment Manual*. Toronto: University of Toronto Press.

Ladd, H.W. and Simard, T.G. (1972) Bilateral controlled neuromuscular acitivitry in congenitally malformed children – an electromyographic study. *Inter-Clinic Inf.*, **11**, 5, 9.

McCredie, J. (1974) Embryonic neuropathy. An hypothesis of neural crest injury as the pathogenesis of congenital malformation. *Med. J. Aust.* **1**, 6, 159.

Roskies, E. (1972) *Abnormality and Normality: The Mothering of Thalidomide Children*. Ithaca, NY: Cornell University Press.

Sanders, G.T. (1986) *Lower Limb Amputations: A Guide to Rehabilitation*. Philadelphia, PA: F.A. Davis.

Swinyard, C.A. (1969) *Limb Development and Deformity: Problems of Evaluation and Rehabilitation*. Illinois: Thomas.

Whatley, E. (1962) The reactions of parents of handicapped babies. *Mental Health*, **21**, 93.

Section IV

Disorders of bones, joints, muscles and skin

17 Introduction
18 Muscle disorders (myopathies)
19 Torticollis
20 Structural scoliosis
21 Inflammatory disorders of soft tissues and joints
22 Burns in childhood

Introduction

The chapters in this section describe the disorders of bones, joints, muscles (excluding those of congenital origin) and skin suffered by children, and seen most commonly by the physiotherapist.

The role of the physiotherapist in the treatment of children with orthopaedic disorders has shifted emphasis considerably over the years. Much time used to be spent in treating children with knock knees, bow legs and flat feet, and children with Perthes disease and tuberculosis of the hip and spine, who spent a considerable part of their childhood immobilized on frames. Now *knock knees*, *bow legs* and *flat feet* are recognized as being usually only transient stages in the development of the normal postural mechanism. Diseases such as *tuberculosis* are disappearing, although not in underdeveloped countries. *Perthes disease* is now treated by allowing early ambulation in ambulatory braces or surgically, rather than by long-term immobilization on a frame. *Poor posture*, commonly a combination of kyphosis, lordosis and round shoulders, is seen as a mostly transient stage in some adolescents, physical treatment drawing attention to a child already discomforted by constant nagging on the part of parents and teachers. For these children swimming, gymnasium and other activities are more acceptable than exercises which they will be poorly motivated to perform at home.

Apart from congenital orthopaedic disabilities, the major part of musculoskeletal physiotherapy is concerned with the treatment and motor training of children with muscular dystrophy, inflammatory joint disorders, torticollis and scoliosis. Children with disorders including Legg–Calvé–Perthes disease, coxa vara, leg length discrepancy and fractures may also need physiotherapy to improve performance of walking while in and after removal of various forms of orthosis.

Fractures

Children's bones respond to trauma with a pattern of injuries quite different from that of adult bones, except where osteoporosis is the predisposing factor. They are more pliable and therefore subject to greenstick fractures. However, if a fracture in a child *is* complete, the periosteum, which is very strong, frequently remains intact, thus aiding both reduction and repair.

Fractures in children are typically classified as *buckle* fractures caused by compression of the bone; *bending* or *bowing* fractures which are not true fractures; *greenstick* fractures in which one side of the shaft fractures and the other bends; and *complete* fractures.

As a general rule, the younger the child is the more rapidly the fracture will heal. Children with muscle paralysis, such as those with myelomeningocele or poliomyelitis, and those who have had a prolonged period of immobilization, may develop osteoporosis. In children with rheumatoid arthritis there may also be an associated osteoporosis. These children may have an increased tendency to fracture even though the bones may only be subjected to minimal stress. Other children are born with multiple fractures and continue to suffer fractures on slight trauma, due to the familial disorder called *osteogenesis imperfecta. Epiphyseal separation* occurs only in childhood, and an injury which may cause a dislocation or a soft tissue tear in an adult may produce in the child the separation of an epiphysis, a few of which will result in growth arrest if uncorrected.

The physiotherapist may be required to apply the fixation for a child following a fracture – a fully enclosed plaster cast for a fracture involving a limb, traction for a femoral fracture, or a figure-of-eight bandage for a fracture of the clavicle. Except in the case of a child with multiple injuries, rehabilitation of full function upon removal of splinting proceeds in most cases quite naturally and requires little assistance. Most children progress their activities spontaneously, as their strength and mobility improve. The exception may be the child with a stiff elbow following a supracondylar fracture of the humerus. Recovery of movement at this joint usually proceeds slowly, but the physiotherapist can devise ways of improving mobility which the child can practise at home. It is most important that all movement is within a pain-free range, and that no attempt is made to force the joint which will react by increased stiffness and permanent disability (Watson-Jones 1960, Sharrard 1971). Swimming and ball games will encourage the child to regain movement, and are more suitable techniques for a home programme than exercises for the elbow itself, avoiding the irresistible tendency on the part of some parents, as well as physiotherapists, to force the elbow into a greater range. Some children after lower limb fractures need gait retraining.

Legg–Calvé–Perthes disease

Most cases of Perthes disease, occur between 3 and 10 years of age. It is more common in boys than girls, and is usually unilateral. From onset to healing is typically 4 years.

Children with Perthes disease, in which there is a self-limiting vascular necrosis of the femoral epiphysis, present with a history of limp and pain.

A review of histological findings (Catterall 1982) has reported avascular necrosis with revascularization, areas of normal bone alternating with areas of necrosis, and active osteoblastic activity with new bone being laid down. Adaptive changes in the acetabulum have been noted with the acetabulum shaping to the deformed femoral head. The histological and radiological variability suggests an incomplete ischaemic necrosis that does not occur necessarily at one time (Lloyd-Roberts and Fixsen 1990).

On examination the hip is found to lack full range of movement with reduced abduction with the hip in flexion and reduced hip rotation. In more severe cases, a positive Trendelenburg sign may be present with some leg length discrepancy. Orthopaedic treatment is controversial and there have been difficulties in testing the effectiveness of different methods, partly due to the variability of the pathology. Abduction of the hip and containment of the femoral head within the acetabulum are considered necessary and this is achieved by abduction cast or orthosis, for example, broomstick plaster, Toronto brace (Fig. 17.1), Scottish rite orthosis (Fig. 17.2) or surgery (femoral or pelvic osteotomy) followed by full mobility.

Early treatment may involve rest, sometimes in skin traction, followed by ambulation in an abduction orthosis. Treatment is completed when the radiograph shows revascularization of the femoral head. Physiotherapy involves

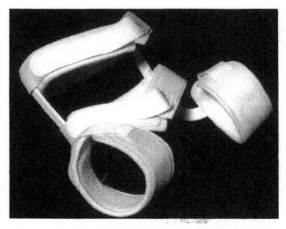

Figure 17.1 Modified Toronto brace. (Courtesy of the Orthotics Department, Prince of Wales Hospital, Sydney, Australia.)

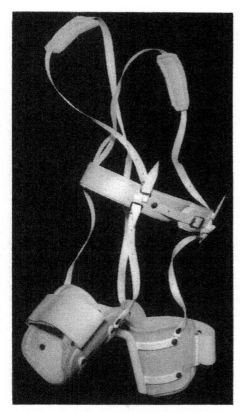

Figure 17.2 Scottish Rite orthosis. (Courtesy of the Orthotics Department, Prince of Wales Hospital, Sydney, Australia.)

walking training, both in the orthosis and after its removal.

Knock knees, bow legs, flat feet

Although these disorders usually do not require physical treatment, they are common disorders in childhood and therefore seen frequently by the physiotherapist in patients attending for treatment of some other unrelated problem. In the course of assessment of a child, a severe degree of knock knee may be noted, and the child should be referred to a medical practitioner.

Genu valgum (knock knees)

Most children between the ages of 2 and 5 years have some degree of knock knee, many with associated flat feet, the latter due to the altered line of weight-bearing. The deformity seems more common in children who are overweight and in children who persist in sitting between their feet, a position which may stretch the medial knee ligaments. The severity of knock knee lessens as the child grows, although a small degree of valgus is normally present at the knee due to the relationship of the femur to the pelvis and the angle at which the femur joins with the tibia.

The degree of genu valgum is estimated by measuring the distance in centimetres between the medial malleoli with the child in supine and the medial sides of the knees in contact with each other. A measurement of more than 10 cm at the age of 3 years requires radiological investigation to exclude bony abnormality (Sharrard 1971).

Genu valgum may also occur secondary to paralysis of the lower limbs. It occurs when there is paralysis of the quadriceps and hamstrings due to the inability of these muscles to control the weight-bearing alignment of the knee. Adequate splinting will prevent the knee being forced by the weight of the body into a valgus position.

Few orthopaedic surgeons prescribe splinting for children with knock knees, except where the condition is secondary to paralysis and likely to progress, in which case some form of bracing may be necessary. Significant valgus deformities may be corrected by osteotomy.

Some surgeons treat the associated flat feet, recommending a medial raise and elongation of the heel of the shoe, with the aim of transferring weight-bearing more laterally. Others recommend no treatment, and advise parents that the stage is normal and transient, and that no treatment is required. In a small percentage of children the deformity does persist, probably due to an underlying growth disturbance (Ferguson 1968).

Where persistent knock knee of greater than 10 cm intermalleolar space exists in a child within 2 years of skeletal maturity, stapling of the lower medial femoral epiphysis may be necessary (Lloyd-Roberts and Fixsen 1990).

Genu varum (bow legs)

In this deformity there may be lateral curvature of the tibia alone, or of both the femur and the tibia. Some degree of bow legs with flat feet is seen in small children when they first begin to walk, the whole leg being bowed outwards; the bowing is more apparent than real. The deformity in this case is developmental and disappears within a short time, being replaced usually by a degree of genu valgum by the age of 3 years (Salenius and Vankka, 1975). However, genu varum may also be due to rickets, and is found in children with achondroplasia, osteogenesis imperfecta and Blount's disease. There may also be an apparent rather than a true deformity in children with genu recurvatum (hyperextended knees) and those with medial rotation of the legs due to anteversion of the femoral neck.

The degree of bowing is measured with the child in supine and the medial malleoli in contact with each other. The distance between the medial femoral condyles is measured in centimetres. If the deformity is very severe it may need to be corrected surgically by osteotomy or by stapling of the lateral side of the femoral or tibial epiphysis. Otherwise no treatment is needed where the deformity is developmental – a fact which needs to be carefully explained to the child's parents.

Flat feet

There are several types of flat feet seen in children. The difference between these types needs to be established, as management will vary according to the causal mechanism.

Pes planovalgus (developmental or inherited flat foot)

Some degree of flat-footedness is seen in all infants when they first begin to stand and walk, as a normal stage in the development of the postural mechanism. It may persist, and in these children it is frequently of familial origin, and remains asymptomatic. It is generally accepted that restoration of the longitudinal arch when the child stands on tiptoe or on extension of the great toe is the most reliable indicator of a normal, even though flat, foot (Rose *et al.* 1985).

The foot muscles in pes planovalgus are not weak, nor is the foot lacking in mobility, and exercises designed to strengthen or mobilize the foot are unnecessary. Some surgeons recommend that the shoes be built up on their medial side in order to prevent excess wear on that side, but neither this build-up, nor the arch supports sometimes recommended are likely to influence the flat feet (Wenger *et al.* 1989; Lloyd-Roberts and Fixsen 1990).

Secondary flat feet

Flat feet may be secondary to genu valgum and varum, or to medial rotation of the legs due to anteversion of the femoral neck.

Flat feet may also be secondary to contracture of the calf muscles. Prolonged weight-bearing on a foot in which the calcaneus is held in equinus by shortening of the calf muscles may cause the foot to 'break' at the mid tarsal joints, the foot being made plantigrade by dorsiflexion at these joints rather than at the ankle joint. This is relatively commonly seen in children with cerebral palsy or after head injury, and although the foot is unaesthetic in appearance it is surprisingly asymptomatic in childhood. If there is pain, it is usually due to the great toe being pushed into a valgus position by the medial weight-bearing. Nevertheless, the soft tissue contracture should be corrected as soon as possible, both to improve function in weight-bearing activities (e.g. sit-to-stand, walking) and to prevent abnormal bone development as musculoskeletal growth proceeds.

This deformity is best prevented by serial plasters and exercise to lengthen the calf muscles and increase control of the muscles linking the foot to the shank.

Flat feet may also be secondary to muscle weakness such as may follow poliomyelitis, when the tibialis anterior and posterior, both essential to maintenance of the medial longitudinal arch, are weak or paralysed. The foot will be more stable and there will be less likelihood of strain to the medial ligament of the ankle if the child wears an arch support.

Where there is insufficient tone to maintain the normal foot posture, the foot will collapse into a valgus position as soon as the child bears weight. This is seen in children who have hypotonia due, for example, to Werdnigg–Hoffmann's disease or benign hypotonia. An arch support inside the shoe may be helpful. However, surgery such as talar arthrodesis may eventually be necessary in a very unstable foot.

Peroneal spasm causing flat feet

Peroneal spasm appears to be caused either by irritative lesions of the tarsus (as in juvenile rheumatoid arthritis) causing a localized painful spasm of the peroneal muscles, or by congenital tarsal anomalies such as the presence of a talo-calcaneal or a calcaneo-navicular bar, with associated shortness of the peroneal muscles.

Treatment in the latter case may not be necessary as the painful symptoms tend to disappear. If they persist, surgery in the form of a triple arthrodesis or excision of the bar may be necessary when the child is old enough.

Painful flat feet

These are sometimes seen in adolescence, perhaps due to overstretching of the plantar ligaments during the final growth and weight gain (Lloyd-Roberts and Fixsen 1990).

Wedging of the heels of the shoes is probably not acceptable cosmetically at this stage, but an arch support inside the shoe may help relieve symptoms, which will soon disappear anyway.

References

Catterall, A. (1982) *Legg-Calvé-Perthes' Disease.* Edinburgh: Churchill Livingstone.

Ferguson, A.B. (1968) *Orthopaedic Surgery in Infancy and Childhood.* Baltimore, MD: Williams & Wilkins.

Lloyd-Roberts, G.C. and Fixsen, J.A. (1990) *Orthopaedics in Infancy and Childhood,* 2nd edn. Oxford: Butterworth-Heinemann.

Rose, G.K., Welton, E.A. and Marshall, T. (1985) The diagnosis of flat foot in the child. *J. Bone Joint Surg.,* **67-B**, 71–78.

Salenius, P. and Vankka, E. (1975) The development of the tibiofemoral angle in children. *J. Bone Joint Surg.,* **57-A**, 259–261.

Sharrard, W.J.W. (1971) *Paediatric Orthopaedics and Fractures.* Oxford: Blackwell.

Watson-Jones, R. (1960) *Fractures and Joint Injuries.* Edinburgh: Livingstone.

Wenger, D.R., Mauldin, D., Speck, G., Morgan, D. and Lieber, R.L. (1989) Corrective shoes and inserts as treatment for flexible flatfoot in infants and children. *J. Bone Joint Surg.,* **71-A**, 800–810.

Further reading

Asher, C. (1975) *Postural Variations in Childhood.* London: Butterworth.

Farrier, C.D. and Lloyd-Roberts, G.C. (1969) The natural history of knock knees. *Practitioner,* **203**, 789.

Meyer, J. (1977) Legg–Calvé–Perthés' disease. A study of the efficacy of three methods of treatment. *Acta Orthop. Scand. Suppl.* 167.

Rang, M. (1983) *Children's Fractures,* 2nd edn. Philadelphia, PA: J.P. Lippincott.

Rose, G.K. (1986) *Orthotic Principles and Practice.* Oxford: Butterworth-Heinemann.

18

Muscle disorders (myopathies)

There are a number of myopathic disorders affecting children. Those classified as the muscular dystrophies all have in common a progressive degeneration of striated muscle with no associated abnormality of central nervous system, spinal cord, anterior horn cell, peripheral nerve or neuromuscular junction (Fig. 18.1). Other groups of myopathies are associated with peripheral neuropathy (e.g. Charcot–Marie–Tooth disease), anterior horn cell neuropathy (the progressive spinal atrophies –

```
┌─────────────────────────────────────────────────┐
│ X-Linked Recessive                                │
│        Duchenne Muscular Dystrophy                │
│        Becker Muscular Dystrophy                  │
│        Emery-Dreifuss Muscular Dystrophy          │
│                                                   │
│ Autosomal Recessive                               │
│        Limb Girdle Muscular Dystrophy             │
│        Congenital Muscular Dystrophy              │
│                                                   │
│ Autosomal Dominant                                │
│        Facioscapulohumeral Dystrophy              │
│        Myotonic Dystrophy                         │
└─────────────────────────────────────────────────┘
```

Figure 18.1 Classification of the muscular dystrophies according to pattern of inheritance. (Adapted from Swaiman K.F. and Smith, S.A. (1989) Progressive muscular dystrophies. In: *Pediatric Neurology. Principles and Practice*, edited by K.F. Swaiman. St Louis, MO: C.V. Mosby, pp. 1139–1163, and Dubowitz, V. (1989) *A Colour Atlas of Muscle Disorders in Childhood*. Ipswich: Wolfe Medical.)

Werdnig–Hoffmann disease and Kugelberg–Welander disease) or disease of the neuromuscular junction (e.g. myasthenia gravis). Others are classified as congenital (e.g. myotonia congenita or Thomsen's disease) or metabolic myopathies. Classification of these disorders is not precise since many of the specific biochemical, physiological and structural defects are still unknown (Swaiman and Smith 1989). These disorders can often be divided into distinct syndromes according to the pattern of inheritance and characteristics of muscle weakness (see Dubowitz 1989).

The most common of the disorders affecting muscle is Duchenne muscular dystrophy (DMD), which is described in this chapter since it exemplifies the problems seen in children with progressive muscle weakness. Characteristics of other myopathic disorders can be found in several texts (e.g. Swaiman and Smith 1989; Dubowitz 1989).

Description

DMD was first described by Duchenne, the French neurologist, in 1868. It is characterized by progressive weakness and wasting of muscles. It is seen almost entirely in males, and is transmitted as a sex-linked recessive characteristic with a high mutation rate. Clinical features are usually evident within the first 5 years of life, and the disease progresses until the patient is unable to walk, which may occur between 7 and 13 years. The child may die as a result of respiratory failure some time in his second or third decade.

The deterioration of muscle strength is relatively symmetrical and begins proximally in the pelvic girdle, shoulder girdle and trunk. The hands usually maintain some useful function until the later stages of the disease, although the extreme weakness of the arms and the muscles around the shoulder girdle makes it very difficult for the child to make use of his hands without mechanical assistance. Pseudohypertrophy is seen to some extent in almost every affected individual, in the calf muscles, quadriceps, gluteal and deltoid muscles, and occasionally in other muscle groups (Fig. 18.2).

Progressive muscle weakness, muscle imbalance and the effect of gravity, result in soft tissue contracture. Eventual restriction to a

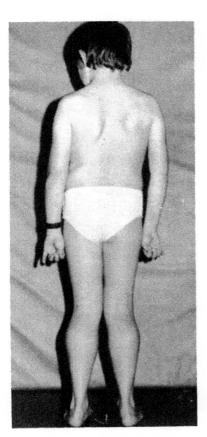

Figure 18.2 Boy with Duchenne muscular dystrophy. Note the apparently hypertrophied calf muscles and the valgus feet.

wheelchair hastens the development of contractures and deformity. Contractures of the hip flexors, iliotibial tract and calf muscles occur relatively early and result in the typical posture and gait. Once confined to a wheelchair, hip and knee flexion contractures, and inverted, plantarflexed feet causing an equinovarus deformity may become very marked. As the respiratory muscles weaken, coughing becomes ineffective and pulmonary infections may be more frequent. Weakness of trunk muscles plus the effect of gravity in the sitting position causes the spine to telescope into a scoliotic deformity which may become extreme, further interfering with respiratory function. These deformities, although not preventable, do not need to occur to such a gross extent as is unfortunately sometimes seen.

In the past the intelligence of these children was thought to be unaffected, but several authors have described cognitive impairment and apathy in a significant number of children (Worden and Vignos 1962, Walton 1981). The mean IQ of children with DMD has been reported as 80, with 25% having a frank mental retardation (Huttenlocher 1987). Some authors comment that in those children who are retarded, evidence of intellectual impairment may precede the onset of weakness, which suggests that the intellectual impairment may not be related to the physical handicap.

Pathology

There is some doubt about the most significant pathological changes. There is a decrease in the number of muscle fibres, enlargement and atrophy of fibres, necrosis, signs of phagocytosis, infiltration by fat cells and increase in connective tissue. The muscles are eventually reduced to fat and connective tissue. In the later stages, some degree of osteoporosis of the long bones is found, probably due to disuse.

Theories of the underlying primary mechanism have included a neurogenic basis, a vascular abnormality and an intrinsic abnormality within muscle fibres, possibly related to an abnormality in enzyme metabolism or structural protein defects (Swaiman and Smith 1989). In terms of the latter, a protein termed dystrophin has recently been identified, the product of the gene affected in DMD, and known to be absent in children with DMD (Hoffman *et al.* 1987; Rowland 1988). The function of dystrophin in normal muscle is unknown; however, dystrophin has been localized to the sarcolemma, the muscle surface membrane (Zubrzycka-Gaam *et al.* 1989).

Type II muscle fibres have been found to have a severe deficit of glycogenolytic enzymes. Since type II fibres are critical in the generation of muscle force, this deficit has considerable clinical significance (Chi *et al.* 1987). There is also some evidence of alterations in the structure of the brain, including low brain weight and microgyria.

Diagnosis

Diagnosis is made on the basis of the clinical manifestations and knowledge of the family history, and is confirmed by the results of certain tests, including DNA analysis and a dystrophin electrophoresis.

In an estimation of *serum enzymes*, serum creatine kinase is found to be elevated, not only in the affected child but also in the asymptomatic carriers. *Muscle biopsy* demonstrates the typical changes seen in myopathy, including degeneration and regeneration, variation in fibre size, and proliferation of adipose and connective tissue (Dubowitz 1989). *Electromyographic studies* demonstrate a characteristic pattern common to all forms of myopathy. An increased echo is found on *ultrasound*.

It is usual to offer genetic counselling to parents of a dystrophic boy. Gardner-Medwin (1977) points out that the mother is a carrier of the gene in two-thirds of all cases and will have a one in four chance of producing an affected child in each subsequent pregnancy.

Clinical features

A delay in motor milestones in infancy is often evident. The child presents to the physician, usually by the age of 3, with a history of frequent falls, of difficulty walking up stairs and running. When he gets up from the floor he does so in a characteristic way first described by Gower, rolling to one side, pushing up to four-foot kneeling, extending the legs, finally pushing the body to the erect position by walking the hands up the legs. This manoeuvre is

due to weakness of the extensor muscles, particularly the gluteals, and is also seen in other myopathic disorders.

Gait alters as muscle weakness progresses. An early change is an increased lumbar lordosis with the shoulders and upper trunk thrust backwards (Fig. 18.3). Gait becomes high-stepping and eventually the typical waddling gait is evident, with increasing difficulty maintaining balance. Recently, biomechanical studies of gait in children with DMD have clarified many of the clinical observations (Schultz 1981).

Sutherland and colleagues (1989) describe the progressive pathomechanics of the gait of 21 children with DMD, following a study using data from film, forceplate and electromyography (EMG). They noted that the equinus foot position which becomes so marked as the disease progresses is not necessarily due to calf

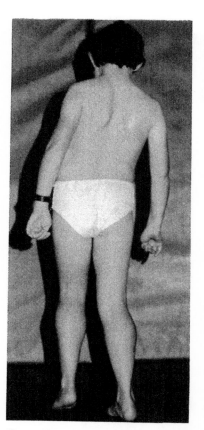

Figure 18.3 Note: a downwards tilt of the pelvis to the left side with a compensatory lean of the upper body to the right when his right leg is in stance phase; lack of hip extension on the right.

muscle contracture. They found a lack of calf muscle contracture in some children who walked in equinus, with an increase in calf muscle EMG activity in the stance phase and the centre of foot pressure concentrated at the front of the foot.

From their data it was evident that the key functional deficit in walking is quadriceps insufficiency. They proposed that the child uses a forceful contraction of the calf muscles to provide a joint moment of force to compensate for the tendency to knee flexion in stance caused by the quadriceps weakness. The quadriceps weakness also necessitates an increase in anterior pelvic tilt and decrease in hip extension in order to move the force line in front of the knee joint, the progressive equinus being associated with this posture.

The investigators point out the distinction between the lumbar lordosis, which occurs early, and the anterior pelvic tilt, which occurs later in the progression. The lordosis seen in standing and walking is caused by the relative posterior alignment of the upper body, not by abdominal weakness. As pointed out by others (e.g. Johnson 1977), lordosis is the first observable alteration in body alignment, developed, as the biomechanical analysis shows, in order to keep the force line behind the hip.

Other abnormal features of gait which develop as muscle weakness progresses include a lateral sway of the trunk and abduction of the ipsilateral arm as compensations for gluteus medius weakness (Siegel 1972; Johnson 1977, Sutherland *et al.* 1989). An increase in hip flexion in swing phase is an adaptation necessary for clearing the foot from the ground due to ankle dorsiflexor weakness and lack of hip extension at the end of stance phase.

As muscle weakness increases, stability in single support is threatened, leading to a decrease in step length. The child must maintain a balance between competing adaptive motor behaviours in compensation for hip and knee extensor weakness. This results in an increase in effort, falls and fear of falling (Sutherland *et al.* 1989). Without bracing of the legs, ambulation will cease around this point.

Management

The principal aims for all concerned with this child are to enable him to live a satisfactory and happy life, avoiding loneliness and boredom, and to ensure a means of education and an interesting, active childhood. Respiratory infections must be avoided, as also must fractures which may occur as a result of trauma to osteoporotic bones. Treatment should mean giving support to the parents as well as to the child, giving both practical assistance and emotional support when they are needed.

No exercise programme, surgery or bracing will reverse the progression of this disease. It has been shown, however, that muscle stretching, regular periods of walking and the provision of long leg calipers at the appropriate time will delay the loss of ambulation and reliance on a wheelchair.

The exercise and stretching can be done at home with the child and parents seeing the physiotherapist periodically for evaluation, feedback, motivation and revision to the programme. In order to encourage enthusiasm for the programme, instructions should be simple, numbers of exercises a few and, where possible, linked to an activity the child enjoys. Positive feedback and encouragement need to be given frequently, which can be by telephone between periodic visits to the physiotherapist.

Treatment is therefore partly *preventive* and partly *supportive*. It should be kept in mind that it is probably impossible to prevent either respiratory illness or deformity in the later and terminal stages of the disease. The word 'preventive' is used to indicate the importance of preventing such secondary complications from occurring in the younger child, causing him distress and making him immobile before he need be.

Assessment

It is necessary to assess the child regularly as a guide to possible apparatus and to treatment, but the assessment should not be done in a way that might depress or upset the child. It should not appear a confirmation of increasing weakness and disability.

Functional testing

A method of testing has been suggested by Vignos *et al.* (1963a), which is done at 3-monthly intervals (Fig. 18.4). It may be used as a guide to treatment and splinting and as a

Grade 1.	**Walks and climbs stairs without assistance.**
Grade 2.	**Walks and climbs stairs with aid of a railing.**
Grade 3.	**Walks and climbs stairs slowly with the aid of a railing (over 25 seconds for eight standard steps).**
Grade 4.	**Walks unassisted and rises from chair but cannot climb stairs.**
Grade 5.	**Walks unassisted but cannot rise from chair or climb stairs.**
Grade 6.	**Walks only with assistance or walks independently with long leg braces.**
Grade 7.	**Walks in long leg braces but requires assistance for balance.**
Grade 8.	**Stands in long leg braces but unable to walk even with assistance.**
Grade 9.	**Is in wheelchair. Elbow flexors more than antigravity.**
Grade 10.	**Is in wheelchair. Elbow flexors less than antigravity.**

Figure 18.4   Test for functional ability based on ability to walk. (Adapted from Vignos, P.J., Spencer, G.E. and Archibald, K.C. (1963a) Management of progressive muscular dystrophy of childhood. *J.A.M.A.*, **184**, 2, 89.)

method of testing the effectiveness of intervention (e.g. Scott *et al.* 1981). In addition to this test, the physiotherapist should make periodic observations of the child's functional ability, in addition to discussing with school teachers the use of standing apparatus and checking that parent and child are carrying out the stretching procedures and other exercises correctly.

Joint range testing

Lower-limb joint range of motion (i.e. muscle length) is tested periodically using a goniometer (American Academy of Orthopedic Surgeons 1965). Any method of measuring joint range which does not take account of the force applied cannot be expected to be particularly reliable for sequential measurements. Goniometry has been shown to have high intratester reliability but variable intertester values (Pandya *et al.*, 1985). Nevertheless, either method will give a reasonable estimate, and ankle dorsiflexion, knee and hip extension are the principal measurements to take. Periodic joint range testing may be necessary once the child is in a wheelchair as a means of determining the need for augmented muscle stretching or Achilles tenotomy. Tenotomy is performed for cosmesis, to enable the boy to select the shoes he wants to wear and to maximize the use of the feet to assist moving about in the chair.

Muscle strength testing

Manual muscle testing is controversial. It is inherently subjective with poor reproducibility and poor intertester reliability (Brooke *et al.* 1983). Weakness of fixator and synergist muscles makes the testing of specific prime mover muscles inaccurate. Although it is difficult to quantify muscle strength by manual muscle testing, a method of grading some muscles using an 11-point scale has been developed (Ziter *et al.* 1977). A myometer in the form of a hand-held dynamometer has been suggested as a means of obtaining quantitative data on muscle force production, although there are some disadvantages (Edwards and Hyde 1977; Stuberg and Metcalf 1988). An electronic strain gauge is reported as being more effective and reliable as a measure of isometric force (Brussock *et al.* 1992).

Some authors suggest quantified muscle strength testing is important as a means of measuring muscle deterioration (Allsop and Tecklin 1989; Brussock *et al.* 1992). Nevertheless, even if such measurements are quantified and reliable, their value is questionable since the results do not necessarily give any relevant information about functional abilities. In a progressive disease such as DMD, biochemical tests which give an indication of changes in total functional muscle mass can be used to trace the development of the disease without the child having to spend time having muscle strength tests and avoiding the need to confront him with further evidence of his gradual deterioration. Of the physical measures, functional testing and measurement of joint range are probably useful guides to treatment and indicators of a child's status.

Respiratory function tests

Respiratory function tests have an important place in the management of these children. The strength and fatigability of respiratory muscles, as well as variations in vital capacity, may be measured. Peak expiratory flow rate is measured by a peak flow meter and forced vital capacity with a spirometer. (Normal values have been produced for children; Godfrey *et al.* 1970; Polgar and Promadhat 1971.) Maximum expiratory pressure is measured by manometer (Florence *et al.* 1978; Alison 1992).

Preventive treatment

Prevention of respiratory illness

Rationale

Respiratory failure is a common cause of death in these children. Weakness and paralysis of the accessory muscles of respiration, particularly the abdominal muscles, latissimus dorsi and sternomastoid, make effective inspiration and expiration and, as a result, expulsion of mucus from the airways difficult or impossible. Little can be done to avoid this in the terminal stage of the disease, when the child is confined to bed with little muscle power. At this stage, the only voluntary muscles capable of active contraction may be the diaphragm and facial muscles. Careful preventive measures in the early stages, however, will prevent the child from developing severe infections which would require bed rest with subsequent deterioration in general condition. Due to the rapid deterioration which always follows periods of immobility, the dystrophic child will not be confined to bed during such childhood illnesses as chickenpox or measles, unless this is considered by the physician to be essential.

Methods

Daily breathing exercises for about 5 minutes, attempting to obtain good expansion of the lungs, may be done at home under some super-

vision. An incentive spirometer may have a motivating effect. There is evidence that swimming and breathing exercises increase or maintain ventilatory function (Adams and Chandler 1974; Siegel 1975).

In the early stages, adequate ventilatory function may be gained by swimming, and by games such as blowing a ping-pong ball around obstacles, in which case it is important that the child makes long controlled expirations. The child may be encouraged to play a wind instrument. Instruction in methods of postural drainage, chest percussion and assisted coughing is given to the parents, to be done when necessary. The criteria for necessity, the development of a cough or an upper respiratory tract infection, are carefully explained to the child and parents. The length of time for postural drainage should be approximately 5–10 minutes, although it is done for longer if necessary, and it may be done three or four times a day, depending also on necessity. The child is positioned in prone and in side lying, in the manner described in Chapter 27, for drainage of the lower lobes, unless specific segments need to be drained separately. Vibrations and breathing exercises with emphasis on full expiration will help to clear the secretions from the airways. In the later stages, the child may need routine daily postural drainage, a portable suction apparatus for the removal of secretions from the pharynx and a portable intermittent positive pressure breathing apparatus.

Nocturnal hypoxaemia may occur in the presence of respiratory muscle weakness even when there is only moderate impairment of respiratory function while awake. Nocturnal ventilation which can be managed independently at home improves ventilation during sleep and results in the restoration of more normal sleep patterns. Subjectively, patients report feeling refreshed on awakening (Ellis *et al.* 1987). Intermittent positive pressure ventilation through a nose mask, which stabilizes the upper airway, appears preferable to negative pressure (e.g. by cuirass ventilator), which can cause upper airways obstruction (Ellis *et al.* 1987).

Chronic alveolar hypoventilation has been reported in children with muscular dystrophy (Buchsbaum *et al.* 1968). Hypoxaemia, retention of carbon dioxide and respiratory acidosis lead to confusion, blurred vision and headache.

Prevention of soft tissue contracture and deformity

Rationale

One of the greatest problems facing the child is the rapidity with which contractures progress once they have reached a certain point. Muscle weakness occurring in one group of muscles leaves the opposing group free to pull the joint or limb into a deformed position. Since they are acting in a relatively unopposed manner, these muscles eventually adapt and become shortened. Muscle length changes, once started, progress very rapidly as the position of the limb becomes more mechanically favourable to the unopposed muscle group. Gravity and positioning favour the flexors in upright positions, and the weakness of the lower-limb extensors, which occurs early in the development of the disease, increases the tendency towards flexion deformity. If the child is not encouraged to move about and to stand for periods of the day, time spent in sitting will also add to the tendency of the lower-limb flexors to contract. So there is a trio of circumstances – unopposed muscle action, gravity and position – which, acting together, rapidly produce soft tissue shortening and deformity.

Unfortunately some children in the early stages develop soft tissue contractures which may become severe enough to limit activity even before muscle weakness is marked. However, provided the child is kept mobile and upright during the early stages, it is possible to delay the early development of disabling deformity, although eventually as the disease progresses it becomes unpreventable.

It is difficult, even in the early stages, to maintain soft tissue length in these children. Muscles may adapt so slowly and relentlessly that the therapist may not notice that less range is being gained as the weeks pass. This is the reason why periodic tests of joint range with a goniometer are useful as a guide to the progress of deformity.

Whether or not it is of benefit to stretch shortened soft tissues manually once these adaptations have become well-established is controversial. It is doubtful that anything is achieved, and the procedures are time-consuming and painful. If the physiotherapist has the strength to affect the soft tissues, it is more likely that they will rupture before they will elongate. The soft tissue which is contracted is only partly muscle fibre. It is also composed to a greater or lesser extent of fibrous tissue, which has no elastic properties.

Methods

Activities which encourage the fullest range of movement possible plus the maintenance of an erect posture for as long as possible during the day will delay the development of muscle length changes and deformity. The therapist guides the child's choice of activities and makes sure the limbs are moved to the limits of their range. Movements should involve active contraction of the muscles antagonistic to the predicted short soft tissues, and movements involving extension are emphasized. Exercises with adapted gymnasium equipment and participation in exercises with a parent may be the most acceptable means of maintaining soft tissue length and promoting mobility.

Since calf muscles start to shorten early in the disease, stretching should start as soon as the condition is diagnosed. Night splints (thermo-plastic or plaster of Paris) are recommended (Dubowitz 1977) to help prevent calf muscle shortening. It has been shown that a programme of systematic passive stretching and below-knee night splints in the early stages delayed the development of calf muscle contracture and increased the time that a group of boys were able to walk independently (Scott *et al.*, 1981). Hamstring and hip flexor stretching can start once there is evidence that muscle length is decreasing.

The child is taught to stretch calf muscles, by standing with the pelvis forwards, arms on a desk or on the wall, making sure heels remain on the ground with knees fully extended (Fig. 18.5). A period is spent at home lying in prone, which will help to maintain the length of the hip flexors (Fig. 18.6). The older child may need to spend some time at home standing in an upright tilt table or frame in order to provide some stretch to the lower-limb flexors after spending the day at school sitting in a wheelchair.

Parents are taught how to maintain length of muscles. The iliotibial band is stretched in prone, the hip being maintained in full extension while the leg is adducted (Vignos *et al.* 1963a; Fig. 18.7). The hamstrings are

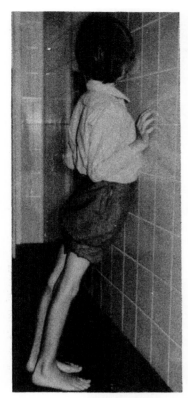

Figure 18.5 A method of maintaining length in the calf muscles. The child should push his pelvis forwards as far as possible, with his heels on the ground.

stretched with the child in sitting supine. The knee is kept extended as the hip is flexed to approximately 60° (Fig. 18.8).

Prevention of immobility and inactivity, both mental and physical

Rationale

It is probably possible to gain some increase in strength and activity when treatment first begins, as the child may have some disuse weakness if not referred to the physiotherapist until weakness is noticeable. The habit of exercising should be developed early in life. The child is kept as active as possible without causing fatigue. Games and activities need to be carefully thought out so they will be a challenge to the child. Inactivity is detrimental, and a bored disillusioned child tends to be inactive, especially if it is also an effort to move.

It is essential that the child develops varied interests and an enthusiasm for hobbies which can be continued once activities are severely limited.

Methods

Swimming and games in the pool are activities which encourage mobility, endurance and respiratory control. The child's time in the pool is carefully planned to include the necessary activities without the element of fun being excluded. A group of children can play ball games with a ping-pong ball which is blown towards the goal. Flippers on the feet provide assistance to the knee extensors. Kicking practice with a board encourages spinal extension as well as active movement of the legs.

Tunbridge and Diamond (1966) have suggested sandhill climbing as a means of develop-

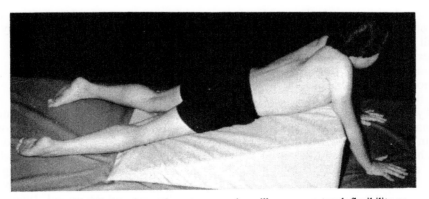

Figure 18.6 Modified push-ups done over a wedge will encourage trunk flexibility as well as lengthening the hip flexors.

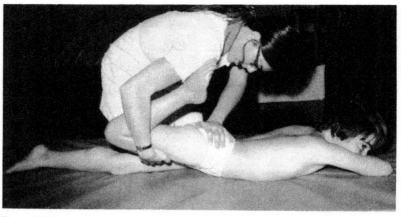

Figure 18.7 A method of stretching the iliotibial tract by adducting the extended hip. Firm pressure should be given downwards on the pelvis to minimize movement at the lumbar spine.

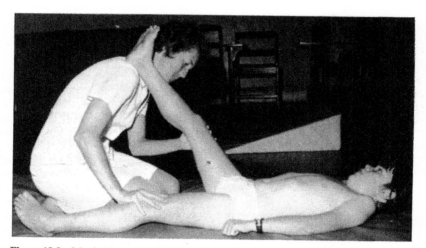

Figure 18.8 Maximal contraction of the hamstrings followed by relaxation in an attempt to maintain their length.

ing endurance. Activities with the assistance or resistance of a pulley system or with small weights will exercise the abdominal muscles, the trunk extensors and lower-limb extensors. Wrestling on mats on the floor can be enjoyed by even a moderately disabled child, and boxing a punching bag encourages balance in sitting or standing. Tying knots with the guidance of a scout manual keeps the fingers dextrous, and modelling in clay or plasticine can be encouraged at school. Some children enjoy video games and developing their computing skills. Wheelchair sports are encouraged.

Part of each day – at least 30 minutes – should be set aside at home or at school for vigorous games and activities to encourage strength, mobility and respiratory function.

Orthoses

Regular walking is encouraged since there is evidence that this will maintain muscle strength and retard contracture formation (Ziter and Allsop 1976). There is also evidence that the provision of long leg calipers when the child starts falling a lot will prolong independent walking in many children (Vignos *et al.* 1963a; Tunbridge and Diamond 1966). However, in terms of the amount of additional walking time, variability in the response of individual children (from 2 to 5 years after start of bracing) has led to a search for the variables which can be used as predictors of outcome. Vignos and colleagues (Vignos *et al.* 1963b) found the most influential predictor appeared to be residual muscle strength. The subjective manual muscle test can be validated objectively by a creatinine coefficient test which gives a biochemical measure of total functional muscle mass.

It has been suggested that the criteria for bracing are the inability to walk for more than 1 hour a day with external support (Ziter and Allsop 1976). Percutaneous tenotomy of the tendo Achilles, followed within 24 hours by remobilization in plaster casts and subsequently light-weight long leg calipers (Dubowitz 1989) may enable a boy to resume independent walking or at least regain the ability to stand (Spencer and Vignos 1962; Siegel 1975; Vignos 1975; Allsop and Ziter 1981). In a child who does not yet need a caliper, an orthosis (a light sleeve support) which assists knee extension in walking when the quadriceps becomes too weak to extend the knee independently can be made from closed-cell nitrogen neoprene rubber with anterior steel stays (Siegel *et al.* 1982). A parapodium-type device or swivel walker may be useful for some children as they require less energy (Sibert *et al.* 1987). It is evident that the success of a remobilization programme depends considerably on the child's level of motivation (Vignos *et al.* 1963b).

Once the effort to stay on the feet becomes too much of a struggle, a wheelchair will increase the child's mobility (Gardner-Medwin 1977). The child should play a part in selecting the wheelchair and the necessary additions to it. Apart from the size and colour of the chair, additions may include a desk top, special seat and swing-away elevating leg rests to allow the legs to be elevated at intervals during the day. A relatively narrow chair makes propulsion easier. An electric-powered wheelchair is essential for a child who lacks the upper-limb strength needed to propel a chair. The control switch may need to be positioned in the centre of the tray in order to avoid an asymmetrical sitting position and early onset of scoliosis.

A spinal support (Vignos *et al.* 1963a; Tunbridge and Diamond 1966; Sharrard 1971) may prevent the development of severe scoliosis once the child is confined to a wheelchair. It is also important to ensure that the seat of the chair is very firm to prevent lateral tilting of the pelvis. Dubowitz (1977) suggests that the back rest should be angled backwards 5 or 10°. This presumably prevents gravity exerting a directly vertical force upon the spine. Gibson and Wilkins (1975) suggest that a lumbar lordotic posture helps to prevent lateral curvature of the spine by locking the posterior intervertebral facets. They therefore recommend fitting moulded inserts to the wheelchair in order to induce this posture. However, there is some evidence that no support or alteration to the seat will affect the development of scoliosis. Surgical intervention, such as posterior spinal fusion with Luque rods, may be advised in boys approaching puberty.

Supportive treatment

For parents

The physiotherapist tries to establish a good relationship with the child's parents as soon as possible after treatment is started. It makes a considerable difference if the parents feel there is one person, outside their circle of family, friends and neighbours, to be contacted about problems which may arise. Many of the practical problems can be dealt with by the physiotherapist, or by an occupational therapist. However, there may be other problems, both social and economic, and in this case, the parents are referred by the therapist to the social worker. Emotional problems stemming from guilt at being a carrier affect many parents, and these feelings may need to be talked out with the social worker or physician.

Home visits will be made at intervals to determine what mechanical aids may be needed to solve practical problems. If it is possible these problems should be anticipated. Parents often have a tendency to endure what there is no need to endure. This occurs either because they are not aware of the facilities available, or because problems arise long before they are noticed to be such. For example, the parents of a 12-year-old had been lifting him in and out of the bath daily for some time and without complaint before anyone thought to ask how the child was being washed. Only when a hydraulic hoist was made available did the parents, looking back over the preceding weeks, remember how difficult the situation had been.

Parents need guidance about the child's diet and this guidance should begin in infancy. Inactivity, overeating and an inappropriate diet are probably the principal causes of the obesity frequently encountered in these children. Where an older child has already developed obesity, consultation with a dietician should be advised.

What the child does for pleasure at home will depend to some extent on the nature of recreation within the family. It is sometimes necessary to give some guidance in suitable activities for the child to pursue. Whatever activities the child does engage in at home, he should not remain long in one position but should be as mobile as possible. However, the physiotherapist must be careful not to interfere in the life of the family, remaining available to answer questions rather than giving advice where it may not be wanted. Families differ in their needs for help and the therapist must not be so insensitive as to ignore cries for help or to intrude unnecessarily upon the family's privacy.

For the child

The child requires encouragement. He may be negative and uncommunicative and may become depressed if little is being achieved despite hard work. What is achieved may depend on how the physiotherapist organizes the physical programme. Assistance and resistance are graded in such a way that the child feels he is doing his best and sees that he is accomplishing something at the same time. The therapist should know the child's abilities well enough, through continuing reassessment, to be able to avoid a situation in which he has to struggle. He may, for example, be given passive stretching on a low bed rather than on a mat on the floor, as this will make it easier for him to stand up. The dystrophic child is often faced with failure and the physiotherapist should try to demonstrate to him for as long as possible what he *can* do rather than what he cannot. Confidence should be encouraged, and this can be discussed with the school teacher, who will be in a position to give the boy the necessary support at school. He should not be overprotected either at home or at school, and should be helped to be as independent as possible.

When the issue of sexuality is raised, the boy is given the opportunity for discussion on the topic. Many organizations run sessions on sexuality for both disabled and able-bodied adolescents.

Adolescents are encouraged to continue their education beyond school as a means of intellectual satisfaction and a preparation for a career. Advances in computer technology, in particular, make a career a real possibility, even in very disabled individuals.

Summary

The child with Duchenne-type muscular dystrophy faces a childhood and adolescence of gradually developing disability. The muscle weakness in this disease is unpreventable and irreversible (Walton 1981). However, it has been shown that deformity and weakness can be minimized in the early stages by keeping the child erect and active. In general, the best the physiotherapist can hope to do is to keep the child as happy and as active as possible, in the hopeful expectation that the disease will one day become curable.

References

Adams, M.A. and Chandler, L.S. (1974) Effects of a physical therapy program on vital capacity of patients with muscular dystrophy. *Phys. Ther.*, **54**, 494–496.

Alison, J. (1992) Pulmonary function tests: performance and interpretation. In: *Key Issues in Cardiorespiratory Physiotherapy*, edited by E. Ellis and J. Alison. Oxford: Butterworth-Heinemann, pp. 24–55.

Allsop, K. and Tecklin, J.S. (1989) Physical therapy for the child with myopathy and related disorders. In: *Pediatric Physical Therapy*, edited by J.S. Tecklin. Philadelphia, PA: J.P. Lippincott.

Allsop, K.G. and Ziter, F.A. (1981) Loss of strength and functional decline in Duchenne's dystrophy. *Arch. Neurol.*, **38**, 406–411.

American Academy of Orthopedic Surgeons (1965) *Joint Motion: Method of Measuring and Recording*. London: E. & S. Livingstone.

Brooke, M.H., Fenichel, G.M., Griggs, R.C., Mendell, J.R., Moxley, R., Miller, A.B. and Province, M.A. (1983) Clinical investigation in Duchenne dystrophy, II: determination of the 'power' of therapeutic trials based on the natural history. *Muscle Nerve*, **6**, 91–103.

Brussock, C.M., Haley, S.M., Munsat, T.L. and Bernhardt, D.B. (1992) Measurement of isometric force in children with and without Duchenne's muscular dystrophy. *Phys. Ther.*, **72**, 2, 105–114.

Buchsbaum, H.D. *et al.* (1968) Chronic alveolar hypoventilation due to muscular dystrophy. *Neurology*, **18**, 319–327.

Chi, M.M., Hintz, C.S., McKee, D. *et al.* (1987) Effect of Duchenne muscular dystrophy on enzymes of energy metabolism in individual muscle fibers. *Metabolism*, **36**, 761.

Dubowitz, V. (1977) Analysis of neuromuscular disease. *Physiotherapy*, **63**, 2, 38–46.

Dubowitz, V. (1989) *A Colour Atlas of Muscle Disorders in Childhood*. Ipswich: Wolfe Medical.

Edwards, R.H.T. and Hyde, S. (1977) Methods of measuring muscle strength and fatigue. *Physiotherapy*, **63**, 2, 52–55.

Ellis, E.R., Bye, P.T.B., Bruderer, J.W. and Sullivan, C.E. (1987) Treatment of respiratory failure during sleep with neuromuscular disease: positive pressure ventilation through a nose mask. *Am. Rev. Respir. Dis.*, **135**, 148–152.

Florence, J.M., Brooke, M.H. and Carroll, J.E. (1978) Evaluation of the child with muscular weakness. *Orthop. Clin. North Am.*, **9**, 409–430.

Gardner-Medwin, D. (1977) Management of muscular dystrophy. *Physiotherapy*, **63**, 2, 46–56.

Gibson, D.A. and Wilkins, K.E. (1975) The management of spinal deformities in Duchenne muscular dystrophy. A new concept of spinal bracing. *Clin. Orthop.*, **108**, 41–51.

Godfrey, S., Kamburoff, P.L. and Nairn, J.R. (1970) Spirometry, lung volumes and airways resistance in normal children aged 5 to 18 years. *Br. J. Dis. Chest*, **64**, 15.

Hoffman, E.P., Brown, R.H. and Kunkel, L.M. (1987) Dystrophin: the protein product of the Duchenne muscular dystrophy locus. *Cell*, **51**, 919–928.

Huttenlocher, P.R. (1987) Diseases of muscle. In: *Nelson Textbook of Pediatrics*, 13th edn., edited by R.E. Behrman and V.C. Vaughan. Philadelphia, PA: W.B. Saunders.

Johnson, E.W. (1977) Pathokinesiology of Duchenne muscular dystrophy: implications for management. *Arch. Phys. Med.*, **58**, 4–7.

Pandya, S., Florence, J.M., King, W.M., Robison, J.D., Oxman, M. and Province, M.A. (1985) Reliability of goniometric measurements in patients with Duchenne muscular dystrophy. *Phys. Ther.*, **65**, 1339–1342.

Polgar, G. and Promadhat, V. (1971) *Pulmonary Function Testing in Children: Techniques and Standards*. Philadelphia, PA: W.B. Saunders.

Rowland, L.P. (1988) Dystrophin. A triumph of reverse genetics and the end of the beginning. *N. Engl. J. Med.*, **318**, 21, 1392–1394.

Schultz, P. (1981) The pathomechanics of gait in Duchenne muscular dystrophy. *Dev. Med. Child Neurol.*, **23**, 3–22.

Scott, O.M., Hyde, S.A., Goddard, C. and Dubowitz, V. (1981) Prevention of deformity in Duchenne muscular dystrophy. *Physiotherapy*, **67**, 6, 177–180.

Sharrard, W.J.W. (1971) *Paediatric Orthopaedics and Fractures*. Oxford: Blackwell.

Sibert, J.R., Williams, V., Burkinshaw, R. and Sibert, S. (1987) Swivel walkers in Duchenne muscular dystrophy. *Arch. Dis. Child.*, **62**, 741.

Siegel, I.M. (1972) Pathomechanics of stance in Duchenne's dystrophy. *Arch. Phys. Med. Rehabil.*, **53**, 403–406.

Siegel, I.M. (1975) Surgery in the management of Duchenne muscular dystrophy. In: *Recent Advances in Myology*, edited by W.G. Bradley, D. Gardner-Medwin and J.N. Walton. Amsterdam: Excerpta Medica.

Siegel, I.M., Silverman, O. and Silverman, M. (1982) Quadriceps femoris muscle assist orthosis in Duchenne muscular dystrophy. *Phys. Ther.*, **62**, 9, 1296.

Spencer, G.E. and Vignos, P.J. (1962) Bracing for ambulation in childhood muscular dystrophy. *J. Bone Joint Surg.*, **44A**, 234–242.

Stuberg, W.A. and Metcalf, W.K. (1988) Reliability of quantitative muscle testing in healthy children and in children with Duchenne muscular dystrophy using a hand-held dynamometer. *Phys. Ther.*, **68**, 977–982.

Sutherland, D.H., Olshen, R., Cooper, L., Wyatt, M., Leach, L., Mubarek, S. and Swaiman, K. (eds) (1989) *Paediatric Neurology. Principles and Practice*. St Louis, MO: C.V. Mosby.

Swaiman, K.F. and Smith, S.A. (1989) Progressive muscular dystrophies. In: *Pediatric Neurology. Principles and Practice*, edited by K.F. Swaiman. St Louis, MO: C.V. Mosby, pp. 1139–1163.

Tunbridge, P.B. and Diamond, S. (1966) Recent treatment of progressive muscular dystrophy. *Med. J. Aust.*, **1**, 962.

Vignos, P.J. (1975) The comprehensive management of Duchenne muscular dystrophy. In: *Recent Advances in Myology*, edited by W.G. Bradley, D. Gardner-Medwin and J.N. Walton. Amsterdam: Excerpta Medica.

Vignos, P.J., Spencer, G.E. and Archibald, K.C. (1963a) Management of progressive muscular dystrophy of childhood. *J.A.M.A.*, **184**, 2, 89–96.

Vignos, P.J., Wagner, M.B., Kaplan, J.S. and Spencer, G.E. (1963b) Predicting the success of reambulation in patients with Duchenne muscular dystrophy. *J. Bone Joint Surg.*, **65-A**, 6, 719–728.

Walton, J. (1981) *Disorders of Voluntary Muscle*, 4th edn. Edinburgh: Churchill Livingstone.

Worden, D.K. and Vignos, P.J. (1962) Intellectual function in childhood progressive muscular dystrophy. *Paediatrics*, **29**, 968.

Ziter, F.A. and Allsop, K.G. (1976) The diagnosis and management of childhood muscular dystrophy. *Clin. Pediatr.*, **15**, 540–548.

Ziter, F.A., Allsop, K.G. and Tyler, F.H. (1977) Assessment of muscle strength in Duchenne muscular dystrophy. *Neurology*, **27**, 981–984.

Zubrzycka-Gaam, E., Bulman, D.E., Karpati, G. *et al.* (1989) The Duchenne muscular dystrophy gene product is localized in the sarcolemma of human muscle skeletal fibers. *Nature*. In press.

Further reading

Archibald, K.C. and Vignos, P.J. (1959) A study of contractures in muscular dystrophy. *Arch. Phys. Med.*, **40**, 150.

Banker, B.Q., Victor, M. and Adams, K.D. (1957) Arthrogryposis multiplex due to congenital muscular dystrophy. *Brain*, **80**, 319.

Bishop, A., Gallup, B., Skeate, Y. and Dubowitz, V. (1971) Morphological studies on normal and diseased human muscle in culture. *J. Neurol. Sci.*, **13**, 333.

Goldspink, G. and Williams, P. (1990) Muscle fibre and connective tissue changes associated with use and disuse. In: *Key Issues in Neurological Physiotherapy*, edited by L. Ada and C. Canning Oxford: Butterworth-Heinemann, pp. 197–218.

Herbert, R. (1988) The passive mechanical properties of muscles and their adaptations to altered patterns of use. *Aust. J. Physiother.*, **34**, 3, 141.

Hosking, G.P., Bhat, U.S., Dubowitz, V. and Edwards, R.H.T. (1976) Measurements of muscle strength and performance in children with normal and diseased muscles. *Arch. Dis. Child.*, **51**, 957–963.

Inkley, S.R., Oldenburg, F.C. and Vignos, P.J. (1974) Pulmonary function in Duchenne muscular dystrophy related to stage of disease. *Am. J. Med.*, **56**, 297.

Kakulas, B.A., and Adams, R.D. (1985) *Diseases of Muscle*, 4th edn. Philadelphia, PA: Harper & Row.

Kottke, F.J., Pauley, D.L. and Ptak, R.A. (1966) The rationale for prolonged stretching for correction of shortening of connective tissue. *Arch. Phys. Med.*, **47**, 45, 345.

Scott, O.M., Hyde, S.A., Goddard, C. and Dubowitz, V. (1981) Prevention of deformity in Duchenne muscular dystrophy. *Physiotherapy*, **67**, 6, 177–180.

Siegel, I.M. (1975) Pulmonary problems in Duchenne muscular dystrophy. *Phys. Ther.*, **55**, 2, 160–162.

Vignos, P.J. and Watkins, M.P. (1966) The effect of exercise in muscular dystrophy. *J.A.M.A.*, **197**, 11, 121.

19

Torticollis

The terms muscular torticollis and congenital torticollis are used to indicate the 'wry neck' associated with fibrosis of the sternomastoid muscle found in infants and young children. This condition needs to be differentiated from torticollis associated with other factors, whether neurological (spasmodic torticollis), structural (congenital hemivertebrae) or associated with parodiditis.

The infant with torticollis lies with the head flexed to one side and rotated to the other (Fig. 19.1). It is normally possible to rotate the head of a newborn baby through 180° from side to side. The infant with torticollis, however, may be unable to rotate the head in the opposite direction beyond the midline. In many cases, but not in all, a sternomastoid nodule is evident. If it is present, it is noticed as an elongated swelling in the belly of the muscle, becoming obvious usually in the second or third week after birth, and usually disappearing before 5 or 6 months of age (Fig. 19.1) A degree of facial asymmetry will usually be present, and in some cases cranial asymmetry is severe enough to develop into plagiocephaly, although plagiocephaly is present at birth in a small percentage of these infants. This asymmetry may be very noticeable in the older baby or child, causing considerable anxiety to the parents.

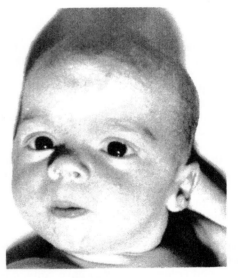

Figure 19.1 Infant with left torticollis and a nodule in the left sternomastoid.

Aetiology

The cause of torticollis is unknown, but there have been several theories advanced. One hypothesis is that of intrauterine malpositioning of the neck with resultant local ischaemia of the sternomastoid (Adams *et al.* 1962).

Birth trauma is typically implicated (Suzuki *et al.* 1984), and torticollis has been noticed to follow after breech delivery (Ferguson 1968; Suzuki *et al.* 1984). Suzuki and colleagues

(1984) found that an intrauterine posture with knees and cervical spine extended appeared to be closely related to the development of torticollis. They suggested that a direct cause may be stretching of the sternocleidomastoid during delivery. The authors also found that 51% of the 43 babies studied had an obstetrical paralysis and most of these were ipsilateral to the torticollis.

However, the fact that torticollis has also been found in babies delivered by caesarean section (Coventry and Harris 1959) suggests an alternative prenatal cause. Familial factors (Thompson *et al.* 1986) and the concurrence of torticollis and other congenital anomalies, particularly hip dysplasia (Weiner 1976; Canale *et al.* 1982; Binder *et al.* 1987), have also been cited. Jones (1968) describes in detail the various theories of aetiology.

Pathology

There is considerable confusion about the pathology of torticollis. Jones (1968) points out that the most constant finding is fibrosis of the sternomastoid which may be present with or without a nodule. He also considered the nodule to be a localized phenomenon in an already fibrosed sternomastoid muscle.

Sanerkin and Edwards (1966) describe an autopsy they performed on a 2-day-old premature infant with a sternomastoid nodule. In the muscle they found haemorrhage, rupture and fragmentation of the muscle fibres with necrosis of some of the fibres, and disruption of the endomysial sheaths. This latter disruption is followed in experimental animals by a proliferative fibroblastic reaction.

Adams and colleagues (1962) have commented that as the endomysial sheaths are destroyed there is fibrous tissue proliferation which prevents effective regeneration.

Differential diagnosis

In all babies with torticollis, but particularly those without an evident sternomastoid nodule, the following diagnoses will be excluded by the baby's physician:

1   Painful septic deep glands which will cause the baby to hold the head to one side.

2   Orthopaedic abnormalities, such as subluxation of the atlanto-axial joint, Klippel–Feil syndrome and congenital hemivertebrae, which will result in a side-flexed head posture.
3   Visual defects such as diplopia due to strabismus, causing an ocular torticollis.
4   Plagiocephaly, in which the shape of the infant's head causes it to be held in an asymmetrical posture without actual contracture of the sternomastoid.
5   Brain injury or developmental abnormality may be suggested in the young infant by persistent rotation to one side of the head and neck, either as part of an asymmetrical tonic neck reflex or due to hypotonia or dystonia.

Prognosis

Although most of the cases of torticollis seen are infants, the onset of this deformity may develop or become accentuated at any age during early growth. Correction occurs in the majority of infants who have conservative treatment (stretching and exercises) by 12 months of age.

Binder and colleagues (1987) suggest that specific physiotherapy is necessary in all but the very mildest cases, and leads to excellent cosmetic and functional results, even when the torticollis is moderately severe. Key predictors for good outcome following conservative management, they propose, are the severity of torticollis and the age at which treatment is begun. Canale and colleagues (1982), however, report poor results from conservative methods in moderately and severely involved children. Leung and Leung (1987), using the modified criteria of Canale and colleagues, reported satisfactory results in 90% of subjects, although they noted a persistent head tilt in 42% of subjects and poor cosmetic results. Differing outcomes may well reflect the type of conservative therapy given in different centres.

If the contracture persists, as it does in a small number of children, or if it is first seen in an older child, the surgeon performs a tenotomy of the sternomastoid and adjacent tight soft tissues. This procedure is usually not done before 1 year of age, and treatment is usually conservative until then. Surgery gives a successful result in most cases.

Once the head position has been corrected the facial asymmetry usually resolves. The baby's head moulds normally once it is free to rotate from side to side. Parents, often very anxious about this, may be reassured.

Treatment

Assessment

An initial assessment is made by the physiotherapist along the following lines.

The general appearance of the baby is noted, particularly the position of the head in relation to the trunk and limbs. The presence and extent of a sternomastoid nodule are palpated. The range of movement at the neck is tested by passively moving the baby's head in all directions and by attracting attention to estimate the amount of active correction obtainable.

A Myron goniometer can be used to measure the passive and active ranges of cervical lateral flexion and rotation so that progress can be objectively evaluated and recorded. Since the pressure generated by the tester can vary from one measurement to another, causing goniometric measures to be inaccurate, care should be taken in the passive test to place the infant's head gently at the end of range and not to apply overpressure. The physiotherapist should note any apparent pain on movement or on palpation of the nodule. The degree of facial and cranial asymmetry is assessed with the baby's head in the mid-position with the face upwards.

General development should be tested briefly, with note taken particularly of any persistent asymmetry of the limbs or trunk, any asymmetrical or abnormal reflex activity, such as presence of an asymmetrical tonic neck reflex, or asymmetry of a Moro, Galant or grasp reflex. If there is any doubt about development or progress, this should be reported to the baby's doctor, and a more thorough assessment made. This procedure is particularly necessary in those babies with no history of a sternomastoid nodule. The physiotherapist will occasionally find signs of neural or more extensive musculoskeletal abnormality in babies referred for treatment of what appears to be torticollis and it is important that the findings are made known to the doctor so that treatment of what may prove to be cerebral palsy or some other disorder is begun early.

Rationale for treatment

It is difficult to devise a rational method of conservative treatment while the nature of the pathological process remains so uncertain. However, it is obvious that treatment should principally be directed towards ensuring full extensibility of the affected sternomastoid muscle and adjacent neck muscles and soft tissues, and preventing adaptive skull, face, eye and trunk asymmetries. In a young infant with a sternomastoid nodule but with little or no contracture of the sternomastoid, the purpose of treatment is to *prevent*, by stimulation of full-range active neck movement, the contracture of the muscle which may result from the fibrosis of the muscle fibres in the vicinity of the nodule. Where contracture is already established, the object is to gain full-range movement of the cervical spine by lengthening the sternomastoid and by encouraging active correction by the baby. It is usually unnecessary to use splintage to hold the baby's head in a corrected position. However, a baby with plagiocephaly may require splinting by a cap and jacket (see Fig. 19.8) for a short period in order to prevent the head rolling on to its flattened lateral surface.

Passive muscle lengthening

Technique

The baby is placed on a padded surface in supine with the affected side away from the physiotherapist, who sits facing the table with the baby's legs and body under one arm. One hand holds the shoulder, thereby fixing the sternoclavicular attachment of the sternomastoid and allowing the side flexion of the head to perform the stretch. The other hand holds the baby's head, taking care not to press on the ear, and pulls it into as much side flexion as possible (Fig. 19.2). The stretch is repeated, this time with the addition of rotation (Fig. 19.3). Head rotation is encouraged by the parent, who should talk to the baby from one side.

The stretches may be done as one movement, rotation and side flexion together, as described above. However, it is suggested that side flexion also be done as a separate stretch, as it gives the baby a rest from rotation, which is often very uncomfortable, yet still allows the muscle to be stretched to some extent. It is sometimes suggested that flexion should be added to the passive stretch (Hulbert 1950; Canale *et al.* 1982).

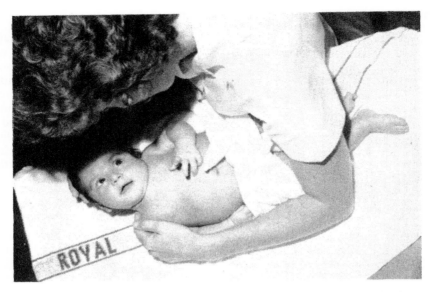

Figure 19.2 Lengthening the right sternomastoid muscle by side flexion of the head.

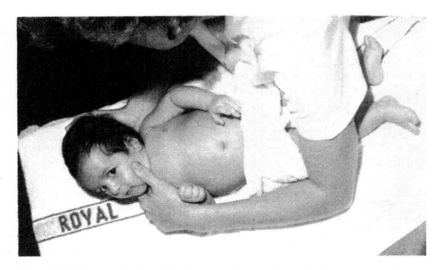

Figure 19.3 Lengthening the right sternomastoid muscle by side flexion and rotation of the head.

However, the added discomfort caused to the baby, especially if there is a large sternomastoid nodule, makes the addition of the flexion element unjustified.

Others (Behrman and Vaughan 1987) suggest that the neck be extended as well as rotated and side-flexed. It is not certain that the extension element will add any significant stretch to the muscle and, given that passive neck extension, even in skilled hands, carries an element of risk in relation to the cervical spine, it hardly seems justified and may well be contraindicated.

Precautions

It has been noted in some infants that the sternomastoid nodule appears painful within the first few weeks after birth; the baby cries when the swelling is palpated or the muscle stretched. The neck should therefore be handled gently, and the stretching done with minimal disturbance to the baby.

The physiotherapist need not give a maximum stretch to the muscle immediately, but should instead move the head until the baby resists the movement, then wait for the muscle to relax, when it will be possible to move it a little further. It is certainly not necessary for the muscle to be held on the stretch with the baby crying and struggling. If the baby is about to cry, the stretch can be relaxed a little, allowing the baby to move. The parent's help can be enlisted in calming and distracting the infant, then the stretch can be reapplied. By doing this, a 5-minute stretch may take much longer, but the delay is worthwhile as the baby will stay relatively contented and unafraid. Furthermore, stretching a strongly contracting muscle is probably ineffective.

The shoulder on the side of the contracture must be held gently on to the bed, and not forcibly depressed. A strong pull between the head and shoulder girdle may cause traction sufficient to injure the brachial plexus.

Stretching should not proceed to the point where the infant is crying and cyanosed. In some infants a large sternomastoid nodule would press against the blood vessels in the neck during rotation, causing pain and cyanosis. With these infants the amount of rotation

gained should only gradually be increased as the nodule becomes smaller.

Recently Leung and Leung (1987) published the follow-up results of 206 infants with torticollis who had conservative treatment, which included muscle stretching, called manipulation. The authors reported that 15% of infants suffered complications: rupture of the sternomastoid muscle, bruising, fractured clavicle.

Duration of passive muscle lengthening

Each stretch is done several times a day for approximately 5 minutes, but will probably take longer if the baby is allowed to move around and if the physiotherapist tries to keep the infant relaxed and happy. The baby should be seen by the physiotherapist several times in the first few weeks, until the parents are confident about their ability to continue treatment at home, with fortnightly or monthly supervision by the physiotherapist.

Active correction

Either before or after the passive lengthening has been done, the physiotherapist shows the parents how to play with the baby in order to encourage active full-range movements of the head and neck (Fig. 19.4) and to achieve extensibility of the neck muscles.

As head control develops in the erect position, lateral head-righting is stimulated by mov-

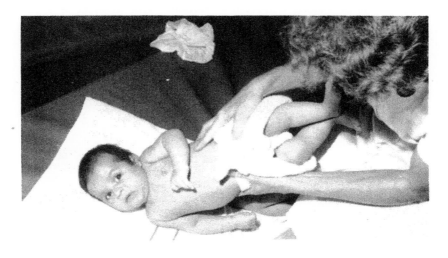

Figure 19.4 A method of lengthening the right sternomastoid which can be done by the parents while playing with the baby.

ing the baby to encourage rotation and side flexion. Rotation is trained with the baby in prone and supine, as well as in the upright position. As the baby is tilted to one side, the head will rotate and side-flex, especially if the stimulus of a parent's face on that side is added (Fig. 19.5). Once the head can be rotated to the midline, the baby may be placed in prone with brightly coloured toys hanging on one side to attract attention, and a parent may talk to him or her from this side. There are other ways of handling the infant in order to gain active correction and the physiotherapist should explore these with individual babies.

In the author's opinion treatment may well consist only of these techniques of training head and neck movement, passive stretching of the sternomastoid being carried out as the baby is handled and moved about. However, the value of passive lengthening as described above has not yet been measured against the value of active lengthening and this should be a subject for further investigation.

It must be stressed that methods of encouraging active full-range neck movement need to be practised by the parents with all infants who have a sternomastoid nodule, not only those with a recognizable torticollis.

Home treatment

It is important for the physiotherapist to talk to the baby's parents on their first visit, and explain not only the purpose of treatment, but also some practical ways of making treatment at home as enjoyable as possible. Unfortunately, in a busy department, torticollis can be regarded as a relatively unimportant complaint, and the anxiety of the baby's family may be overlooked. Some parents are nervous of handling their young infants, and may, when they leave the physiotherapist, be very anxious about the stretching of the sternomastoid and the training which they are required to do at home (Davids 1989).

The baby's parent is taught how to lengthen the sternomastoid, and how to encourage the necessary movements. The parents should demonstrate the stretches and exercises at every visit until it is certain that they are confident and skilful. The parents will require sympathetic understanding, for they may think they will hurt the baby when stretching, and if the baby cries, their fears will be realized. If this part of the treatment becomes too upsetting it is probably better to discontinue the stretching and to put more emphasis on attempts at active correction.

On rare occasions parents react by giving overzealous stretches which do hurt the baby, and soon a cycle develops in which the baby begins to cry before the stretches are started. In this case it is better if the stretching is omitted from the home routine, and the baby taken more frequently to the physiotherapist, or again this part of the treatment may need to be discontinued altogether.

Parents are encouraged to give the baby exercises at least three times daily for about 10 minutes, and to make it a time to play and

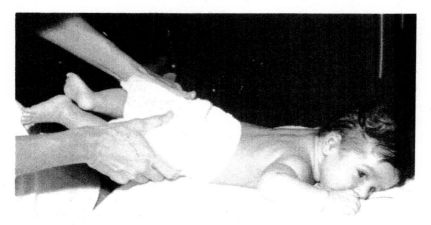

Figure 19.5 Another method of lengthening the right sternomastoid muscle with the baby in prone.

talk. A simple mobile (e.g. aluminium foil which catches the light) suspended above the head, and other toys, will keep the baby amused at other times and encourage the necessary head movements.

How treatment is fitted into the daily routine of the household may be left to the parents. If the baby is bottle-fed, the bottle can be offered in such a way as to encourage active head-turning. However, it is better not to time the passive movements around mealtimes. If it does cause pain or anxiety for the baby, there is no need to make mealtimes miserable too, and the baby will soon learn to associate eating with the discomfort of passive movements.

If the baby reacts badly to the stretch as it is described above, an alternative method can be used by parents. The baby is held with the unaffected side uppermost, facing a mirror. The shoulder and head are held in the same way as in the original stretch, but it is the baby's body weight which applies the stretch. The advantage here is that the baby can be moved about gently and encouraged to relax, making it easier to lengthen the sternomastoid without too much discomfort. The mirror serves two purposes. The baby can recognize him- or herself, and if too young to do this, the light on the mirror may attract attention. The mirror also enables the parent to see clearly the baby's position. (Fig. 19.6). The baby can be carried around the house and garden in this way, increasing the time spent providing the opportunity to lengthen the shortened muscles.

When the baby is in the cot, brightly coloured toys or foil shapes can be hung in front and to one side to encourage looking around and reaching. The cot should be placed in such a position that the baby can see what is happening in the room. The baby should be carried in a way which encourages head turning in the direction opposite to the abnormal posture, and may be nursed in a position similar to that suggested for stretching (Fig. 19.7).

Cap and jacket splinting

Rationale

This method of splinting is no longer in use in most centres except occasionally for those babies with severely asymmetrical skulls, when it is useful to optimize head-moulding. In most

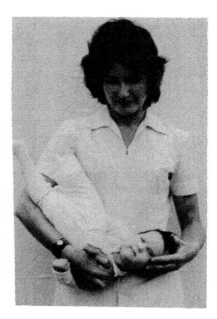

Figure 19.6 Method of lengthening the left sternomastoid while carrying the baby. (Courtesy of J. Harrison.)

babies with torticollis, the value of splinting is doubtful. It is said to hold the baby's head in a corrected position, and this it does to some extent, but it is doubtful that the amount of correction gained is worth the distress caused to the baby's parents, who resent such an overt demonstration of abnormality. Its advantage is that it does persuade the baby to look in a direction muscle shortness would otherwise prevent, but it is better that this should be gained if possible by more active means. The cap is sometimes prescribed by the surgeon following tenotomy of the sternomastoid, when it is worn for a short period until the child can hold the head in a symmetrical position (Fig. 19.8). Alternatively, a soft collar may be worn postoperatively for a few weeks to discourage the child from reverting to a habitual asymmetrical head posture.

Materials

The cap is made from preshrunk webbing and can be kept in place by non-allergenic strapping. It must fit firmly or it will slip about on the head. Three webbing straps are attached. The anterior two control the position of the head and the posterior one prevents the cap

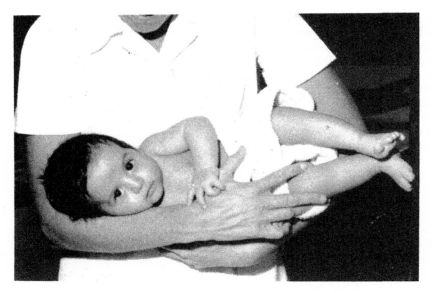

Figure 19.7   Another method of carrying an infant with right torticollis.

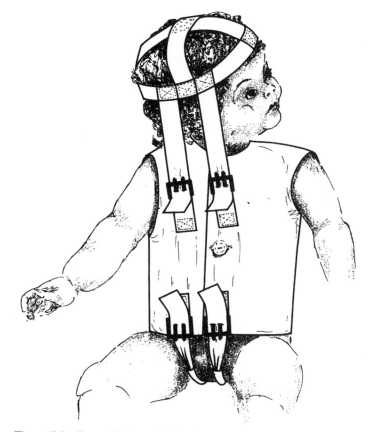

Figure 19.8   Cap and jacket splinting. Alternatively, the jacket may be pinned to the baby's nappy.

being pulled down anteriorly. Velcro is attached to a jacket, two pieces on the front and one on the back. The front Velcro is attached in such a way as to gain the most correction from the two straps which come one in front of and the other behind the ear. The type of correction required can be altered by changing the position of the Velcro and therefore of the straps. The buckle for the posterior strap is placed anywhere in the midline at the back of the jacket; its function is merely to prevent the cap being pulled down anteriorly.

Surgical treatment

If the contracture persists despite conservative treatment and if the child is older than 1 year, a surgical release of tight structures may be necessary (Morrison and MacEwen 1982). It is usually performed just above the attachment of the muscle to the clavicle. Sharrard (1971) and Lloyd-Roberts and Fixsen (1990) describe the procedures.

Postoperative physiotherapy

Immediately following surgery, the child lies without a pillow, a sandbag preventing the head from returning to the asymmetrical position. The surgeon may prescribe cap and jacket splinting or a soft collar to be worn until the child can hold the head in the midline.

Active correction is started approximately 36 hours after surgery, with the aim of maintaining the length of muscle gained at operation. A child who is old enough to cooperate may assist by actively moving the head into side flexion and rotation as far as possible. Full-range neck movement can often be gained in this manner without having to use passive lengthening procedures. Lying in supine with the physiotherapist holding the head and shoulder, the child tries to move the head as far as possible against gentle resistance applied by the therapist, without causing pain. The therapist helps by holding the head in this position until the child is ready to try to move it a little further. The two movements may be done separately. By attempting this active correction, which should result in relaxation and lengthening of the sternomastoid, painful passive stretches against the resistance of an upset child are avoided. These movements must be done gently as the sutures will not be removed for several days, and a cosmetic well-healed scar is important.

After surgery, the child's bed, chair, and television should be positioned in the ward so that the head will be rotated in the direction required.

As soon as the child is allowed out of bed, the physiotherapist gives exercises and games to gain full-range active head and neck movement in the erect position. There is no difficulty in overcoming the rotation element of the torticollis usually, unless the child has a visual defect, as the face will be brought forward as soon as possible. However, the side flexion element may persist for longer.

The feeling of holding the head erect may be reinforced for the older child if, sitting on a stool in front of a mirror, he or she stretches up as tall as possible against the firm pressure of the physiotherapist's hand on the top of the head. The child may also like to practise walking with an object balanced on the head.

If the child persists in holding the head to one side despite treatment, the possibility of an acquired visual defect should be considered; this may only become evident when the head is held in the altered position. In this case the child should be referred back to the physician for investigation.

Summary

Torticollis is a disorder of which the aetiology and pathology are not fully understood. The effectiveness of physiotherapy in the treatment of infants with this deformity is generally accepted (Binder *et al.* 1987), although it seems equally certain that the type of physiotherapy given may determine the degree of success. Emphasis in conservative treatment is on careful explanation of techniques of passive muscle lengthening to the parents, plus discussion of the ways in which they may encourage active correction. Passive movement should not leave the infant distraught and exhausted, or the parent guilty and anxious, but should be gently performed, with time allowed for the infant to become accustomed to this way of being handled. Physiotherapy following surgery is necessary and the combination usually effective.

References

Adams, R.D., Denny Brown, D. and Pearson, C.M. (1962) *Diseases of Muscle. A Study in Pathology*. London: Kimpton.

Behrman, R.E. and Vaughan, V.C. (1987) *Nelson Textbook of Pediatrics*, 13th edn. Philadelphia, PA: W.B. Saunders.

Binder, H., Eng, G.D., Gaiser, J.F. and Koch, B. (1987) Congenital muscular torticollis: results of conservative management with long-term follow-up in 85 cases. *Arch. Phys. Med. Rehabil.*, **68**, 222.

Canale, S.T., Griffin, D.W. and Hubbard, C.N. (1982) Congenital muscular torticollis: a long-term follow-up. *J. Bone Joint Surg.*, **64A**, 6, 810.

Coventry, M.B. and Harris, L.E. (1959) Congenital muscular torticollis in infants. *J. Bone Joint Surg.*, **41A**, 815.

Davids, L.M. (1989) Congenital muscular torticollis: a preliminary survey. *Physiotherapy*, **43**, 2, 45–46.

Ferguson, A.B. (1968) *Orthopaedic Surgery in Infancy and Childhood*. Baltimore, MD: Williams & Wilkins.

Hulbert, K.F. (1950) Congenital torticollis. *J. Bone Joint Surg.*, **32B**, 1, 50.

Jones, P.G. (1968) *Torticollis in Infancy and Childhood*. Illinois: Thomas.

Leung, Y.K. and Leung, P.C. (1987) The efficacy of manipulative treatment for sternomastoid tumours. *J. Bone Joint Surg.*, **69B**, 3, 473–476.

Lloyd-Roberts, G.C. and Fixsen, J.A. (1990) *Orthopaedics in Infancy and Childhood*, 2nd edn. Oxford: Butterworth-Heinemann.

Morrison, D.L. and MacEwen, G.D. (1982) Congenital muscular torticollis: observations regarding clinical findings, associated conditions, and results of treatment. *J. Pediatric Orthopedics*, **2**, 500–505.

Sanerkin, N.G. and Edwards, P. (1966) Birth injury to the sternomastoid. *J. Bone Joint Surg.*, **48B**, 441.

Sharrard, W.J.W. (1971) *Paediatric Orthopaedics and Fractures*. Oxford: Blackwell.

Suzuki, S., Yamamuro, T. and Fujita, A. (1984) The aetiological relationship between congenital torticollis and obstetrical paralysis. *Int. Orthop.*, **8**, 175.

Thompson, F., McManus, S. and Colville, J. (1986) Familial congenital muscular torticollis. In: *Clinical Orthopaedics and Related Research*, edited by M.R. Urist. Philadelphia, PA: J.B. Lippincott, pp. 193–196.

Weiner, D.S. (1976) Congenital dislocation of the hip associated with congenital muscular torticollis. In: *Clinical Orthopaedics and Related Research*, edited by M.R. Urist. Philadelphia, PA: J.B. Lippincott, pp. 163–165.

Further reading

Chandler, F.A. (1948) Muscular torticollis. *J. Bone Joint Surg.*, **30A**, 556.

Chandler, F.A. and Altenburg, A. (1944) Congenital muscular torticollis. *J.A.M.A.*, **125**, 476.

Lee, E.H., Kang, Y.K. and Bose, K. (1986) Surgical correction in muscular torticollis in the older child. *J. Pediatr. Orthop.*, **6**, 585.

Ling, C.M. and Low, Y.S. (1972) Sternomastoid tumour and torticollis. *Clin. Orthop. Rel. Res.*, **86**, 144.

Macdonald, D. (1969) Sternomastoid tumour and torticollis. *J. Bone Joint Surg.*, **51B**, 3, 432.

20

Structural scoliosis

Structural scoliosis is a serious, progressive and disabling condition, which may be uncorrectable by any but surgical means. It is clearly distinct from the correctable, non-structural but postural lateral curvature of the spine. This latter may be found in some adolescents whose postural mechanism has suffered a temporary set-back due to a rapid growth spurt, and in children with one leg shorter than the other. This asymmetry is corrected when the legs are made an equal length by the addition of a raise to the shoe, or by leg-lengthening (Sharrard 1971) or leg-shortening surgery.

Structural scoliosis does not just involve a lateral curvature of the spine, but also rotation within the spine itself. A simple test makes the difference between the two easily distinguishable. When the child with a postural lateral curvature bends forwards to touch the toes in standing, the lateral curve disappears. In marked contrast, the child with a structural scoliosis continues to demonstrate a lateral curvature and the rotation element will be evident as a bony prominence on the side of the convexity (Fig. 20.1). This prominence is caused by the posterior displacement of the ribs on that side due to the rotation of the bodies of the vertebrae towards the side of the convexity. This causes the transverse processes on that side to be angled posteriorly. The ribs, because of their articulation with these processes, project backwards on the side of the convexity (Fig. 20.2). It is this rotational element that causes to a

large extent the typical deformity. The rib cage deformity becomes increasingly severe as the scoliosis progresses. The ribs on the concave side are prominent anteriorly and flattened posteriorly, while on the convex side they are flattened anteriorly and project posteriorly. The lateral curvature in which the rotation element is present is called the primary curve (Fig. 20.3). Above and below the primary curve are compensatory curves, which do not clinically contain a rotation element on forward flexion of the spine (Sharrard 1971). The compensatory curves are adaptive, serving to centre the body mass over the base of support and hold the head vertical with eyes horizontally aligned.

Where deformity is severe the trunk muscles on the side of the convexity are at a mechanical disadvantage, and the degree of deformity is probably increased by the mechanical advantage of the spinal muscles on the concave side. Secondary complications eventually arise as the child grows if the scoliosis remains uncorrected. Severe thoracic curves are associated with cardiopulmonary complications. Lung growth can be affected with considerable lung deformity and a permanent reduction in vital capacity. Torsion of the pulmonary arteries and aorta may occur where the curve is severe: these factors may cause cardiac anomalies in later life (Sharrard 1971). There is a relatively higher incidence of back pain in this group than in the normal population (Weinstein *et al.* 1981).

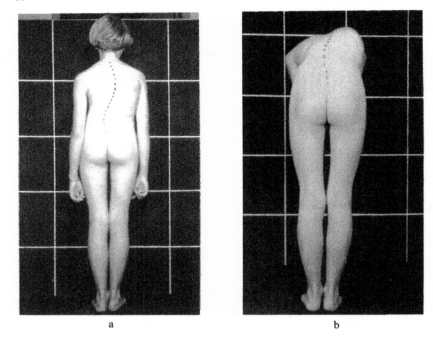

a   b

Figure 20.1 (a) Structural scoliosis with the primary curve convex to the right in the thoracic spine. (b) Bending forwards. Note the prominence of the ribs on the right side of the thorax.

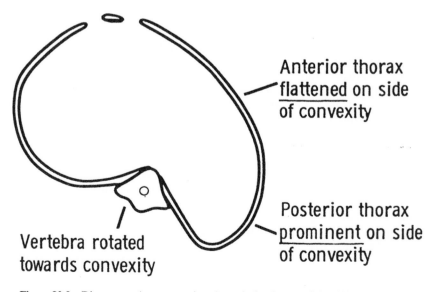

Anterior thorax
flattened on side
of convexity

Posterior thorax
prominent on side
of convexity

Vertebra rotated
towards convexity

Figure 20.2 Diagrammatic cross-section through the thorax of the child shown above, demonstrating the rib distortion.

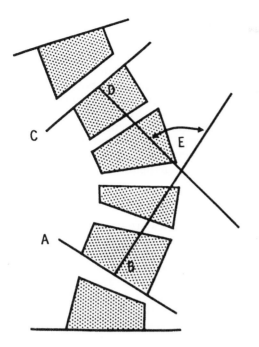

Figure 20.3 Cobb's method of measuring the primary curve. A = Lowest vertebra whose inferior surface tilts to the side of the concavity. B = Perpendicular drawn from the inferior surface of the distal vertebra. C = Highest vertebra whose superior surface tilts to the side of the concavity. D = Perpendicular drawn from the superior surface of the proximal vertebra. E = Intersecting angle measurement.

Aetiology

Scoliosis may be *idiopathic*, inferring the cause to be unknown. In a review article, Taylor *et al.* (1982) point out that the prevalence of adolescent idiopathic scoliosis is considerably greater in girls than in boys and that it is estimated that 2 per 1000 adolescents of those screened at school require active treatment. Idiopathic scoliosis is generally considered to be familial, inherited as a multifactorial genetic disorder (Filho and Thompson 1971; Nachemson and Sahlstrand 1977). Whether the primary pathology is a skeletal growth disturbance (Burwell and Dangerfield 1977) or due to a central nervous system dysfunction affecting motor control mechanisms remains unresolved, although theories abound. Asymmetrical growth at growth plates between the vertebral arches and vertebral bodies could lead to scoliosis (Knutsson 1963; Taylor 1980).

Children with idiopathic scoliosis have been found to have a greater postural sway pattern in standing (as measured by changes in centre of pressure) compared with healthy children (Sahlstrand *et al.* 1978). There have been other reports of disorders of balance mechanisms (e.g. Yamada *et al.* 1974). An association between idiopathic scoliosis and vestibulo-ocular reflex dysfunction has been postulated (Yamada *et al.* 1969) and the postural instability may be explained, therefore, by a conflict between visual and vestibular information within the brain centres which integrate and calibrate converging sensory data for the control of postural movement. The neurological picture suggests a functional involvement of the brainstem in the integration of afferent information from different sources essential for balance control (Nachemson and Sahlstrand 1977). More recent work suggests the muscle spindles in the paraspinal muscles may be implicated in idiopathic scoliosis (Low *et al.* 1983; Ford *et al.* 1988).

Scoliosis may be *congenital* in a baby born with such congenital spinal defects as hemivertebrae. It is termed *paralytic* when it is due to spinal muscle imbalance such as may occur as a result of myelomeningocele or poliomyelitis. In one study of the natural history of paralytic spinal deformity associated with myelomeningocele (Raycroft and Curtis 1972), 52% of 103 children with no vertebral anomaly apart from spina bifida developed scoliotic curves by the age of 10 years.

Paralytic scoliosis is an almost constant finding in the later stages of progressive muscular dystrophy, causing further respiratory complication. The spine in these dystrophic children collapses due to gradually increasing muscle weakness plus the effect of gravity, and eventually may become so misshapen that pressure areas are formed between the bony protuberances of the lower ribs and the pelvis. Cerebral palsied children with severe asymmetrical tonic spasms or hemiplegia and children with neurofibromatosis may also demonstrate scoliosis.

Assessment and treatment

The introduction of school screening programmes in many countries has decreased the percentage of children requiring surgery while increasing the use of spinal bracing and exercise in the management of the deformity (Torell *et al.* 1981; Liston 1981). Screening programmes are directed towards the early diagnosis of adolescent idiopathic scoliosis in the age group in which it typically develops – between 10 and 14 years of age (Taylor *et al.* 1982).

Screening assessment typically involves the forward-bending test (Fig. 20.1). Subsequent radiographic tests allow the calculation of the extent of lateral curvature using the Cobb method (Fig. 20.3).

It is not possible to predict with any accuracy which idiopathic scoliotic curves will increase in severity and which will not. A small proportion of adolescent curves less than 25° may regress spontaneously and the majority of the milder curves do not progress (Torell *et al.* 1981). However, curves greater than 25° frequently progress (Winter 1975) and the risk for progression is considered to be greatest in girls whose spinal curvature is detected before menarche (Lonstein and Carlson 1984) and in children whose initial degree of curvature was greatest (Bunnell 1983).

In the past claims have been made that certain methods of physical treatment have an effect upon the scoliotic deformity, either halting or slowing its progression, or correcting the deformity. None of these has been proved effective; the curvature in most cases relentlessly progresses, although it may become benign at adolescence. Bracing and surgery hold out the best hope for most children with scoliosis, and appear to correct the deformity in many cases. However, scoliosis remains a potentially disabling and sometimes fatal disorder.

Physiotherapy alone does not appear to be effective in preventing the deformity progressing when the curve has been established at 30–40°. However, it is suggested that exercise to maintain a full range of movement may prevent the subsequent development of deformity in children with delayed development (Lloyd-Roberts and Fixsen 1990).

The physiotherapist has a part to play in developing an exercise programme while the child is wearing a brace, in maintaining adequate respiratory function, particularly in those children with progressing paralytic curves, and in giving advice to parents and child about physical activities such as swimming. Such activities maintain as much mobi-

lity as possible, not only in the spine, but in the whole musculoskeletal system. It is probably true that activity helps maintain the child in the best possible general health. That the child should be kept as fit as possible, both physically and emotionally, is particularly important if surgery is likely, as most methods involve considerable insult to the system. Postoperatively the physiotherapist is responsible for the child's respiratory function, and for eventual mobilization and rehabilitation.

Bracing

Children whose curves are greater than 25° are usually given a spinal brace to wear. The goal of bracing is to use three-point fixation – one point at the apex of the curve, the others at two points of counterforce. The brace is typically worn for 23 hours a day. The Boston and Milwaukee braces are the most commonly used, with the Boston jacket and the electrospinal orthosis used in some centres. This latter involves transcutaneous electrical stimulation of muscle, applied while the child is asleep.

Plaster of Paris casts

The modified Risser localizer plaster (Risser 1955, 1964) is used in the treatment of younger children or milder curves in older children. The modification, the Cotrel EDF localizer cast (Cotrel and D'Amore 1966), includes traction (elongation), derotation and flexion of the lumbar spine. Casts are used to provide support for the growing spine to prevent further deformity, or, in the very young child, to maximize potential for spontaneous correction (Mehta and Morel 1979). They are also used preoperatively and before the application of a brace.

Seat moulds and other methods of splinting chair-bound scoliotic children are briefly described in Chapter 18.

Milwaukee brace

The brace described by Blount (1958) is, with some modifications, still in use, particularly where the curve has its apex at T8 or above. The brace provides longitudinal distraction and lateral pressure to correct the deformity and prevent progression. The traction element, together with pressure over the point of maximum convexity, corrects the curvature to some extent and prevents secondary contracture of the spinal muscles on the side of the concavity (Fig. 20.4). Distraction is exerted between the skull and the pelvis. The brace must be applied so that when pressure is on the occiput the mandible is free, therefore allowing the child to move the head, although in a limited way, and to eat comfortably. The degree of distraction can be increased by increasing the length of the anterior and posterior rods, and adjustment for growth is made in the same manner.

Early models of the Milwaukee brace caused lower-jaw deformities and dental problems. However, modifications to the headpiece have overcome this problem (Mellencamp *et al.* 1977).

Boston brace

This brace (Fig. 20.5), described by Watts *et al.* (1977), consists of pads applied laterally below the apex of each curve. It has been found to be effective in treating most curves. It is often preferred to the Milwaukee brace as it does not have the superstructure with headpiece and it can be worn under the clothes. When upper thoracic curves are present, a superstructure can be added.

Denis Browne splint

Scoliosis developing in the first year of an infant's life tends to resolve in the majority of cases (Lloyd-Roberts and Pilcher 1965). Browne (1956) designed a splint in which the infant could lie with the spine curved in the direction opposite the deformity.

Surgery

Surgical intervention consists of spinal fusion and is generally the treatment of choice when a curve is greater than 35–40° and brace treatment has failed or when curvature is greater than 50°. The spine is fused posteriorly in most cases, with Harrington or Luque rods (Harrington and Dickson 1973; Luque 1982). When scoliosis results from neuromuscular disease, an anterior fusion may be performed using the Dwyer (Dwyer 1969) or Zielke procedures. Surgery may be followed by early bracing or restricted activity.

Physical treatment

The aim of physiotherapy is the prevention, as far as possible, of those secondary problems

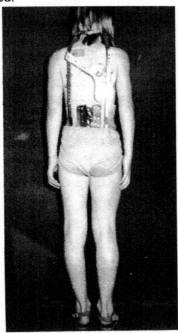
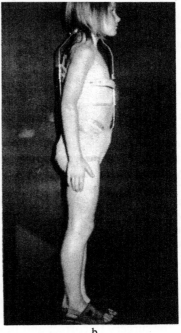

a
b

Figure 20.4 Milwaukee brace. (a) Note the pad over the convexity of the primary curve. (b) Traction is applied between the occiput and the pelvis.

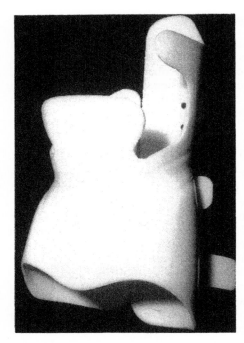

Figure 20.5   Modified Boston brace. (Courtesy of the Orthotics Department, Prince of Wales Hospital, Sydney, Australia.)

which may arise as a result of the skeletal deformity – poor respiratory function and lack of general mobility.

Respiratory function

Poor respiratory function is common and is due to the deformity of the thoracic cage and consequent poor rib mobility and lung expansion. The object of breathing exercises, which can be done daily by the child at home, is to develop respiratory function as effectively as possible despite the deformity of the thorax – that is, to mobilize the thorax and to obtain the most efficient ventilation possible. Parents are taught how to give the child postural drainage should a respiratory tract infection develop. Swimming or similar activities will also improve respiratory function and may be sufficient treatment for many children. This routine is, in addition, preoperative as some children will eventually be candidates for surgery to correct and fuse their spines. Respiratory function should be assessed at intervals (Chapter 27).

General mobility and strength

A daily exercise programme is an essential adjunct to bracing (Nash 1980). Exercises are typically performed both in and out of the brace. The major aims of exercise are to promote strength and control in trunk muscles and muscles linking limbs to the trunk, to maintain effective lung function and to encourage cardiovascular fitness. General mobility and strength are frequently poor, particularly in children whose scoliosis is due to muscle weakness or paralysis. However, children with severe idiopathic scoliosis are seldom energetic, and suffer a secondary lack of mobility and strength due to their deformity. It must be emphasized that no amount of enthusiasm on the part of the physiotherapist will mobilize the spine of a child with structural scoliosis where the loss of mobility is due to the skeletal deformity, but a programme of activity designed to maintain mobility in a general sense is of benefit to most children. Swimming is recommended as one of the best ways of combining mobility and improved respiratory function with sport and pleasure, and children can be taught how to swim different strokes, and how to swim under water. The therapist teaches the child exercises which will strengthen the trunk muscles, particularly the abdominals, as well as the muscles which link the limbs to the trunk. As in any strength-training programme, the number of repetitions and the weight lifted can be gradually increased. Exercises can be performed in two or three sets of the maximum repetitions. A child in a brace is encouraged to be as active as possible, and at periods during the day to stretch up in the brace to be as tall as possible. A daily stretching routine should also be established to maintain optimum muscle length, particularly in hamstrings, hip flexors and shoulder adductors and flexors.

Pre- and postoperative treatment

Preoperatively the physiotherapist measures the child's respiratory function and gives intensive breathing exercises with postural drainage if necessary for the few days before surgery. This is in order to maintain a clear airway and to ensure the child will be able to resume effective ventilation and an effective cough after surgery. The postoperative treatment depends upon the surgery performed. In general, an intensive period of breathing exercises is given for the first few days. If necessary, a respirator may be used to aid ventilation. As soon as possible the child is mobilized within the prescribed limits. It is not until all splinting is finally removed that the child can be fully rehabilitated, and this may be achieved by a period of exercise aimed at increasing mobility, strength, coordination and endurance, most of which can be accomplished by swimming practice and other activities which the child finds enjoyable.

Summary

Scoliosis may be a severely disabling progressive deformity, with distortion of the thoracic cage caused by rotation within the laterally curved spine. Treatment consists of casting or bracing, which correct the deformity by applying traction to the spine, followed by surgery, which gains further correction by internal devices and maintains correction by spinal fusion. Physical treatment has no effect on the scoliotic deformity, but is an important adjunct in improving respiratory function and general mobility.

References

Blount, W.P. (1958) Scoliosis and the Milwaukee brace. *Bull. Hosp. Joint Dis.*, **19**, 152.

Browne, D. (1956) Congenital postural scoliosis. *Proc. R. Soc. Med.*, **49**, 395.

Bunnell, W. (1983) A study of the natural history of idiopathic scoliosis. *Orthop. Trans.*, **7**, 6.

Burwell, R.G. and Dangerfield, P.H. (1977) Anthropometry and scoliosis. In: *Scoliosis: 5th Symposium*, edited by P.A. Zorab. London: Academic Press, pp. 123–164.

Cotrel, Y. and D'Amore, M. (1966) Spinal traction in scoliosis. In: *Proceedings of a Second Symposium on Scoliosis*, edited by P.A. Zorab. Edinburgh: Livingstone, pp. 37–43.

Dwyer, A.F. (1969) Experience of anterior correction of scoliosis. *Clin. Orthop.*, **62**, 192.

Filho, N.A. and Thompson, M.W. (1971) Genetic studies in scoliosis. *J. Bone Joint Surg.*, **53A**, 199.

Ford, D.M., Bagnall, K.M., Clements, C.A. and McFadden, K.D. (1988) Muscle spindles in the paraspinal musculature of patients with adolescent idiopathic scoliosis. *Spine*, **13**, 5, 461–465.

Harrington, P.R. and Dickson, J.H. (1973) An eleven-year clinical investigation of Harrington instrumentation. A preliminary report on 578 cases. *Clin. Orthop.*, **93**, 113–130.

Knutsson, F. (1963) A contribution to the discussion of the biological cause of idiopathic scoliosis. *Acta Orthop. Scand.*, **33**, 98.

Liston, C.B. (1981) An evaluation of school screening for scoliosis in Western Australia. *Aust. J. Physiother.*, **27**, 37.

Lloyd-Roberts, G.C. and Fixsen, J.A. (1990) *Orthopaedics in Infancy and Childhood*, 2nd edn. Oxford: Butterworth-Heinemann.

Lloyd-Roberts, G.C. and Pilcher, M.F. (1965) Structural idiopathic scoliosis in infancy. *J. Bone Joint Surg.* **47B**, 520.

Lonstein, J.E. and Carlson, J.M. (1984) The prediction of curve progression in untreated idiopathic scoliosis during growth. *J. Bone Joint Surg.*, **66A**, 1070.

Low, W.D., Chew, E.C., Kung, L.S., Hsu, L.C.S. and Leong, J.C.Y. (1983) Ultrastructure of nerve fibres and muscle spindles in adolescent idiopathic scoliosis. *Clin. Orthop.*, **174**, 217–221.

Luque, E.R. (1982) Postural curve correction. *Spine*, **7**, 3, 270–275.

Mehta, M.H. and Morel, G. (1979) The non-operative treatment of infantile idiopathic scoliosis. In: *Scoliosis*, edited by P.A. Zorab and D. Siegler. London: Academic Press, pp. 71–84.

Mellencamp, D.D., Blount, W.P. and Anderson, A.J. (1977) Milwaukee brace treatment of idiopathic scoliosis: late results. *Clin. Orthop. Rel. Res.*, **126**, 47.

Nachemson, A. and Sahlstrand, T. (1977) Etiologic factors in adolescent idiopathic scoliosis. *Spine*, **2**, 3, 176–184.

Nash, C.L. (1980) Scoliosis bracing. *J. Bone Joint Surg.*, **62A**, 5, 848.

Raycroft, J.F. and Curtis, B.H. (1972) Spinal curvature in myelomeningocele: natural history and etiology. In: *The American Academy of Orthopedic Surgeons Symposium on Myelomeningocele*, St Louis, MO: C.V. Mosby, pp. 186–201.

Risser, J.C. (1955) Application of body casts. *Instruction Course Lectures: American Academy of Orthopedic Surgery*, **12**, 255.

Risser, J.C. (1964) Scoliosis: past and present. *J. Bone Joint Surg.*, **46A**, 1.

Sahlstrand, T., Ortengren, R. and Nachemson, A. (1978) Postural equilibrium in adolescent idiopathic scoliosis. *Acta Orthop. Scand.*, **49**, 354.

Sharrard, W.J.W. (1971) *Paediatric Orthopaedics and Fractures*. Oxford: Blackwell.

Taylor, J.R. (1980) Vertebral genesis of scoliosis. *J. Anat.*, **130**, 197.

Taylor, J.R., Liston, C.B. and Twomey, L.T. (1982) Scoliosis: a review. *Aust. J. Physiother.*, **28**, 3, 20.

Torell, G., Nordwall, A. and Nachemson, A. (1981) The changing pattern of scoliosis treatment due to effective screening. *J. Bone Joint Surg.*, **63A**, 337.

Watts, H.C., Hall, J.E. and Stanish, W. (1977) The Boston brace system for the treatment of low thoracic and lumbar scoliosis by the use of a girdle without superstructure. *Clin. Orthop. Rel. Res.*, **126**, 87.

Weinstein, S.L., Zavala, D.C. and Ponseti, L.V. (1981) Idiopathic scoliosis. Long-term follow-up and prognosis in untreated patients. *J. Bone Joint Surg.*, **63**-A, 5, 702–711.

Winter, R.B. (1975) Scoliosis and other spinal deformities. *Acta Orthop. Scand.*, **46**, 401.

Yamada, K., Ikata, I., Yamamoto, H. *et al.* (1969) Equilibrium function in scoliosis and active plaster jacket for the treatment. *Tokushima J. Exp. Med.*, **16**, 1–7.

Yamada, K., Yamamoto, H., Tamura, T. *et al.* (1974) Development of scoliosis under neurological basis, particularly in relation with brain-stem abnormalities. *J. Bone Joint Surg.*, **56**-A, 1764.

Further reading

Cassella, M.C. and Hall, J.E. (1991) Current treatment approaches in the nonoperative and operative management of adolescent idiopathic scoliosis. *Phys. Ther.*, **71**, 12, 897–909.

Cobb, J.R. (1948) Outline for study of scoliosis. *Instruction Course Lectures: American Academy of Orthopedic Surgery*, **5**, 261.

James, J. (1956) Paralytic scoliosis. *J. Bone Joint Surg.*, **38B**, 660.

Moe, J.H. (1980) Modern concepts of treatment of spinal deformities. *Clin. Orthop. Rel. Res.*, **150**, 137.

21

Inflammatory disorders of soft tissues and joints

Rheumatic diseases are characterized by inflammation of connective tissue with arthritis or inflammation of a joint a frequent manifestation. Juvenile chronic or rheumatoid arthritis (JCA) is the most common type of chronic arthritis in children (Cassidy and Petty 1990). Other diseases in this group of disorders include dermatomyositis, scleroderma, juvenile ankylosing spondylitis and systemic lupus erythematosus. Children affected with any of the disorders in this group suffer loss of function due to the inflammatory process involving the soft tissues, and in the case of rheumatoid arthritis, the bones and articular cartilages as well.

The loss of function is due to loss of range of movement which occurs as the result of pain, protective muscle spasm, contracture of soft tissues surrounding the joint, and in some cases of chronic arthritis and haemophilia, to ankylosis of the joint. Loss of function is also due to muscle weakness and loss of coordinated movement of the limbs and trunk, due principally to disuse, but in some cases to emotional disturbances in an anxious child who feels an invalid.

It is in order to minimize or prevent loss of function that children are referred to the physiotherapist for treatment.

The terminology and classification of the chronic arthropathies of childhood are more difficult than they are in adult rheumatoid arthritis and they vary throughout the world. The condition called JCA is one of a diverse collection of chronic arthropathies (Fig. 21.1) manifesting themselves in many different ways.

```
JUVENILE CHRONIC ARTHRITIS (Still's Disease)
        Systemic onset
        Polyarticular
                Seronegative
                Seropositive
        Pauciarticular
                Early onset
                Late onset

SPONDYLARTHROPATHY
        Juvenile ankylosing spondylitis
        Reiter's syndrome
        Psoriatic arthropathy
        Reactive arthropathy
        Enteropathic arthropathy

OTHER RHEUMATIC DISEASES IN CHILDHOOD
        Systemic lupus erythematosus
        Vascular syndromes
        Dermatomyositis
        Scleroderma
```

Figure 21.1 Types of chronic arthritis in childhood.

Juvenile chronic arthritis (Still's disease)

JCA differs from adult chronic arthritis in several respects, including the occurrence of secondary growth disturbance, the frequent absence of pain and stiffness in the presence of impaired function, the rapid development of fixed soft tissue contractures, and involvement of the eye. In addition, most children have a negative blood test for rheumatoid factor (Brewer *et al.* 1982).

JCA manifests itself in children as either a generalized systematic disease involving many joints, or as a disease apparently localized to a few joints with few systemic symptoms.

Three subtypes are usually described:

1 Systemic, with multiple joint involvement.
2 Polyarticular, with five or more joints involved with a symmetrical distribution.
3 Pauciarticular, with four or less joints involved, usually with asymmetrical involvement. The knee is the most commonly affected joint, then the ankle and the elbow in this latter subtype.

Those children with a generalized disease may present with more obviously systemic symptoms than arthritic, with pyrexia, rash, general malaise, anaemia, and occasionally pericarditis, as well as the peripheral symptoms of warm swollen joints, tenderness, muscle spasm, pain, tenosynovitis, muscle weakness and wasting.

JCA is rarely seen in children of less than 1 year of age. Its aetiology is unknown. Possible factors implicated include a genetic predisposition, autoimmunity (Brewer *et al.* 1982), infection and trauma (Cassidy 1982). There is also some question whether it may be based on psychodynamic factors (Rimón *et al.* 1977). Onset may be a gradual development of symptoms, or a sudden acute flare-up. Symptoms may exacerbate and remit throughout the course of the disease. In a large percentage of affected children stress, trauma, infection or inoculation can reactivate the disease, even in adult life (Stoeber 1977).

Prognosis in uncontrolled cases may be poor, with the child progressing to a stage where ill health, blindness, deafness and eventually death occur. In the majority of cases, however, the disease eventually becomes inactive.

No single laboratory test confirms the diagnosis of JCA. In the acute systemic form, anaemia, elevated erythrocyte sedimentation rate and leukocytosis are prominent findings.

Pathology

The pathophysiological mechanism involves a chronic non-suppurative inflammation of the synovium. The earliest changes are periarticular oedema with little synovial reaction or joint effusion. However, synovial inflammation soon becomes apparent. The thickened synovium protrudes into the joint space, and may result in erosion and eventual destruction of the articular cartilage. If the disease progresses, synovial tissue will fill the joint space causing narrowing and fibrous ankylosis, and bony fusion may eventually destroy the joint (Behrmann and Vaughan 1987; Cassidy and Petty 1990).

Thus the swelling – a constant finding in affected children – is due to periarticular oedema, joint effusion and synovial thickening. The loss of movement found on examination may be due in the early stages to protective muscle spasm, but eventually to actual joint destruction and ankylosis. The inflammatory process extends to the tendons and tendon sheaths, and to the muscles. Osteoporosis may occur in the vicinity of the involved joints. Growth may be interfered with, being either slowed or hastened, and this is due to involvement of the epiphyseal centres, which may prematurely fuse (Ansell 1977). Any joint may be involved, but the most commonly affected in children are the wrist, metacarpophalangeal, ankle, subtaloid, knee, hip and temporomandibular joints, and the joints of the cervical spine.

Uveitis, a potentially scarring eye disease, is an insidious complication, usually associated with early-onset pauciarticular JCA. Early recognition and treatment are essential to the preservation of vision.

Joint destruction once it occurs has generally been considered to be irreversible, partly because early studies (Bywaters 1937) showed cartilage to exhibit very limited powers of repair. There is some evidence that this may not be so. Bernstein *et al.* (1977) described 6 children with long-standing rheumatoid arthritis and radiological evidence of severe hip joint damage, who were found to have radiological evidence of widening of joint space and remodelling of articular surfaces. The authors consider that control of the inflammatory disease was a necessary prerequisite for the apparent hip joint restoration. A common factor was vigorous physiotherapy with emphasis on increasing muscle strength and ambulation and on avoiding inactivity. There is evidence from animal experiments (Thompson and Bassett 1970; Kirivanta *et al.* 1987) that joint immobility results in degeneration and necrosis of cartilage in areas of articular compression and in the contact-free area.

Bernstein *et al.* (1977) suggested that there may be an equilibrium between reparative processes and destructive processes, and that the growth potential of children may be the principal factor in shifting the balance towards repair if vigorous medical and physical measures are used.

Dermatomyositis

This disease is also characterized by a non-suppurative inflammatory process, involving widespread vascular changes in the connective tissue of skin, muscle, fat and small nerves. It is rarely seen before the age of 2 years. Its aetiology is not well-defined. A variety of causes are implicated, including viral agents. A genetic predisposition is likely. The disease may develop slowly, with the usual presenting symptoms being a symmetrical muscle weakness which develops insidiously in the proximal muscles of the extremities, trunk and neck muscles, with some children experiencing pain and tenderness. Children may demonstrate difficulty climbing stairs, standing up without using their arms, as well as difficulty lifting heavy objects and combing their hair.

Weakness may also involve palatal, pharyngeal and oesophageal musculature. The clinical picture may be very varied, and include a rash or dry scaly areas usually on the face, extensor surface of knees and elbows and dorsal surface of hands, and subcutaneous calcifications. All muscles may eventually be affected. Involvement of respiratory and swallowing muscles may lead to death.

Pathology

Behrmann and Vaughan (1987) describe the most prominent lesion in children as a vasculitis involving capillaries, arterioles and venules in the connective tissue of the skin, subcutaneous tissue, muscles and gastrointestinal tract. In the affected muscles, cells show features of both degeneration and regeneration:

variation of fibre size, fibre necrosis and basophilia of some fibres with centralis of nuclei. Fibre atrophy may be severe at the periphery of the muscle fascicule.

In the affected skin there is a thinning of the epidermis, oedema and vasculitis in the dermis. Soft tissue calcification occurs in approximately one-third of affected children. Calcium may extrude through the skin, producing painful sores.

The skin over the affected parts appears tight and shiny. Eventually it may atrophy and become bound down to subcutaneous tissues. The progress of the disease eventually slows, but although it may become inactive, the child may be left with marked residual disability due to contractures and deformity. It is to prevent or minimize this disability that the child is referred for physiotherapy. Muscles are tender and painful when the disease is active and exercise cannot be started until pain and tenderness have subsided.

There is evidence of improved prognosis following corticosteroid therapy (Sullivan *et al.* 1972). The improvement which follows the initially high dosage allows the child to participate more actively in physiotherapy. Thoracic expansion exercises will be necessary if there is intercostal muscle involvement.

Scleroderma (systemic sclerosis)

This uncommon condition is a chronic inflammatory disorder of unknown aetiology affecting the small blood vessels and connective tissue. It may affect the skin alone or involve internal organs as well. It is characterized by typical skin lesions called morphea. These lesions are at first either erythematous or atrophic, but later become indurated and may enlarge to involve an extensive area of the body. Inflammatory changes may occur and the skin may be bound down to subcutaneous tissues, with resultant contractures of the affected part. Fibrosis may also involve the heart, lungs, kidneys, gastrointestinal tract and synovium.

A child with scleroderma may develop Raynaud's phenomenon and will need to minimize exposure to cold in order to control the tendency to vasospasm. The active disease may spontaneously arrest or continue as a chronic state for a long time. In some children it may be rapidly fatal. Physiotherapy is important in the early stages of the skin lesions to minimize contractures and loss of function. Facial muscle exercises may be necessary to minimize contracture of soft tissues of the face which restrict mouth-opening and facial expression.

Juvenile ankylosing spondylitis

Ankylosis of the spine with thoracic kyphosis commonly occurs as a result of the spondyloarthropathy (Schaller 1977). Additional involvement of sternal and costovertebral joints and more proximal limb joints also occurs.

Maintenance of normal postural alignment, particularly of the spine and hips, is the major goal of physiotherapy. Activities such as swimming (crawl, breaststroke, backstroke) can be enjoyable ways of exercising spinal and lower-limb extensor muscles with the joints aligned in extension. Such activity also promotes deep breathing with increased thoracic expansion. Table and chair heights at school and for school homework should be monitored as the child grows to ensure appropriate spinal alignment.

Management of inflammatory disorders

The overall goals of the health care team in a child afflicted with one of these disorders are to decrease joint inflammation, relieve pain, optimize function and fitness, and provide support and information for the child and family. All treatment is directed to this end, and it is hoped that the child will be referred to the physiotherapist in time for an attempt at prevention to be made. In severe manifestations of these disorders it may be difficult to prevent some degree of disability occurring, because of the rapidity with which the inflammatory process may progress. Nevertheless, the various members of the health care team must strive for a positive attitude towards treatment, aiming for normal function and not setting limitations, either consciously or unconsciously, for the child.

Anti-inflammatory drugs, such as the salicylates, are prescribed for these children. Corticosteroids are only given in certain circumstances, their side-effects making them a contraindication for all but the most severe and uncontrollable cases. Pain as a warning signal may not be felt by the child following drug therapy and the therapist must bear this in mind during treatment. Pain is not a prominent feature in JCA, and severity of pain is therefore not a good indicator of the severity of this disease or the activity of the disease process (Scott *et al.* 1977).

Physiotherapy varies according to whether or not pain and inflammation are controlled by medication. For example, during stages of acute illness as yet uncontrolled by medication, rest, heat or cold applications and encouragement of relevant functional activities of daily life may be all the child can tolerate. However, once the acute illness is controlled, the child can begin an active exercise programme to increase function and fitness.

Physical treatment, for convenience of description, is discussed under three headings:

1 Relief of pain.
2 Optimization of mobility, strength, function and fitness.
3 Teaching of a home programme.

Rest is important, particularly during exacerbations in children with rheumatoid arthritis, but rest does not mean immobilization. Periods of inactivity are not advisable. They are instead encouraged to lead active lives with appropriate periods of rest, with the intention of preventing loss of mobility. Children with arthritis complain of stiffness and a feeling of 'seizing up' when they get up in the morning, and after any period of prolonged immobility. Most physicians are in agreement that the child should spend as little time in bed, especially in hospital, as possible. Similarly, if splinting is used, it is to rest a painful limb, not to immobilize it, and splints must be designed so they can easily be removed.

These can be depressing disorders, and a concerted effort must be made to prevent the affected child from lapsing into a state of emotional invalidism out of proportion to the physical disability. Pain and the fear of it plus muscle weakness, combine to increase anxiety. Well-planned treatment, practical advice to parents, and an encouraging approach from the physiotherapist will help the child be active and to develop emotionally and physically. Where pain and protective spasm are inhibiting movement they must be relieved. Where a child is too anxious to move freely, the physiotherapist will find ways of encouragment. As much treatment as possible should be done at home, the parents being supervised by the physiotherapist at regular intervals.

Assessments are important in establishing the child's particular problems. The American Rheumatism Association (1982) has defined four categories that describe the various degrees to which musculoskeletal difficulties may interfere with function. Joint range is measured with a goniometer. Muscle strength is tested by charting of individual muscles where there is evidence of weakness, with emphasis on antigravity muscles.

The Schober test of lumbosacral mobility, which gives normative values (Cassidy and Petty 1990), gives information about maximum linear excursion between two identified points 5 and 10 cm above a surface landmark as the child flexes fowards maximally in standing.

Posture in sitting and standing can be recorded for comparative evaluation by photographing the child in a standardized manner. Similarly, critical functional activities such as sit-to-stand, reaching for an object, walking and stair-climbing, can be recorded on videotape using standardized procedures. A checklist of critical biomechanical characteristics (for example, see Chapter 3) can be used to provide informative details of such actions. The attachment of body markers over joints before videotaping will allow objective measures such as joint angular displacements, to be taken off either on a sheet of transparency paper or using a digitizing tablet. Significant differences in velocity, cadence and stride length compared to normal have been found in walking (Lechner *et al.* 1987). Of particular interest was the significant decrease in hip extension and ankle plantarflexion at toe-off, which is a major factor interfering with stride length, resulting in an adaptive forward-tilt pelvic position.

It has been suggested that functional actions should be tested on the basis of ability to perform independently, speed of performance and endurance (the capacity to perform multiple repetitions of the action (DeNardo *et al.* 1990; Rhodes 1991)). It should also be noted whether or not the child utilizes adaptive behaviours such as using hands for support in standing or to increase propulsive effort in standing up.

Objective testing as an indication of progress and the effects of treatment or training is critical (MacBain and Hill 1973; Coulton *et al.* 1987; Rhodes *et al.* 1988; Lovell *et al.* 1989).

Relief of pain

Pain is not a constant finding in these conditions, but it does occur at one time or another, and in varying degrees of severity in most cases.

Pain results in protective spasm of the muscles surrounding the painful area, and because it is usually the flexors rather than the extensors which protectively spasm, the part involved is held in a position of flexion. Due to the inability of these muscles to relax and lengthen in reciprocation, movement is inhibited, the child being unable to move or wary of moving the part. Pain, or fear of pain, results in protective spasm and loss of movement. It follows that all physical treatment must be painfree if the aim of treatment is to encourage the fullest, most functional movement possible.

Pain during or immediately after treatment may indicate overstretching and damage to soft tissues, and this also causes a limitation rather than the hoped-for gain in range of movement. Moreover, painful treatment will certainly alienate the child, who can hardly be blamed for rejecting further attempts of the physiotherapist at treatment.

Methods for the relief of pain and protective muscle spasm, apart from drug therapy, include rest, heat in the form of warm packs and wax, and cold in the form of ice packs.

Superficial heating does not appear to raise intra-articular temperature (Hollander and Horvath 1949) nor affect inflammatory processes (Mainardi *et al.* 1979). Both heat and cold have been shown to raise the pain threshold (Lehmann *et al.* 1958; Benson and Copp 1974). Ultrasound raises intra-articular temperature and, since it appears to increase the plastic extensibility of ligamentous structures, may be a useful adjunct to stretching exercises (Lehmann *et al.* 1970). Rhodes (1991) suggests the use of transcutaneous electrical nerve stimulation (TENS) for children with one or two painful joints. TENS appears to provide pain relief, allowing gentle active exercise during an exacerbation of symptoms.

Rest

It has been suggested above that rest does not mean immobilization. Where there is pain the child may need periods of bed rest. A limb or part of a limb may be rested effectively in a light splint, which will help maintain the optimum position of the limb. Splints may be of plaster, aluminium or thermoplastic material. They should be padded and well-fitting, light and as simple as possible. When making splints, it should be remembered that there will be a tendency to flex a painful joint. The ankle joint tends to fall into plantarflexion, and will need to be splinted in a plantigrade position. The knee is splinted in extension, although not hyperextension. A knee flexion deformity is easily acquired in rheumatoid arthritis and causes great handicap. The foot must not be allowed to flex at the mid tarsal joints or metatarsophalangeal joints. When the hips are involved, the child may spend part of a rest period in prone. It is important that the feet are over the end of the bed to ensure a good position for knees and ankles. The wrist is rested in an extended position and is not allowed to fall into ulnar deviation; the thumb in abduction with some opposition; the fingers in slight flexion. No joint is allowed to remain splinted day and night. It cannot be stressed enough that splinting is a means of resting a painful part of a limb. A splint is made so it fulfils this requirement yet does not allow the joint to become stiff or to assume an unnatural position. Once pain is no longer a problem the splint can be removed.

Heat

Care must be taken during any application of heat not to burn the delicate and sometimes atrophic skin. It is a good precaution to test temperature sensation before the application of either heat or cold. *Warm packs* are probably the most practical and most effective form of applying heat. They can be applied at home to relieve pain and protective spasm and should precede the active part of treatment. Towels may be heated in the oven or in hot water, in which case they must be thoroughly wrung out, and they are wrapped around the part of the limb involved. They are changed every few moments as the heat soon dissipates, and the total period of application need not exceed 7–10 minutes, although this depends on the effect.

Heated wax is a useful means of applying heat to the hands, particularly in children with dermatomyositis, and the wax has the added effect of being a lubricant for the skin. This also can be easily done at home. The wax remains on the hands for approximately 10 minutes, and is followed by active movement.

Cold

For some children, cold is more effective for relieving pain and protective spasm in inflammatory disorders than heat, although care should be taken that the application of cold is not intolerable and that it does not cause the child to feel stiff. In a child with residual deformity due to soft tissue contracture, cold may be a useful means, if combined with mobilizing techniques, of gaining more range of movement.

Cold is applied by towelling which has been soaked in flaked ice and water and wrung out to remove as much moisture as possible. The towels are reapplied every minute for approximately 5–10 minutes, in such a way that the part is kept constantly cold. If they are left on for too long they absorb heat from the body and the required effect is lost. The towels are wrapped around the part to be treated. In the case of hamstrings, for example, care is taken to apply the cold to the entire length of the muscle, and not just to the part nearest the joint. For the use of cold to be effective, gentle peripheral joint mobilizing techniques, or active exercises to increase muscle length and joint range must be done either during the application of the towels, or immediately afterwards, before the effect of the cold has been dissipated.

Optimization of mobility, strength, function and fitness

For both their physical and emotional development these children need to participate as fully as possible in normal daily activities. This means that parents need to be aware of what their child can do.

No matter how local and peripheral the inflammatory process may be, the physiotherapist must remember to treat the child as an individual whose entire function as a child is disturbed because of this one part which cannot perform normally.

Pain and protective spasm must be relieved, joint range increased and muscles strengthened, and all by specific techniques directed locally at the affected part. All these techniques are a way of enabling the child to move more normally. Treatment ends prematurely if it consists only of warm packs and techniques directed at the affected limb. The effect of mobilizing and strengthening techniques becomes consolidated if the child is encouraged to use the affected limb in conjunction with the rest of the body in some appropriate functional action (see Chapter 3).

Techniques such as contract–relax may be effective for lengthening shortened muscles in the short term. It is likely, however, that a combination of active stretching during practice of specific functional activities will have a more long-term effect. Muscles adapt their length to the demands placed upon them and this is typical of non-disabled as well as disabled individuals. Length of calf muscles can be maintained (or increased) by a combination, for example, of sit-to-stand and step-up-and-down exercises, together with passive stretching in standing (see Figs 3.19 and 3.20). These exercises utilize body weight to apply stretch. In addition, the active stretch is applied during the first two actions by angular displacement at the ankle imposed by the requirements of the actions themselves. It is necessary for some supervision of practice or a feedback device to ensure the necessary angular displacements take place.

Take, for example, a child with rheumatoid arthritis affecting a knee. Warm packs or ice may relieve protective spasm in hamstrings, plus techniques to gain full-range flexion and extension of the knee and to strengthen flexors and extensors. These modalities are very specific. The child will also be encouraged to use the knee in as normal a manner as possible in everyday actions. Activities such as those described below may form part of an exercise programme:

1   Sitting on a stool, moving around the stool as quickly as possible to face the other direction. Feet must be on the floor during weight shift (to encourage weight-bearing and the ability to coordinate movement of limbs and trunk).

2   Sitting on a stool to standing (to lengthen calf muscles and strengthen lower limb extensors, as well as to train effective sit-to-stand). If this action is too difficult because of decreased muscle strength and/or range of movement at lower-limb joints, the child can practise from a higher than normal seat. The action should be done with multiple repetitions in order to increase muscle strength and provide active stretch to muscles with a tendency to shorten.

3   Walking in footsteps drawn on the floor (for a gait with even steps and to encourage hip extension/ankle plantarflexion plus equal weight-bearing on each foot).

4   Walking in the rungs of a ladder laid on the floor (for balance and controlled walking).

5   Treadmill walking.

These activities are merely suggestions to illustrate how a child may be persuaded to use the knee in movements which involve the whole body. They can be made simpler or more complex depending on the age of the child, the number of joints affected and the severity of the involvement. Activities should be designed to encourage the child's best effort and they should be fun. Feedback devices already exist and can be designed to be entertaining and to encourage the best effort. The child may need to be shown what he or she is capable of doing, that is, he or she may need to be surprised by what is possible. However, whatever activity is given, it should not produce pain.

For the child with pain, or for the very anxious child, *hydrotherapy* and swimming make useful adjuncts to treatment. Water temperature should not exceed 34°C or it will be too enervating, and the child should not stay in the water longer than 15–20 minutes. Activities again will need to be adjusted according to the child's disability, age and temperament. Movements and games in a pool can be great fun and are better if treated more as a swimming lesson than as treatment. The child is taught simple swimming techniques, kicking with a board and dog paddle, and these can be progressed to breast-stroke swimming and the crawl, and to backstroke. By this stage the child should be attending the heated pool nearest home for professional instruction, or just to practise. Swimming with the face in the water, ducking under the water to retrieve a toy, blowing a ping-pong ball along the surface all improve breathing control in children with some thoracic involvement. Children who experience pain in weight-bearing joints on walking and who are otherwise confined to bed may be able to stand and walk with the help of the buoyancy of the water. Games with other children can be devised to encourage certain movements which need to be practised. The Halliwick method of swimming (Reid Campion 1991) provides an enjoyable combination of water activities and group involvement.

Splinting may sometimes be necessary to increase range and may be in the form of serial plaster splints or wedged plaster cylinders.

Assistive devices, such as walkers, crutches or sticks, may be necessary in the short term for a child with severe involvement. However, care needs to be taken that such an aid does not impose abnormal weight-bearing stress on the upper-limb joints. Dynamic splinting may be used to reduce contractures if static splinting is ineffective. Surgery, such as hip adductor and psoas muscle tenotomies (Swann 1990), may be necessary if soft tissues over a joint become severely contracted. Total hip or knee arthroplasty may be necessary for some children (Ruddleston *et al.* 1986; Scott 1990).

Hand function

Where part of the hand is involved, particular care must be taken to preserve or regain full wrist extension, thumb abduction, pincer, palmar and ulnar grasp and release. Such activities as described below may be used:

1 Playing with plasticine (emphasis on making different objects).
2 Squeezing a plastic ball with retractable knobs (for pincer grasp).
3 Hammering wooden pegs (for palmar grasp and radial extension).
4 Screwing and unscrewing wooden nuts and bolts (for palmar and pincer grasp combined with forearm movement).
5 Dressing and undressing dolls (for dexterity).

Manipulative activities are given according to the child's age and preference, as well as disability. They should not be aimless, and the child should see a definite result for the effort. Peripheral mobilizing techniques, such as those described by Kaltenborn (1980) and Maitland (1991), may be useful in preventing loss of function. Where the physiotherapist and the occupational therapist work together, as they should with the management of a child with this type of disability, the development or restoration of hand function may be their joint responsibility.

Postural development should be carefully assessed as the child grows, and deviations corrected by muscle-lengthening or strengthening techniques, relaxation techniques and by methods of improving postural awareness.

Respiratory function

It has been pointed out above that disorders of growth may occur in children with severe arthritis, and these children, as well as those suffering from dermatomyositis and scleroderma will benefit from exercises and activities designed to increase the mobility and expansion of the thorax as well as increasing respiratory efficiency. Some children, especially those with generalized disease, require regular testing of their ventilatory efficiency, and this may be done as described in Chapter 27. For these children, and for those who tend to be inactive, breathing exercises directed at expanding the lower ribs and the ribs laterally and apically are done at home each day. Should infection of the lower respiratory tract occur, parents will have been taught techniques of postural drainage and so will be able to commence them as soon as necessary.

Rhodes (1991) refers to two unpublished studies on fitness in children with JCA. In one study which examined the maximal oxygen uptake of a group of children, these children were found to be significantly less fit than a group of their peers without JCA (Jasso *et al.* 1986). Another study investigated the effect of aerobic exercise in a pool in a small group of children with JCA compared to a group who had non-aerobic exercise in the pool. The authors found that the subjects in the aerobic exercise programme showed a significant decrease in resting heart rate and no signs of deterioration in JCA-related measures such as sedimentation rate and morning stiffness. It seems very likely, therefore, that children with JCA would benefit from exercising for fitness three or four times a week, either in a pool or on a bicycle.

Teaching of a home programme

The child should spend as little time as possible in hospital and this applies also to visits to the physiotherapist. Treatment is planned so it can be carried out at home with a minimum of effort for the parents and with maximum amount of effect and pleasure for the child. The physiotherapist assesses the child at regular intervals, plans treatment, teaches the parents how to carry out treatment at home, and regularly supervises this. It is sometimes necessary for the child to be treated by the physiotherapist more frequently when in hospital or if developing contractures or any other specific difficulty, but outpatient visits should be kept to a minimum. It has to be remembered that none of these disorders occurs briefly, and that it is unrealistic to expect parent and child to attend for treatment frequently over a prolonged period. Similarly, this is kept in mind when planning home treatment, which should be short and to the point, with the possibility of some variation to prevent the child becoming bored.

The child should sleep on a firm mattress with a small pillow, especially with cervical rheumatoid arthritis. Desk and chair should be of appropriate height so the child can sit with flat feet on the floor and thighs and back supported. The desk should be high enough to allow the forearms to rest on it comfortably. The child should be encouraged to be as active as possible, but to take periods of rest when necessary.

Parents are shown how to apply any necessary splinting, how to give wax to the hands, warm or cold packs, breathing exercises and postural drainage if necessary. They are encouraged to take the child swimming in the local heated pool. Riding a tricycle or bicycle will also help the child keep mobile. The child must be allowed to dress himself, including buttons and shoelaces, even if it does take a little longer than necessary.

One of the major problems for the child, particularly approaching adolescence, is difficulty relating a desire to lead a 'normal' life with the need to exercise caution in everything that is done. The outward appearance of normalcy makes this task even more difficult. In adolescence, the capacity to control one's own body is threatened. The child may have difficulty developing independence. Encouragement to play sport (e.g. swimming, water polo), develop hobbies and interests (e.g. birdwatching, bicycling) and to join clubs may help at this time.

Haemophilia

This is a chronic, hereditary and incurable disease resulting from a congenital deficiency in blood coagulation factors. It is a sex-linked recessive disorder affecting males. The first signs of haemophilia do not appear until the third trimester of infancy, and sometimes not until the second or third year.

Haemorrhage occurs recurrently within any part of the body, but it is haemorrhages into the joints and soft tissues of the limbs which cause the most disability, and it is the weight-bearing joints, particularly the knee, elbow or ankle, that are most commonly the sites of repeated haemarthroses.

Mechanism of haemarthrosis

When trauma occurs in or around a joint, haemorrhage may be severe, causing rapid onset of local swelling, pain, heat and tension, and pressure on nerves and soft tissues. As a result of repeated episodes the synovial lining cells and the connective tissue in the joint capsule proliferate. There will eventually be a lack of nutrition to the articular cartilage, the surface of which becomes irregular and pitted. There is a risk of ultimate subluxation, instability and loss of range of movement and function, as occurs in the end-stage of any destructive arthropathy (Harris and Saidi 1988). Muscles become fibrosed and with other soft tissues may contract. The most commonly involved nerve is the femoral, which is associated with haemorrhage into the sheath of the iliacus muscle (Goodfellow *et al.* 1967), and which takes several months to recover function.

Treatment

It seems that joint destruction and deformity can be prevented or minimized in many cases by prompt recognition of an episode of bleeding and early replacement of the missing clotting factor, which involves the child's parents, as well as the physician and physiotherapist. The parents will have to be educated about the dangers to their child even in earliest infancy, and will have to exercise care in the selection of toys, and supervise activities more than normal. Emphasis is on strengthening muscles surrounding the at-risk weight-bearing joints, with the intention of minimizing the likelihood of trauma to the area and of protecting the joints. Cryoprecipitate is frequently given as a prophylactic, enabling greater continuity of rehabilitation.

The child may be hospitalized after severe intra-articular haemorrhage. During this acute period of anti-inflammatory measures, replacement of deficient clotting factor, cold packs and, in the case of weight-bearing joints, bed rest are instituted, with immobilization in a plaster back slab or compression bandage, which is continued until pain, effusion and protective spasm have subsided.

Joint aspiration may be necessary if effusion is very tense. The joint is rested in a functional position, the knee, for example, in extension. Active remobilization begins as soon as an acute phase subsides. Isometric contractions are effective for regaining some control over a muscle group prior to active movement. Mobilizing techniques are used carefully in a pain-free range. Treatment in a pool is a useful adjunct for mobilizing and ambulation.

The child should be encouraged to be active in non-body-contact sports and to carry out exercises and activities designed to strengthen muscles and increase movement control, particularly of the lower limbs.

Summary

Inflammatory diseases affecting soft tissues and joints interfere with movement by causing pain and protective muscle spasm, soft tissue contracture and, in some cases, ankylosis. Physical treatment is aimed at enabling the child to grow and develop with a minimum of musculoskeletal deviation and deformity. It consists principally of methods of relieving pain and protective spasm, of strengthening muscles, increasing flexibility, encouraging movement and of training functional movement and physical fitness.

References

American Rheumatism Association (1982) *Dictionary of the Rheumatic Diseases*, vol. 1: Signs and symptoms. New York: American Rheumatism Association, p. 71.

Ansell, B.M. (1977) Joint manifestations in children with juvenile chronic polyarthritis. *Arthritis Rheum.*, **20**, 204–206.

Behrmann, R.E. and Vaughan, V.C. (1987) *Nelson Textbook of Paediatrics*, 13th edn. Philadelphia, PA: W.B. Saunders.

Benson, T.B. and Copp, E.P. (1974) The effect of therapeutic forms of heat and ice on the pain threshold of the normal shoulder. *Rheum. Rehabil.*, **13**, 101.

Bernstein, B. *et al.* (1977) Hip joint restoration in juvenile rheumatoid arthritis. *Arthritis Rheum.*, **20**, 5, 1099–1104.

Brewer, E.J., Giannini, E.H. and Pearson, D.A. (1982) *Juvenile Rheumatoid Arthritis*. Philadelphia, PA: W.B. Saunders.

Bywaters, E.G.L. (1937) The metabolism of joint tissues. *J. Pathol. Bacteriol.*, **44**, 247–268.

Cassidy, J.T. (1982) *Textbook of Pediatric Rheumatology*. New York: John Wiley.

Cassidy, J.T. and Petty, R.E. (1990) Juvenile rheumatoid arthritis. In: *Textbook of Rheumatology*, edited by J.T. Cassidy and R.E. Petty. 2nd edn. New York: Churchill Livingstone.

Coulton, C.J., Zborowsky, E., Lipton, J. *et al.* (1987) Assessment of the reliability and validity of the arthritis impact measurement scales for children with juvenile rheumatoid arthritis. *Arthritis Rheum*, **30**, 819–824.

DeNardo, B.S., Rhodes, V.J., Gibbons, B. *et al.* (1990) *Physical Therapy Standards of Care for Children with Chronic Arthritis*. Boston, MA: The Affiliated Children's Arthritis Centers of New England.

Goodfellow, J., Fearn, C.B. and Matthews, J.M. (1967) Iliacus haematoma. A common complication of haemophilia. *J. Bone Joint Surg.*, **49B**, 748.

Harris, E.D. and Saidi, P. (1988) Hemophilic arthropathy. In: *Primer on the Rheumatic Diseases*, edited by H.R. Schumacher. 9th edn. Atlanta, GA: Arthritis Foundation.

Hollander, J.L. and Horvath, S.M. (1949) The influence of physical therapy procedures on intra-articular temperature of normal and arthritic subjects. *Am. J. Sci. Med.*, **218**, 543–548.

Jasso, M.S., Protas, E.J., Giannini, E.H. *et al.* (1986) Physical work capacity (PWC) in juvenile rheumatoid arthritis (JRA) patients and healthy children. Presented at the *Annual Meeting of the American Rheumatism Association/American Health Planning Association*. New Orleans, LA.

Kaltenborn, F.M. (1980) *Mobilisation of the Extremity Joints*, 3rd edn. Oslo: Olaf Norlis Bokhandel.

Kirivanta, I., Jurvelin, J., Tammi, M. *et al.* (1987) Weightbearing controls glycosaminoglycan concentration and articular cartilage in the knee joints of young beagle dogs. *Arthritis Rheum.*, **30**, 801–808.

Lechner, D.E., McCarthy, C.F. and Holden, M.K. (1987) Gait deviations in patients with juvenile rheumatoid arthritis. *Phys. Ther.*, **67**, 1335–1341.

Lehmann, J.F., Brunner, G.D. and Stow, R.W. (1958) Pain threshold measurement after therapeutic application of ultrasound microwaves, and infrared. *Arch. Phys. Med. Rehabil.*, **39**, 560–565.

Lehmann, J.F., Masock, A.J., Warren, C.G. *et al.* (1970) Effect of therapeutic temperatures on tendon extensibility. *Arch. Phys. Med. Rehabil.*, **51**, 481–487.

Lovell, D.J., Howe, S., Shear, E. *et al.* (1989) Development of a disability measurement tool for juvenile rheumatoid arthritis. *Arthritis Rheum.*, **32**, 1390–1395.

MacBain, K.P. and Hill, R.H. (1973) A functional assessment for juvenile rheumatoid arthritis. *Am. J. Occup. Ther.*, **26**, 6, 326–330.

Mainardi, C.L., Walter, J.M. and Speigel, P.K. (1979) Rheumatoid arthritis: failure of daily heat therapy to affect its progression. *Arch. Phys. Med. Rehabil.*, **60**, 390–392.

Maitland, G.D. (1991) *Peripheral Manipulation*, 3rd edn. Oxford: Butterworth-Heinemann.

Reid Campion, M. (1991) *Hydrotherapy in Paediatrics*, 2nd edn. Oxford: Butterworth-Heinemann.

Rhodes, V.J. (1991) Physical therapy management of patients with juvenile rheumatoid arthritis. *Phys. Ther.*, **71**, 910–919.

Rhodes, V.J., Pumphrey, K.F. and Zemel, L. (1988) Development of a functional assessment tool for children with juvenile rheumatoid arthritis. *Arthritis Rheum.*, **31** (suppl 4), S151.

Rimón, R., Belmaker, R.H. and Ebstein, R. (1977) Psychosomatic aspects of juvenile rheumatoid arthritis. *Scand. J. Rheumatol.*, **6**, 1–20.

Ruddleston, C., Ansell, B.M., Arden, G.P. *et al.* (1986) Total hip replacement in children with juvenile rheumatoid arthritis. *J. Bone Joint Surg.*, **68-B**, 218–222.

Schaller, J.G. (1977) Ankylosing spondylitis of childhood onset. *Arthritis Rheum.*, **20**, 398–401.

Scott, R.D. (1990) Total hip and knee arthroplasty in juvenile rheumatoid arthritis. *Clin. Orthop.*, **259**, 83–91.

Scott, P.J., Ansell, B.M. and Huskisson, E.C. (1977) Measurement of pain in juvenile chronic polyarthritis. *Ann. Rheum. Dis.*, **36**, 186–187.

Stoeber, E. (1977) Juvenile chronic polyarthritis and Still's syndrome. Basle: *Documenta Geigy*.

Sullivan, D.B., Cassidy, J.T., Petty, R.E. and Burt, A. (1972) Prognosis in childhood dermatomyositis. *J. Pediatr.*, **80**, 555.

Swann, M. (1990) The surgery of juvenile chronic arthritis. *Clin. Orthop.*, **259**, 83–91.

Thompson, R.C. and Bassett, C.A.L. (1970) Histological observations on experimentally induced degeneration of articular cartilage. *J. Bone Joint Surg.*, **52A**, 435–443.

Further reading

Ansell, B.M. (1965) Rheumatoid disorders in childhood. In: *Physical Medicine in Paediatrics*, edited by B. Kiernander. London: Butterworth.

Blom, G.E. and Nicholls, G. (1954) Emotional factors in children with rheumatoid arthritis. *Am. J. Orthopsychiatry*, **24**, 588.

Chaplin, D., Pulkki, T., Saarimaa, A. *et al.* (1969) Wrist and finger deformities in juvenile rheumatoid arthritis. *Acta Rheum. Scand.*, **15**, 206.

Cole, S. and Jones, P. (1976) Physiotherapy in haemophilia. *Physiotherapy*, **62**, 7, 217.

Edmonds, J. and Hughes, G. (1985) *Lecture Notes on Rheumatology*. Oxford: Blackwell.

France, W.G. and Wolf, P. (1965) Treatment and prevention of chronic haemorrhagic arthropathy and contractures in haemophilia. *J. Bone Joint Surg.*, **47B**, 247.

Greenberg, R.S. (1972) The effects of hot packs and exercise on local blood flow. *Phys. Ther.*, **52**, 273.

Kass, H., Hanson, V. and Patrick, J. (1966) Scleroderma in childhood. *J. Pediatr.*, **68**, 243.

Kelley, W.N., Harris, E.D., Ruddy, S. and Sledge, C.B. (1989) *Textbook of Rheumatology*, 3rd edn. Philadelphia, PA: W.B. Saunders.

Nordemar, R., Berg, U., Ekblom, B. and Edström, L. (1976) Changes in muscle fibre size and physical performance in patients with rheumatoid arthritis after 7 months of physical training. *Scand. J. Rheumatol.*, **5**, 233–238.

Schumacher, H.R. (ed) (1988) *Primer on the Rheumatic Diseases*, 9th edn. Atlanta, GA: Arthritis Foundation.

Scull, S. (1989) Juvenile rheumatoid arthritis. In: *Pediatric Physical Therapy*, edited by J.S. Tecklin. Philadelphia, PA: J.B. Lippincott, pp. 217–236.

22

Burns in childhood

'Few accidents can match a major burn in the speed with which the unlimited possibilities of youth are shrivelled and handicap replaces promise' (Cosman 1974). Cosman goes on to note: 'burn is one of the most severe traumas that the body can survive and one of the most painful it can endure'. The extent of the disability may be wide-ranging, affecting a great deal more than the dermal covering of the body, and resulting in functional, cosmetic and psychiatric disability. The importance of skin should be carefully considered. Not only does it give protection and appearance; its integrity and elasticity are essential for all physical activity.

Children form a large part of the burn population, burns being a common form of injury during childhood. The causes include domestic accidents (electrical burns, hot-water scalds, flame burns due to burnt clothing), the so-called battered baby syndrome, and attempted suicide.

Electrical burns and hot-water scalds are most common in infancy. *Electrical burns* may occur when a toddler is left alone in a room with a radiator. The child may chew the cord or touch the bright element. *Hot-water scalds* are sometimes referred to as the hot-teapot syndrome and usually occur when a toddler pulls a pot of boiling water down from the stove. The sites of injury in these cases are usually typical, and include the upper arm, forearm, neck and chest, and may result eventually in contractures of the anterior axillary fold, elbow and anterior surface of the neck. *Flame burns* due to ignited clothing principally affect legs and lower trunk but may be more extensive. *Abused children* may demonstrate hot-water scalds or localized cigarette burns combined with evidence of other forms of assault. The majority of burns are said to involve 'the interaction of a poorly supervised child with a poorly supervised environment' (Cosman 1974).

Depth of burn wound

A burn may extend through the entire thickness of skin or damage or destroy only part of the skin. Burns are classified according to the depth of tissue injured. A third-degree burn is a full-thickness injury. First- and second-degree burns are partial-thickness injuries.

A *first-degree burn* is characterized by erythema and involves only the surface epithelium. It will heal within a few days. A *second-degree burn* may be superficial or deep. The *superficial* burns are characterized by erythema, oedema, blistering and pain, and will also heal within 2 weeks, although with minor scarring. *Deep* second-degree burns may result in destruction of the epidermis and upper levels of corium. These may heal without grafting in a few weeks provided no infection occurs. However, scarring may be considerable. Pain is experienced in both first- and second-degree burns, although there will be little pain with deep second-degree burns where there is destruction of superficial nerve endings. *Third-degree burns* involve the destruction of the skin with its appendages (hair follicles, sweat glands and sebaceous glands). Peripheral nerve endings are also destroyed. These burns will not heal spontaneously and will therefore require grafting.

Estimation of burn size

Burns in children encompassing more than 10% of the body area are said to be severe, and survival beyond 60% is uncertain. Estimation of the percentage of total body surface involved is usually based on the 'rule of nines', in which the body surface is divided into anatomical areas, each constituting 9% or a multiple of 9% of the total body surface. This requires some modification for small children who need a greater percentage allowance for the head compared to the trunk and extremities.

Burn physiology

A large burn loses a considerable amount of fluid (in the form of water, electrolytes and serum proteins) both externally and internally through the walls of damaged capillaries. Oedema occurs initially at the site of injury and becomes generalized within a few hours. Loss of fluid into the interstitial and intracellular spaces results in elevated haematocrit and haemoglobin (called haemoconcentration).

Fluid loss leads to shock with vasodilation, increased capillary permeability, increased fluid loss and diminished urine output. Eventually renal shutdown may occur. Hypotension and tachycardia may result finally in cardiopulmonary arrest. The severity of burn shock is related to the size of the burn area rather than its depth. However, overall prognosis depends on depth.

A burn imposes an increased caloric loss upon the child. One of the causes for this is destruction of the protective epithelium with increased fluid loss. It is said that between 2000 and 3350 calories may be lost in evaporation from a burn of 1 m². Wound-healing also places a greater demand on calories than normally required for growth and development. Added to this is the sick child's reluctance to eat.

While the wound lacks skin cover there is great risk of sepsis. The necrotic mass of burned tissue, called the eschar, is bound by collagen fibres to the viable tissue below. Eventually, these two layers will separate, but until they do the space between them allows bacteria to proliferate.

If a burn is circumferential around a limb, the eschar may act as a tourniquet as oedema develops. Decreased arterial blood supply will result in pallor, numbness and inability to move the fingers or toes. Interrupted venous return results in swelling, cyanosis and pain as well as difficulty in moving.

Healing will eventually take place by scar tissue formation, which has a tendency to contract. It is generally considered that early skin coverage combined with the early resumption of normal activity and continuous pressure, is the best means of controlling excessive scar tissue formation and contraction.

Respiratory complications

Inhalation of hot air may burn the mouth, nose, pharynx and larynx as far as the upper trachea. However, heat is effectively removed from the air by the nose and larynx in most cases, so damage is rarely seen beyond the upper respiratory tract.

Nevertheless, smoke and fumes, especially in confined spaces, may injure the lower airways. The mucosal lining may be inflamed or destroyed, in which case it will eventually slough off. The child may cough up the plugs of necrotic tissue or they may block small airways.

Respiratory complications may include bronchospasm caused by inhaled smoke debris, dyspnoea, consolidation or collapse. In certain types of burns, respiratory damage may lead to severe and rapidly progressive bronchopneumonia. Infection may occur due to blood or air-borne bacteria. An increased metabolic rate may add to the already present ventilatory inadequacy. If the chest is burnt, a tight eschar around the circumference of the chest may restrict breathing.

Care of the child in the post-burn period

The post-burn period can be divided into three stages according to Cosman (1974):

1 Initial shock and resuscitation (first 2–4 days).

2 Wound débridement and coverage (3–6 weeks).
3 Skin restoration and reconstruction (several years).

Growth and development of the child impose ever-changing requirements for both function and appearance. Hence the third stage will continue for a lengthy period.

In all stages, the prevention of complications is essential. Hence, nutritional support, antibacterial measures and physical treatment to ensure effective ventilatory function and effective movement of the limbs, trunk and head, must be carried out throughout the entire period.

Aggressive resuscitation, replacement plasma therapy, nutritional supplement, topical antibiotics, surgical débridement and early skin grafting are resulting in the survival of many burned children, including those with a large percentage of body area burned. A comprehensive burn management programme, to be effective in ensuring survival of the child and some quality in that survival, requires a team effort from parents, nurse, physiotherapist, occupational therapist, psychologist, social worker and medical practitioner working together with a mutual understanding of the child's needs.

Immediately post-burn

Treatment consists of prevention of shock or resuscitation if shock is present, fluid replacement therapy, antibiotics and nutritional supplement. Maintenance of a good airway will be a major consideration, particularly in burns of face, neck and chest and where there is actual airway damage. Intubation may be necessary and in some cases tracheostomy may be performed, although this is a controversial point.

Bladder catheterization may be required to allow monitoring of urine concentration and output. Blood pressure and pulse are monitored frequently. Escharotomy may be required to relieve constriction of a limb or of the thorax.

Physical treatment consists of treatment of already existing problems and prevention of suspected future problems. Techniques of treatment for specific ventilatory problems will be as described in Section V. However, there are some points specific to the care of the burnt child which should be mentioned.

Where *nasopharyngeal suction* is necessary to remove secretions, particular care must be taken to maintain a sterile procedure and to pass the tube gently because of the damaged mucosal lining. Where suction is performed via a tracheostomy, care must be taken not to dislodge any slough into the airway.

The intensive treatment, which may be necessary in the so-called inhalation burns, is adjusted according to the extent and site of all burnt areas. If secretions must be cleared from the chest, *vibrations* are necessary and if the chest skin is burnt, the therapist wears sterile gloves. The pain caused by vibrations may actually inhibit respirations, so they should be avoided where possible.

Postural drainage may be necessary to mobilize secretions. Unless there is a specific lung area involved, elevation of the foot of the bed with breathing exercises and instructions to cough may be sufficient. If the child needs to be positioned for a particular lobe, sufficient people should be present to enable the child's position to be shifted with a minimum of trauma. Posturing with the legs higher than the head may have to be avoided if neck and facial oedema is present.

Where possible, *burnt limbs are elevated* to help disperse oedema. The arm is elevated on pillows and the end of the bed is elevated if the legs are involved. Unfortunately, the position of comfort will usually be conducive to contracture, so the child must be positioned to minimize this risk. If the neck is burnt, for example, the head is extended over a foam block. If the axilla is involved, the arm may be positioned above the head. Splinting may be necessary for particular segments of the limbs.

Active movement with assistance from the therapist is begun as soon as the child is admitted. These movements are also performed in the daily bath. On the whole the child will move little unless encouraged to do so. The combination of lying still and sepsis may cause significant bone decalcification (Koepke and Feller 1967). Lack of movement will also result in wound contracture and joint stiffness, disuse muscle weakness and depressed respiratory function. It is therefore essential that the therapist is able to encourage the child to move. Reassurance may need to be given that the skin will not be damaged by moving. The child may be allowed out of bed and to walk if the general condition allows. If the hands are burnt, the child may be allowed to remain independent in activities such as feeding if the hands are encased in sterile plastic bags.

Preparation for skin grafting

The main *objectives* at this stage are to prevent infection and encourage wound-healing – in other words, to promote the best possible functional cosmetic skin covering. Infection will prevent successful skin grafting, and it must also be remembered that infection can threaten the child's life until the wound is completely healed.

Débridement, which involves separation and removal of remnants of dead tissue, is carried out if necessary as soon as the child's general condition is stabilized. It may be done non-traumatically in a bath as well as surgically.

Daily or twice daily *active movements* in water and whirlpool baths help to separate remnants of dead tissue non-traumatically, reduce bacterial infection and stimulate capillary ingrowth, as well as facilitating dressing changes. An antibacterial agent, such as chlorhexidine, is added to the water, and the temperature should be approximately 35°C. The child spends 15–30 minutes in the bath. Room temperature should be warm, and after the bath the child may be dried under heat lamps. It is generally considered impractical to maintain sterility of the bath but some suggest the use of disposable plastic liners, and certainly the bath should be cleaned after use.

The child may resist hydrotherapy. Anxiety may be relieved if the child is encouraged to become involved in the various procedures, such as filling the bath, and if interesting bath toys are provided. A television in the room may also divert attention.

Following the bath, the burn eschar may be probed with forceps and trimmed. An antibacterial cream such as silver sulphadiazine, or embryonic membrane, is applied directly to the wound, sealing it from the air.

Early *surgical débridement*, followed by skin grafting, is said by its advocates to minimize sepsis, provide early skin cover, allow early resumption of normal activity and decrease time spent in hospital.

If the burn does not involve the full thickness of skin, granulation tissue will form on the surface of the wound as the burn eschar separates. If epithelium has survived, it will grow to the surface and across the granulation tissue and this results in wound-healing.

Skin grafting

Skin grafting will be necessary in the case of a full-thickness burn. Autogenous split-thickness skin is taken from an unburned part of the child's body, called the donor site. The graft tissue is placed over the wound, either completely covering it in the case of a relatively small area, or in strips a few millimetres apart in the case of a larger area. Meshed grafts with multiple perforations are also used, and are said to allow the skin to stretch. Further skin grafting will be necessary as the child grows because scar tissue and skin grafts do not grow at the same rate as the child. Elastic pressure supports are applied as soon as healing and graft take permit. They are worn at first in conjunction with splinting.

Physical treatment following skin grafting

Deep breathing and *coughing* must be stimulated following surgery. If the chest skin is involved, the therapist must wear sterile gloves. Posturing and turning a child with extensive burns may require three or four people in order that sufficient care can be taken of the newly grafted areas and the donor sites. Pain will inhibit respirations so vibrations are only given if really essential for clearing the chest. *Nasopharyngeal suction* will stimulate the cough reflex and eliminate secretions if the child is reluctant to cough or expectorate, but it should not be done unless really necessary as it adds to the child's discomfort and fear. Elevation of the foot of the bed must be avoided if neck and facial oedema are present.

No movement of the newly grafted area is allowed for several (5–10) days. Immobilization is gained by thermoplastic splinting or skeletal traction. When the donor sites have healed (in approximately 7–10 days) *hydrotherapy* may recommence. Movements should not be too vigorous. It is suggested (Koepke and Feller 1967) that movement may, in some cases, stimulate contracture band formation on flexor surfaces, resulting in a band of scar tissue. The extremities should not be dependent too soon after grafting or microhaemorrhage will occur beneath the graft. Standing can be gradually assumed with elastic supports if the legs are involved, and the child should have the legs elevated when resting.

Burns to the hand

Burns to the thin elastic skin on the dorsum of the hand present a particular problem as the extensor mechanism and joint capsules are very vulnerable. The common deformity following a burn to this area results from hyperextension of the metacarpophalangeal joints and flexion of the interphalangeal joints. As soon as possible after admission, the hand is splinted to a functional position. The thumb should be in an opposed position with a large web space, the wrist extended 30°, metacarpophalangeal joints flexed 70°, proximal and distal interphalangeal joints extended. The arm is elevated to relieve oedema, and active movement is encouraged several times a day. Following skin grafting the hand is immobilized for 7–10 days before movement can be recommenced and then splinting will need to be continued at night and when the child is resting during the day. Activities with relevance for the individual may be preferable to exercises. The child should be encouraged to be independent in eating and dressing and to use the hands. Excess stretch to the extensors should be avoided as it may cause the tendons to rupture.

Wound-healing, hypertrophic scarring and contracture

Two of the most frustrating sequelae of burns are contractures and hypertrophic scars. A child may demonstrate a satisfactory appearance upon discharge, following either spontaneous healing or skin grafting, yet only a few weeks later scar hypertrophy may already be leading to severe deformity.

Joint contracture and *scar contracture* both pose a serious problem during the healing stage which commences immediately after injury and continues throughout the entire post-recovery period for a minimum of 6 months. Both are facilitated by a number of factors, including the child's preference for certain 'comfortable' positions and reluctance to move. Scars anterior to the flexor surface will, if uncontrolled, lead to severe contracture.

Scar hypertrophy occurs anywhere except those areas of the body in which the skin is splinted by its attachment to underlying structures. It tends to form a bridge across the crease lines of the body.

Hypertrophy occurs following both spontaneous healing and skin grafting. Skin grafting actually decreases hypertrophic scar formation but scarring will still develop between the normal skin and the graft, or between adjacent grafts. The graft limits the excessive proliferation of connective tissue and by its natural pressure prevents to some extent the formation of the whorl-like or nodular arrangement of collagen fibres characteristic of a hypertrophic scar (Larson 1973) and unlike the normal parallel arrangement of collagen fibres.

The risk of scar contracture and hypertrophy will be present throughout the phase of scar maturation, during which the scar is actively growing.

Both hypertrophic scarring and joint contracture are frequently accepted as the natural course of events following burns. However, it is becoming apparent that these sequelae can be significantly altered and controlled with special techniques involving continuous controlled pressure with custom-made splints and anti-burnscar elastic supports. These give non-surgical control of scar contracture and hypertrophic scar formation.

Custom-made splints

Splints (usually of thermoplastic material) are applied soon after admission to maintain the appropriate body position for function. The position of uninvolved as well as involved joints must be considered in order to prevent soft tissue shortening. Unfortunately, the child's preferred position will be one of flexion, and splinting must be used to maintain the extension necessary to prevent contracture and to allow function to be eventually regained. Such splinting is particularly important where burns involve the hands, axilla and neck. Once wound coverage has been attained, appropriate positioning is maintained by splinting and pressure garments (elastic supports).

Anti-burnscar elastic pressure supports (Jobst)*

These are worn for 24 hours a day until the scars are mature (approximately 6–12 months).

**Jobst anti-burnscar. Available from Jobst Institute Inc., PO Box 653, Toledo, OH 43694, USA.

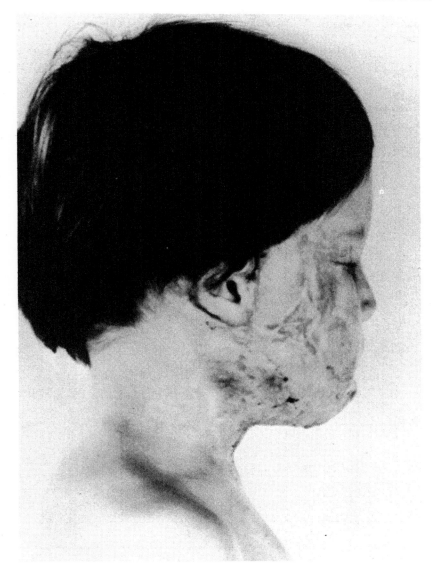

Figure 22.1 A burned child before wearing the Jobst anti-burnscar support. (Courtesy of the Jobst Institute.)

They promote flatness and smoothness of the healing tissue (Figs 22.1–22.5). They are usually applied a few weeks after skin grafting before scars begin to form.

Emotional and behavioural complications

Pain and increasing perception of the extent of the injury usually become most evident after the fourth day and are then present constantly. In this early stage, the child's relative isolation and the continuous interruptions of treatment procedures may be confusing. How the child copes with the mental and physical agony following the burn depends partly on his or her pre-burn personality, and partly on how parents and care-givers can cope with their own feelings and give encouragement and motivation. The child may develop stress ulceration of the stomach or duodenum or bizarre signs such as amnesia or opisthotonos. Behaviour may regress.

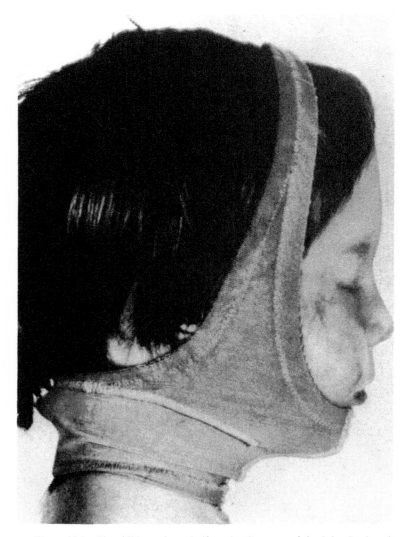

Figure 22.2 The child wearing a half-mask. (Courtesy of the Jobst Institute.)

The hospital staff also suffer emotional distress and this, combined with anger at having to cause pain, may cause them to withdraw from the close contact with the child which is so necessary. The nurse and therapist must be able to gain the child's cooperation in painful treatment and cope constructively with the child's response to pain. Changing a dressing or encouraging active movements with a hysterically screaming child, knowing that one is increasing the pain, requires that the nurse and therapist understand fully the reasons for the treatment being given. If they also realize that fear and anxiety increase pain, they can divert their own thoughts to ways of easing these in the child.

The therapist should be firmly reassuring to the child and make sure to explain each step of treatment so the child will know what is happening. The establishment of a daily routine of therapy often gives emotional support and helps to allay anxiety. Excessive staff changes should be avoided as the child may react badly to this, thinking bad behaviour has driven the therapist away.

Savedra (1977) studied the coping strategies of 5 children aged 6–9 years, hospitalized with severe burns. They included the following:

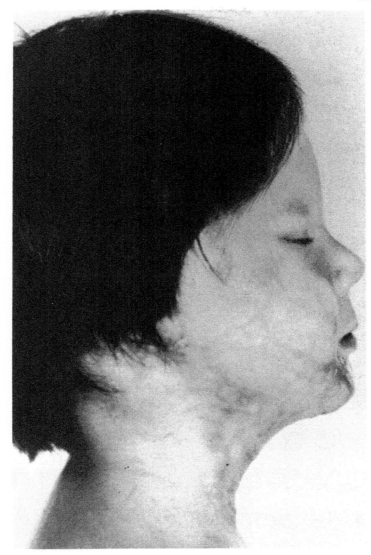

Figure 22.3 After wearing the half-mask for 1 year. (Courtesy of the Jobst Institute.)

1 Reduction of threat with efforts made to lessen the expected pain ('Don't hurt me').
2 Postponement (asking that another child could have his bath first).
3 Bypassing the procedure (asking nurse to pretend to do the dressing).
4 Creating a distance between the child and the threat (kicking legs to keep the nurse or therapist away).
5 Dividing attention (having the hand held, story reading, talking).
6 Sleep.
7 Responses to crying of others (intolerance of other children crying).

Shorkey and Taylor suggested in 1973 that more attention should be paid to behaviour modification techniques in the management of social and emotional behaviour of severely injured children.

Leaving hospital is a major hurdle for the burnt child and the family, and efforts must be made by the parents, with help from the

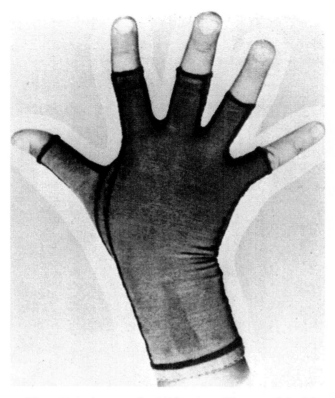

Figure 22.4 A custom-fitted Jobst glove. (Courtesy of the Jobst Institute.)

social worker, child guidance counsellor and therapist, to re-establish family routine as soon as possible.

The child's skin must be protected from the sun as it will burn and blister easily. The skin should be patted dry after a bath rather than rubbed. The importance of pressure garments must be impressed upon the parents before the child leaves hospital. Parents and child are taught how to care for these garments and avoid staining and other damage. Parents may need to encourage the child to be active, by playing active games or doing exercises. The child's progress will depend a great deal on the motivation, help and encouragement given by the family.

Summary

Burns constitute a severe and common trauma in childhood. The sequelae may be long-lasting and may affect the child's motor function, personality and general development. Emphasis in physical treatment is on the prevention of permanent disability by the encouragement of active functional movement, by splinting and pressure supports, and by careful advice to parents and child.

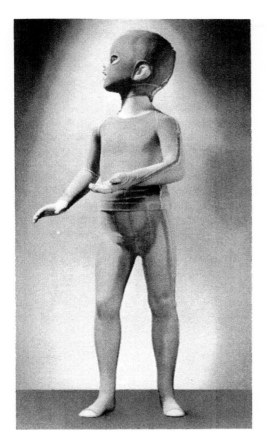

Figure 22.5   Custom-made Jobst anti-burnscar supports.
(Courtesy of the Jobst Institute.)

References

Cosman, B. (1974) The burned child. In: *The Child with Disabling Illness. Principles of Rehabilitation.* Philadelphia: W.B. Saunders.

Koepke, G.H. and Feller, I. (1967) Physical measures for the prevention and treatment of deformities following burns. *J.A.M.A.*, **199**, 127.

Larson, D.L. (1973) *Prevention and Correction of Burn Scar Contractures and Hypertrophy.* Shriners Burn Institute, University of Texas Medical Branch, Galveston, TX.

Savedra, M. (1977) Coping with pain. Strategies of severely burned children. *Can. Nurs.*, Aug., 28–29.

Shorkey, C.T. and Taylor, J.E. (1973) Management of maladaptive behavior of a severely burned child. *Child Welfare*, **52**, 8, 542–547.

Further reading

Alhopuro, S., Sundell, B. and Ritsila, V. (1976) Late complications of scalding in children. Treatment and prevention. *Ann. Chirurg. Gynaecol.*, **65**, 151–153.

Behrman, R.E. and Vaughan, V.C. (1987) *Nelson Textbook of Pediatrics*, 13th edn. Philadelphia, PA: W.B. Saunders.

Brown, J.M. (1977) Respiratory complications in burnt patients. *Physiotherapy*, **63**, 5, 151–153.

Burke, J.F. (1971) Isolation techniques and their effectiveness. In: *Contemporary Burn Management*, edited by H.C. Polk and H.H. Stone. Boston, MA: Little, Brown.

Eckhauser, F.E., Billote, J., Burke, J.F. and Quinby, W.C. (1974) Tracheostomy complications in massive burn injury. *Am. J. Surg.*, **127**, 418–423.

Evans, E.B., Larsen, D.L., Yates, S. (1968) Preservation and restoration of joint function in patients with severe burns. *J.A.M.A.*, **204**, 91.

Gilder, N. (1977) Treatment of burns in a general hospital. *Fisioterapie*, Sept., 5–7.

Hales, M. (1977) Physical treatment and rehabilitation for burns. *Physiotherapy*, **63**, 5, 157–158.

Malick, M.H. (1975) Management of the severely burned patient. *Br. J. Occup. Ther.*, **38**, 4, 76–80.

Newton, W. and Bubenickova, M. (1977) Rehabilitation of the autografted hand in children with burns. *Phys. Ther.*, **57**, 12, 1383–1387.

Quinby, S. and Bernstein, N.B. (1971) Identity problems and adaptation of nurses to severely burned children. *Am. J. Psychiatry*, **128**, 1, 90–95.

Van der Spuy, J.W. (1977) The changing face of burns. *Fisioterapie*, Sept., 3–4.

Willis, B.A. (1973) *Burn Scar Hypertrophy.* Toledo, OH: Jobst Institute.

Section V

Disorders of the respiratory system

23 Introduction
24 The development and mechanics of respiration
25 Respiratory disorders in the neonatal period and infancy
26 Respiratory disorders in childhood
27 Physical evaluation and treatment

Introduction

Infants and children with respiratory disorders are referred to the physiotherapist in order to improve their pulmonary function. The treatment of most of these children involves three basic aims – to clear airways obstructed by accumulated secretions or aspirated material, to re-expand a collapsed segment of lung, and to improve the mechanism and control of breathing. These aims are directed at fulfilling the major objective of ensuring adequate transmission of gases to and from vital organs such as the brain. There are certain specific techniques used by the physiotherapist in the treatment of these problems of increased secretions and inefficient ventilation, and these are described in Chapter 27. The treatment of children with cystic fibrosis and asthma is described separately and in detail as the problems to be handled by the physiotherapist are complex.

In treating both infants and children, the anatomy of the bronchial tree must be carefully considered, plus the effect of the child's habitual posture upon the siting of accumulated secretions. For example, an infant or a bed-ridden child with pneumonia will be more likely to develop pooling of the secretions in the right upper lobe, although this may also occur elsewhere. The child who is upright is more likely to aspirate secretions into the right lower lobe, the right main bronchus being straighter than the left. The development of the respiratory tract must also be considered. The infant with a relatively undeveloped bron-

chial tree may suffer far more serious consequences of infection or aspiration than the older child or adult. For example, a small obstruction will cause a large reduction in cross-sectional area of the lumen of the airway because of the small size of the airway.

There is an important element of prevention involved in the physical treatment of these infants and children (Fig. 23.1). Diseases such as bronchiolitis, aspiration, bacterial and viral pneumonia may be complicated by atelectasis and the retention of infected secretions if the obstruction caused by the secretions becomes complete. These complications may also occur following attacks of asthma in which mucus plugs may effectively obstruct airways. Bronchiectasis may develop as the result of the effect of infected mucus secretions on the walls of the bronchioles if these secretions are allowed to remain. The child with cystic fibrosis may develop atelectasis, pneumonia or bronchiectasis as a result of a failure on the part of the clearing mechanism to remove tenacious secretions. Emphysema may develop in children, as in adults, as a result of chronic respiratory disability. Figure 23.2 lists the various causes of increased mucus secretions and Figure 23.3 the causes of airways obstruction.

There is another aspect of prevention involved in the physical treatment of all children who are at risk of developing disorders of the lower respiratory tract, and who may be seen by the physiotherapist for other reasons. The child who suffers recurrent upper

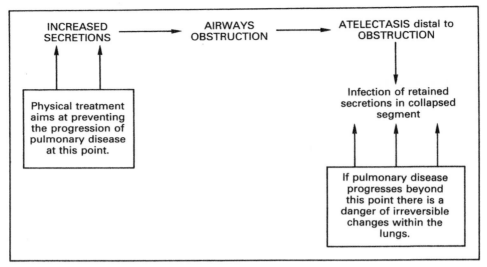

Figure 23.1   Preventive role of physical treatment.

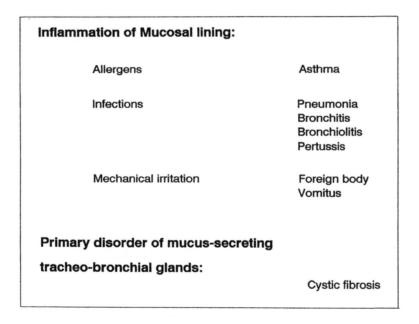

Figure 23.2   Causes of increased mucus secretions.

respiratory tract infections may be prevented from developing bronchitis as a recurrent sequela by the use of postural drainage and breathing exercises designed to maintain clear airways. The child with weakness or paralysis of the muscles involved in respiration and the child who is bed-ridden also need treatment to prevent the hypostatic pneumonia and segmental collapse which will result if obstruction of the airways by secretions is allowed to occur. The child with severe deformity involving the thorax, such as occurs in scoliosis and in thoracic myelomeningocele, also requires treatment to maintain the best possible thoracic expansion plus clear airways, and therefore maximum respiratory efficiency.

Children who have general surgery usually do not require pre- and postoperative treatment to prevent respiratory complications as do adults in a similar situation, unless they have pre-existing lung disease. However, the child who undergoes pulmonary or cardiac surgery will require physiotherapy to prevent respiratory complications, and to regain full and effective use of the lungs.

Increased mucus secretions

Abnormal viscosity of secretions

Aspirated material:

    Foreign body
    Vomitus
    Upper respiratory tract secretions

Tuberculosis

Bronchospasm

Figure 23.3   Causes of airways obstruction.

24

The development and mechanics of respiration

One of the commonest causes of death in the newborn is respiratory failure. An understanding of the differences between the fetal, neonatal and adult lung is essential for the physiotherapist giving treatment to infants and children.

The lungs are not fully developed when the infant cries for the first time. The number of airways and alveoli and the diameters of the alveoli increase until the child is approximately 8 years old. There is some evidence that the number of alveoli increases until 12 years of age (Doershuk *et al.* 1975) and normal growth and remodelling of the ventilatory system continue into adult life (Thurlbeck 1975; Reid 1977; Kendig and Chernick 1977). This is important to remember when treating infants and small children with respiratory disease since the development of the airways and air spaces is dependent to some extent on the demands made upon them. The presence of disease or the retention of secretions may result in abnormal development since, during the period of alveolar increase, any destructive process will limit the potential for the development of an adult number of pulmonary alveoli (Polgar and Weng 1979). Similarly, the therapist must also take care that treatment directed at such immature and small airways does not cause damage which will affect the future development and growth of lung tissue.

The embryonic and fetal lung

The embryonic development of the lungs is summarized in Table 24.1

The respiratory system arises as a median ventral diverticulum of the foregut called the laryngotracheal groove at about the middle of the fourth week of embryonic life. The lower end of the diverticulum divides into two lung buds. The median stalk of the diverticulum becomes the trachea. The two lung buds will develop into the bronchial tree and respiratory epithelial lining of the lungs. The right lung bud will divide into three branches and the left into two branches. Thus the right lung bud will eventually develop three lobes and the left two lobes (Langman 1969).

The size difference between the two lungs is due to the shift of the embryonic heart to the left side of the pleural cavity. The heart's position produces the cardiac notch in the left lung. The relative proportions of larynx and trachea change from the embryonic period to adult life. While the trachea is short and narrow, the larynx is relatively large, and it is not until several months after birth, when the trachea grows at a faster rate than the larynx, that the two structures attain the relative proportions seen in the adult.

The infant's larynx is not a miniature of its adult form. Its relatively high position enables the neonate to breathe and swallow simultaneously up to approximately 3–4 months of age (Laitman and Crelin 1980). The subglottic

Table 24.1 The development of the lungs

Time	Development
24 days	Outpouching of gut
26–28 days	Two primary branches appear – the two main bronchi
8 weeks	Paratracheal mucous glands forming
10 weeks	Cartilage deposition begins
12 weeks	Lobes well-demarcated Elastic fibres in walls of main bronchi and trachea Cartilaginous rings present in lobar and segmental bronchi Further formation of mucus-secreting glands
16 weeks	Formation of bronchial divisions nearly completed
18–20 weeks	Septa now recognizable Cilia appear on epithelial cells of trachea and main bronchi, and spread towards the periphery
20 weeks	Cannulization of airways
24 weeks	Bronchi now the same as at term Cartilage formed Alveolar formation commences
26–28 weeks	Capillary network proliferates close to the developing airways
28 weeks	Lung now the most vascular organ in the body. Maintenance of extrauterine life as depending upon gas exchange is possible at this stage
28 weeks to term	Terminal alveoli appear as outpouchings of bronchioles, and from now to term increase in numbers to form common chambers called alveolar ducts
Birth	Terminal bronchioles are smooth. Terminal air sacs are shallow and wide-mouthed Pulmonary blood flow increases due to mechanical lung expansion Respiratory passages elongate 20 million alveoli now present. They become dilated and expand at onset of respiration
6–8 weeks	Typical sharply curved alveoli can be identified
Several months	Terminal air sacs assume cup-like configuration New alveoli appear proximal to terminal air spaces by transformation of pre-existing bronchioles
Up to 8 years approximately	Lung growth proceeds with increase in number of bronchiolar divisions, alveoli, alveolar diameters and surface area for gas exchange Numbers of alveoli and airways increase 10 times from infancy to adulthood Lung surface area increases 20 times. Alveoli number 300 million in adult life
Up to 40 years	Further increase in dimensions of terminal air spaces Bronchiolar and tracheal diameters increase

Details from Avery, M.E. (1975) *The Lung and its Disorders in the Newborn Infant*. Philadelphia, PA: W.B. Saunders; Langman, J. (1969) *Medical Embryology*. Baltimore, MD: Williams & Wilkins; Hamilton, W.J., Boyd, J.D. and Mossman, H.W. (1972) *Human Embryology*. Cambridge: Heffer.

cavity below the vocal cords extends backwards as well as downwards in the neonate. In older children and adults it is almost vertical. An intubation tube must therefore not only be small but also correctly shaped for the airway and introduced correctly. The mucosal lining of the infant's larynx becomes oedematous on minimal irritation and air flow may easily be obstructed.

The lung is a glandular organ with no air spaces in the period before the fetus becomes viable at the 28th week (Avery 1975). In the fetus the placenta is the organ of gas exchange. On ventilation of the lungs at birth a new vascular bed replaces the vascular bed of the placenta. The presence of fetal breathing has been recorded in animals and also in humans. Fetal breathing is reported to be state-dependent, in contrast to the need for sustained inspiratory effort after birth (Henderson-Smart 1984). In the absence of air, the potential airways of the fetus are in contact with a fluid which is partly amniotic, inhaled during *in utero* respiratory movements, and partly the secretions of submucous glands and goblet cells of the respiratory epithelium. Although respiratory-type movements of the thorax occur in the fetus, this does not occur as a means of gas exchange (Avery 1975). Before birth, the diaphragm is capable of vigorous contraction in a form of hiccup.

The lung at birth

The changeover at birth from dependence on placental gas exchange to air-breathing is a critical event. Following birth, breathing efforts are regulated to meet the metabolic demands (Henderson-Smart 1984), and this is dependent on many factors, including the level of neural maturation. The first breath is a gasp, a contraction of the diaphragm which is probably triggered by tactile and thermal changes (Avery 1975; Henderson-Smart 1984). As the infant takes the first breaths, the alveoli open one after the other in proximal to distal sequence. Good inflation of the lungs occurs with the first loud cry, although for the first 7–10 days small areas of lung may remain uninflated. As the infant takes these first breaths, air replaces the fluid in the airways. Some of this fluid is extruded from the mouth and nose, but most of it is absorbed into the intestinal tissue by the lung, and subsequently removed by the lymphatic system.

This transition from fluid-filled airways to air-filled airways is potentially hazardous and the principal cause of death in the perinatal period is the respiratory system's failure to function adequately. Success of this transition depends largely on both the presence and the quality of pulmonary surfactant, a phospholipid material secreted by cells lining the pulmonary alveoli. Surfactant lowers the surface tension within the alveolus, allowing it to inflate with smaller pressure and less work by the infant than if surfactant were deficient. Before the first breath, the surface tension of the partially collapsed alveoli holds the alveolar walls together. Hence a very great effort is needed for the alveoli to inflate.

As air fills the alveoli, surfactant is rapidly released into the alveolar space, forming an interface between the fluid which remains and the newly entered air. Surfactant maintains low alveolar surface tension, and its presence allows air to remain in the alveoli at all times, preventing airway collapse.

In neonates whose lungs are deficient in quality or quantity of surfactant, more inspiratory effort is needed to produce the appropriate negative pressure within the airways, in other words to retain air at the end of expiration. This extra effort is physically exhausting even for a full-term infant. Respiratory distress syndrome in premature infants is caused by surfactant not having reached the correct chemical composition because of the infant's immaturity. The baby may not be able to maintain alveolar expansion due to the ineffective sufactant and would die without mechanical ventilation to support breathing.

At birth the alveoli are not present in adult number, nor are they fully developed. The diameter of the alveoli at 2 months is approximately 60–130 μm, increasing to 100–200 μm in older children and 200–300 μm in adults (Doershuk *et al.* 1975). However, the airways have a greater relative diameter and the anatomical dead space is correspondingly larger than that of the adult. This is the reason for the preference for administration of oxygen by intubation rather than by tent, taking the gas directly to the respiratory epithelium thus bypassing the dead space of the non-respiratory airways.

There is a relative weakness of bronchiolar walls up to age 3–4 years while development of smooth muscles is occurring. This structural weakness may contribute to airway collapse and air-trapping in very young children. In addition to lack of structural support in small airways, collateral ventilation via pores of Kohn and Lambert's canals is limited (Murray 1976). This predisposes to a greater susceptibility of young children to the development of atelectasis and infection.

Small airways size and small distal bronchiolar diameter cause a high resistance to air flow and greater work in breathing. The respiratory rate of a child also differs from that of an adult (Fig 24.1), gradually approximating to the adult rate during the second decade.

It is possible that muscle fatigue could lead to respiratory failure in the newborn (Muller *et al.* 1979). Type 1 slow-twitch, fatigue-resistant high oxidative muscle fibres are not present in adult proportions in the diaphragm and other ventilatory muscles until 8 months. The diaphragm of premature infants contains as little as 10% of type 1 fibres, neonates 25% and adults 50% (Keens *et al.* 1978; Muller and Bryan 1979).

NORMAL RESTING RESPIRATORY RATE PER MINUTE		
AGE (YEARS)	BOYS MEAN ± SD	GIRLS MEAN ± SD
0 - 1	31 ± 8	30 ± 6
1 - 2	26 ± 4	27 ± 4
2 - 3	25 ± 4	25 ± 3
3 - 4	24 ± 3	24 ± 3
4 - 5	23 ± 2	22 ± 2
5 - 6	22 ± 2	21 ± 2
6 - 7	21 ± 3	21 ± 3
7 - 8	20 ± 3	20 ± 2
8 - 9	20 ± 2	20 ± 2
9 - 10	19 ± 2	19 ± 2
10 - 11	19 ± 2	19 ± 2
11 - 12	19 ± 3	19 ± 3
12 - 13	19 ± 3	19 ± 2
13 - 14	19 ± 2	18 ± 2
14 - 15	18 ± 2	18 ± 3
15 - 16	17 ± 3	18 ± 3
16 - 17	17 ± 2	17 ± 3
17 - 18	16 ± 3	17 ± 3

Figure 24.1 Normal resting respiratory rate from birth to 18 years. SD = One standard deviation of the mean. (From Iliff, A. and Lee, V.A. (1952) Pulse rate, respiratory rate and body temperature of children between 2 months and 18 years of age. *Child Dev.*, **23**, 237.)

As a consequence of a relatively low proportion of type 1 fibres, muscles fatigue quickly. Diaphragmatic fatigue has been reported as occurring in preterm babies during sleep and in babies with respiratory failure (Muller *et al.* 1979).

The mechanics of ventilation

For air to be inhaled into the lungs and exhaled from them, the thorax must increase and decrease in size. This alteration in thoracic volume occurs because of the coordinated contraction and lengthening of the muscles encompassing the thorax. This mechanism is complex and incompletely understood.

The diaphragm is not indispensable in adult ventilation, although it usually functions for waking respiration. Adequate ventilation in adults is possible in spite of diaphragmatic paralysis by the use of the accessory muscles of inspiration and the intercostal muscles (Steindler 1955), although activity is very restricted. The diaphragm is, however, essential during deep anaesthesia and sleep when the other muscles of respiration are inactive

(Kendig and Chernick 1977). In the normal person it is the most important of the respiratory muscles, normal resting inspiration being almost entirely due to diaphragmatic contraction. When on inspiration it contracts and descends, the vertical diameter of the thorax is increased.

It is now well-established that the intercostal muscles move the ribcage (Loring and de Troyer 1985). It is commonly held that the external intercostals and interchondral part of the internal intercostal muscles (parasternal muscles) are inspiratory and raise the ribs, whereas the interosseus part of the internal intercostals is expiratory and lowers the ribs (Loring and de Troyer 1985). Contraction of the external intercostal muscles pulls the upper ribs down and the lower ribs up, thus facilitating expansion of the lungs during inspiration. Their downward pull on the upper thorax is counteracted by the contraction of the scalene muscles. During forced inspiration, such as occurs during effort, the sternomastoid and scaleni muscles contract to elevate the sternum and ribs. On inspiration the descent of the diaphragm tends to pull the lungs downwards and the levator costae and suprahyoid muscles seem to stabilize the trachea and larynx.

The accessory muscles have not been extensively studied. Trapezius and serratus superior may have an inspiratory role, serratus inferior an expiratory one. The abdominal muscles, internal and external obliques, transversus abdominis and rectus abdominis are powerful expiratory muscles. The obliques and transversus pull the abdominal wall inwards and increase intra-abdominal pressure. However, the abdominal muscles also assist inspiration. By contracting, they lengthen the inspiratory muscles to a more advantageous operating length. They also store elastic energy in the chest wall during expiration, which is then used during inspiration. In addition, resistance to air flow in the upper airway is decreased on deep inspiration by the dilation of the nostrils and by movement of the muscles of the cheek, of the platysma, and of the tongue.

Inspiration requires muscular effort to overcome resistance in the airways and lung elasticity. Normal resting expiration, however, is thought to be a passive process as the muscles of inspiration relax and the lungs recoil. The walls of the thorax relax against the pressure of gravity and the elastic lungs pull inwards on them. The alveoli are prevented from collapsing at the end of expiration by the presence of the fluid surfactant which lines their walls. During forced or difficult expiration the abdominal muscles contract strongly, increasing intra-abdominal pressure and thereby aiding elevation of the diaphragm. These muscles are a powerful effector of forced expiration and are used strongly on coughing.

A cough can result from irritation of the nerve endings in the proximal airways by a foreign body or by accumulated secretions. The diaphragm and intercostals contract, the lung fill with air and the glottis closes. Air is expelled forcefully by relaxation of the diaphragm and contraction of the abdominal muscles, combined with opening of the glottis. The diaphragm and abdominal muscles are therefore essential for an effective cough. The production of mucus is a normal function of the bronchial tree and it is produced by the tracheobronchial glands. It is the action of the cilia in the normal lung which moves this thin layer of mucus upwards to where it can be coughed out. There is a greater density of mucus glands in relation to size of bronchial surface in young children. In the infant up to the age of 4 months the mucus appears to be more viscid than in the older child and adult.

The infant's pattern of breathing shows some mechanical differences compared to that of the adult. The relatively horizontal alignment of the ribcage, the rounded configuration of the thorax, the cartilaginous nature of the thoracic skeleton and the horizontal angle of diaphragm insertion provide a poor mechanical advantage to the intercostal and accessory muscles. These factors result in less efficient ventilation and a tendency towards distortion of chest wall shape on inspiration. In the neonate the diaphragm is therefore particularly important for ventilation, especially in the first few days after birth. As the thoracic skeleton contains so much flexible cartilage and lacks rigidity, contraction of the accessory muscles has little effect. The thorax tends therefore to collapse inwards (retract) with each inspiration, particularly during sleep (Henderson-Smart and Read 1978). Consequently anything that impedes diaphragmatic movement will cause respiratory distress (Roberts and Edwards 1971). In the premature infant this tendency is much greater and may seriously impede ventilation.

Summary

The development of the lungs in the embryonic, fetal and neonatal periods, with their continuing development through childhood is briefly described, as are the mechanics of ventilation. It is essential for the physiotherapist to understand the process of development in order to appreciate the significance of physical measures in the prevention and treatment of respiratory disorders in infancy and childhood.

References

Avery, M.E. (1975) *The Lung and its Disorders in the Newborn Infant*, 2nd edn. Philadelphia, PA: W.B. Saunders.

Doershuk, C.F., Fisher, B.J. and Matthews, L.W. (1975) Pulmonary physiology of the young child. In: *Pulmonary Physiology of the Fetus, Newborn and Child*, edited by E.M. Scarpelli. Philadelphia, PA: Lea & Febiger.

Hamilton, W.J., Boyd, J.D. and Mossman, H.W. (1972) *Human Embryology* Cambridge: Heffer.

Henderson-Smart, D.J. (1984) Regulation of breathing in the perinatal period. In: *Sleep and Breathing*, edited by N.A. Saunders and C.E. Sullivan. New York: Marcel Decker.

Henderson-Smart, D.J. and Read, D.J. (1978) Depression of intercostal and abdominal muscle activity and vulnerability to asphyxia during active sleep in the newborn. In: *Sleep Apnea Syndromes*, edited by C. Guilleminault and W. Dement. New York: A.R. Liss.

Keens, T.G., Bryan, A.C., Levison, H. and Ianuzzo, C.D. (1978) Developmental pattern of muscle fibre types in human ventilatory muscles. *J. Appl. Physiol.*, **44**, 909–913.

Kendig, E.L. and Chernick, V. eds (1977) *Disorders of the Respiratory Tract in Children*. Philadelphia, PA: W.B. Saunders.

Laitman, J.T. and Crelin, E.S. (1980) Developmental change in the upper respiratory system of human infants. *Perinatol. Neonatol.*, **4**, 15.

Langman, J. (1969) *Medical Embryology*. Baltimore, MD: Williams & Wilkins.

Loring, S.H. and de Troyer, A. (1985) Actions of the respiratory muscles. In: *The Thorax*, edited by C. Roussos and P.T. Macklem. New York: Marcel Dekker.

Muller, N.L. and Bryan, A.C. (1979) Chest wall mechanics and respiratory muscles in infants. *Pediatr. Clin. North Am.*, **26**, 503.

Muller, N., Gulston, G., Cade, D. *et al.* (1979) Diaphragmatic muscle fatigue in the newborn. *J. Appl. Physiol*, **46**, 688–695.

Murray, J.F. (1976) *The Normal Lung*. Philadelphia, PA: W.B. Saunders.

Polgar, G. and Weng, T.R. (1979) The functional development of the respiratory system. *Am. Rev. Respir. Dis.*, **120**, 625–695.

Reid, L. (1977) The lung: its growth and remodeling in health and disease. *Am. J. Roentgenol.*, **129**, 777.

Roberts, K.D. and Edwards, J.M. (1971) *Paediatric Intensive Care*. Oxford: Blackwell.

Steindler, A. (1955) *Kinesiology of the Human Body*. IL: Thomas.

Thurlbeck, W.M. (1975) Postnatal growth and development of the lung. *Am. Rev. Respir. Dis.*, **111**, 803.

Further reading

Bucher, U. and Reid, L. (1961) Development of the intrasegmental bronchial tree. *Thorax*, **16**, 207.

Bucher, U. and Reid, L. (1961) Development of the mucus-secreting elements in human lung. *Thorax*, **16**, 219.

Burns, B.D. (1963) The central control of respiratory movements. *Br. Med. Bull.* **19**, 7.

Comroe, J.H. (1974) *The Physiology of Respiration*, 2nd edn. Chicago, IL: Year Book.

Cotes, J.E. (1975) *Lung Function*, 3rd edn. Oxford: Blackwell.

Crelin, E.S. (1975) *Development of the Lower Respiratory Tract*. New Jersey: Ciba-Geigy.

de Rueck, A.V.S. and Porter, R. (1967) *Development of the Lung*. Ciba Foundation Symposium. London: Churchill.

Emery, J. (1969) Embryogenesis. In: *The Anatomy of the Developing Lung*. Oxford: Butterworth-Heinemann.

Iliff, A. and Lee, V.A. (1952) Pulse rate, respiratory rate and body temperature between 2 months and 18 years. *Child Dev*, **23**, 237.

Karlberg, P. and Koch, G. (1962) Respiratory studies in newborn infants. III. Development of mechanics of breathing during the first week of life. *Acta Paediatr. Suppl.*, **135**, 121.

Polgar, G. and Promadhat, V. (1971) *Pulmonary Function Testing in Children: Techniques and Standards*. Philadelphia, PA: W.B. Saunders.

Strang, L.B. (1977) Growth and development of the lung. *Ann. Rev. Physiol.*, **39**, 253.

West, J.B. (1985) *Respiratory Physiology – The Essentials*, 3rd edn. Baltimore, MD: Williams & Wilkins.

25

Respiratory disorders in the neonatal period and infancy

Respiratory abnormalities comprise some of the commonest causes of death in the newborn. Several structural and metabolic factors associated with immaturity predispose the infant to acute respiratory failure:

1 The high incidence of respiratory tract infection due to decreased immunological defences.
2 Small airway size.
3 Poor mechanical advantage of the respiratory muscles (absence of fatigue-resistant fibres, poor development of abdominal muscles, horizontal alignment of the ribcage, lack of rigidity of costosternal cartilage, the predominantly supine position with the abdominal viscera impeding the full descent of the diaphragm).
4 High metabolic rate.
5 Small glycogen support (Pagliara *et al.* 1973).

Respiratory abnormalities result from varying causes: from infection as in staphylococcal and streptococcal pneumonia and bronchiolitis, from congenital abnormalities such as tracheo-oesophageal fistula and congenital heart disease, and from such genetically determined diseases as cystic fibrosis. Premature babies may suffer respiratory distress syndrome and other respiratory abnormalities arising from their immature respiratory and circulatory systems.

Generalized atelectasis is seen frequently in premature infants and may be due to a defi-ciency of the normal alveolar lining layer resulting from the immaturity of lungs which have not progressed to the stage of adequate alveolar formation (Avery 1975). Segmental atelectasis is a more common complication in infants with respiratory infection than in older children (Kendig and Chernick 1977), because of the relatively undeveloped state of the lungs and the small diameter of the airways. It is difficult for an infant to clear bronchial obstruction because of the hypermobile thorax and undeveloped muscular control. Atelectasis results most commonly from obstruction by mucus secretions in such diseases as bronchiolitis and pneumonia. However, obstruction can also be caused by the inhalation of a foreign body. Young infants have an immature swallowing pattern which allows aspiration of feeds with the possibility of airways obstruction. Atelectasis may result from lack of alveolar patency as seen in infants with respiratory distress syndrome, in which there is no control over surface tension, resulting in retraction of the alveolar walls. Obstructive atelectasis is preventable if postural drainage is efficiently and frequently performed on all infants with increased mucus secretions from whatever cause.

It is essential in the treatment of infants with respiratory disorders for the physiotherapist to consider the brain's need for oxygen, that is, the relationship between brain function and respiration. This consideration is essential in the treatment of premature and full-term neonates and infants. It appears that acidosis and anoxia may be important factors in the production of lesions of the central nervous system and that there may be some correlation between the severity of these lesions and the length of survival under anoxic and acidotic conditions. The combination of apnoea, cyanosis, hypotension and a sudden drop in haematocrit is recognized as often correlating in preterm infants with severe intracerebral haemorrhage (Grunnet *et al.* 1974).

Several investigators (e.g. Finer and Boyd 1978) have studied the effects of chest physiotherapy on neonates with various pulmonary disorders, with the specific aim of determining its effect on arterial blood gases. Appropriate physiotherapy was found to lead to an increase in arterial pO_2 which was sustained.

Bronchiolitis

This is an acute viral infection which affects infants during their first 6 months of life.

Pathophysiology

Inflammation of the small airways occurs due to the infection, which causes oedema of the bronchial walls, the lumen of which becomes further obstructed by the excessive secretions from the mucosal lining. If the obstruction is not removed air becomes trapped distally, and atelectasis occurs if this air is completely absorbed. The trapped secretions in the collapsed segment may also become infected. Contraction of the smooth muscles of the bronchiolar walls occurs and airways narrowing is more marked on expiration. Difficulty in expiring air causes hyperinflation of the lungs, and the diaphragm becomes flattened, moving little on inspiration or expiration. When hypoxaemia becomes severe, carbon dioxide retention can occur.

Clinical features

The infection begins in the upper respiratory tract. A paroxysmal cough develops. The respiratory rate increases, and being distressed, the infant uses the accessory muscles of respiration. The chest wall, very mobile in infants, retracts on inspiration because the already flattened diaphragm cannot descend any further and acts paradoxically to retract the lower ribs. Upper thoracic movement is obvious. Crepitations can be heard on auscultation, both on inspiration and expiration, and wheezing is evident on expiration due to airways narrowing. If the decrease in oxygen is marked the infant will appear cyanosed, becoming very distressed, with flaring of the nostrils on inspiration, restlessness and opisthotonus. Feeding is usually difficult and insufficient intake of fluid increases the risk, already present, of dehydration.

Treatment

The infant is given oxygen therapy through a plastic head box or a small tent or by endotracheal intubation, and the air is humidified. If there is bronchospasm a bronchodilator is administered before postural drainage is given. Postural drainage with squeezing of the chest wall, vibrations and clapping are done as often as necessary, in order to dislodge obstructive secretions and prevent atelectasis (Chapter 27). The infant may need to be tube-fed, as respiratory difficulties will increase the likelihood of aspiration of feeds.

Pneumonia

This is frequently a fatal condition in the young infant. It may be caused by the aspiration of material such as meconium which may occur just before birth, by the aspiration of regurgitated feeds, or by the inhalation of air-borne bacteria or viruses. Regurgitated milk, if aspirated by a newborn baby, particularly if premature, may cause severe obstruction of the airways, which may be followed by secondary bacterial pneumonia. Aspiration probably occurs because of the uncoordinated swallowing mechanisms in the infant, and is particularly likely to occur in premature infants and in infants with brain damage. Aspiration also occurs as a result of the defect in tracheo-oesophageal fistula, and is sometimes the result of the forced feeding of crying infants.

Pathology

Inflammation of the bronchial, bronchiolar and alveolar walls occurs with resultant increase in mucus secretions and exudate. Where obstruction is marked, atelectasis occurs. Aspiration pneumonia occurs most commonly in the posterior segments of the lungs, particularly of the right upper lobe in infants due to the anatomy of the airways and the habitual horizontal posture. Pneumonia from inhalation of bacteria and viruses is usually diffusely spread throughout the lungs.

Clinical features

The neonate who has aspirated material before birth is slow to establish respiration, will have a low Apgar rating, and will probably need to be resuscitated. The infant who develops pneumonia later will demonstrate signs of respiratory difficulty, with rapid, shallow, grunting breaths, flaring of the alae nasi and rib recession. The baby may become cyanosed or have periods of apnoea.

Treatment

This infant must be promptly and vigorously treated. Medical treatment involves the administration of antibiotics and, if necessary, oxygen therapy. Physical treatment is directed at clearing the airways by postural drainage and pharyngeal aspiration (see Chapter 27).

Tracheo-oesophageal fistula with oesophageal atresia

The mechanisms of these malformations are still unclear. They are frequently associated with muscular and skeletal anomalies, cardiac lesions and gastrointestinal abnormalities. The insult to the embryo probably occurs between the second and fourth week of gestation. Oesophageal atresia and tracheo-oesophageal fistula may occur as separate defects but maldevelopment of the trachea and oesophagus in its commonest form results in the oesophagus ending in a blind pouch with a fistula passing between the trachea and the lower oesophagus (Fig. 25.1). There are other forms of the defect (Ashcraft and Holder 1976). Mucus secretions and feeds pour into the upper oesophageal pouch, and overflow into the trachea. Gastric contents may also reflux through the distal fistula into the lungs. Crying contributes to this as

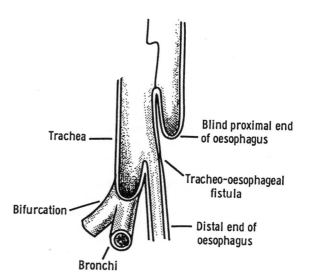

Figure 25.1 One type of tracheo-oesophageal fistula with oesophageal atresia.

the closure of the glottis forces air through the tracheo-oesophageal fistula and into the stomach. This allows reflux of the chemical contents of the stomach into the airway, causing a chemical pneumonitis usually located in the right upper lobe.

Treatment

The infant will die in the neonatal period if the condition is not recognized and treated very early after birth. Early treatment is necessary to avoid aspiration and regurgitation pneumonitis. The therapist must report any neonate who appears to have excessive mucus, who coughs, chokes, regurgitates and becomes cyanotic when being fed. This apparently excessive mucus is regurgitated saliva which cannot be swallowed.

Urgent surgical treatment to divide the fistula and anastomose the oesophagus is essential. The infant is referred to the physiotherapist pre- and postoperatively to aid drainage of aspirated material and mucus secretions, and to improve aeration of the lungs (Chapter 27).

Preoperative treatment is essential to improve the infant's chance of surviving surgery and the postoperative period. It includes gastrostomy for gastric decompression and continuous suction of the blind upper pouch. The infant is nursed in semi-Fowler's position.

Following the thoracotomy there is a tendency for right upper lobe collapse. Castilla *et al.* (1971) have suggested nursing the infant in prone following surgery to repair oesophageal atresia, and described a special frame to facilitate nursing care.

Idiopathic respiratory distress syndrome (hyaline membrane disease)

This disease is one of the commonest causes of respiratory symptoms and a relatively common cause of death in newborn premature infants. The aetiology is unclear, although there are several theories (Avery 1975). It occurs in premature infants and in infants with diabetic mothers. Its occurrence in premature infants is related to surfactant deficiency. However, other factors, including development of asphyxia in the perinatal period (with resultant damage to the respiratory mucosa), may contribute. At birth these babies typically have a low Apgar rating and require resuscitation. They may demonstrate the flaccid posture of the premature infant. Respiratory failure may cause death, and cerebral haemorrhage is not uncommon. This syndrome is a major cause of death in premature neonates. However, early intensive care can significantly reduce morbidity and mortality.

Pathophysiology

The pathology of this disease is little understood. The appearance of the lungs at autopsy differs according to whether the infant was still- or live-born and to the length of time survived. The lungs usually appear underinflated with areas of atelectasis. Alveoli are often filled with fluid of a high protein content resembling a hyaline membrane. In this case the infant is said to have suffered hyaline membrane disease. There is a decreased amount of surfactant. Surfactant, a lipoprotein which normally binds to the internal walls of alveoli, equalizes the forces of surface tension in the alveoli and is a potent factor in preventing atelectasis.

The infant shows hypoxaemia and hypercapnia with poor peripheral blood flow (Fig. 25.2). The impairment of gas exchange is due to poor perfusion/ventilation matching. The deficiency in the surfactant allows the alveoli to collapse

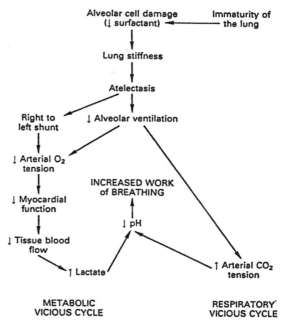

Figure 25.2 Aetiology and consequences of respiratory distress syndrome. (Adapted from Jones, R.S. and Owen-Thomas, J.B. (1971) *Care of the Critically Ill Child.* London: Arnold.)

because of lack of control over the surface tension which it normally provides.

Bronchopulmonary dysplasia, a form of chronic obstructive lung disease, has been described (Reilly *et al.* 1973) in infants treated for respiratory distress syndrome. It is manifested by bronchospasm, cyanosis, pneumonitis and bronchitis and the infants may have atelectasis, focal air-trapping and fibrosis. The pathogenesis is controversial but the condition is considered to result from factors arising from mechanical ventilation, high concentrations of oxygen and endotracheal intubation. Philip (1975) comments that immature lungs may develop bronchopulmonary dysplasia when they are exposed to inspired oxygen concentrations over 40% for as little as 3 days via positive pressure ventilation. In other words, it appears that immature lungs react differently from mature lungs in this situation.

Mikity–Wilson syndrome, or pulmonary dysmaturity, has a clinical course comparable with bronchopulmonary dysplasia. The syndrome occurs in very premature infants and its cause is unknown (Klaus and Fanaroff 1979).

Clinical features

Gradually increasing respiratory insufficiency occurs within a few hours of birth. Breathing is difficult and laboured, and the infant demonstrates rapid, shallow, grunting respirations. The intercostal and subcostal spaces are retracted. There are apnoeic periods and central cyanosis, with a tendency to hypothermia. There may be a build-up of secretions.

Treatment

There is considerable controversy about the aetiology and pathology of respiratory distress syndrome, and therefore about the management of these infants.

In general, treatment in intensive care is directed towards improving ventilation, giving thermal protection, providing for metabolic needs and supporting circulation.

Physiotherapy in the form of bronchial drainage is designed to clear airways and aerate the atelectactic lungs (Finer and Boyd 1978). Treatment is largely supportive, the infant being given oxygen in the incubator. As with all premature infants, the body temperature must not be allowed to fall as this will increase the need for oxygen.

The use of respirators for these infants is controversial (Avery 1975). Some surviving infants show the harmful effects of high oxygen and low nitrogen concentrations in inspired air, of endotracheal intubation and positive pressure ventilation (Jones and Owen-Thomas 1971; Philip 1975). The inhalation of a high oxygen concentration by premature infants will lead to retrolental fibroplasia and may cause permanent blindness. It is considered that the early use of continuous positive airways pressure may be protective of the lungs of many infants. Kronskop *et al.* (1975) have suggested that it may prevent the inactivity of surfactant in those infants who weigh 1500 g or more at birth.

Summary

Some respiratory disorders seen in infants are described. These disorders may be due to the infant's immaturity, or to infection; in rare cases there may be a congenital cause. As more neonates of low gestational age survive the perinatal period and intensive care facilities improve, the physiotherapist's role in neonatal pulmonary care increases, as does the need for the physiotherapist to be well-informed about that role and the effects of immaturity on lung function. The major objectives of physiotherapy in neonates with pulmonary dysfunction are to improve clearance of airways, enhance ventilation and decrease the work of breathing (Crane 1990). Early, frequent, and vigorous physical treatment is essential in infants with respiratory disorder if permanent lung damage or permanent retardation of lung development is to be avoided.

References

Ashcraft, K.W. and Holder, T.M. (1976) Esophageal atresia and tracheoesophageal fistula malformations. *Surg. Clin. North Am.*, **56**, 2, 299.

Avery, M.E. (1975) *The Lung and its Disorders in the Newborn Infant*, 2nd edn. Philadelphia, PA: W.B. Saunders.

Castilla, P., Irving, I.M., Jackson Rees, G. and Rickman, P.P. (1971) Posture in management of esophageal atresia. *J. Pediatr. Surg.*, **6**, 6, 709.

Crane, L.D. (1990) Physical therapy for the neonate with respiratory disease. In: *Cardiopulmonary Physical Therapy*, edited by S. Irwin and J.S. Tecklin. St Louis, MO: C.V. Mosby.

Finer, N.N. and Boyd, J. (1978) Chest physiotherapy in the neonate: a controlled study. *Pediatrics*, **61**, 282.

Grunnet, M.L., Curless, R.G., Bray, P.F. and Jung, A.L. (1974) Brain changes in newborns from an intensive care unit. *Dev. Med. Child Neurol.*, **16**, 320.

Jones, R.S. and Owen-Thomas, J.B. (1971) *Care of the Critically Ill Child*. London: Edward Arnold.

Kendig, E.L. and Chernick, V. (eds) (1977) *Disorders of the Respiratory Tract in Children*, 2nd edn. Philadelphia, PA: W.B. Saunders.

Klaus, M.H. and Fanaroff, A.A. (1979) *Care of the High-Risk Neonate*, 2nd edn. Philadelphia, PA: W.B. Saunders.

Kronskop, R.W., Brown, E.G. and Sweet, A.Y. (1975) The early use of C.P.A.P. in the treatment of idiopathic respiratory distress syndrome. *Pediatrics*, **87**, 2, 263.

Pagliara, A.S., Karl, I.E., Haymond, M. and Kipnis, D.M. (1973) Hypoglycemia in infancy and childhood. *J. Pediatr.*, **82**, 365–379.

Philip, A.G.S. (1975) Oxygen plus pressure plus time: the etiology of bronchopulmonary dysplasia. *Pediatrics*, **55**, 44.

Reilly, B.J., Bryan, M.H., Hardie, M.J. and Swyer, P.R. (1973) Pulmonary function studies during the first year of life in infants recovering from the respiratory distress syndrome. *Pediatrics*, **52**, 169.

Further reading

Behrmann, R.E. and Vaughan, V.C. (1987) *Nelson Textbook of Pediatrics*. 13th edn. Philadelphia, PA: W.B. Saunders.

Farrell, P.M. and Avery, M.E. (1975) Hyaline membrane disease. *Am. Rev. Respir. Dis.*, **3**, 657.

Schaffer, A.T. and Avery, M.E. (eds) (1977) *Diseases of the Newborn*, 4th edn. Philadelphia, PA: W.B. Saunders, pp. 122–126.

26

Respiratory disorders in childhood

The commonest respiratory disorders of childhood seen by the physiotherapist are asthma, bronchitis, bronchiectasis, asthmatic or allergic bronchitis and cystic fibrosis, and only these will be described at any length in this chapter. There are, however, other respiratory disorders for which children will be referred to the physiotherapist for treatment. For example, physiotherapy has a preventive role in ensuring clear airways and improving ventilation in children with immunosuppression associated with acquired immunodeficiency syndrome (AIDS) or bone marrow transplantation. Children who have thoracic or abdominal surgery require pre- and postoperative physiotherapy. Atelectasis or pneumonia is seen in children who have inhaled a foreign body, following pertussis (whooping cough) and as a complication of other respiratory disorders, such as cystic fibrosis. Atelectasis and pneumonia have been described in Chapter 25.

The infant leads a relatively protected life, hence it is common for respiratory infections to begin when the child first goes to school, and the infections may be recurrent through the early school-going years while immunological defences develop.

Pertussis (whooping cough)

This is a common infectious disease of childhood, and although it usually runs an uncomplicated course, it may be followed by extensive lung collapse or bronchopneumonia. The child will be referred to the physiotherapist for treatment to clear the airways and to assist in re-expansion of the lungs.

Inhalation of a foreign body

The embryonic right bronchus is slightly larger than the left and more vertically oriented. These differences become more pronounced as the bronchi mature, and foreign bodies are therefore more likely to enter the right bronchus than the left.

Inhalation of foreign bodies such as peanuts and small toys is common throughout infancy and childhood. If the foreign body is not immediately coughed up it will lodge in the airway, causing obstruction.

The foreign body irritates the wall of the airway, causing inflammation and mucosal oedema, and eventually air absorption and collapse of that part of the lung. Air is trapped distal to the obstruction and the area becomes atelectatic. The accumulated secretions become infected and the child develops the signs of pneumonitis, a fever and cough.

The child will be referred for physiotherapy to clear the airways and regain full lung expansion immediately following bronchoscopic removal of the foreign body. Postural drainage given before this may result in obstruction of a vital airway when the foreign body shifts positions, and it has been recommended that bronchial drainage should be carried out in the presence of resuscitative equipment (Law and Kosloske 1976).

Bronchitis

Clinically, bronchitis means many things, and occurs in conjunction with many varied clinical features. It may be more a symptom than a disease entity in itself, occurring, for example, as part of pertussis or cystic fibrosis. The primary problem may exist in the upper respiratory tract with infection spreading from a chronic sinus infection, or from the nose following a common cold. It may also exist in the lower respiratory tract, following on from infection of the trachea, or accompanied by wheezing, or occurring as part of a generalized inflammation of the airways.

It is the acute bronchitis which occurs recurrently in some children, and which may follow on from an upper respiratory tract infection, from measles or another infectious disease, which is described here. It is caused by viral or bacterial infections.

Clinical features

The child develops a cough which may be dry, hacking and painful in the beginning with some fever. Later the cough becomes productive of purulent sputum. Coarse crackles or wheeze may be present. If uncontrolled, pneumonia may develop.

Treatment

Antibiotic therapy and postural drainage are the usual means of treatment. Postural drainage need not be specific for certain segments. The child is drained as for the lower lobes (Chapter 27), at an angle of 45° from the horizontal, in prone and side lying, with percussion, vibrations and breathing exercises emphasizing full expiration. Parents are taught how to carry out treatment at home three to four times daily, and it is suggested that this routine be recommended on any subsequent occasion when the child develops a cough following an upper respiratory tract infection.

This is also an excellent opportunity for teaching nasal hygiene. It is surprising how many older children are incapable of blowing their noses thoroughly, and it is important to spend some time in giving this instruction to any child presenting with a respiratory disorder.

Bronchiectasis

This disease has not been commonly seen in children during the last decades (Illingworth 1971, Kendig and Chernick 1977). It is suggested that this may be due to the decrease in numbers of children having pertussis and measles and other childhood diseases which were frequently associated with the development of bronchiectasis, plus the effectiveness of antibacterial drugs in preventing and controlling respiratory tract infections.

Bronchiectasis may occur following infectious diseases such as bronchiolitis and pneumonia, as part of Kartagener's syndrome of sinusitis, bronchiectasis and situs inversus, or as part of a genetically determined disease such as cystic fibrosis.

Pathology

An infective episode results in a severe inflammatory reaction within the bronchi. The mucus-secreting glands produce exudate and viscous secretions accumulate, blocking the distal airways. Atelectasis will occur if obstruction is complete and the bronchus proximal to the obstruction dilates, causing cylindrical or saccular dilations (see Fig. 27.1). Typically, large amounts of exudate accumulate. A cycle then occurs in which secondary infections of the accumulated secretions occur with increased exudate and accumulation of secretions. The dilated bronchial walls show, depending on the stage of progression of the disease, loss of elastic tissue and damage to the muscular and cartilaginous walls. This results in loss of the flexibility of the bronchial walls.

Clinical features

The child presents with a chronic cough which is productive of copious amounts of mucus, especially in the morning. In children with severe chronic disease, dyspnoea on minimal exertion, anorexia and haemoptysis may be evident. Clubbing of the fingers is common in long-standing cases.

Treatment

Medical treatment is aimed at controlling the infection by the use of antibiotics. These children are referred to the physiotherapist for removal of secretions by postural drainage, percussion, forced expiratory technique (FET) and effective coughing, and for instruction to the child's parents in the techniques to be used at home (Chapter 27). Medical and physical treatment will be successful in most cases, but if not, it may be necessary for surgical removal of the involved section of the lung.

Asthma

Asthma is a disorder characterized by hyperreactivity of smooth muscles of the bronchial walls in response to a variety of internal and external factors. Children with asthma experience repeated attacks of difficulty with breathing, frequently with considerable respiratory embarrassment. The severity of an attack may range from a mild wheezing to a fatal asphyxia. The aetiology is not clear as it appears there may be many causes, even for one individual. Factors such as change in temperature, stress, inhaled allergens, infection, exercise, exposure to bronchial irritants and fatigue may precipitate an asthma attack. Attacks may come on at night, with little or no warning, or may occur as an obvious result of one of the above factors. During these attacks there is an urgent need for air which varies in degree, and it is not surprising that the child appears very anxious. There is wheezing on expiration, a tight cough and laboured breathing. When the cough becomes productive, as it may when the airways resistance is less severe, the sputum is seen to be sticky and tenacious, although it may be coughed up in small plugs. A child whose asthma attack remains unresponsive to treatment after a period of some hours is said to be in status asthmaticus. It should be noted that wheezing does not occur only in asthma, but may be heard in children with obstruction due to an inhaled foreign body, when it is usually heard as an inspiratory wheeze, or with bronchiolitis.

Pathology

An asthma attack is the result of a widespread decrease in airway calibre caused by contraction of the bronchial smooth muscle. During an attack there is gradually increasing obstruction of the peripheral airways. Obstruction is rarely complete and it has been suggested (Gandevia 1959) that the term airways resistance is more accurate. This airways resistance is caused by oedema of the inflamed mucous membrane. Spasm of the smooth muscles of the bronchi further decreases the lumen, and increased mucus secretions from the tracheobronchial glands cause mucus plugging and further obstruction. The lungs become hyperinflated with air, which is gasped by the child and which cannot be completely exhaled due to further airway narrowing during expiration. If obstruction of a bronchus or a bronchiole becomes complete, atelectasis or complete collapse of a segment may occur.

Physiology

The physiological changes underlying asthmatic signs and symptoms are thought to be initiated by release of chemical mediators from mast cells within the airways (e.g. histamine). These stimu-late a parasympathetic nervous system response. Contraction of smooth muscles leads to increased mucus secretions from goblet cells of the bronchial epithelium, leading to oedema of the bronchial vasculature, obstruction of airways, decreased expiratory air flow, increased lung volume and airways resistance, decreased airway conductance, ventilation/perfusion inequality and arterial hypoxaemia. The forced expiratory volume in 1 second (FEV_1) is markedly decreased as demonstrated by the result of pulmonary function tests.

In the lungs of children in status asthmaticus, so little air is moving in either direction that carbon dioxide retention becomes marked. Carbon dioxide is the normal stimulus to respiration, acting upon the respiratory centre in the brainstem. When carbon dioxide is retained the respiratory centre adapts and responsiveness is reduced. Respiration is then regulated by oxygen lack, which is detected by the carotid bodies and the aorta. It is this that gives the patient the desperate need for air called air hunger. At this stage, when it is the lack of oxygen only that is driving the patient to breathe, care must be taken in the administration of oxygen, as this may remove the stimulus to breathe.

Allergy

There is said to be an allergic factor present in many cases of asthma in children. It seems that certain substances cause an allergic reaction in the air passages, the allergens having a special affinity for the mucous membranes of the respiratory tract.

Allergic children are rarely allergic to only one substance, but are usually found to react to substances as varied as house dust, food and pollen. Some children appear to be prone to allergy from birth, suffering eczema and rhinitis for a few years until they have their first attack of asthma. There are some children whose asthma appears to be due to other than allergic reactions, seeming more related to infection, although this also may involve an immunological reaction.

Exercise-induced asthma

For some children, asthma is induced by exercise. After a few minutes of exercise, there is a sudden onset of symptoms and the child develops dyspnoea and wheezing. It is thought that the increased ventilation during exercise results in heat and water loss from the respiratory mucosa. The water loss increases the osmolarity of the respiratory tract and decreases the temperature. This results in a release of mediators from mast cells in the airway lumen, which causes contraction of bronchial smooth muscle and oedema of the bronchial vasculature (Anderson 1988).

Clinical features

During an asthma attack the child demonstrates signs and symptoms that result from increased airways resistance causing interference with air exchange. There is a cough which is paroxysmal and non-productive. Breathing becomes progressively more laboured with shallow inspirations and prolonged wheezing expirations. The child tries to fix the shoulder girdle by bracing the arms and hunching the trunk, in this way increasing the effectiveness of the accessory muscles of respiration. Hyperinflation causes the respiratory mus-

cles to be at a mechanical disadvantage, which puts a further strain on the respiratory system. The child may appear cyanosed, the chest distended in an anteroposterior direction, and showing little movement. Breathing is mostly upper chest and the lower ribs, already elevated, suck in on inspiration. If the attack becomes more severe, breath sounds are almost inaudible and the cough is suppressed.

At this stage the child is liable to asphyxiate. Signs of right-sided heart failure may be evident. However, the severity of the attack usually decreases and as it does the cough becomes productive.

Between asthma attacks the child may appear to have normal respiratory function, although dyspnoea may be experienced on minimal exertion. Some children appear in poor health, fail to put on weight, and have poor exercise tolerance. Some may become habitual 'upper chest breathers' due to chronic hyperinflation if their asthma is not well-controlled. Some children demonstrate distortions of the chest due to the pressure changes brought about by forced inspiration and expiration. This deformity may be produced early before ossification of cartilaginous junctions occurs.

Treatment

The aims of treatment depend on the problems with which each child presents, but the following aims will probably require to be fulfilled with most asthmatic children.

1 To remove as far as possible any predisposing factors and to minimize sensitivity to particular allergens.
2 To decrease bronchial obstruction due to oedema or bronchial smooth muscle spasm.
3 To improve exercise tolerance.
4 To remove excessive secretions from the lungs.

Medical treatment

A child may undergo hyposensitization to minimize sensitivity to particular allergens, although the effectiveness of this is controversial. In order to avoid the predisposing causes of attacks the child may have to sleep in a dust-free room.

Corticosteroid therapy will be necessary for some children with intractable asthma in order to control mucosal oedema that predisposes to frequent attacks. Antibiotics may be prescribed to counteract infection. Otherwise bronchodilator drugs are prescribed to be taken orally or by spray inhalation when necessary, as well as a mast cell stabilizer (disodium cromoglycate). Long-term management involves pharmacological, environmental and immunological interventions.

Physical treatment

The place of the physiotherapist in the treatment of the asthmatic child is sometimes misunderstood. There have been dogmatic claims made in the past about the effectiveness of certain methods of treatment, although there are probably no completely effective techniques. However, the skilful physiotherapist should be able to work out with each child the most effective assistance. There may be a few children who are not helped by physical treatment. Most children, however, will derive some benefit from a carefully planned programme of treatment, particularly in improved breathing control, improved exercise tolerance, and in the prevention of thoracic and spinal deformity. It is also important to remember two factors. The first is that the lungs of a young child are developing during growth and secondly, a large number of children with asthma appear to grow out of it by the time they reach adolescence. It is therefore important that the child's breathing control and respiratory efficiency are maintained at as normal a level as possible during these years of development.

The experienced physiotherapist can also offer considerable psychological support to the child and family. As Hinshaw and Garland (1965) stated: 'Treatment that serves to quiet fear ... is good treatment'. There is probably considerable value in asthma holiday camps, where a physiotherapist is able to be with the child during attacks and is able to calm fear and encourage relaxation.

Outpatient physiotherapy may include controlled breathing techniques, exercises for thoracic mobility, relaxation and conditioning exercises (Seligman *et al.* 1970; De Cesare and Graybill 1990). The physiotherapist should discuss with the child and parent an emergency plan for use during an acute attack. Postural drainage with percussion and vibrations may help to clear secretions after bronchodilation.

Some of the techniques of treatment which may be of use in overcoming the problems of these children are described below.

To decrease bronchial obstruction and remove excessive secretions from the air passages

Bronchodilator drugs (e.g., salbutamol or isoprenaline)

These are prescribed by the physician for the relief of bronchospasm. They are administered from a hand-held apparatus, via a nebulizer attached to an air pump or via intermittent positive pressure breathing apparatus.

Hand-operated aerosol dispenser

Use of the dispenser must be carefully taught to the child and parent. This method can only be effective if the child is old enough to coordinate an effective inhalation with the operation of the spray mechanism, otherwise the spray will penetrate no further than the mouth. The prophylactic use of disodium cromoglycate (Intal) via a spinhaler enables many children with asthma to lead relatively normal lives. Children over 3 years can inhale effectively, as can some children even younger. A very young child can be taught on a spinhaler. The child must be supervised in the use of the spray, as overuse may result in chemical irritation of the airways and other severe complications. There is a limit to the number of times the bronchodilator may be used each 24 hours, and this limit must be carefully adhered to.

Nebulizer with mouthpiece

Webber *et al.* (1974) suggested that in the stage of recovery from status asthmaticus, the bronchodilator response is as good using a simple nebulizer as with intermittent positive pressure breathing. It is also less frightening for young children, and can be used by a young child who cannot yet cope with a spinhaler or metered aerosol.

Intermittent positive pressure ventilators

The two machines in common use are the Bennett and the Bird ventilators. This method of inhalation is used in some instances to deliver bronchodilator aerosols.

Postural drainage

Coughing and postural drainage may aggravate bronchospasm. However, once bronchospasm has been sufficiently relieved, excessive mucus secretions are removed from the lungs by postural drainage. Unless there is a specific area of a lung to be drained, as would occur if there was an area of collapse or infection present, it is usually sufficient to drain the patient in side lying (prone if it is easily tolerated) as for the lower lobes (see Fig. 27.16). Supine is not usually well-tolerated. There is a tendency for the diaphragm to elevate in supine, due to movement of the abdominal viscera and this increases the patient's breathing difficulties. If the child cannot tolerate the deeply tipped position it may be modified as in Fig. 26.1 which is a position of relaxation. Breathing exercises encouraging expansion of the lower part of the thorax are given. Vibrations on expiration with encouragement to cough are given if they cause no tension or increase in wheezing. Many children find percussion effective in loosening secretions.

Postural drainage techniques are taught to the parents and should be carried out by the child after each asthma attack until the cough is unproductive. There is usually little to be gained from giving postural drainage to a

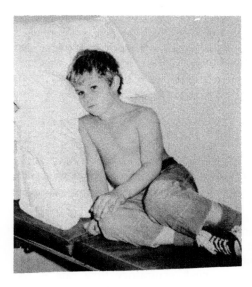

Figure 26.1 Position designed to promote relaxation and the elimination of secretions when the child cannot tolerate the horizontal position.

child with unrelieved severe bronchospasm, as the airways obstruction caused by the bronchospasm will not allow the free passage of secretions and the techniques used may increase the child's respiratory difficulty. However, there are some children who gain relief while lying in a tipped position, and each child must be evaluated individually.

Some asthmatic children, especially those whose asthma is related to recurrent attacks of bronchitis, require postural drainage as a daily routine at home in order to keep the airways free from excessive secretions. Others need drain only when necessary following an upper respiratory tract infection, or bronchitis, or an asthma attack. Toddlers may object strongly to the discipline of postural drainage, particularly when performed at home. It is better for the therapist to suggest to the parents of a 'chesty' infant that establishing during infancy a routine of daily postural drainage for 5 minutes will enable the toddler to accept drainage as part of the daily routine of eating, bathing and sleeping.

One 2-year-old who had been on this routine since the age of 8 months, would ask his mother for postural drainage whenever he felt he needed it. He seemed to have developed some understanding of the importance of drainage to his subjective well-being. Although he had several attacks of bronchitis and bronchospasm during this period, they cleared up rapidly and he required no further periods of hospitalization.

It is necessary to teach young children how to blow their noses efficiently, one nostril at a time. Allergic rhinitis and sometimes sinusitis are seen in asthmatic children. Mouth-breathing should be discouraged.

To improve breathing control and exercise tolerance, and to prevent deformity

During an asthma attack

The child is shown what to do to alleviate respiratory distress during an asthma attack. The success of this depends largely on the physiotherapist's ability to get the idea of self-help across to the child, on the child's age and therefore ability to understand the situation, and lastly on the ability of the family to control their own anxieties and negative feelings.

The time for the child to start on the emergency plan is when an attack feels imminent. While waiting for an administered bronchodilator to take effect, the child may find it useful to lean forwards in a relaxed position with the arms supported on a table, the edge of a bed or railing, attempting to breathe quietly with emphasis on depth of inspiration followed by a relaxed expiration (Figs 26.2 and 26.3). It is not advisable to attempt to alter the rate of breathing as such. The respiratory centre adjusts the rate and depth of breathing to obtain the best ventilation most economically (Gandevia 1959). However, the rate of breathing is also affected by the child's fear, and if this fear can be allayed the respiratory rate may become more efficient. The advantage of suggesting to the child that he or she can breathe more quietly lies in the allusion to relaxation and in the fact that the child is given something positive to think about. If the physiotherapist sees the child during the early stages of an attack, and if by attitude and conversation any fears can be dispelled, the child may be convinced of the usefulness of this approach. If a parent can give similar support at home, the child may be helped considerably. It is probable that this routine has little effect directly upon the respiratory pathophysiology – at

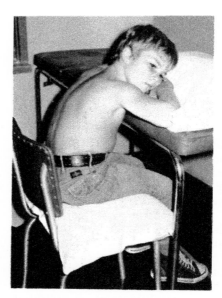

Figure 26.3 Position to promote relaxation and control of breathing.

least, there is no proof that it has. However, if the physiotherapist can teach the child to relax emotionally, the extra workload which is put on the respiratory system by the tense elevated shoulders and strong contraction of the accessory muscles will be relieved, and this will have an effect on the ventilatory system, even if not directly upon the pathophysiology within the lungs themselves. Treatment is an attempt to dispel fear and utilize the individual child's capacity to control to some extent his or her own body. In the author's opinion, it is always worthwhile attempting this approach. With some children, circumstances beyond the control of the physiotherapist and the child may render it useless.

Between asthma attacks

It is important that the asthmatic child learns how to avoid dyspnoea on exertion, as this may trigger an asthma attack. However, exercise and sport should not be avoided unless it is really necessary. The child needs to understand how to use drug therapy to block exercise-induced asthma, and the importance of not exercising if FEV_1 or peak expiratory flow rate is too low, so exercise can be carried out safely. The child can be taught to lean against a wall and relax breathing if dyspnoeic (Fig. 26.4). When

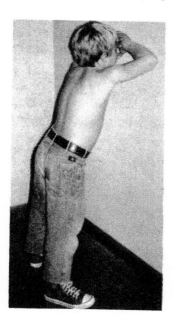

Figure 26.2 Position to promote relaxation and control of breathing.

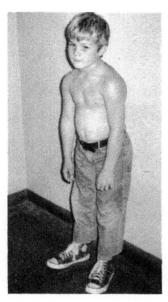

Figure 26.4 Position to promote relaxation and control of breathing.

possible, the child should be taught to swim, and encouraged to swim with the face in the water, to duck-dive in shallow water to pick up objects from the floor of the pool, and to swim underwater. Swimming has been shown to be preferable to running and bicycling as an exercise, as it results in significantly smaller falls in FEV_1 (Fitch and Morton 1971). Not only does swimming, if properly done, probably improve coordination in breathing, it also improves the child's physical development, helps prevent secondary deformity, such as kyphosis, rounded shoulders with contracted pectoral muscles, and improves thoracic expansion. Singing lessons accomplish similar aims in some children.

Sly and colleagues (Sly *et al*. 1972) report that a swimming programme resulted in fewer days on which wheezing occurred in the group of children who attended (from 31 days before the programme to 6 days during the programme). Fitch and colleagues (Fitch *et al.* 1976) reported on another group of children who attended a 5-month swimming programme. The children showed a marked improvement in asthma score (wheeze, cough, sputum), drug score (amount of medication) and physical work capacity. However, the authors found no change in FEV_1 or in the severity of exercise-induced asthma.

It may be necessary, if swimming is impractical, to give the child one or two exercises to be done at home, which will gain full extension of the thoracic spine, and full length of the pectoral muscles. These exercises will need to be changed before they become boring. It is important to remember that the asthmatic child has ahead several years of development, and that development cannot proceed normally in the presence of deformity and contracture.

Breathing exercises

The child is taught how to localize breathing and is discouraged from expanding only the upper thorax. Each day breathing exercises should be practised for 5 minutes, getting as full and efficient expansion as possible, in a relaxed manner. The aim is that the child practises the normal pattern of breathing in preparation for attempting it when respiratory function is threatened. Breathing exercises which emphasize long, forced expiration have no place in the treatment of the asthmatic child. A forced expiratory volume test of a normal person indicates that nearly all the air is exhaled within 2 seconds. Breathing exercises should stress relaxation, an effective deep inspiration concentrating on the diaphragm, which should be followed automatically by a passive relaxed expiration.

Classwork

Once a child and parents have been taught a home programme and the child is beginning to cope, visits to the physiotherapist can be decreased and on these visits the child could join a small group of 4 or 5 other children. In this way the physiotherapist is able to see how the child is coping with exercise and activities with other children, and can judge the effectiveness of attempts at controlling breathing in what is a more normal environment than may be present during individual treatment. The children practise their breathing exercises together, demonstrate their ability to breathe in a relaxed, normal manner between exercises and games, and there will be time for the physiotherapist to talk to the parents and hear about any difficulties at home. This treatment in a class is not suitable for some children who may need to have more individual contact with the therapist. Gaskell and Webber (1977) suggest the precautionary measurement of FEV_1 or peak flow rate of each child who attends. The child with low readings would have individual treatment, the administration of a bronchodilator and breathing exercises, with postural drainage if indicated.

The child in status asthmaticus

A child is said to be in status asthmaticus when asthma is still unrelieved despite usual therapy. Emergency treatment is necessary, and bronchospasm must be relieved as quickly as possible. A child may develop a dangerous degree of hypoxaemia within a few minutes, may quickly asphyxiate, and must not be left unattended while so acutely ill.

The administration of a bronchodilator by intermittent positive pressure breathing or nebulizer with mouthpiece or a mask is often very effective. Treatment is given 4-hourly during the acute phase. A peak flow chart filled in before and 15–30 minutes after treatment gives a picture of the effect of the bronchodilator upon lung function. Postural drainage can be instituted as soon as airway resistance is decreased sufficiently to allow drainage of secretions. The positions used will need to be modified if the child is not able to tolerate a deeply tipped position. Figure 26.1 shows a possible modification. Medical management includes corticosteroids or aminophylline administered intravenously.

Cystic fibrosis

This is an inherited, generalized disorder affecting the exocrine glands. It is inherited as a Mendelian recessive trait, and is now found to be fairly common in the community (perhaps 1:2000). The incidence varies within families. For example, in a family of four children, three may be affected, while in a family of seven only one may be affected. Some of the

children in both families will be carriers, but there is no positive method at the present time for determining which members of the community are carriers. For a child to be born with cystic fibrosis, both parents must be carriers (Fig. 26.5).

Pathology

The exocrine glands most frequently and significantly involved are those of the pancreas and of the tracheobronchial tree. Glandular secretions are of abnormal viscosity and readily cause obstruction. The salivary glands, nasal sinuses, intestinal and sweat glands are also involved.

The *pancreatic defect*, which is due to obstruction of the ducts, results in failure of the pancreas to secrete the enzymes trypsin, lipase and amylase, which are necessary for the breakdown of fats. Eventually, destruction of the enzyme-producing cells occurs. Interference with fat absorption within the intestine results.

The *pulmonary defect* is the most serious and difficult to control. Bronchial mucus secretions are normally produced by mucus and serous cells of the submucosal glands, but in the case of cystic fibrosis, in abnormally large quantities. The abnormally thick and sticky mucus causes obstruction of the airways. Pneumonia and recurrent attacks of bronchitis are common and the child may develop a chronic cough. Impacted mucus becomes infected, causing further obstruction by producing oedema and stimulating further increase of mucus secretions. Ciliary action is impaired and the normal clearing mechanism in the lungs is ineffective. Obstruction of the smaller airways, if it is complete, will result in atelectasis distal to the obstruction. Bronchospasm may occur with an effect similar to that seen in asthma. If respiratory disease is controlled, the pulmonary changes are reversible (see Fig. 23.1). If disease continues unchecked, bronchiectasis may

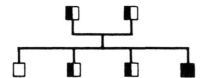

 ◨ Normal but Carrier
 ☐ Normal non-Carrier
 ■ Cystic fibrotic

Figure 26.5 Diagram showing the mode of inheritance of cystic fibrosis.

develop due to progressive weakness of the bronchiolar walls. Pockets of mucus in the bronchiectatic sacs are prone to reinfection and lead to further pulmonary damage. The pulmonary lesion may progress to obstructive emphysema and eventual right-sided heart failure. The failure to shift mucus will therefore be responsible for severe progressive and irreversible changes within the lungs.

The *sweat gland defect* results in the excessive secretion of sodium and chloride in the sweat.

Clinical features

The earliest manifestation of the disorder may be meconium ileus in the neonate. Immediately after birth the large intestine is found to be obstructed by thick viscid meconium. In most children the signs of pancreatic insufficiency appear before those of pulmonary insufficiency. The infant passes large quantities of foul-smelling fatty stools and is slow to thrive and gain weight. The pancreatic defect may cause recurrent abdominal pain and constipation.

The respiratory signs vary according to the pathology present at the time. Where there is chronic infection within the lungs the child will fail to thrive, and this failure may be augmented by malabsorption of food within the intestine. If bronchitis or bronchiectasis is present the child will have a cough productive of thick, tenacious and purulent sputum. If infection has caused pneumonia, the cough may be paroxysmal, the breathing rapid and shallow, with the accessory muscles of respiration elevating the thorax on inspiration. If bronchospasm is present, wheezing will be heard. As emphysematous changes develop the thorax may become hyperinflated. Dyspnoea may be severe. The child is prone to dehydration and heat exhaustion in hot weather because of the sweat gland defect.

The disease varies a great deal in severity. Some infants manifest severe symptoms at an early age and the disease proceeds rapidly to death. In others the disease starts in a similar manner, but their condition improves and they manage to live relatively normal lives.

As management of these children improves, more are growing to adolescent and adult life. Their prognosis seems to depend to a large extent on the quality of treatment they receive. If the airways can be kept clear, and if irrever-sible damage to the lungs can be prevented or kept to a minimum, the prognosis becomes much more optimistic.

Diagnosis

The most reliable test is of the sweat electrolytes. The sweat is obtained by iontophoresis, and sodium and chloride concentrations are estimated. A sodium content in excess of 60 mmol/l indicates the presence of cystic fibrosis.

Treatment

There is no cure for this disease. Treatment is symptomatic and consists of the substitution of animal extract for the absent pancreatic enzymes, the prevention of irreversible pulmonary changes, the prevention of heat exhaustion by the addition of adequate salt to the diet, and the maintenance of good general health and a sound emotional state in both the child and family. The main aim of all treatment is to enable the child to live as normal a life as possible. Single- and double-lung transplants are now proving successful in these children.

Management of the obstructive pulmonary lesion

Sputum culture and sensitivity tests enable the particular pathogens to be identified and the appropriate drugs to be administered. Treatment must be adapted to whatever is the stage of pulmonary involvement, but basically it is directed towards the clearing of excessive mucus secretions from the airways. This aim should be uppermost in the physiotherapist's mind when treating these children. Irreversible changes in the lungs must be prevented if possible, but if they have already occurred, treatment aims at maintaining optimum respiratory function. The fact that irreversible lung changes seem to occur more readily in infants and young children is due to the effect of infection and retained secretions upon the relatively undeveloped lungs (Chapter 24).

Methods of clearing secretions

The usual methods of postural drainage alone are not effective in the treatment of children with cystic fibrosis. The secretions are thick and tenacious, and therefore difficult to dislodge. Sputum viscosity is decreased by aerosol or oral medications. This facilitates removal. The infant who cannot cough effectively must be stimulated to do so.

Inhalation therapy

The viscosity of the bronchial secretions may be decreased by several methods.

Intermittent aerosol therapy is given via mouthpiece or mask. The mouthpiece is considered to be the more effective but a mask may be necessary for small children and infants. Secretions can be liquefied via a nebulizer attached to a source of compressed air, such as a portable air pump (Fig. 26.6). This is also a satisfactory method for use at home. A liquefying agent is used. The child is given this therapy three times a day or as required, and the liquefying of the secretions must be followed by postural drainage. If bronchospasm is present, a bronchodilator is added to the nebulizer. If infection is present, an antibiotic may be given via the nebulizer, but in this case, *after* the postural drainage.

Another method of intermittent inhalation is via an *intermittent positive pressure ventilator*. Its use is controversial and some authorities consider it to be a contraindication in the treatment of most infants and children with cystic fibrosis, due to the possibility of rupture of the overdistended alveoli in those children with emphysematous changes. It may be used where there is segmental collapse, in which case the flow rate should be low initially, and only gradually increased. Positioning with the appropriate part of the lung uppermost is also necessary. Intermittent positive pressure therapy has been found to increase residual volume after prolonged treatment. For this reason some authors have suggested short periods of treatment, with a maximum of 14 days (Matthews *et al.* 1964).

Postural drainage with percussion and/or FET

This is an essential method of removing secretions from the lungs and should be accurately and thoroughly done. It should commence as a daily routine as soon as the infant is diagnosed as having cystic fibrosis. This is considered the best way to prevent a build-up of secretions which will gradually lead to deteriorating respiratory function. Tecklin and Holsclaw (1975), in a study on the effects of bronchial drainage on a group of 26 cystic fibrosis patients, found significant increases in peak expiratory flow rate, forced vital capa-

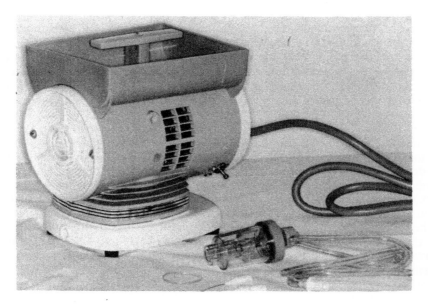

Figure 26.6 The Maxi-Myst compressor with nebulizer. (Courtesy of Mead Johnson, Crow's Nest, Sydney, Australia.)

city, expiratory reserve volume and inspiratory capacity. Feldman and colleagues (Feldman *et al.* 1979) showed improvement in flow rates at low lung volumes 45 minutes after drainage. If the lungs can be kept clear the child will thrive. It may be necessary to concentrate on a particular focal area, but all segments will need to be drained at each session. This is time-consuming but essential if the child is to be kept healthy. The child's parents are taught the techniques of postural drainage, percussion and breathing and the use of the necessary equipment so they will be efficient at home treatment. For the parents to be effective they must understand the child's problems, and some details of respiratory anatomy and physiology should be explained to them. Postural drainage is given twice daily at home with regular visits to the physiotherapist for supervision. Infants in particular should be drained *before* feeds. The methods of drainage are described in Chapter 27. Each segment is drained every day and the child has vigorous percussion. The upper lobes may be drained in the morning, the lower lobes and the right middle lobe in the evening. The amount of time spent in drainage must be increased during periods of infection. The upper lobes are the most vulnerable in an infant, the lower in a small child.

When the child reaches adolescence, the need for independence will require the therapist to initiate a discussion on the importance of postural drainage, and the best way this can be organized. The child may prefer a good friend to assist with the daily programme, or more frequent visits to the therapist may be preferred.

Effective nose-blowing is practised as part of the postural drainage routine. Vigorous active exercise is given before and during postural drainage to help loosen secretions. Haemoptysis, provided it is only small, is not a contraindication to postural drainage. However, percussion and vibration techniques should be avoided until the risk of haemoptysis has passed, when it is vigorously restarted in order to remove old blood which would otherwise cause obstruction.

Specialized breathing techniques such as the forced expirator technique (FET) and autogenic drainage are described briefly in Chapter 27 and in more detail by De Cesare and Graybill (1990) and Pryor (1992).

Breathing exercises

These are given during postural drainage with emphasis on full expansion and expiration, in order to facilitate drainage of secretions. The aims of breathing exercises are to improve breathing control by encouraging gentle breathing using the lower chest with relaxation of the upper chest and shoulders (so-called diaphragmatic breathing). The child is also given breathing exercises in half lying, sitting or standing after active exercise. Serial chest measurements may be a means of motivating a child who is reluctant to do breathing exercises at home.

General activities

Ventilatory muscle training has been shown to improve maximum sustainable ventilatory capacity more than 50%. A general physical activity programme at summer camp resulted in a similar improvement (Keens *et al.* 1977). Parents usually need to be given advice about their child's need for exercise and physical activity. Running about and playing active games are useful ways of loosening secretions and stimulating a productive cough. Swimming probably improves breathing control and in the growing child it stimulates skeletal development and coordinated muscular action. Infants too small to be active can have their relationship to gravity changed by frequent alteration of bed position.

Methods of treating pancreatic insufficiency and disorder of the digestive tract

The child requires a nutritious diet, with sufficient protein and adequate calories. The physician may refer the parents to a dietitian for advice. A substitute for the pancreatic enzymes is taken daily. Good nutrition is also maintained by control of the pulmonary problems. A child with excessive mucus secretions which are allowed to build up will have, understandably, a poor appetite and little interest in food.

Methods of treating the sweat gland defect

The parents supervise the child's daily salt intake, especially during hot weather. If insufficient salt is taken with the food, salt tablets are given.

Psychosocial care

A disease of this nature causes considerable emotional and social problems for parents and child. For the parents there will be anxiety about the genetic nature of the defect, with the risk of subsequent diseased children. There is a large expense involved due to periodic hospital admissions and the cost of equipment for home use. The parents have to bear the burden of the child's home treatment, which is time-consuming and sometimes difficult if the child is rebellious. The child has to endure the visits to the doctor and physiotherapist, the occasional periods of time spent in hospital, interference with school and social life, as well as the discomforts of respiratory insufficiency. The emotional support for these children and their parents will be similar to that needed whenever a child suffers a chronic disability. Cystic fibrosis support groups are often a valuble resource for these families.

Summary

Some common respiratory disorders seen in children are described in this chapter. In the case of cystic fibrosis and asthma, where the physiotherapist may be called upon to take a relatively complex role in the management of the child, details of treatment are given. For specific techniques of physical therapy, the reader is referred to Chapter 27.

References

Anderson, S. (1988) Exercise-induced asthma. In: *Allergy Principles and Practice*, 3rd edn, edited by E. Middleton. Washington: C.V. Mosby, pp 1156–1175.

De Cesare, J.A. and Graybill, C.A. (1990) Physical therapy for the child with respiratory dysfunction. In: *Cardiopulmonary Physical Therapy*, 2nd edn, edited by S. Irwin and J.S. Tecklin. St Louis, MO: C.V. Mosby.

Feldman, J., Traver, G.A. and Taussig, L.M. (1979) Maximal expiratory flows after postural drainage. *Am. Rev. Respir. Dis.*, **119**, 239–245.

Fitch, K.D. and Morton, A.R. (1971) Specificity of exercise-induced asthma. *Br. Med. J.*, **4**, 577.

Fitch, K.D., Morton, A.R. and Blanksby, B.A. (1976) The effect of swimming training on children with asthma. *Arch. Dis. Child.*, **51**, 190–194.

Gandevia, B. (1959) Pulmonary function and physiotherapy. *Aust. J. Physiother.*, **5**, 87.

Gaskell, D.V. and Webber, B.A. (1977) *The Brompton Hospital Guide to Chest Physiotherapy*, 3rd edn. Oxford: Blackwell.

Hinshaw, H.C. and Garland, L.H. (1965) *Diseases of the Chest*. Philadelphia, PA: W.B. Saunders.

Illingworth, R.S. (1971) *Common Symptoms of Disease in Children*. Oxford: Blackwell.

Keens, T.G., Krastins, I.R.B., Wannamaker, E.M. *et al.* (1977) Ventilatory muscle endurance training in normal subjects and patients with cystic fibrosis. *Am. Rev. Respir. Dis.*, **116**, 853–860.

Kendig, E.L. and Chernick, V. (eds) (1977) *Disorders of the Respiratory Tract in Children*. Philadelphia, PA: W.B. Saunders.

Law, D. and Kosloske, A.M. (1976) Management of tracheobronchial foreign bodies in children: a reevaluation of postural drainage and bronchoscopy. *Pediatrics*, **58**, 362.

Matthews, L.W., Doershuk, C.F., Wise, M., Eddy, G., Nudelman, H. and Spector, S. (1964) A therapeutic regime for patients with cystic fibrosis. *Pediatrics*, **65**, 558.

Pryor, J. (1992) Mucociliary clearance. In: *Key Issues in Cardiorespiratory Physiotherapy*, edited by E. Ellis and J. Alison. Oxford: Butterworth-Heinemann.

Seligman, T., Randel, H.O. and Stevens, J.J. (1970) Conditioning program for children with asthma. *Phys. Ther.*, **50**, 641.

Sly, R.M., Harper, R.T. and Rosselot, I. (1972) The effect of physical conditioning upon asthmatic children. *Ann. Allergy*, **30**, 86–94.

Tecklin, J.S. and Holsclaw, D.S. (1975) Evaluation of bronchial drainage in patients with cystic fibrosis. *Phys. Ther.*, **55**, 10, 1081.

Webber, B.A., Shenfield, G.M. and Paterson, J.W. (1974) A comparison of three different techniques for giving nebulised albuterol to asthmatic patients. *Am. Rev. Respir. Dis.*, **109**, 293.

Further reading

Ellis, E. and Alison, J. (eds) (1992) *Key Issues in Cardiorespiratory Physiotherapy*. Oxford: Butterworth-Heinemann.

Irwin, S. and Tecklin, J.S. (eds) (1990) *Cardiopulmonary Physical Therapy*, 2nd edn. St Louis, MO: C.V. Mosby.

Motoyama, E.K., Gibson, L.E. and Zigas, C.J. (1972) Evaluation of mist tent therapy in cystic fibrosis using maximum expiratory flow volume curve. *Pediatrics*, **50**, 299.

Reid, L. and de Haller, R. (1964) *Lung Changes in Cystic Fibrosis*. London: Chest and Heart Association.

27

Physical evaluation and treatment

Methods of assessment

Assessment of the respiratory system involves observation, the use of manual techniques such as palpation and percussion, and listening to breath sounds (auscultation), usually with a stethoscope. This chapter presents a broad outline of the information to be collected and the techniques in common use by physiotherapists. Other texts describe assessment in more detail (Crane 1990; De Cesare and Graybill 1990; Kigin 1992).

Each child is assessed and a history taken by the physiotherapist on the first visit, and re-evaluation is carried out on subsequent visits. Taking a history from the parent enables the physiotherapist to know the answers to questions such as these: Is there a productive cough, and if so are secretions copious, infected or tenacious? Is the cough present constantly, is it worse in the morning or does it recur at intervals? Does the child suffer from recurrent respiratory tract infections or rhinitis? Does a cough develop immediately following an upper respiratory tract infection? Does the child have dyspnoea, and if so, when? Is the child as active as other children of the same age? Are there attacks of wheezing or difficulty with breathing? Do these occur as a result of exertion, emotional strain, or do other factors appear to precipitate these attacks? Do they occur at night or at school? What are the effects of these difficulties on home life?

The physiotherapist must know what drugs have been prescribed and what advice has already been given to the family by the physician. The radiographs and the radiologist's reports are examined to see any focal areas of collapse or consolidation, or any other relevant abnormality (Figs 27.1–27.4).

The assessment includes an examination of the shape of the child's chest, noting the presence of flared lower ribs, whether the chest is barrel-shaped or asymmetrical, or whether the upper part of the sternum is prominent. The pattern of thoracic expansion is noted, particularly the presence of upper chest movement and whether the subcostal margins move closer together on inspiration. If the subcostal margins do move closer together this is an indication that the diaphragm is already relatively flattened and on inspiration is moving paradoxically. Whether the child is a mouth-breather is noted, and if so, whether the child can breathe through the nose when asked. The resting respiratory rate is noted once the therapist has gained the child's confidence and the child is not tense or anxious. On coughing, whether this causes any respiratory embarrassment is noted – whether the cough is paroxysmal, or productive. Accurate and, if possible, first-hand information about the nature and quantity of sputum is required.

A hand placed on the chest wall will pick up vibrations due to bronchospasm or accumulated secretions, and will help the physiotherapist to localize areas requiring postural

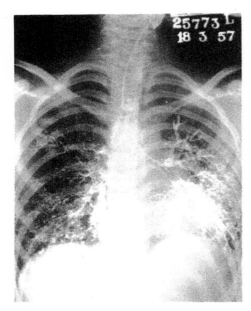

Figure 27.1 Bronchogram of a child with bronchiectasis. Note the crowding of the bronchi in the right lower lobe adjacent to the heart, and the cylindrical dilation of the more distal bronchi, which should normally be narrowing as they reach the pleura. (Courtesy of the Royal Alexandra Hospital for Children, Sydney, Australia.)

drainage. A stethoscope is used to localize areas with retained secretions, but the therapist needs a great deal of practice in listening to normal breath sounds before the use of a stethoscope will be of any value (Baskett 1971; Kigin 1992).

A frightened nervous child may be better assessed on the parent's knee rather than sitting alone on a treatment bed. It is important that the chest be uncovered for assessment and it is usually less frightening for the child to be undressed by a parent.

Measurement of thoracic expansion

Measuring thoracic expansion is a method of assessing the range of movement in the thorax. It is important as a means of assessing progress in children with chronic respiratory diseases such as bronchiectasis and cystic fibrosis in whom thoracic expansion may become limited. It may provide incentive for an older child. However, it is probably not necessary as a record in a number of children seen by the physiotherapist, as it does not provide any information about ventilation distribution, only about ribcage mobility (Grimby 1974). In many children, for example those with asthma,

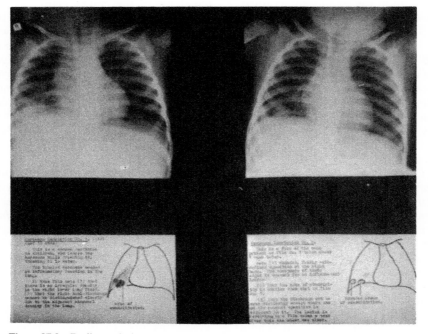

Figure 27.2 Radiograph demonstrating the effects of kerosene inhalation in an 18-month-old child. (Courtesy of the Royal Alexandra Hospital for Children, Sydney, Australia.)

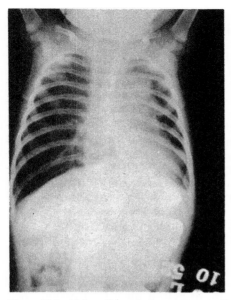

Figure 27.3 This radiograph demonstrates collapse of the left lower lobe with emphysema of the remainder of the lungs. Note that the heart and mediastinum have shifted towards the collapse, and the left diaphragm is elevated towards the collapse. (Courtesy of the Royal Alexandra Hospital for Children, Sydney, Australia.)

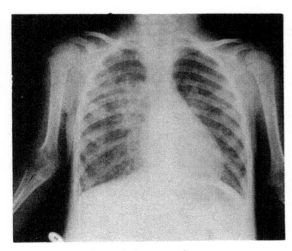

Figure 27.4 Radiograph demonstrating bronchopneumonia in the lungs of a child with cystic fibrosis. There are patchy increased densities scattered throughout both lungs. (Courtesy of the Royal Alexandra Hospital for Children, Sydney, Australia.)

it is the way in which they breathe that needs to be assessed and the physiotherapist should record observations in detail.

Measurements are taken using a tape measure, with the child in the same position each time, half lying, sitting or standing, at the fourth rib (at the level of the axillae), at the ninth rib (three fingers' breadth below the tip of the xiphoid process), and subcostally. The measurements are taken for a full inspiration and expiration, with the average taken of three attempts.

Sputum collection

The physiotherapist records the amount of sputum at each visit, and the type, whether frothy, tenacious or purulent. The type of cough is also recorded, whether dry and hacking, or paroxysmal, and whether or not it is effective.

If it is necessary to collect a sputum specimen for pathological investigation, the child is asked to cough and spit some sputum into a sterilized glass jar, with the name and date printed on it. If the child is too young to cooperate, a specimen of sputum can be collected from the back of the throat on the cotton-wool tip of a swab stick. A small catheter is inserted to stimulate the cough reflex, the child's cheeks are pressed inwards to prevent swallowing and the sputum is removed with a swab stick which is put into a sterilized test tube. Care must be taken not to contaminate the specimen or the collecting device and sterile gloves should be used. A more effective method involves the use of a small plastic sputum trap attached to a suction apparatus (Fig. 27.5). The container should be labelled with the baby's name, date, time of collection and type of specimen, for example, endotracheal tube or oropharyngeal aspirate. It should be sent to the bacteriology department as soon as possible. The sputum can be collected effectively even from an infant in this manner. These are uncomfortable and frightening manoeuvres for an infant or small child, and should be accurately done on the first attempt if possible.

Assessment of exercise tolerance

The parent will give an indication of exercise tolerance if asked whether or not the child can keep up with other children the same age in play activities and in sport. In the case of an asth-

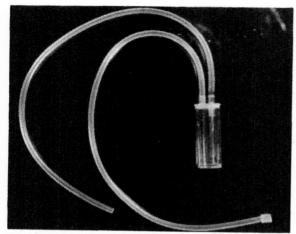

Figure 27.5 Mucus extractor. (Courtesy of Pharma-Plast.)

ond (Kendig and Chernick 1977). This test is commonly used in children with asthma to estimate the degree of airways resistance, in which case the FEV_1 in these children is tested before and after the administration of a bronchodilator. One machine in use for this test is the bellow-type spirometer, the Vitalograph (Fig. 27.6).

In addition to measuring FEV_1, two other measurements can be made from the output of the spirometer (Fig. 27.7): the maximum mid-expiratory flow rate (MMEFR or $FEF_{25-75\%}$), which is the flow rate over the middle half of the expiratory curve; and the total volume of air that can be exhaled after a maximum inspiration – vital capacity (VC; Alison 1992).

matic child, a distinction should be made between exercise tolerance when free of bronchospasm as well as when bronchospasm is present. Skipping or jumping on a trampoline is an effective way of assessing exercise tolerance in children with bronchiectasis, cystic fibrosis or asthma. Following 2 minutes of such activity, the child's respiratory rate, pulse rate, use of accessory muscles of respiration, and any increase in cough or wheeze are noted. If laboratory facilities are available, ventilation, heart rate, respiratory rate and workload achieved can be measured during an exercise test on a bicycle ergometer, treadmill or by step test before and after a training programme (Alison and Ellis 1992). In children who suffer from bronchospasm, more specific exercise testing may be necessary as a diagnostic tool. Godfrey (1974) describes the details of this procedure. Children with asthma may be shown how an aerosol bronchodilator and/or sodium cromoglycate can block exercise-induced asthma.

Pulmonary function tests

Measurement of 1 second forced expiratory volume (FEV_1)

This test measures the percentage of vital capacity which can be expired by maximum effort in 1 second. Children can usually expire more than 90% of the total vital capacity in the first sec-

Method The child is instructed to take a deep breath, to hold it for a brief period, then to exhale fully through a disposable mouthpiece attached to the tubing of the machine. As the child exhales, a line is traced on graph paper indicating the volume of air exhaled. If the child's FEV_1 is also required after bronchodilator therapy, the solution is given via a hand-held aerosol spray, and the child is tested again approximately 10 minutes later.

The degree of accuracy of this type of test depends upon the child's ability to concentrate and cooperate, and the skill of the therapist in persuading the child to perform the test as well as possible. It may provide incentive if the child is shown how a breath out moves the tracing pen. A small child may try hard if told that there is a large balloon inside the machine which must be blown up. Polgar and Promadhat (1971) suggest that the child may be asked to blow out the candles on an imaginary birthday cake, trying to blow out as many as possible in one breath.

The results of the test are recorded on a card (Fig. 27.7). The predicted vital capacity (PVC) for a child of this age is taken from a chart and forced vital capacity (FVC) is noted from the graph. The percentage of PVC is then calculated: FVC/PVC. FEV_1 is noted from the graph and is measured against vital capacity (FEV_1/FVC). This should be $\geq$ 90%.

In the example given (Fig. 27.7), the child demonstrated a change in FVC and FEV_1 following the administration of the bronchodilator.

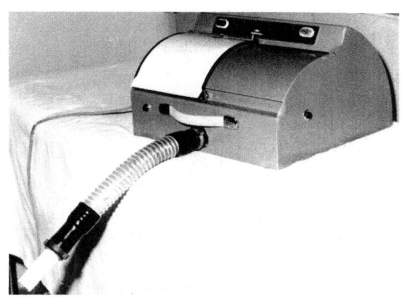

Figure 27.6 Vitalograph machine. (Courtesy of Vitalograph, Buckingham, England.)

Measurement of Peak Expiratory Flow Rate (PEFR)

A peak flow meter can be used to measure maximum flow over 10 ms at the beginning of expiration. This is a simple portable device which can be used to give information about the reversibility of airways obstruction following administration of a bronchodilator. It does not measure accurately changes in small airways, hence, when this information is required, spirometry is the preferred test. Children as young as 3 years can be taught to use this apparatus.

Method The child takes a deep breath and gives a short fast blow into the mouthpiece. The test is repeated three times and the best attempt is recorded. The PEFR value is given by the meter in litres per minute. Normal values for children have been reported by Godfrey and colleagues (1970).

There are other pulmonary function tests, including tests which measure the diffusing capacity of the lung. These are described by Alison (1992).

Gravity-assisted drainage

This is a means of removing excessive secretions from the air passages, and employs the use of gravity to facilitate drainage. Positions are employed which promote the most effective drainage of specific segments of the lungs. These positions are shown in Figures 27.8–27.16. However, although each segment should be drained in the prescribed manner, there are times when the postural drainage position should be adjusted slightly in order to drain the secretions effectively. Thacker (1971) comments that the direction of the airways may be altered by disease.

Drainage may be done on a bed with the necessary elevation gained by lying the child on pillows or by tilting the bed, or over a chair (Fig. 27.17). The procedure must be taught to the child's parents as many children will need to carry out this drainage several times a day at home. It is not a good idea to suggest the child hang over the end of the bed. Drainage positions must be as accurate as possible for the particular segments to be drained, and the child should be comfortable in the position in order to cooperate with breathing exercises and coughing. Hanging over the end of the bed is

H.M.O. ....   NAME

WARD .... Ht. 130 cm   IDENT. NO.

DATE 7.12.78 Wt. ....   BIRTH DATE 2.7.70   SEX. M

Provisional diagnosis:

	Pre-Bronchodilator (B.D.)			Post-Bronchodilator (B.D.)	
	Observed A.T.P.S.	Predicted B.T.P.S.	% Predicted	Observed A.T.P.S.	% Predicted
FEV₁	950	1750	54 %	1500	86 %
V C	1400	1875	75 %	1800	96 %
FEV₁ : VC ratio	68 %	/////	/////	83 %	/////
MMEFR	34	132	26 %	86	65 %
PEFR	—	—	—	—	—

(Left margin: RESULT OF SPIROMETRY)

Explanation of Terms:

V C   = Vital capacity = Litres

FEV₁   = Forced expiratory volume in 1 second = Litres per second

MMEFR = Maximum mid-expiratory flow rate = Litres per second

PEFR   = Peak expiratory flow rate = Litres per minute

Interpretation:

Figure 27.7 The result of ventilatory tests done before and after administration of a bronchodilator. (Courtesy of the Royal Alexandra Hospital for Children, Sydney, Australia.)

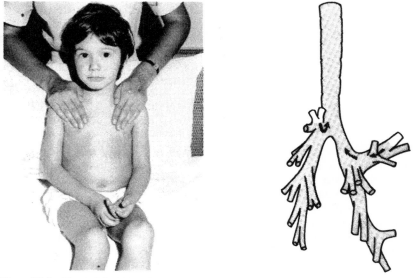

Figure 27.8 Upper lobes: apical segments. The child may lean forwards or backwards to drain the more anterior and posterior areas.

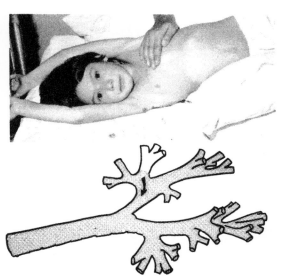

Figure 27.9 Right upper lobe: posterior segment. Quarter-turn from prone. A pillow prevents the child rolling into prone. To drain the posterior segment of the *left* upper lobe, the child is placed in a similar position but with two pillows elevating the head and shoulders on the left side.

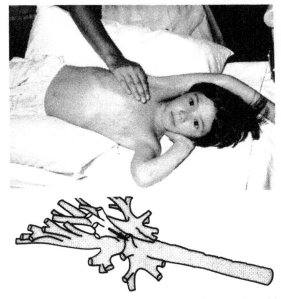

Figure 27.11 Left upper lobe: lingular segment. Quarter-turn from supine with left side uppermost, two pillows under the lower trunk and another pillow to prevent the child from rolling into supine. The thorax should be at an angle of 30° from the horizontal. Alternatively, the bed may be elevated 12°.

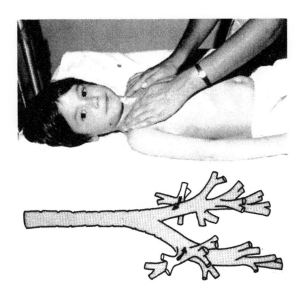

Figure 27.10 Upper lobes: anterior segments. Supine, pillow under knees.

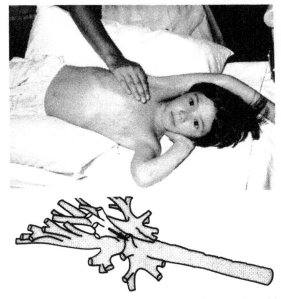

Figure 27.12 Middle lobe. Quarter-turn from supine with right side uppermost, two pillows under the lower trunk and another pillow to prevent the child from rolling into supine. The thorax should be at an angle of 30° from the horizontal. Alternatively, the bed may be elevated 30 cm.

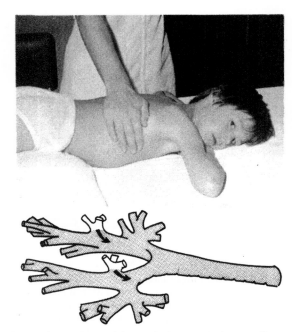

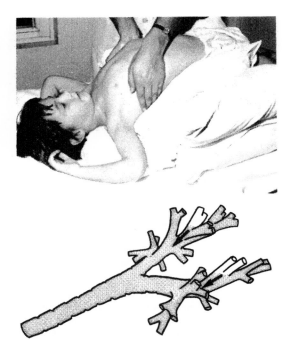

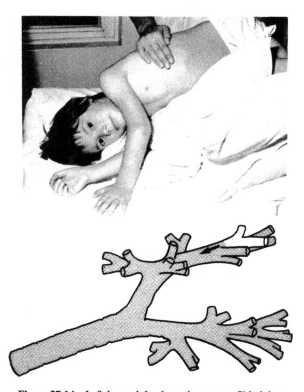

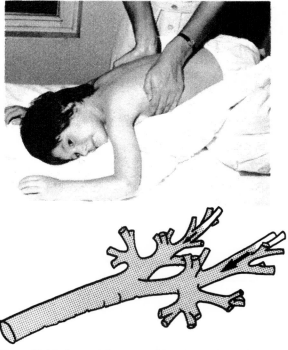

Figure 27.13 Lower lobes: apical segments. Prone, pillow under the abdomen.

Figure 27.15 Lower lobes: anterior segments. Supine, thorax at an angle of 45° from the horizontal. This child should have another pillow to support the pelvis and take the strain from the abdominal muscles. Alternatively, the bed may be elevated 25–30 cm.

Figure 27.14 Left lower lobe: lateral segment. Side lying, thorax at an angle of 45° from the horizontal. Alternatively, the bed may be elevated 25–30 cm.

Figure 27.16 Lower lobes: posterior segments. Prone, thorax at an angle of 45° from the horizontal. This child should have an extra pillow under his pelvis. Alternatively, the bed may be elevated 25–30 cm.

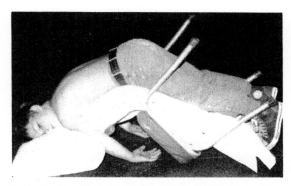

Figure 27.17 Alternative method of draining the posterior segments of the lower lobes, which may be more conveniently used at home.

neither accurate nor comfortable. An infant may be drained by tilting the cot or incubator. Alternatively, drainage for an infant may be done on the physiotherapist's lap, or as shown for the older child. The former may not be satisfactory as the supporting surface is not firm enough.

Where appropriate, postural drainage can be preceded by games or exercise. Vigorous exercise, such as swimming or static bicycle riding and exercise programmes, has been shown to increase clearance of excessive secretions (Pavia 1984; Dodd 1991). Activity may need to be modified or eliminated if the child's condition contraindicates such exercise.

Each segment in which there is a focus of infection, a collapse or a build-up of secretions, is drained separately until clear. This applies particularly in conditions such as cystic fibrosis, bronchiectasis and pneumonia. Children with bronchitis and asthma, in which there may be no particular focus, can be drained as for the posterior segments of the lower lobes (Fig. 27.16). Secretions tend to accumulate towards the bases of the lungs in children who spend their day in an upright position. Infants and bed-ridden children with respiratory disorders tend to accumulate secretions in the upper lobes (particularly the posterior and lateral segments) because of the dependent position of these lobes in the horizontal position, and attention must be paid to clearing these areas. Castilla *et al.* (1971) found that a contrast medium instilled into the trachea of an infant lying supine passed first into the right upper lobe. They also found that the

angle between the right main bronchus and the right upper lobe bronchus is different in neonates compared to adults. Attention should therefore be paid in particular to the right upper lobe in infants lying supine, and where possible this position should be avoided where the infant is at risk of aspiration.

Children with bronchospasm frequently cannot tolerate a position with head down. The position can be modified as in Figure 26.1. It is of little use to attempt drainage of secretions from the lungs of a child with unrelieved bronchospasm, as the airways are not patent enough to allow the free passage of mucus. These techniques are used more successfully following the administration of a bronchodilator, by aerosol spray, nebulizer or by intermittent positive pressure respirator.

Drainage will not be effective if the child is merely placed in the appropriate position and left alone. The child can be percussed and vibrated over the thorax, and be given localized breathing exercises by the physiotherapist or by a parent while in the drainage position. It is better for this to be done for a short period of time thoroughly than for the child to be left alone for a longer period. A reminder to cough usually needs to be given while draining, and to blow the nose when necessary.

The physiotherapist will decide with each particular child and parent the best time of day for drainage to be done, but on waking in the morning and before dinner at night will be the most usual times. This will be decided by the times at which the child is most productive, but the routine of the family should be taken into consideration. The child's chest should be drained until it seems clear.

Percussion and vibration techniques

These techniques, although applied externally to the bony thorax, help loosen secretions within the air passages, and if the child is tilted at the correct angle and coughs effectively the secretions will be removed.

Percussion is the transmission of mechanical energy through the chest wall to the airways. The resultant increase in intrathoracic pressure is considered to loosen bronchial secretions and aid in their clearance (Pryor 1992). Percussion is done manually or with a mechanical device. Done manually it involves clapping the chest, through clothing or a sheet, with a cupped hand and loose wrist movements.

There is no evidence that in individuals with chronic chest disease percussion alone will increase the clearance of secretions (Webber *et al.* 1985; van der Schans *et al.* 1986). However, it has been shown to increase the rate of sputum removal, and will enhance removal of secretions, if they are copious, when used in conjunction with postural drainage and forced expiratory technique (FET); (Webber 1988; Gallon 1991, 1992). Percussion has been said to decrease FEV_1 (Campbell *et al.* 1975), to increase FVC (Tecklin and Holsclaw 1975) and to cause hypoxia (McDonnell *et al.* 1986). It has been shown, however, that percussion does not cause hypoxia if interspersed with thoracic expansion exercises (Pryor *et al.* 1990). Similarly, percussion does not decrease FEV_1 if the individual is premedicated with a bronchodilator, which is essential in order to maximize the effect of a mucus clearance technique.

Percussion can be done to older children using a high-frequency mechanical percussor (Pryor 1992) or, in the case of neonates, contact-heel percussion or cupping, using a Bennett facemask (Parker 1985). An electric toothbrush has been advocated (Curran and Kachoyeanos 1979); however this has been shown in one study (Tudehope and Bagley 1980) to be ineffective in raising arterial Po_2. In addition, 6 of the 15 infants in this study became agitated and developed a dusky appearance or bradycardia. It is possible that mechanical vibration to the ribcage of a certain frequency may have an inhibitory effect on the phrenic nerve which would cause apnoea in preterm infants. The use of contact-heel percussion involves applying pressure through the heel of the hand at right angles to the chest wall at a frequency of approximately 40 per min (Finer and Boyd 1978).

Vibrations are done, either unilaterally or bilaterally, towards the end of expiration. They involve fine, rapidly oscillating movements of the chest wall with most of the force given through the fingers during expiration. For neonates, manual vibration is given by placing two fingers on top of each other and doing anteroposterior oscillatory movements at right angles to the chest wall (Finer *et al.* 1978).

Compression involves relatively constant compressive force to the thorax during expira-

tion. It aids in increasing expiratory force (Pryor 1992).

Shaking is a large-amplitude, vigorous movement of the chest wall with pressure given mostly through the palm of the hand.

After each bout of shaking or vibration the child is asked to cough. These techniques are interspersed with localized breathing exercises. A small child may have to be taught how to cough. If a hand is placed in front of the mouth the sensation of expelled air on the hand may help the child to learn the technique. Emphasis must be on a deep inspiration followed by a series of explosive expirations. A child of 2–3 years can usually be taught to expectorate. Pharyngeal 'tickling' with a small-bore catheter will stimulate coughing in infants and young children, as the cough reflex is a protective one. Crying is sometimes an advantage provided it is not prolonged, as it ensures the infant takes deep breaths. In the author's opinion the therapist should work hard at treating the infant and young child without provoking crying, and this strategy should be discussed with the parents. Talking to the infant, a reassuring manner, combined with percussion which starts off very gently, will enable the infant to accept more vigorous percussion. Parents should also be shown ways of comforting the infant by talking, putting a hand on the chest, holding the hands gently to help the infant quieten.

Chest compression may also provoke a cough from an infant (see below). Care should be taken by the physiotherapist to avoid being directly in front of the child during a cough, as this may result in inhalation of infected material.

Percussion and vibrations are given to small infants with care not to use too much force or pressure. In the treatment of a small premature baby one finger on top of another will give sufficient vibration. However, treatment must still be vigorously done. It is important to remove secretions quickly from an infant's lungs, as obstruction of the tiny airways occurs rapidly with subsequent deterioration in the infant's condition. The physiotherapist must take care not to be ineffectual in these treatments.

Vibrations and percussion are contraindicated in infants and children with tuberculosis, a tendency to haemorrhage, osteoporosis or certain cardiac conditions, such as arrhythmias.

Breathing exercises and coughing

Deep breathing or thoracic expansion exercises are done with the child in the required drainage position. This is used, for example, in the case of excessive secretions in the right lower lobe, when the child is encouraged during postural drainage by the pressure of the physiotherapist's hands to localize breathing to the lower thorax. As full an expiration as possible without effort is done, as this will facilitate further drainage. A few breaths are followed by a cough and by a short rest. A deeper inspiration may be encouraged in an infant or unconscious child by manual compression on the thorax. In the infant whose ribs have not yet developed the normal bucket-handle action, compression is done more horizontally.

Clearing the upper respiratory tract

If the child is to breathe in through the nose, the nose must be clear. When necessary the child must be taught to blow the nose correctly, one nostril at a time. Most children need to be reminded of this.

Teaching parents

At the first visit, parents are shown the methods required, and the mechanism of drainage and the reasons for the techniques are explained. The parent practises the techniques in front of the physiotherapist. Most parents feel clumsy on attempting vibrations, percussion and breathing exercises for the first time, and the physiotherapist needs to be encouraging. Percussion can be practised on a pillow if necessary. At each subsequent visit the parent does some of the treatment with the physiotherapist, who can then judge how successful the teaching has been. A printed sheet with pictures of the various drainage positions and some details of the other techniques used should be available for parents.

In summary, postural drainage involves tilting of the thorax to facilitate drainage from a particular segment of a lung, plus breathing exercises, effective coughing, percussion and vibration techniques to loosen the secretions. It *must be noted that merely tilting the thorax does not imply that drainage will take place*.

Breathing exercises

Breathing exercises may be given with any one of several objectives. They may be given in order to maintain or restore a more normal breathing pattern, to aid in the expulsion of excessive secretions from the lower airway, and to maintain or regain thoracic mobility. They are usually done voluntarily by the child with the physiotherapist or parent guiding the thoracic movement, or in the case of the infant or unconscious child techniques are used which facilitate better expansion. For whatever reason breathing exercises are being given, the method is similar, involving expansion of the lungs in as normal a pattern as possible.

Breathing control (Webber 1988)

Traditionally the physiotherapist has guided rib movement in order to expand particular areas of the thorax either unilaterally or bilaterally by upper costal, lateral basal or posterior basal as well as diaphragmatic breathing. However, increasing thoracic and diaphragmatic expansion affects ribcage and diaphragm mobility and increases ventilation, although it does not alter the distribution of ventilation. Breathing control is the term given to gentle breathing using the lower chest with relaxation of the upper chest and shoulders, often referred to as diaphragmatic breathing. If an attempt is being made to restore more normal breathing in, for example, a child who has excessive movement of the upper thorax or who pulls the abdomen in on inspiration, emphasis may be on relaxation, a quiet inspiration with shoulders relaxed, followed by a relaxation of the respiratory muscles. This will result in expiration.

Thoracic expansion or deep breathing exercises

These are considered to augment the normal 'milking' effect of inspiration and expiration on mucous material (Pryor 1992), as well as bringing in alternative pathways for air flow, the collateral channels (Menkes and Traystman 1977).

When breathing exercises are being used as an adjunct to drainage of secretions, emphasis is on deep breathing since this has an expulsive effect.

Specialized breathing techniques

Positive expiratory pressure (PEP) mask therapy

This technique consists of self-applied PEP produced by breathing through a mask designed to create some expiratory resistance (Stafanger *et al.* 1983). It is considered to allow more air to enter peripheral airways via collateral channels and prevent the alveoli from collapsing. The air allows pressure to build up behind plugs of sputum, moving them towards larger airways where they can easily be expelled (Falk *et al.* 1984).

A study by Hofmeyr and colleagues (1986) which examined the use of the PEP mask in conjunction with postural drainage and breathing techniques, including FET, found no significant difference in the clearance of bronchial secretions when PEP was used. Postural drainage with and without PEP was found to produce more sputum than PEP given in the sitting position (see Davidson *et al.* 1988).

Forced expiratory technique (FET)

This technique involves a forced expiration or huff following a small breath (i.e. from mid to low lung volume), combined with breathing control (Thompson 1978). One or two huffs are followed by 15–30 seconds of relaxation with gentle breathing using the lower chest. When secretions are felt in the large upper airways, a huff or cough should expel them. FET has been shown to improve pulmonary function in cystic fibrosis (Webber *et al.* 1986) and to be an effective means of mobilizing and expelling bronchial secretions without increasing air flow obstruction (Pryor and Webber 1979).

Autogenic drainage (AD)

This technique involves the use of breathing at various levels of lung volume in order to obtain maximum expiratory flow in the different generations of bronchi (Schoni 1989). It has been claimed that AD is an effective means of mobilizing and evacuating mucus in cystic fibrosis but there has been as yet little research (Davidson *et al.* 1988).

Breathing exercises may need to be avoided or modified in the presence of certain conditions. A child with emphysema can be given breathing exercises by blowing bubbles, the

expiration against some resistance maintaining airways patency more effectively in emphysematous lungs than the normal relaxed breathing exercises.

If the patient is an infant or young child, or is unconscious and unable to cooperate, voluntary breathing exercises cannot be given. However, movement of air through the lungs can be encouraged by firm manual pressure on the chest during the expiratory phase. In the case of a small infant, it is necessary to give stability to the thorax with one hand in order to give pressure over a particular area of the lung. This is also done in the appropriate postural drainage position if it is also required to aid expulsion of excess mucus from the airways.

Breathing exercises will be done as part of home treatment where appropriate, the child's parent or care-giver being taught the necessary techniques.

Intensive care

Infants and children are placed in an intensive care unit if they are unconscious, or in respiratory distress, if in the case of neonates they are of low birth weight, and following thoracic or cranial surgery. Intensive care implies a situation in which special and continuous care is given the child by physician, nurse and therapist. Temperature, pulse and respiratory rate are recorded more frequently than usual and technical tests to determine the oxygen and carbon dioxide concentrations of the blood will be carried out as often as necessary.

The seriously ill infant or child is nursed in the horizontal position if comatose or receiving positive pressure ventilation. If there is respiratory failure and the child is breathing without mechanical assistance, or if there is a tracheo-oesophageal fistula or gastro-oesophageal reflux, the child is nursed with head and shoulders elevated. If nursed horizontally, the child is turned from side to side approximately every 2 hours (Jones and Owen-Thomas 1971). The infant may be nursed in an incubator or a tent. Both the infant and child may be tracheostomized and ventilated via a positive pressure ventilator or ventilated by endotracheal intubation. However, such continuous respiratory assistance may not be required. Instead, frequent visits are made by the physiotherapist to drain excess secretions from the lungs and to improve aeration by breathing exercises and in some cases by the administration of bronchodilator or mucolytic substances via an aerosol apparatus.

As a result of the anatomical and physiological immaturity of the growing lungs, infants and children have a lack of pulmonary reserve during stress. The resultant relatively easy fatigability means that physiotherapy sessions usually have to be shorter and more frequent than in adolescents and adults.

Due to the frequency of medical intervention needed in caring for an acutely ill child, attempts may be made to protect the child from unnecessary disturbance using a structured intervention schedule allowing periods of rest. Physiotherapy will need to be coordinated within this approach (De Cesare and Graybill 1990).

The effect of body positioning on arterial blood gases and lung mechanics in neonates has been the subject of several studies (e.g. Stark *et al.* 1984) and there appear to be some benefits in the prone position (Martin *et al.* 1979; Wagamen *et al.* 1979; Lioy and Maninello 1988).

Handling of sick neonates for either diagnostic or therapeutic procedures has been shown to cause a fall in P_aO_2. Although recovery is usually spontaneous, it is possible that repeated handling may cause a prolonged fall, necessitating respiratory support (Speidel 1978). Many neonatal intensive care units as a result have a policy of minimal handling with remote monitoring techniques to record heart rate, respiratory rate and blood pressure (Long *et al.* 1980).

One factor to be remembered during treatment of infants with respiratory distress is the effect of cooling on oxygen consumption, which is said to be lowest when the abdominal skin temperature is 36°C (Silverman *et al.* 1966). The therapist must therefore take care not to allow the infant's skin to cool during treatment. This applies particularly to the treatment of an infant in an incubator.

There is considerable stress for children undergoing cardiothoracic surgery and for those who are admitted into an intensive care unit. The problems of the child in hospital are discussed briefly in Chapter 1.

It is the author's opinion that infants and children requiring intensive care should be treated only by physiotherapists with experience in this field, and that until physiotherapists become proficient they should only work under the guidance of someone who has the necessary expertise.

Care of the infant or child following surgery

Infants and children undergoing surgery to thoracic or abdominal regions benefit from pre- and postoperative physiotherapy to mobilize secretions, clear airways and improve ventilatory capacity (Kigin 1981). Children have surgery, for example, to correct cardiac anomalies (Rockwell and Campbell 1976; Sade *et al.* 1977) and for organ transplantation (De Cesare and Graybill 1990). Common respiratory complications include depressed central respiratory drive caused by fluid retention or nasogastric drainage; lobar atelectasis caused by bronchial oedema and decreased diaphragmatic excursion and upward displacement of the diaphragm; pulmonary oedema associated with blood transfusion; and pleural effusion.

Cardiac surgery

Infants and children undergo cardiac surgery for such congenital defects as Fallot's tetralogy, transposition of the great arteries, persistent patent ductus arteriosus, coarctation of the aorta or septal defects.

Preoperatively the physiotherapist may need to institute treatment to clear the airways, as infants and children requiring cardiac surgery can have excessive secretions. Also important are the explanations and demonstrations to the child and parents which will prepare them for the immediate postoperative period. The therapist must build up a good relationship with the child and parents at this stage.

Modified postural drainage, gentle percussion and vibrations and stimulation to cough are given when necessary. By clearing the chest in this way the therapist is aiming to decrease the risk of postoperative complications (Thoren 1954), thereby decreasing the time the child will need to be hospitalized.

Even at 16–18 months, many children can be taught deep breathing by blowing balloons, paper toys and pinwheels. This will prepare the child for the breathing exercises to be done postoperatively.

Rockwell and Campbell (1976) stress the importance of preoperative family education in anticipating and avoiding the detrimental effects of hospitalization and surgery on children who are unprepared. They describe a preoperative visit to the intensive care unit, and aids such as tape recordings, glove puppets and colouring books.

Postoperatively the child in the intensive care unit may be intubated using intermittent positive pressure ventilation or continuous positive airways pressure (CPAP).

On CPAP the infant breathes spontaneously against positive pressure. This appears to assist the airways to remain patent, and to increase the functional residual capacity or FRC (Gregory *et al.* 1975). When moving the child, care is taken to ensure the tubing remains in a dependent position behind the child's head. Otherwise condensation from the humidified air could drain into the respiratory tract.

An infant after hypothermia will be kept warm by an overhead radiant heat warmer. Pericardial drains carry blood to underwater seal drainage bottles. Frequent checks of blood gases and electrolytes are made to assess progress.

Should physiotherapy be necessary to clear the chest, the child is turned into side lying and given gentle percussion or vibrations. In infants, even a small amount of mucus can block off a large amount of lung.

Effective and regular suction may be necessary, and the physiotherapist needs to be very alert to changes in the infant's condition.

Removal of secretions may be difficult and *manual hyperinflation* or 'bag squeezing' may be necessary. The tracheostomy or endotracheal tube is disconnected from the ventilator; one operator, who must be highly skilled in the technique, squeezes the bag slowly, then releases it quickly. The bag should be squeezed during inspiration or the air will inflate the stomach. The other operator compresses the chest manually just before the bag is released. The combination of high expiratory flow rate and chest compression assists movement of secretions towards the main airways where they can be coughed up or suctioned.

The chest incision should be 'splinted' when the child coughs by holding the thoracic cage firmly with the hands or with a soft doll or animal (De Cesare and Graybill 1990). Coughing may need to be stimulated by the therapist, by either a soft tube down through the nose and into the larynx, or by gentle lateral pressure on the trachea (which is soft and pliant in infants and young children) to bring the walls into apposition.

Following extubation, physiotherapy may be given several times a day for a couple of days, with the aim of clearing the airway. Not all children require this treatment but the therapist should check the child's condition regularly as changes may occur rapidly.

Children who are not intubated are also turned into side lying and the chest is cleared as above.

Where there are no complications, children are usually allowed out of bed soon after surgery and go home in approximately 1 week, with instructions to continue deep-breathing exercises and active play. Some children need stimulation to move; others do not, and run around freely as soon as they are allowed up.

Emergency care

Changes in the infant or child's condition may be sudden and the physiotherapist must be observant of the patient's respiratory rate and colour at all times during treatment. Deterioration may be rapid in the small child and collapse quickly occurs. Should a cardiorespiratory arrest occur, and this will be evidenced by the absence of pulse and respiration, the physiotherapist must remain calm, lying the child flat, and calling medical or nursing help by whatever means are used in the unit. There are certain procedures which the experienced physiotherapist will use, including suction of the airway if blockage by secretions appears the cause of respiratory arrest, administering oxygen, and commencing external cardiac massage if there is cardiac arrest. It is not within the scope of this book to describe these procedures in detail.

Care of the infant in an incubator

Infants are nursed in incubators (Fig. 27.18) if they are premature, or if they are neonates of

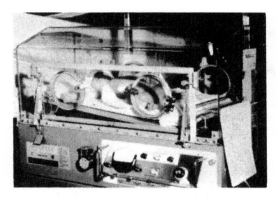

Figure 27.18 Baby nursed in an incubator. Note the portholes through which the baby may be handled. (Courtesy of R. Samios.)

low birth weight or with any acute respiratory illness. The advantages of an incubator are the maintenance of even temperature, the ease with which the infant can be observed, and by which an oxygen–air mix can be circulated. Humidity is provided and may be added to by the nebulization of water. The disadvantages are the ease with which the incubator becomes contaminated, both by the infant and by the arms and sleeves of staff handling the baby through the portholes. An added problem with infants in incubators is their isolation from the outside world and the unrelenting nature of the bright environment to which they are exposed for 24 hours a day.

The physiotherapist should avoid undue handling of the infant, and take care not to contaminate the incubator when the hands and arms are placed through the portholes. Opening the incubator causes a loss of heat and oxygen and allows pathogenic organisms to enter. The infant is nursed uncovered so that respiratory rate and depth and colour can be easily observed. Chilling must be avoided as it may lead to sclerema and, as described above, a lowering of the temperature will cause an increase in the need for oxygen. Similarly, overheating will also lead to an increase in oxygen consumption. The amount of oxygen is carefully monitored by the physician, particularly in low-birth-weight premature babies, who may develop retinopathy and blindness as a result of an excessive oxygen intake.

Postural drainage is given by elevating the mattress within the incubator. Percussion is given by the fingers rather than with the whole hand if the infant is very small. Gentle overpressure is given on expiration to aid the elimination of secretions (see p. 375).

Ventilation therapy

Artificial ventilation may be given by an intermittent positive pressure or an intermittent negative pressure apparatus.

Positive pressure devices

Intermittent positive pressure breathing (IPPB) is the maintenance within the airways of a positive pressure throughout inspiration, typically via a pressure-cycled ventilator (Fig. 27.19). IPPB may be given via a mouthpiece, a face mask, a tracheostomy tube or an oral or nasal endotracheal tube. Positive pressure ventilation may be used to administer drug therapy direct to the airways or to administer humidified air/oxygen to a respiratory-distressed child. However, a metered dose inhaler, or a mask if the child is too distressed to coordinate the release of the dose with inhalation, is considered to be as effective in administering a bronchodilator as IPPB (Cayton *et al.* 1978).

The value of IPPB in infants and young children is controversial and considered by some to be positively harmful. It is generally considered to be contraindicated in the treatment of children with cystic fibrosis, except in selected cases, due to the possibility of rupture of over-

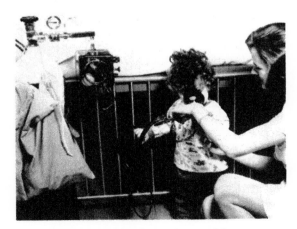

Figure 27.19 Child being shown the use of the intermittent positive pressure respirator. (Courtesy of R. Samios.)

distended alveoli. However, this form of ventilation is commonly used to maintain ventilatory function in a child with paralysis of the respiratory muscles, following poliomyelitis, polyneuritis or curare paralysis in the treatment of tetanus, or a flail chest due to multiple rib fractures.

Alternatively, the child with paralysis of the respiratory muscles may be ventilated by *intermittent negative pressure* in a tank respirator or in a cuirass-type ventilator.

One disadvantage of negative pressure ventilators is that they can cause upper airway obstruction. Severe nocturnal hypoxaemia may occur in patients with respiratory muscle weakness associated with neuromuscular disorders and intermittent positive pressure ventilation through a nose mask seems preferable to negative pressure.

A study of 5 patients with neuromuscular disorders (Ellis *et al.* 1987a) reported that negative pressure ventilation improved non-rapid eye movement (REM) ventilation in all patients but did not prevent severe oxyhaemoglobin desaturation which occurred during REM sleep. The authors found that negative pressure ventilation appeared to contribute to upper airways obstruction during REM sleep. In contrast, positive pressure ventilation through a nose mask was highly effective as it stabilized the oropharyngeal airway. Ellis and colleagues (1987b) also report the effects of intermittent positive pressure ventilation through a nose mask in a 6-year-old girl with alveolar hypoventilation.

IPPB has been shown to increase tidal volume (Sukumalchantra *et al.* 1965) and decrease the work of breathing (Ayres *et al.* 1963). It has been shown to be an effective alternative to physiotherapy in sputum elimination in patients who are unable to do active breathing exercises (Pavia *et al.* 1988). It is typically used in conjunction with postural drainage, breathing exercises and FET.

Positive expiratory pressure (PEP) Applied via a mask, PEP provides positive expiratory pressure during expiration. Its use is described on page 376.

Periodic continuous positive airway pressure (PCPAP) This involves the periodic use through inspiration and expiration of positive pressure in the airways in the spontaneously breathing child. It is derived from a high-flow generator and is administered in sitting or in a postural drainage position via a mask or mouthpiece and nose clip (Pryor 1992). PCPAP is used in the presence of atelectasis or a collapsed segment and has been shown to increase FRC and decrease the work of breathing (Gherini *et al.* 1979). PCPAP is followed by breathing exercises, including FET.

Incentive spirometry Incentive spirometry involves the use of visual feedback about inspiratory flow rate or tidal volume (Pryor 1992). It is considered to be a useful adjunct to breathing exercises, providing motivation and encouraging thoracic expansion. Although incentive spirometry has been shown in adults to be no more effective than deep-breathing exercises in preventing postoperative respiratory complications and in clearing excess secretions (Celli *et al.* 1984; Stock *et al.* 1985), it can be a useful means of providing motivation and interest for children.

Some specific points in management

Application by facemask or mouthpiece
If a facemask is used it must be a good fit (there are several sizes available) and must be held firmly over the child's mouth and nose in order to prevent leakage of air around the sides of the mask (Figs 27.19 and 27.20). If a mouthpiece is used, the child must be old enough to understand the need for firm lip closure, again to prevent the leakage of air (Fig. 27.21). Humidification of air, normally performed by the upper respiratory tract, is provided by the fluid in the nebulizer, either sterile water or a mucolytic or bronchodilator substance prescribed by the physician. The child may sit in a chair, or lie in a position which will facilitate postural drainage. The airways of small children are narrow, and where there is bronchospasm they are narrower still, so a low flow rate is used and pressure over 15 cm of water is usually not prescribed. The upper limits of pressure which are safe to use in all circumstances are not known. The child, who preferably has already been taught breathing exercises, may be given these exercises while using the ventilator, but if inexperienced, the child must be encouraged to take deep breaths with the machine.

The tracheostomized or intubated child

Endotracheal intubation involves the insertion of a tube into the trachea via the nose or mouth (Fig. 27.22). It is usually inserted via the nose in infants and children to avoid the tubing being bitten. Tracheostomy, which involves the passage of a tube directly into the trachea, is the preferred method of providing an artificial airway if this airway will be required for any length of time, for example, longer than 1 week. It is performed under general anaesthesia, a tube is inserted into the trachea and held in place by tapes around the neck. The advantages of artificial ventilation by these means include the enabling of any upper airways obstruction to be bypassed, the reduction of anatomical dead space thereby reducing the amount of respiratory effort necessary, an increase in alveolar ventilation, the facilitation of aspiration of secretions and the passage of bronchodilators, oxygen and moisture. The negative features include lack of natural humidification, inability to cough effectively, inability to speak, which is particularly frightening for a child, increased risk of infection, and asphyxia if the tube becomes blocked. Following tracheostomy incoordination of the larynx may occur (Roberts and Edwards 1971).

Importance of artificial humidification or nebulization

This is required whenever the nose is continually bypassed during artificial ventilation, whether by an endotracheal tube or a tracheostomy. The nose normally heats air to approximately 35°C, and adds water vapour to it. A humidifier is a device that produces water vapour. A nebulizer is a device that breaks water down into small particles suspended in a stream of gas. If a humidifier is not added to the circuit of the ventilator, bronchial secretions become thick and inspissated, the cilia of the cells of the bronchial mucosa cease working and sputum retention occurs (Roberts and Edwards 1971). Postural drainage and, if possible, FET, preceded by 5 minutes' inhalation of nebulized normal saline has been shown to increase mucociliary clearance (Sutton *et al*. 1988).

The efficiency of the humidifier must be checked by the physiotherapist on each visit, to ensure that it is filled with water and that the temperature is correct.

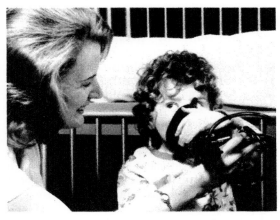

Figure 27.20 The child is encouraged to hold the mask firmly over his mouth and nose. (Courtesy of R. Samios.)

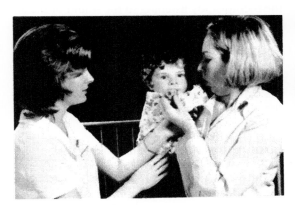

Figure 27.21 The child's mother encourages him to hold the mouthpiece firmly between his lips. (Courtesy of R. Samios.)

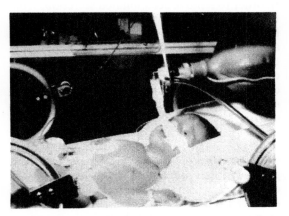

Figure 27.22 Nasal endotracheal intubation of an infant in an incubator following cardiac surgery. (Courtesy of R. Samios.)

Postural drainage

It is most important that secretions are not allowed to accumulate in the lower airways. Postural drainage is given to children on continuous artificial ventilation either to drain specific segments of the lungs or by elevating the foot of the bed in order to get a more overall drainage. Following cardiac or cranial surgery, drainage may have to be given in the child's nursing position as elevation of the foot of the bed may be contraindicated. Consideration should be given to the child's position throughout the day. Secretions will accumulate in the posterior segments if the child is nursed in supine, and in the lateral segments if in side lying. Side lying with 2-hourly turning is a position frequently adopted for nursing, and postural drainage may be given if necessary 2-hourly to whichever side the child is turned. Vibrations and percussion are given, with pressure on expiration, and secretions are removed by aspiration, as described below.

Throughout treatment the condition of a child on a ventilator is checked by observing colour, respiration rate and depth, and pulse rate. If the child's condition is being monitored, the physiotherapist must be experienced enough to interpret the signs shown by the monitors. When the child is removed from artificial ventilation, usually slowly weaned from this, the main aim of the physiotherapist is to restore normal respiratory function.

Techniques of aspiration or suction

In order to remove accumulated secretions from the airway, which will be necessary if only because of the child's depressed cough reflex, a catheter is inserted into the airway and suction employed. This must be done at all times quickly and gently. The catheter must be the correct size for the child's airway, that is, not so large that it causes trauma to its walls. Nasal suction should only be done when necessary and not as a routine, as this procedure easily causes trauma to the nose and is most unpleasant. The nasal passage is horizontal and runs parallel to the roof of the mouth, and this is the direction in which the catheter should be passed (Fig. 27.23). It must be emphasized that suction as a general rule is not bronchial. Bronchial suction may need to be performed on some children where blockage is suspected, but will

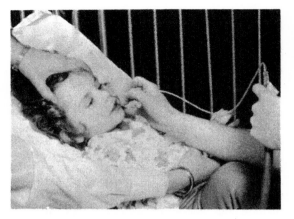

Figure 27.23 Nasopharyngeal aspiration. The child is restrained at the head and hands. (Courtesy of R. Samios.)

only be done as requested by the physician and then only by specially trained staff. Whether the catheter is passed via the nasopharynx or via the tracheostomy, it must not pass down the airway too far, such as to the carina, as damage to the mucosal lining and infection of the lower air passages, especially if the technique is not strictly aseptic, will readily ensue. In most cases it is sufficient for the catheter to be passed only as far as the pharynx, as this will be sufficient to stimulate a cough reflex. There must be one other person present to restrain the child as aspiration is a frightening procedure.

Suctioning is performed only while the catheter is being slowly withdrawn, not while it is being introduced. The routine is repeated until the therapist, by listening to the sound of the air passing through the trachea and pharynx, can be certain that no further secretions remain. This procedure must be strictly aseptic. The physiotherapist must be gowned, gloved, and in some cases masked, and should be sure that the catheter does not touch any object outside the airway as it will then no longer be sterile.

Care of the unconscious child

A child may be unconscious for a significant period of time as a result of head injury, following neurosurgery, encephalitis or meningitis. Under these circumstances special care is required in order to prevent contractures which may occur due to posture, the effects of gravity and immobility. Mobility must be maintained in order to avoid the effects of a relative stagnation of the circulatory system on the nutrition of bones, muscles and viscera. Respiratory efficiency must also be maintained, and the child may need to be artificially ventilated by endotracheal intubation or tracheostomy.

Following neurosurgery, it is important to prevent the build-up of carbon dioxide in the body as this has a harmful effect on brain function, causing dilation of cerebral vessels and an increase in cerebral oedema. The resultant increase in intracranial pressure will jeopardize the child's chances of recovery from the brain injury.

Physiotherapy will include passive movements of trunk and limbs (see Chapter 6), with emphasis on gaining full range, and positioning and frequent turning in order to avoid pressure areas on spine, sacrum, pelvis, elbows, heels and malleoli and to prevent pooling of secretions. The risk of pressure areas may be further minimized if the child sleeps on a water bed or sheepskin. Care must be taken in picking up and handling a paralysed infant or child in order to avoid causing damage to soft tissues.

Specific techniques, such as postural drainage, assisted breathing exercises and pharyngeal aspiration of mucus secretions will be needed on a preventive basis in all these children, but may at times need to be done intensively should respiratory infection or distress supervene.

Particular problems in managing the child with tetanus

There are special problems when a child has tetanus. The voluntary muscular system will be paralysed by the administration of tubocurarine in order to prevent spasm. This will necessitate that the child be tracheostomized and ventilated by positive pressure apparatus dispensing an oxygen–air mix. The main problems at this stage are likely to arise from diminished or absent cough reflex, and the possibility of aspiration of vomitus or saliva. The child will therefore require endotracheal suction at times, and this must be done with great care and only

as necessary, as even this small stimulus may cause an increase in blood pressure and pulse rate, and cardiac irregularities.

Physical conditioning

Children with asthma and cystic fibrosis in particular, but any child with respiratory dysfunction, may be less fit than their peers and need physical training to improve strength and motor control, musculoskeletal flexibility, posture and endurance. Exercise programmes should include exercises and activities directed at lower-limb support and propulsion (e.g. trampolining, bicycle riding, walking). Upper-limb activities will affect the chest wall as well as the arms, promoting thoracic mobility (e.g. shooting in basketball). Walking, jogging, swimming and bicycling will improve endurance. The benefits of jogging for cystic fibrosis (Orenstein *et al.* 1981) and swimming for asthmatic children (Sly *et al.* 1972; Fitch *et al.* 1976) have been reported in the literature. The benefits of exercises to improve thoracic mobility have also been described (Warren 1968; Watts 1968). Children with bronchospasm need to take appropriate medication before they exercise to avoid exercise-induced bronchospasm. Exercises for maintaining length of pectoral muscles, shoulder internal rotators, abdominal and hip flexor muscles are often necessary for avoiding postural malalignment.

Pulmonary limitations to exercise performance are described by Alison and Ellis (1992). Exercise testing and conditioning for children with lung dysfunction is described in detail by Darbee and Czerny (1990).

Summary

This chapter describes the physical methods used by the physiotherapist in the treatment of respiratory disorders in infants and children. Basically these involve techniques for draining excess secretions and for increasing ventilation to the lungs. Some techniques, such as the aspiration of secretions from the trachea of small infants, and the care of infants and children in intensive care units, require considerable skill and experience, and should not be attempted by the inexperienced physiotherapist unless under supervision.

The positive effects of exercise and physical activity on morale as well as on lung function, musculoskeletal flexibility and general fitness are well-documented. Children with respiratory dysfunction should be encouraged to exercise regularly and, if carried out at school and with parents, physical activity should be an enjoyable part of the day.

In the case of the child with chronic respiratory illness, it is essential that parents be taught techniques for draining, and improving ventilation to the lungs and clearing the upper respiratory tract, so treatment commenced and supervised by the physiotherapist continues regularly at home. The teaching of parents is part of the physiotherapist's responsibility. Without their well-trained help no regime of treatment will be successful.

References

Alison, J. (1992) Pulmonary function tests. In: *Key Issues in Cardiorespiratory Physiotherapy*, edited by E. Ellis and J. Alison. Oxford: Butterworth-Heinemann, pp. 24–55.

Alison, J. and Ellis, E. (1992) Pulmonary limitations to exercise performance. In: *Key Issues in Cardiorespiratory Physiotherapy*, edited by E. Ellis and J. Alison. Oxford: Butterworth-Heinemann, pp. 131–157.

Ayres, S.M., Kozam, R.L. and Lucas, D.S. (1963) The effects of intermittent positive pressure breathing on intrathoracic pressure, pulmonary mechanics and the work of breathing. *Am. Rev. Respir. Dis.*, **87**, 370.

Baskett, P.J.F. (1971) The clinical assessment of the respiratory system by the physiotherapist, including reference to the use of the stethoscope. *Physiotherapy*, **57**, 7.

Campbell, A.H., O'Connell, J.M. and Wilson, F. (1975) The effect of chest physiotherapy upon the FEV_1 in chronic bronchitis. *Med. J. Aust.*, **1**, 33.

Castilla, P., Irving, I.M., Jackson Rees, G. and Rickham, P.P. (1971) Posture in management of esophageal atresia. *J. Pediatr. Surg.*, **6**, 6, 709.

Cayton, R.M., Webber, B.A., Paterson, J.W. *et al.* (1978) A comparison of salbutamol given by pressure-packed aerosol or nebulization via IPPB in acute asthma. *Br. J. Dis. Chest*, **72**, 222.

Celli, B.R., Rodriguez, K.S. and Snider, G.L. (1984) A controlled trial of intermittent positive pressure breathing, incentive spirometry, and deep breathing exercises in preventing pulmonary complications after abdominal surgery. *Am. Rev. Respir. Dis.*, **130**, 12.

Crane, L.D. (1990) Physical therapy for the neonate. In: *Cardiopulmonary Physical Therapy*, 2nd edn, edited by S. Irwin and J.S. Tecklin. St Louis, MO: C.V. Mosby.

Curran, R.C. and Kachoyeanos, M.K. (1979) The effects on neonates of two methods of chest physical therapy. *Mothercraft Nurs.*, **4**, 309–313.

Darbee, J. and Czerny, F. (1990) Exercise testing and exercise conditioning for children with lung dysfunction. In: *Cardiopulmonary Physical Therapy*, 2nd edn, edited by S. Irwin and J.S. Tecklin. St Louis, MO: C.V. Mosby.

Davidson, A.G.F. *et al.* (1988) Physiotherapy in cystic fibrosis: a comparative trial of positive expiratory pressure, autogenic drainage, and conventional percussion and drainage techniques. *Pediatr. Pulmonol.*, **4** (suppl. 2), 132.

De Cesare, J.A. and Graybill, C.A. (1990) Physical therapy for the child with respiratory dysfunction. In: *Cardiopulmonary Physical Therapy*, 2nd edn, edited by S. Irwin and J.S. Tecklin. St Louis, MO: C.V. Mosby.

Dodd, M.E. (1991) Exercise in cystic fibrosis adults. In: *Respiratory Care*, edited by J.A. Pryor. Edinburgh: Churchill Livingstone, pp. 27–50.

Ellis, E.R., Bye, P.T.B., Bruderer, J.W. *et al.* (1987a) Treatment of respiratory failure during sleep with neuromuscular disease: +ve pressure ventilation through a nose mask. *Am. Rev. Respir. Dis.*, **135**, 148–152.

Ellis, E.R., McCauley, V.B., Mellis, C. *et al.* (1987b) Treatment of alveolar hypoventilation in a six-year-old girl with intermittent positive pressure ventilation through a nose mask. *Am. Rev. Respir. Dis.*, **136**, 188–191.

Falk, M., Kelstrup, M., Andersen, J.B. *et al.* (1984) Improving the ketchup bottle method with positive expiratory pressure, PEP, in cystic fibrosis. *Eur. J. Respir. Dis.*, **65**, 423.

Finer, N.N. and Boyd, J. (1978) Chest physiotherapy in the neonate: a controlled study. *Pediatrics*, **61**, 282.

Finer, N.N., Boyd, J. and Grace, M.G. (1978) Chest physiotherapy in neonates: a controlled study. *Physiother. Can.*, **30**, 1, 12.

Fitch, K.D., Morton, A.R. and Blanksby, B.A. (1976) Effects of swimming training on children with asthma. *Arch. Dis. Child.*, **51**, 190–194.

Gallon, A.M. (1991) Evaluation of chest percussion in the treatment of patients with copious sputum production. *Respir. Med.*, **85**, 45–51.

Gallon, A.M. (1992) The use of percussion. *Physiotherapy*, **78**, 85–89.

Gherini, S., Peters, R.M. and Virgilio, R.W. (1979) Mechanical work on the lungs and work of breathing with positive end-expiratory pressure and continuous positive airway pressure. *Chest*, **76**, 251.

Godfrey, S. (1974) *Exercise Testing in Children*. New York: W.B. Saunders.

Godfrey, S., Kamburof, P.L. and Nairn, J.R. (1970) Spirometry, lung volumes and airways resistance in normal children aged 5 to 18 years. *Br. J. Dis. Chest*, **64**, 15.

Gregory, G.A., Edmunds, L.H., Kitterman, J.A., Phibbs, R.H. and Tooley, W.H. (1975) Continuous positive airways pressure and pulmonary and circulatory function after cardiac surgery in infants less than three months of age. *Anaesthesiology*, **43**, 426.

Grimby, G. (1974) Aspects of lung expansion in relation to pulmonary physiotherapy. *Am. Rev. Respir. Dis.*, **110** (suppl. 1), 149–153.

Hofmeyr, J.L., Webber, B.A. and Hodson, M.E. (1986) Evaluation of positive expiratory pressure as an adjunct to chest physiotherapy in the treatment of cystic fibrosis. *Thorax*, **41**, 951.

Jones, R.S. and Owen-Thomas, J.B. (1971) *Care of the Critically Ill Child*. London: Arnold.

Kendig, E.L. and Chernick, V. (eds) (1977) *Disorders of the Respiratory Tract in Children*. Philadelphia, PA: W.B. Saunders.

Kigin, C.M. (1981) Chest physical therapy for the postoperative or traumatic injury patient. *Phys. Ther.*, **61**, 1724.

Kigin, C.M. (1992) Assessment of the respiratory system. In: *Key Issues in Cardiorespiratory Physiotherapy*, edited by E. Ellis and J. Alison. Oxford: Butterworth-Heinemann, pp. 5–23.

Lioy, J. and Maninello, F.P. (1988) A comparison of prone and supine positioning in the immediate postextubation period of neonates. *J. Pediatr.*, **112**, 6, 982–984.

Long, J.G., Philp, A.G.S. and Lucey, J.F. (1980) Excessive handling as a cause of hypoxemia. *Pediatrics*, **65**, 2, 203–207.

McDonnell, T., McNicholas, W.T. and Fitzgerald, M.X. (1986) Hypoxaemia during chest physiotherapy in patients with cystic fibrosis. *Ir. J. Med. Sci.*, **155**, 345.

Martin, R.J., Herrell, N., Rubin, D. *et al.* (1979) Effect of supine and prone positions on arterial oxygen tension in the preterm infant. *Pediatrics*, **63**, 4, 528–531.

Menkes, H.A. and Traystman, R.J. (1977) Rationale for physical therapy. *Am. Rev. Respir. Dis.*, **116**, 287.

Orenstein, D.M., Franklin, B.A., Doershuk, C.F. *et al.* (1981) Exercise conditioning and cardiopulmonary fitness in cystic fibrosis. *Chest*, **80**, 392.

Parker, A.E. (1985) Chest physiotherapy in the neonatal intensive care unit. *Physiotherapy*, **71**, 2, 63–65.

Pavia, D. (1984) Lung mucociliary clearance. In: *Aerosols and the Lung*, edited by S.W. Clarke and D. Pavia. London: Butterworths.

Pavia, D., Webber, B.A., Agnew, J.E. *et al.* (1988) The role of intermittent positive pressure breathing (IPPB) in bronchial toilet. *Eur. Respir. J.*, **1** (suppl. 2), 250S.

Polgar, G. and Promadhat, V. (1971) *Pulmonary Function Testing in Children: Techniques and Standards*. Philadelphia, PA: W.B. Saunders.

Pryor, J. (1992) Mucociliary clearance. In: *Key Issues in Cardiorespiratory Physiotherapy*, edited by E. Ellis and J. Alison. Oxford: Butterworth-Heinemann, pp. 105–130.

Pryor, J.A. and Webber, B.A. (1979) An evaluation of the forced expiratory technique as an adjunct to postural drainage. *Physiotherapy*, **65**, 304.

Pryor, J.A., Webber, B.A. and Hodson, M.E. (1990) Effects of chest physiotherapy on oxygen saturation in patients with cystic fibrosis. *Thorax*, **45**, 77.

Roberts, K.D. and Edwards, J.M. (1971) *Paediatric Intensive Care*. Oxford: Blackwell.

Rockwell, G.M. and Campbell, S.K. (1976) Physical therapy program for the paediatric cardiac surgical patient. *Phys. Ther.*, **56**, 670.

Sade, R.M., Cosgrove, D.M. and Castenada, A.R. (1977)

Infant and Child Care in Heart Surgery. Chicago, IL: Year Book Medical Publishers.

Schoni, M.H. (1989) Autogenic drainage: a modern approach to physiotherapy in cystic fibrosis. *J. R. Soc. Med.*, **82** (suppl. 16), 32.

Silverman, W.A., Sinclair, J.C. and Agate, F.J. (1966) The oxygen cost of minor changes in heat balance of small newborn infants. *Acta Paediatr. Scand.*, **55**, 294.

Sly, R.M., Harpe, R.T. and Rosselot, I. (1972) The effect of physical conditioning upon asthmatic children. *Ann. Allergy*, **30**, 86–94.

Speidel, B.D. (1978) Adverse effects of routine procedures on preterm infants. *Lancet* April, 864–865.

Stafanger *et al.* (1983). Longterm study of effect of PEP-mask in cystic fibrosis patients. *Am. J. Dis. Child.*, **96**, 6.

Stark, A.R., Waggener, T.B., Frantz, I.D. *et al.* (1984) Effect on ventilation of change to the upright posture in newborn infants. *J. Appl. Physiol.*, **56**, 64–71.

Stock, M.C., Downs, J.B., Gauer, P.K. *et al.* (1985) Prevention of postoperative pulmonary complications with CPAP, incentive spirometry and conservative therapy. *Chest*, **87**, 151.

Sukumalchantra, Y., Park, S.S. and Williams, M.H. (1965) The effect of intermittent positive pressure breathing (IPPB) in acute ventilatory failure. *Am. Rev. Respir. Dis.*, **92**, 885.

Sutton, P.P., Gemmell, H.G., Innes, N. *et al.* (1988) Use of nebulised saline and nebulised terbutaline as an adjunct to chest physiotherapy. *Thorax*, **43**, 57.

Tecklin, J.S. and Holsclaw, D.S. (1975) Evaluation of bronchial drainage in patients with cystic fibrosis. *Phys. Ther.*, **55**, 1081.

Thacker, E.W. (1971) *Postural Drainage and Respiratory Control*. London: Lloyd-Luke.

Thompson, B.J. (1978) The physiotherapist's role in the rehabilitation of the asthmatic. *N.Z. J. Physiother.*, **4**, 11.

Thoren, L. (1954) Post-operative pulmonary complications: observations on their prevention by means of physical therapy. *Acta Chirurg. Scand.*, **107**, 193.

Tudehope, D.I. and Bagley, C. (1980) Techniques of physiotherapy in intubated babies with the respiratory distress syndrome. *Aust. Paediatr. J.*, **16**, 226–228.

van der Schans, C.P., Piers, D.A. and Postma, D.S. (1986) Effect of manual percussion on tracheobronchial clearance in patients with chronic airflow obstruction and excessive tracheobronchial secretion. *Thorax*, **41**, 448.

Wagamen, M.J., Shutack, J.G., Mommjian, A.S. *et al.* (1979) Improved oxygenation and lung compliance with prone positioning of neonates. *J. Pediatr.*, **94**, 5, 787–791.

Warren, A. (1968) Mobilization of the chest wall. *Phys. Ther.*, **48**, 582–585.

Watts, N. (1968) Improvement of breathing patterns. *Phys. Ther.*, **48**, 563–576.

Webber, B.A. (1988) *The Brompton Hospital Guide to Chest Physiotherapy*, 5th edn. London: Blackwell.

Webber, B.A., Parker, R.A., Hofmeyr, J.L. *et al.* (1985) Evaluation of self-percussion during postural drainage using the forced expiration technique. *Physiother. Pract.*, **1**, 42.

Webber, B.A., Hofmeyr, J.L., Morgan, M.D.L. *et al.* (1986) Effects of postural drainage, incorporating the forced expiration technique, on pulmonary function in cystic fibrosis. *Br. J. Dis. Chest*, **80**, 353.

Zelazo, P.R. (1976) From reflexive to instrumental behavior. In: *Developmental Psychobiology: The Significance of Infancy*, edited by L. Lipsitt. Hillsdale, NJ: Erlbaum.

Further reading

Bozynski, M.E.A., Naglie, R.A., Nicks, J.J. and Johnson, R.V. (1988) Lateral positioning of the stable ventilated very-low-birth-weight infant. *Aust. J. Dis. Chest*, **142**, 200–202.

Ellis, E. and Alison, J. (eds) (1991) *Key Issues in Cardiorespiratory Physiotherapy*. Oxford: Butterworth-Heinemann.

Finer, N.N., Moriartey, R.R., Boyd, J. *et al.* (1979) Postextubation atelectasis: a retrospective review and a prospective controlled study. *J. Pediatr.*, **94**, 1, 110–113.

Fox, W.W., Schwartz, J.G. and Shaffer, T.H. (1978) Pulmonary physiotherapy in neonates: physiologic changes and respiratory management. *J. Pediatr.*, **92**, 6, 977–981.

Kendall, L. (1987) A comparison between adult and paediatric intensive care. *Physiotherapy*, **73**, 9, 495–498.

Prendiville, A., Thomson, A. and Silverman, M. (1986) Effect of tracheobronchial suction on respiratory resistance in intubated preterm babies. *Arch. Dis. Child.*, **61**, 1178–1183.

Upton, C.J., Milner, A.D. and Stokes, G.M. (1991) Apnoea, bradycardia, and oxygen saturation in preterm infants. *Arch. Dis. Child.*, **66**, 381–385.

Vivian-Beresford, A., King, C. and Macauley, H. (1987) Neonatal post-extubation complications: the preventative role of physiotherapy. *Physiother. Can.*, **39**, 3, 184–190.

Appendices

1   Tests for reflexive and prefunctional activity
2   Guide to developmental assessment of the infant
3   The blind infant

Appendix 1

Tests for reflexive and prefunctional activity

The significance of many of the motor behaviours described below is not fully understood. Theoretical concepts regarding reflexes in infancy are currently being re-evaluated (see Chapter 2 for discussion and references). Except where reference is made to a specific author, the references for the following tests are Gesell and Amatruda (1947), André-Thomas *et al.* (1960), Peiper (1963) and Illingworth (1970). Appendix 2 illustrates the times at which these responses can be typically elicited in normal babies.

Amphibian reaction

This is tested with the infant in prone. The examiner rotates the pelvis away from the table a short distance. This is followed by flexion and abduction of the leg on the same side. This reaction can be elicited from birth. It may be absent in babies with brain lesions. Care must be taken not to confuse a passive movement into flexion with the normal active response.

Neonatal standing and stepping

The examiner holds the baby with the feet on a table. The baby responds by extending the legs and standing up, although support is needed as balance has not developed (see Fig. 2.8). If the body is inclined forwards the infant will take a few steps, with marked flexion of hips and knees. These movements are seen in newborn babies, and can be elicited, although with diminishing response in some infants.

It has recently been shown that standing and stepping are maintained in infants who are given practice in these actions (Zelazo 1983). The ability to take weight through the feet and walk at birth is now considered to be prefunctional. These actions may be absent in hypotonic and severely mentally retarded babies.

Crossed extensor response

This is tested with the baby in supine. The examiner holds one leg extended and firmly strokes the sole of the foot from heel towards the toes. The infant responds by flexing the contralateral leg into abduction, then by adducting and extending the leg as though to push the stimulus away. This response is present from birth until 4–6 weeks of age. Absence or persistence may indicate a pathological state. It may be absent or delayed in a baby with other abnormal neurological signs.

Galant reflex

The baby is tested in prone or ventral suspension (Fig. i.i). The examiner runs a finger parallel to the spine from the last rib to the iliac

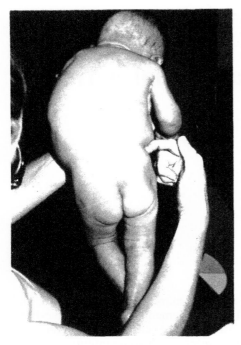

Figure i.i Galant reflex (trunk incurvation reflex) is positive on the right side in this baby with abnormal neurological signs.

crest. The baby responds by side-flexing towards the stimulus. This response is present at birth and can be elicitied for 6–8 weeks. It may be absent in some floppy babies, and may persist, either symmetrically or asymmetrically, in babies with other abnormal neurological signs.

Moro reflex

The examiner holds the baby with the head and trunk supported. Support is withdrawn from the head, letting it drop back into the hand. This sudden loss of head control backwards startles the baby who responds by extending the arms in a wide embracing movement, hands open and fingers abducted. The legs may also extend, although this response varies. The movement often elicits crying. The reflex is present at birth. After the first few weeks the arms extend and abduct less widely, and the reflex can usually no longer be elicited after 2–3 months (Mitchell 1960). This reflex may be absent or diminished in floppy babies.

It may be asymmetrical in a baby with hemiplegia or brachial plexus lesion.

Protective side-turning of the head

This is tested in prone. The examiner holds the baby's head gently face downwards on the table, then releases it. The baby responds by turning the head to one side. This reaction is present from birth. It may be absent in babies with other abnormal neurological signs.

Righting reactions

These are considered to be responsible for the baby's ability to maintain the head and body in relation to space, and to maintain the relationship of various parts of the body to each other (Bobath and Bobath 1955). The baby responds to an externally-imposed change to the position of one body segment (e.g., the head) by moving other segments into line (Milani-Comparetti and Gidoni 1967). Vision probably plays a significant role in the response.

Neck-righting reflex

This is tested in supine. It appears to be a proprioceptive reflex elicited by stretching of the neck muscles. The examiner holds the baby's head and rotates it to one side. The trunk follows the head and the baby may roll over. This response is present at birth and is most evident at 3 months, after which it becomes less reliable, until it can no longer be elicited at 5 months. It may be absent in floppy babies. In babies with cerebral palsy the response may be abnormal. In this case the shoulder girdle may remain retracted and the baby may not bring the arm forwards.

Labyrinthine-righting reaction

This response is tested by observing the position of the baby's head in relation to the body when held in supine and prone and when tilted laterally in the vertical position. A normal newborn baby demonstrates some head lag when pulled to sitting, although some attempt is made to hold the head up. An infant with brain dysfunction may have a marked head lag (see Fig. 5.1). By 4 months the infant holds the head in line with the body when pulled to sitting (see Fig. 2.6). By 5–6 months the head is raised in supine in anticipation of being pulled to sitting (Fig. 2.7). A newborn baby held in ventral suspension will allow the head to fall into some flexion (Fig. i.ii), but not into the completely flexed position of the baby with brain dysfunction (see Fig. ii.iv). By 8 weeks the head will be held in line with the body. By 4 months the head can be held erect when the baby is lying in prone (Fig. 2.1).

Placing reactions

The examiner holds the baby so the dorsum of the foot or anterior aspect of the leg touches the edge of the table. The baby responds by flexing the leg and placing the foot flat on the table. A similar response can be found in the hands, the hand being placed on the table in response to a touch on its dorsal aspect. These responses can be elicited from birth (Zapella 1963). They may, however, be absent in floppy babies, and in babies with cerebral palsy. These responses may be asymmetrical in a baby with hemiplegia or a brachial plexus lesion. The test is useful in detecting lower limb motor dysfunction in a baby who shows few other signs of abnormality.

Landau reaction

This is tested with the baby held in ventral suspension. The normal baby from 4 to 5 months responds to ventral suspension by extending head, trunk, and by 6 or 8 months, the legs. The examiner flexes the baby's head which is followed by flexion of the trunk and legs. When the head is released, the limbs, head and trunk usually return to their extended positions. This response may be absent in babies with cerebral palsy or severe mental retardation, who may maintain a flexed position when held in ventral suspension. In babies with cerebral palsy, there may be no alteration in position when the head is flexed forwards, extension being maintained throughout the head, trunk and lower limbs.

Parachute reaction

The baby is held at the trunk and lowered head-first towards the ground. In response, the arms are extended and the baby reaches out the hands towards the floor. This response can be elicited after 6 months, but is more evident at 9 months, and continues as a protective mechanism. The response may be absent in babies with developmental delay.

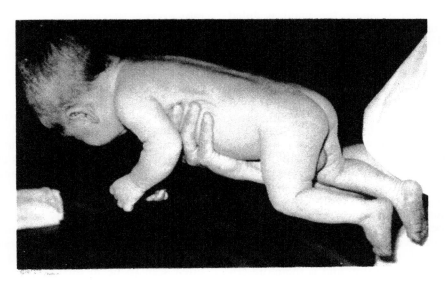

Figure i.ii   Aged 6 weeks, in ventral suspension. Note the head held in line with the body, which is a normal finding at this age. Compare with the baby in Figure ii.iv.

The response is also tested in sitting, when the baby is moved gently forwards, sideways and backwards. In response, the baby puts out one or both hands for support. A normal baby demonstrates this reaction forwards at 6 months, sideways at 8 months and backwards at 12 months.

The parachute reaction has been thought to depend on vestibular control (Paine and Oppé 1966). However, an analysis of the reaction suggests instead that the response is visually controlled (Peters and Walk 1974).

Equilibrium reactions

In the clinic it has been common for the so-called equilibrium reactions to be considered 'postural reflexes', that is, automatic responses to loss of balance. These reactions may be more clearly understood as responses to an external force applied to the body. Unlike the postural adjustments which precede a self-initiated movement, adjustments to externally-imposed forces occur after the perturbation. When these responses are tested in the clinic, perturbation of the body mass is brought about by the therapist either directly (through manual contact) or indirectly (through movement of the support surface).

In *sitting* and *standing* the child is tilted slowly to one side, then forwards and backwards, and, as the body mass is moved towards the limits of stability, the child will move the trunk and limbs in the opposite direction in order to keep the centre of body mass balanced (Figs i.iii and i.iv). These responses appear first in prone and supine at 6 months, in sitting at 9 months and in standing at approximately 14 months. All postural adjustment is specific to the task and the context in which it takes place. Adjustments to external forces have been investigated rather extensively (see Chapter 2). In childhood, responses reflect not only the maturity of the system but also the child's experiences. Although clinically it has been considered that a 'normal' response to external perturbation is reflective of a 'normal' postural reflex mechanism and is therefore critical to the acquisition of 'normal' movement, this is unlikely to be so given the specificity of postural adjustments.

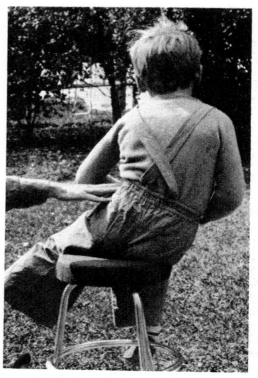

Figure i.iii The response to an externally-imposed perturbation to the body mass in sitting. Note the lateral movement of the head and trunk when the body mass is pushed from over one base of support (both thighs) to another (the right thigh). This response ensures that the centre of body mass is not moved to the point when balance is lost.

Tonic neck reflexes

Asymmetrical tonic neck reflex

This is tested in supine. It is a response apparently elicited by stretch applied to the neck muscles. The baby's head is turned to one side. The examiner both watches and feels the response in the limbs. The arm and leg on the face side are seen to extend while those on the occiput side flex (Fig. i.v). There may not be an actual movement, but only an increase in resistance to passive flexion of the limbs on the face side and to extension on the occiput side. Normal babies in their first 2–3 months are often seen to lie in this 'fencing' position for short periods, but it is a fleeting, not a persistent response, and cannot be regarded as reflexive. If the posture is persistent (after the age of 5

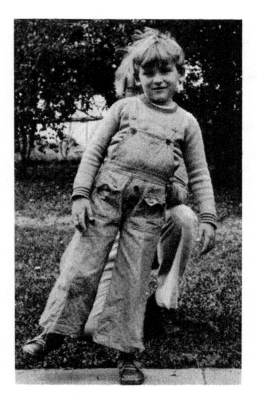

Figure i.iv The response to an externally-imposed perturbation to the body mass in standing. Note the lateral movement of the head, trunk and right leg as the boy balances on the left leg.

months; Bax 1987), or if it is a stereotyped response to rotation of the head, it is considered abnormal. It may dominate the baby's motor function to such an extent that the hand cannot be taken to the mouth.

Symmetrical tonic neck reflex

This may be tested in four-point kneeling. It is apparently elicited by stretch applied to the neck muscles. When the examiner extends the baby's head, the arms will extend while the legs flex. When the head is flexed, the arms collapse into flexion and the legs extend. It is doubtful whether this response is found in normal infants except as a response to a mechanical change in segmental alignment. If it occurs in the stereotyped manner described above it is considered to be abnormal. This reflex is reported to be seen in babies with cerebral palsy (Bobath and Bobath 1955).

References

André-Thomas, Chesni, Y. and Dargassies, S.S.-A. (1960) *The Neurological Examination of the Infant.* Oxford: Butterworth-Heinemann.

Bax, M. (1987) Aims and outcomes of physiotherapy for cerebral palsy. *Develop. Med. Child Neurol.*, **29**, 689–692.

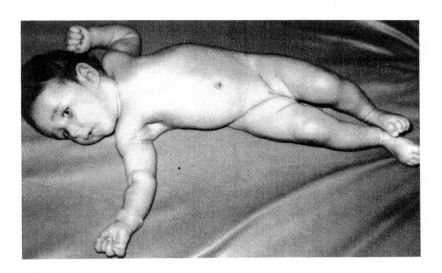

Figure i.v Asymmetrical tonic neck reflex to the right.

Bobath, K. and Bobath, B. (1955) Tonic reflexes and righting reflexes in the diagnosis and assessment of cerebral palsy. *Cerebral Palsy Bull.*, **16**, 5.

Gesell, A. and Amatruda, C.S. (1947) *Developmental Diagnosis*. New York: Hoeber.

Illingworth, R.S. (1970) *The Development of the Infant and Young Child*. London: Livingstone.

Mitchell, R.G. (1960) The Moro reflex. *Cerebral Palsy Bull.*, **2**, 135.

Paine, R.S. and Oppé, T.E. (1966) *Neurological Examination of Children*. Oxford: Butterworth-Heinemann.

Peiper, A. (1963) *Cerebral Function in Infancy and Childhood*. London: Pitman.

Peters, C.P. and Walk, R.D. (1974) Visual placing by human infants. *J. Exp. Child Psychol.*, **18**, 34–40.

Zapella, M. (1963) Placing reactions in the newborn. *Dev. Med. Child Neurol.*, **5**, 497.

Zelazo, P.R. (1983) The development of walking: new findings and old assumptions. *J. Motor Behav.*, **15**, **2**, 99–137.

Zelazo, P.R., Zelazo, N.A. and Kolb, S. (1972) 'Walking' in the newborn. *Science*, **235**, 38–47.

Further Reading

Prechtl, H.F.R. (1977) *The Neurological Examination of the Full-Term Infant*, 2nd edn. Oxford: Butterworth-Heinemann.

Sival, D.A., Prechtl, H.F.R., Sonder, G.H.A. and Touwen, B.C.L. (1993) The effect of intra-uterine breech position on postnatal motor functions of the lower limbs. *Early Hum. Develop.*, **32**, 161–176.

Appendix 2

Guide to developmental assessment of the infant

Neurological assessment of infants is described by several authors (André-Thomas *et al.* 1960; Prechtl 1977; Fiorentino 1980; Milani-Comparetti 1980; Dubowitz and Dubowitz 1981). Behavioural assessment is described by Brazelton (1973).

In testing an infant's responses (see Appendix 1), attention should be paid particularly to persistent asymmetry of posture and movement, and to stereotyped movements.

In supine

Certain signs when persistent may indicate abnormality:

1 Extended, adducted legs with plantarflexed feet; kicking into extension and adduction (Fig. ii.i).

2 Persistent asymmetry of posture. A normal newborn baby lies asymmetrically but can move the head to the opposite side and change position of limbs and trunk (see Fig. i.v).
3 Movement of one arm or leg persistently more than the other.
4 Failure to open one hand more than the other.
5 Persistent adduction of the thumb across the palm, or fisting of the hand (Fig. ii.ii).
6 A frequent Moro reflex on minimal stimulus after the age of 4 months.
7 Stereotyped movements. It is only in the neonate that one sees a relative lack of variety of movement.
8 Tremor on movement after the first few days.
9 Retraction of the head and trunk, or opisthotonus (Fig. ii.i).

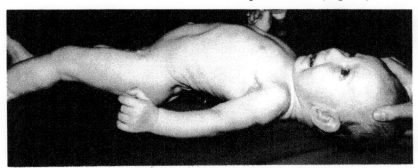

Figure ii.i Infant with opisthotonos. He extends his body so much he cannot remain in supine but rolls to one side.

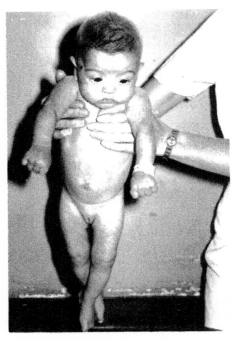

Figure ii.ii Infant with Reye's syndrome. When he is held in standing, he has persistent extension and adduction of the lower limbs and extension of the upper limbs with pronated forearms and fisted hands.

10 Reaching out for an object with the arm always in internal rotation and pronation (Fig. ii.iii).
11 Complete head lag (see Fig. 5.1). Not even a neonate allows the head to fall completely uncontrolled when pulled to sitting.

12 Well-sustained ankle clonus.
13 Immobility.

Actions to observe and analyse:

1 Neck flexion when moved from sitting to supine (see Fig. 2.6).
2 Reaching forwards to an object.
3 Rolling to prone.
4 Lifting the head (see Fig. 2.7).

Responses observed:

1 Crossed extension reflex.
2 Moro reflex.
3 Neck-righting reflex.

In prone

Certain signs when persistent may indicate abnormality:

1 Pelvis flat on bed in newborn period or too high when it should be flat (Fig. ii.iii).
2 Inability to bring arms out from under body.
3 Immobility.

Actions to observe and analyse:

1 Raising the head and upper trunk, resting on forearms and later on hands with extended arms (see Fig. 2.1).
2 Rolling to supine.

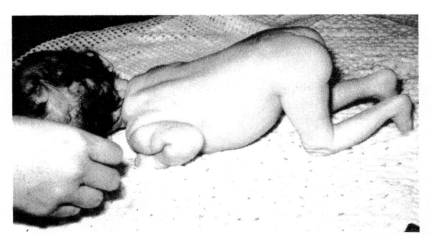

Figure ii.iii Persistent posture of an infant aged 3 months. The pelvis and thighs should be flat on the table in relaxed prone lying at this age.

3 Reaching out with one hand (see Figs 2.2, 2.3).
4 Getting up to four-foot kneeling.
5 Getting to the sitting position.
6 Creeping and later crawling on all fours (see Figs 2.4 and 2.5).
7 Getting to standing.

Responses observed:

1 Protective side-turning of the head.
2 Amphibian reaction.

In sitting

Certain signs when persistent may indicate abnormality:

1 Head and trunk retraction when supported in sitting. The examiner's hand should not be placed behind the head as this may stimulate neck extension, even in normal babies.
2 Adducted legs with feet plantarflexed and knees extended (see Fig. 3.7).
3 Sitting with a wide base (see Fig. 8.1).

Actions to observe and analyse:

1 Independent sitting on the floor; turning the body to look around (see Figs 2.11 and 2.13); reaching out for objects.
2 Support on hands forwards, sideways, backwards (see Figs 2.9 and 2.10).
3 Gets from sitting to sitting sideways on the floor.
4 Gets from sideways sitting to four-foot kneeling and back again.
5 Independent sitting on a seat with feet on floor; turning the body to look around; reaching for objects, down to floor, in front, to the side, behind.
6 Pulls to standing.
7 Gets from sitting on floor to standing through half-kneeling (see Fig. 2.6).
8 Sit-to-stand from a seat.
9 Crouch-to-stand.

Responses observed:

Parachute reaction forwards, sideways, backwards.

Held in ventral suspension

Certain signs when persistent may indicate abnormality:

1 Neck flexion.
2 Extended arms and/or legs (Fig. ii.iv).
3 Persistence of Galant reflex (see Fig. i.i).
4 Flexed-trunk posture (Fig. ii.iv).

Action to observe and analyse:

The ability to extend the head, trunk and hips against gravity.

Responses observed:

1 Galant reflex.
2 Landau reaction.
3 Parachute reaction with arms.

In standing

Certain signs when persistent may indicate abnormality:

1 Flexion of the legs when feet touch the floor.
2 Adducted hips, plantarflexed feet (Fig. ii.iii).

Actions to observe and analyse:

1 Supported standing (see Fig. 2.8).
2 Supported stepping.
3 Walking sideways around the furniture.
4 Walking with hands held.
5 Walking up and down small steps.

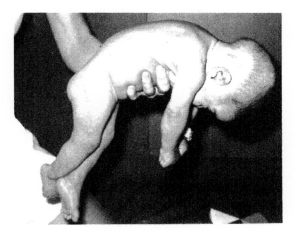

Figure ii.iv Infant with Reye's syndrome. When he is held in ventral suspension, the limbs are stiffly extended.

Response observed:

Placing reaction.

References

André-Thomas, Chesni, Y. and Dargassies, S.S.-A. (1960) *The Neurological Examination of the Infant*. London: Heinemann Medical.

Brazelton, T.B. (1973) *Neonatal Behavioral Assessment Scale*. London: Heinemann Medical.

Dubowitz, V. and Dubowitz, L. (1981) *The Neurological Assessment of the Preterm and Full-Term Infant*. Philadelphia, PA: J.B. Lippincott.

Fiorentino, M.R. (1980) *Normal and Abnormal Development – The Influence of Primitive Reflexes on Motor Development*. Springfield, IL: Charles C. Thomas.

Milani-Comparetti, A. (1980) Pattern analysis of normal and abnormal development: the fetus, the newborn, the child. In: *Development of Movement in Infancy*, edited by D.S. Slaton. Chapel Hill, SC: University of Southern Carolina Press.

Prechtl, H. (1977) *The Neurological Examination of the Full-Term Infant*, 2nd edn. London: Heinemann Medical.

Appendix 3

The blind infant

Blindness may occur as a congenital abnormality or following a variety of causes including injury to the eye. Blindness may also be associated with mental retardation or cerebral palsy, and may also be found in children who are deaf.

Blindness at birth may affect development of spatial perception and form identification, the development of social skills (facial expression, eye contact, eating and drinking, communication) and the development of motor skills. Vision is critical to the development of skill in movement since it normally provides a dominant sensory input for the control of movement, providing critical information as well as feedback about the results of one's actions. Blindness is said to affect the development of certain early learning skills, such as object permanence, the nature of cause and effect, the sorting of objects into categories and imitation (Freeman 1993). The child who is both hearing and vision impaired has serious restrictions placed on the ability to collect information.

The blind infant will usually be seen by the physiotherapist in order to minimize developmental delay, to optimize the infant's ability to develop skill in functional motor actions and to assist the parents to address the infant's needs. Parents need to understand the effects of their behaviour on the infant as their responses influence the infant's future actions (Dubose 1976). One of the parent's tasks is to encourage behaviour which is acceptable to society. Infants normally depend largely on visual cues and imitation for this aspect of learning.

Some specific problems found in blind infants are outlined below. An activities programme begins as soon as possible and aims to minimize these problems in addition to maximizing the infant's functional development. Freeman (1993) gives details of intervention with children with both hearing and visual impairments.

Perseverant or stereotypic behaviours

These consist of actions such as eye poking, rocking, head banging and finger movement. The reasons for such behaviours are not understood. However, there have been several causes suggested, including a response to sensory deprivation and the consequence of emotional disturbance. It has also been suggested that a child with visual impairment may use stereotypic actions in a situation of extreme stress.

Postural adjustments

Many blind infants are slow to develop independent standing and walking, demonstrating the importance of vision both for motor control mechanisms and as a motivating factor in motor behaviour. Touch, hearing and vestibular and proprioceptive inputs need to be substituted for vision in providing information which will elicit and control movement. Fraiberg (1968) suggested that the blind infant demonstrates a readiness for crawling by supporting on hands and knees and rocking back and forth. Similarly, the infant may stand with support some time before being able to walk independently.

Balancing problems may be due to the absence of the optical righting reaction's contribution to orienting the body in space, to difficulties internalizing position in space or to the fact that the infant cannot learn from watching others.

Actions such as crawling, walking, reaching can be encouraged using audible toys. Crawling can be assisted by slinging a towel under the body and giving the infant the feeling of the movement. Reaching toward a sound is normally achieved at around 10 months of age, a developmental step parents need to be made aware of so they are not disappointed when the infant does not do it sooner. Standing unsupported should be encouraged as early as possible since there is a tendency for blind infants to persist in cruising sideways around the furniture. Once independent walking is established, the child needs practice at walking from one surface to another, for example, from floorboards to carpet, since this can be an obstacle to further walking development.

Activities involving total body movement are encouraged early. As the child gets older, activities such as somersaulting, jumping, using playground equipment, swimming, help develop an awareness of self in space, a feeling of confidence and pleasure in movement, and a sense of adventure.

Prehension

Visually-impaired infants tend to keep their arms abducted at shoulder level and are slow to handle objects, to reach, and to perform bimanual actions. The infant is encouraged early to interact manually with objects and people and shown how to seek out what is relevant to the task in hand. Tactile sensitivity is encouraged from an early age as touch will be used in many ways (e.g., in Braille perception, typing) as a substitute for vision. An audible ball and target are used to teach catching and throwing. The child is not protected from making errors during the practice of activities as this is a natural part of motor learning. However, errors may have to be more clearly defined for the child so the necessary corrections can be made.

References

Dubose, R.F. (1976) Development needs in blind infants. *New Outlook*, **Feb.**, 49–52.

Fraiberg, S. (1968) Parallel and divergent patterns in blind and sighted infants. In: *Psycho-analytical Study of the Child.* New York: International University Press.

Freeman, P. (1993) Sensory disorders: the deaf and blind child. In: *Elements of Paediatric Physiotherapy*, edited by P.M. Eckersley. London: Churchill Livingstone, pp. 247–265.

Suggested reading

Adelson, E. and Fraiberg, S. (1974) Gross motor development in infants blind from birth. *Child Develop.*, **45**, 114–126.

Fraiberg, S. (1971) Intervention in infancy. *J. Amer. Acad. Child Psychiatr.*, **10**, 3, 382–404.

Freeman, P. (1985) *The Deaf/Blind Baby.* London: Heinemann Medical.

RESPECT THE CHILD
BE NOT TOO MUCH HIS PARENT
TRESPASS NOT ON HIS SOLITUDE

—*Emerson*

Index

Abnormal posturing
  basal ganglion lesions, 102
  upper motorneuron lesions, 95–96
Anchondroplasia, 278
Aerosol therapy
  asthma, 354
  cystic fibrosis, 360
Agnosia, 157
Airway clearance
  bronchiolitis, 345
  cardiac surgery
    pre-operative, 375
    post-operative, 376
  cystic fibrosis, 359-361
  incubator nursed-infants, 377
  inhaled foreign body, 350
  intensive care, 374
  pertussis (whooping cough), 350
Allergic asthma, 353
Amelia, 261
Amphibian reaction, 387, 395
Ankle-foot orthosis, 192
Anterior floor-reaction ankle-foot orthoses
  (AFO), 254
Anterior horn cell neuropathy, 280
Anteromedial plaster splint, 216, 218
Antibiotic therapy
  bronchiectasis, 352
  pneumonia, 346
Anti-burnscar elastic pressure supports (Jobst),
  326–327
Apert's syndrome, 165
Arch supports, 58
  secondary flat feet, 278
Arnold-Chiari malformation, 241, 243
Arthritic disease, *see* Inflammatory joint/soft tissue
  disorders

Arthrogryposis multiplex congenita, 235–237
  aetiology, 235
  congenital hip dislocation, 229
  description, 235
  management, 235–236
  mobilization, 236
  physical treatment, 236
  splinting, 236
  surgery, 236
  talipes equinovarus, 207, 212, 235, 236
Aspiration
  airway obstruction, 344
  complications, 335
  pneumonia, 345, 346
  poliomyelitis, 188
Assisted coughing, 285
Associated movements, 14–15
  manipulation development, 23, 25
  minimal brain dysfunction, 155
  spastic cerebral palsy, 118
Associated reactions, *see* Associated movements
Asthma, 350, 352–358
  allergic, 353
  breathing techniques, 354, 355, 357
    between attacks, 356–357
    during attack, 355–356
  bronchodilator drugs, 354, 358, 366
    hand-operated aerosol dispenser, 354
    intermittent positive pressure ventilators, 354,
      358
    nebulizer with mouthpiece, 354, 358
  clinical features, 353
  deformity of chest, 353
  exercise tolerance assessment, 365–366
  exercise-induced, 353, 356, 366
  medical management, 353–354
  pathology, 352

Asthma (*continued*)
  physical conditioning, 381
  physical treatment, 354
    classwork, 357–358
  physiology, 352–353
  postural drainage, 354, 355, 371
  respiratory complications, 335
  status asthmaticus, 352, 358
  thoracic expansion measurement, 364
  thoracic mobility/relaxation techniques, 354
Asymmetrical tonic neck reflex (ATNR), 390–391
  environmental modification for head control, 49–50
Ataxia
  acute brain injury, 147
  cerebellar lesions, 101
  cerebral palsy, 115, 119
    postural adjustments, 123
    walking, 121
  minimal brain dysfunction, 155, 157
Atelectasis
  airway obstruction, 344
  asthma, 352
  bronchiectasis, 351
  pre-term infant, 344
Athetosis
  basal ganglia lesions, 102
  cerebral palsy, 114, 118–119
  clumsiness (motor control deficit), 157
Attention control training, 150
Attention deficit disorder, 154, 155
  clinical features, 159–160
  diagnosis, 155, 156
  hyperactive behaviour, 159–160
  learning difficulty, 159
Audiometric testing, 132
Autistic children, 159
Autogenic drainage (AD), 374
Axonal sprouting
  brain injury recovery, 103, 105
  poliomyelitis recovery, 186
Ayres' test, 156

Babbling, 33
Babinski response, 96
Baclofen, 139
Balance
  development, 25–28
    in lower limbs, 17–21
    postural control, 25
  hands support, 18
  proprioceptive role of vision, 27–28
  reflexive aspects, 25
  responsive bracing of body, 26
  righting/equilibrium reactions, 10
  segmental alignment adjustments, 26
  shifting body mass, 21
  support surface perturbation, 26-27
  task-/context-specificity, 26–27

Balance dysfunction, 79–82
  adaptive motor behaviours, 80–82
  cerebellar lesions, 101
  clumsiness (motor control deficit), 157
  congenital limb deficiencies, 262–263, 270
  mental retardation, 168
  minimal brain dysfunction, 158
  myelomeningocele, 252, 255
    with hydrocephalus, 243
  training, 82–84, 263, 270
    environmental modification, 84
    feedback, 82, 84
Ball catching, 25, 32, 69
  minimal brain dysfunction, 158
Ball throwing, 25
  minimal brain dysfunction, 158
Barlow's test, 229, 230
Basal ganglia lesions
  dyscontrol characteristics, 102–103
  involuntary abnormal posturing, 102
  involuntary movements, 102
  training, 102–103
Basic Motor Ability Test–Revised, 156
Bathing aids, 289
Bayley Scale of Infant Development, 166, 252
Bear-walking, 16
Behavioural management
  acute brain injury, 150
  hyperactivity, 161
  mental retardation, 172–173
    eating/drinking training, 181
Behavioural problems, acute brain injury, 147, 150
Bennett ventilator, 354
Bilirubin encephalopathy, 114, 123
Bimanual activity
  blind infant, 398
  brachial plexus lesions, 202
  development, 32
  mirror facilitation, 14
  training, 76–77
Biofeedback, 46–47
  brachial plexus lesions, 202
  sit-to-stand training, 57–58
  withdrawal of device, 47
Bird ventilator, 354
Birth trauma
  brachial plexus lesions, 196
  cerebral palsy, 113
  head injury, 145
  torticollis, 293, 294
Bite reflex, 134
Blind infant, 397–398
  activities programme, 398
  postural adjustments, 397–398
  prehension, 398
  stereotypic actions, 397
Blount's disease, 278
Body mass shift
  lateral, 16

walking, 21, 29
Boston brace, 306, 307
Boston jacket, 306
Bow legs, *see* Genu varum
Brachial plexus lesions, 91, 196–202
    adaptive motor behaviours, 197
    assessment, 198–199
    clinical features, 197–198
    lower roots (Klumpke's paralysis), 196
    Moro reflex, 388
    neglect of affected limb, 201
    orthoses, 202
    pathology, 196–197
    placing reactions, 389
    prognosis, 198
    sensory loss, 198
    soft tissue contractures, 197–198
    treatment, 199–202
        bimanual actions training, 202
        biofeedback therapy, 202
        electrical stimulation, 202
        motor training, 200–202
        passive movements, 199
        restraint of unaffected limb, 75, 201
        splinting, 199–200, 202
    upper roots (Erb's palsy), 196
Brain injury, acute, 91, 145–150
    attention control training, 150
    balance dysfunction, 80
    behavioural management techniques, 150
    causes, 145
    clinical features, 147–148
    medical management, 148
    motor performance evaluation, 149–150
    neurological examination, 148
    pathophysiological mechanisms, 145–146
    physiotherapy, 148–150
    prognosis, 146–147
    recovery processes, 103–105
        age-associated effects, 104–105
        axonal sprouting, 103, 105
        compensation, 103
        diaschisis, 103
        environmental stimulation effects, 103–104
        neuronal supersensitivity, 103
        vicariation/equipotentiality, 103, 104
    respiratory management, 148
    soft tissue contracture prevention, 148
        dynamic splinting, 149
        serial casting, 148–149
    task-/context-specific motor training, 149
Brain tumour, 91
    cerebellar lesions, 100
Brazelton Neonatal Behavioural Assessment Scale
    cerebral palsy, 130
    minimal brain dysfunction, 156
Breathing exercises, 336
    assisted in unconscious child, 381
    asthma, 355, 357

breathing control, 373
    cerebral palsy, 136
    bronchitis, 351
    burns surgery, 325
    cardiac surgery, pre-operative, 375–376
    cystic fibrosis, 361
    Duchenne muscular dystrophy, 285
    inflammatory joint/soft tissue disorders, 318
    intensive care, 374
    myelomeningocele, 257
    postural drainage, 373
    scoliosis, 308–309
    techniques, 373
    thoracic expansion, 373
Bronchial drainage
    cystic fibrosis, 360–361
    inhaled foreign body, 351
    respiratory distress syndrome, 348
Bronchial suction, 380
Bronchiectasis, 335, 350, 351–352
    clinical features, 351
    cystic fibrosis, 358–359
    exercise tolerance assessment, 367
    pathology, 351
    postural drainage, 371
    thoracic expansion measurement, 364
    treatment, 352
Bronchiolitis, 345
    airway obstruction, 344
    bronchiectasis, 351
    clinical features, 345
    complications, 335
    pathophysiology, 345
    treatment, 345
Bronchitis, 350, 351
    clinical features, 351
    cystic fibrosis, 358, 359
    postural drainage, 371
    treatment, 351
Bronchodilator drugs
    asthma, 354
        exercise-induced, 366
        status asthmaticus, 358
    hand-operated aerosol dispenser, 354
    intensive care, 375
    intermittent positive pressure ventilators, 354, 358
    nebulizer with mouthpiece, 354, 358
    postural drainage, 371
Bronchopulmonary dysplasia, 347
Broomstick plaster, 276
Bruininks-Oseretsky Motor Proficiency Scale, 156
Burns, 322–331
    active movements, 324, 325, 328
    anti-burnscar elastic pressure supports (Jobst), 325, 326–327, 330
    causes, 322
    complications prevention, 324
    contractures prevention, 324
    coping strategies, 328–329

Burns (*continued*)
  débridement, 324, 325
  depth of wound, 322–323
  emotional/behavioural complications, 327–336
  eschar-associated restrictions, 323
  escharotomy, 324
  first degree, 320
  hand, 326
  hospital discharge, 329–330
  hydrotherapy, 325
  immediate post-burn care, 323, 324–325
  joint contracture, 326
  limb elevation, 324
  management approach, 323–324
  nutritional support, 324
  pain, 322, 327, 328
  physiology, 323
  respiratory complications, 323
    post-operative, 325
  scars, 322
    contracture, 323, 326
    hypertrophy, 326
  second degree, 322
  size estimation, 323
  skin grafting, 323, 325, 326
    breathing exercises, 325
    physical treatment, 325–326
    preparations, 325
  skin restoration, 324
  splinting, 324, 325, 326
    custom-made splints, 326
  staff reactions, 328
  third degree, 322–323
  ventilatory problem management, 324
  wound healing, 326

Calipers
  Duchenne muscular dystrophy, 283, 288
  myelomeningocele, 254, 255
  poliomyelitis, 192
Canadian parapodium, 254
Cap and jacket splint, 298, 301
  postoperative, 298, 301
  torticollis 298–301
    with plagiocephaly, 295
Cardiac surgery, 375–376
  post-operative physiotherapy, 337, 376
    manual hyperinflation, 376
  pre-operative physiotherapy, 375–376
Cardio-respiratory arrest, 376
Catching, 25, 32, 69
  minimal brain dysfunction, 157–158
Central nervous system
  development, 237
    hierarchical model, 12
  dyscontrol characteristics, 94–103
    basal ganglia lesions, 102–103
    cerebellar lesions, 100–102
    upper motorneuron lesions, 94–100

upper motorneuron syndrome, 96–100
  maturation, 92–94
    fetal/embryonic period, 93
    postnatal, 92, 94
  pathophysiological processes, 94–103
Cerebellar chronic electrical stimulation, 139
Cerebellar lesions
  ataxia, 80, 101
  balance dysfunction, 80, 101
    adaptive motor behaviours, 81
  clumsiness (motor control deficit), 157–158
  dysarthia, 101
  dyscontrol characteristics, 100–102
  dysdiadochokinesia, 101
  dysmetria, 80, 101
  dyssynergia, 80, 101
  gait, 101
  hypotonia, 101
  nystagmus, 101
  rebound phenomena, 101
  signs, 101
  training, 101–102
  tremor, 101
Cerebellar maturation, 92
Cerebral aneurysm, 91
Cerebral contusion/laceration, 145, 146
Cerebral maturation, 92
Cerebral palsy, 91, 110–140
  abnormal movement patterns, 116–117, 126, 130
  adaptive motor behaviours, 127
  aetiology, 112–113
  associated deficits, 123
  ataxia, 115, 119
  athetosis, 114
  bilirubin encephalopathy, 114, 123
  cerebellar lesions, 100
  classification, 114–115
  clinical features, 114, 115–119
  cognitive function testing, 123, 124, 133
  conductive education, 111, 125–126
  crouch-to-stand, 134
  deafness, 123
  developmental assessment, 126–127
  diplegia, 115, 120–121
  drug treatment, 139
  early intervention policy, 127
  environmental stimulation, 127
  functional deficits, 119–123
  grasp, 120, 138
  hemiplegia, 113, 115, 120, 121, 122
    behavioural adaptations, 118
    central motor pathway reorganization, 105
    hand/forearm muscle neuronal pathways, 105
    mirror movements in unaffected hand, 118
  hip dislocation, 139
  historical overview of treatments, 111–112
  history-taking, 127
  hypotonia, 114, 115
  immature motor performance, 123

Landau reaction, 389
learning difficulty, 123
leg movement in supine, 119–120
mental retardation, 113, 123, 165
minimal brain dysfunction, 119
mixed lesions, 102, 115
motor control deficit progression, 110–111
motor performance evaluation, 127–130
   abstract versus concrete tasks, 131
   Brazelton Neonatal Behavioural Assessment
      Scale, 130
   feeding, 129–130
   influence of child-rearing practices, 128, 130
   muscle action analysis, 131
   older infant/child, 130–131
   oral function, 129–130
   parental inputs, 130
   response to passive movement, 128–129
motor training, 133–137
   breathing control, 136
   concrete versus abstract tasks, 48
   context-/task-specific, 100, 111, 124, 133
   floor sitting, 47
   oromotor function optimization, 134–135
   parental involvement, 136–137
   vocalizing, 136
neonatal prefunctional motor patterns, 123
neurodevelopmental therapy (NDT), 111, 123,
   124, 125
neurosurgery, 139–140
orthopaedic surgery, 139
orthotics, 137–139
pathology, 113–114
   haemorrhagic lesions, 113
   hyperbilirubinaema, 114
   hypoxic-ischaemic lesions, 113–114
   nervous system maldevelopment, 114
perceptual function testing, 133
physiotherapy, 123–139
postural adjustments, 122–123
quadriplegia, 115
reaching/manipulation, 72, 118, 119, 120, 133
   thumb (opponens) splint, 78, 138
scoliosis, 139, 305
secondary flat feet, 278
sensory testing, 131–133
   hearing, 132
   joint position sense, 133
   light touch sensation, 132
   stereognosis, 133
   tactile sensation, 132–133
   two-point discrimination, 133
   vision, 132
serial casting, 139
sit-to-stand, 121, 124–125, 130, 131, 134
sitting, 130
   on chair, 121
   on floor, 120-121

soft tissue contractures, 98–99, 116–117, 118, 123,
   139
   prevention, 127, 134
spastic, 98, 100, 113
   abnormal movement patterns, 116–117
   associated movements, 118
   behavioural adaptations, 118
   clinical features, 114, 115–118
   skeletal deformity, 118
speech problems, 123
standing, 130, 133
stepping, 133
tonic neck reflexes, 391
   asymmetrical, 50
visual/visuomotor abnormalities, 123, 127
Vojta method, 111, 125
walking, 61, 62–63, 121–122, 130, 131
   co-activation of leg muscles, 122
   energy cost, 63
   selective dorsal rhizotomy, 139–140
   toe walking, 63
Cerebrovascular accident, 91
   cerebral palsy, 113
   upper motorneuron lesions, 95
Chailey chariot, 245
   congenital limb deficiency, 268
   myelomeningocele, 253
Charcot-Marie-Tooth disease, 280
Chest compression, 372
Chickenpox, 185
Child abuse, 4
   burns, 322
   head injury, 145
   mental retardation, 165
Child-adult communication, 5
Child-rearing practices
   cerebral palsy motor performance evaluation,
      128, 130
   cross-cultural comparisons, 36
   independent sitting, 18
   intra-cultural comparisons, 36
   mental retardation, 181
   motor development, 35, 36
   neonatal standing, 17
   neonatal stepping, 28
   parental expectations, 37
Chorea, 102
Choreiform movements, 155
Claspknife phenomenon, 96
Cleft lip/palate, 242
Clumsiness, 119, 154
   clinical features, 157–158
   manipulation dysfunction, 73
Cognitive function testing
   cerebral palsy, 133
Cognitive impairment, *see* Mental retardation
Cold treatment, arthritic pain relief, 315, 316
Communication
   motor development, 32–34

Communication (*continued*)
  preverbal, 33, 34
Compensation, recovery from brain injury, 103
Computed tomography (CT)
  acute brain injury, 148
  cerebral palsy/perinatal asphyxia, 114
  hydrocephalus with myelomeningocele, 243
  mental retardation, 166
Concussion, 145, 146
Conductive education
  cerebral palsy, 111, 125–126
  mental retardation, 171
Continuous positive airways pressure (CPAP), 376
Cortical blindness, 166
Corticomotoneuronal projection lesions, 73
Contrel EDF localizer cast, 306
Cough mechanism, 342
Covert monitoring, 150
Coxa vara, 275
Cranial ultrasound, 148
Crawling, 11
  blind infant, 397–398
  development, 16
  intra-cultural comparisons, 36
  myelomeningocele, 253
  training, 44
Creeping movement, 16
Crossed extensor response, 387, 394
Crouch-to-stand, 21
  calf muscle length maintenance, 99
  cerebral palsy, 134
  kinematic movement pattern, 52
  talipes calcaneovalgus, 227
  talipes equinovarus, 221
  training, 44–45, 58
  walking training, 65
Crutches, 256
Crying, 33–34
  cerebral palsy, 129
  chest percussion, 372
  mental retardation, 167, 168
Cutaneous reflexes, exaggerated, 96
Cutlery manipulation, 72
Cystic fibrosis, 344, 350, 351, 358, 362
  autogenic drainage (AD), 374
  breathing exercises, 361
  bronchiectasis, 351, 358, 359
  bronchitis, 358, 359
  clinical features, 359
  diagnosis, 359
  exercise tolerance assessment, 366
  meconium ileus, 359
  mode of inheritance, 358
  nose blowing instruction, 361
  pancreatic defect, 358
    management, 361
  pathology, 358–359
  physical activity programme, 361, 381
  pneumonia, 358

postural drainage, 371
psychosocial care, 362
pulmonary defect, 358–359
pulmonary obstruction management, 359–361
  forced expiratory technique (FET), 361
  inhalation therapy, 360
  intermittent aerosol therapy, 360
  intermittent positive pressure ventilators, 360
  percussion, 360, 361
  postural drainage, 359, 360–361
respiratory complications, 335
sweat gland defect, 359
  management, 361
thoracic expansion measurement, 364
ventilation, 377

Dantrolene sodium, 139
Deafness
  cerebral palsy, 123
  clumsiness (motor control deficit), 157
Demonstration, 48
  sit-to-stand training, 56
Denis Browne bootee splints, 221
Denis Browne hip harness, 231, 232, 233
Denis Browne splint
  scoliosis, 307
  talipes equinovarus, 218–220
Denver Developmental Screening Test, 166, 251
Deprivation
  emotional, 4
  mental retardation, 166
  myelomeningocele, 244
Dermatomyositis, 311, 313
  clinical features, 313
  pathology, 313
  physiotherapy, 313
  respiratory function, 318
Developmental assessment, 393–396
  mental retardation, 166
Diaphragm fatigue, 340–341
Diaschisis, 103
Dominance
  handedness establishment, 25
  minimal brain dysfunction, 159
Down's syndrome, 91
  adaptive motor behaviours, 169
  atlantoaxial instability, 166
  eating/drinking training, 179-181
  floor sitting, 178
  hypotonia, 115, 166–167
  learning capacity improvement programmes, 172
  manipulation, 169
  mental retardation, 165
  motor development, 167
  parental attitudes, 181
  physiotherapy interventions, 170, 171
  postural adjustments, 168
    training, 178–179
  supported standing, 173

tongue protrusion, 169
treadmill exercise, 167
vestibular dysfunction, 159
walking, 167–168
Dressing/undressing independence, 25
Drooling control, 135
  cerebral palsy, 135
Duchenne muscular dystrophy, 280–290
  assessment, 283–285
    functional testing, 283–284
    joint range testing, 284, 286
    muscle strength testing, 284–285, 288
    respiratory function tests, 285
  asymptomatic carrier serum enzymes, 282
  bedrest contraindication, 285
  breathing exercises, 285
  chronic alveolar hypoventilation, 285
  clinical features, 282–283
    lordosis, 282, 283
    walking deficit, 282–283
  cognitive impairment, 281
  description, 280–281
  diagnosis, 282
  emotional support for child/adolescent, 291
  games/activities, 287–288, 290
  genetic counselling, 282
  loss of ambulation, 283
  management, 283
  muscle strength deterioration, 281
  muscle stretching exercises, 283, 284, 286–287
  nocturnal ventilation, 285
  obesity, 289
  orthoses, 288–289
  osteoporosis, 283
  parental support, 289–290
  pathology, 281–282
  respiratory problems, 281, 283, 305
    prevention, 283, 285
  scoliosis, 281, 289, 305
    spinal support, 289
    surgical intervention, 289
  soft tissue contracture, 281
    night splints, 286
    prevention measures, 286–287
  wheelchair ambulation, 281, 289
Dynamic splinting
  brachial plexus lesions, 202
  elbow flexors following acute brain injury, 149
  inflammatory joint/soft tissue disorders, 318
Dynamic tripod grasp, 23
Dynamometry
  cerebral palsy, 131
  Duchenne muscular dystrophy, 284
  talipes equinovarus, 212
Dysarthia with cerebellar lesions, 101
Dyscalculia, 156
Dysdiadochokinesia
  cerebellar lesions, 101
  minimal brain dysfunction, 155

Dysgraphia, 156
Dyslexia, 154, 156, 157
Dysmetria
  acute brain injury, 147
  cerebellar lesions, 101
  cerebral palsy, 115
  clumsiness (motor control deficit), 157
Dyspraxia, 157
Dyssynergia
  acute brain injury, 147
  cerebellar lesions, 101
  cluminess (motor control deficit) 157
Dystonia
  basal ganglia lesions, 102
  cerebral palsy, 130
Dystrophin, 281–282

Electroencephalography, 166
Electrogoniometers, 46
Electrospinal orthosis, 307
Emotional environment, 3–4
Encephalitis, 91, 185, 380
  cerebral palsy, 113
  mental retardation, 165
Encephalocele, 165
Encephalomyelitis, 185
Endotracheal intubation, 339, 379
  bronchiolitis, 345
  cardiac surgery post-operative care, 376
  oxygen therapy, 340
Environmental deprivation, 4
Environmental enrichment
  cerebral palsy, 127
  myelomeningocele, 252
  recovery from brain injury, 103–104
Environmental modification, 49–50
  sit-to-stand training, 58
Epidural haemorrhage, 146
Epilepsy, 165
Epiphyseal separation, 276
Equilibrium reactions, 25, 79, 390
  balance dysfunction, 80
Equipotentiality, 103
Exercise tolerance assessment, 365–366
Extensor plantar response, 96
Eye-hand coordination, 15, 22
  reaching/manipulation training, 74, 75

Facilitation method, 5
Family
  assessment, 5
  coping with disability/illness, 6–7
  involvement in treatment, 4–5, 6
  stress, 6, 7
Feedback, 5
  attention control training, 150
  auditory, 44, 45, 48
    hyperactivity, 161
    sit-to-stand training, 57

Feedback (*continued*)
  Down's syndrome learning capacity
      improvement, 172
  hyperreflexia/hypertonus, 100
  inflammatory joint/soft tissue disorders, 317
  poliomyelitis rehabilitation, 190–191
  tactile, 46, 48
    grasp, 71
  verbal, 45, 46, 48, 84
  visual, 44, 45, 46, 48, 84
    balance training, 82, 84
    reaching/manipulation training, 75
    sit-to-stand training, 57
    walking training, 68
Feeding
  cerebral palsy, 129–130
  mental retardation, 167, 179–181
Fetal behaviour, 13, 15
Fingers, independent control, 23
Flail limb
  brachial plexus lesions, 196, 198
  poliomyelitis, 191, 192
Flat feet, 275, 278–279
  painful, 278–279
  peroneal spasm, 279
  pes planovalgus, 278
  secondary, 278
    genu valgum (knock knees), 277
Forced expiratory technique, (FET)
  bronchiectasis, 352
  cystic fibrosis, 361
  technique, 374
Forced expiratory volume in one second (FEV_1),
    366
Forearm weight bearing, 16
Four-point kneeling, 16
Fractionated movements, 14
Fractures, 275–276
  classification, 275
  fixation, 276
Frejka pillow, 231
Frostig Development Test of Visual Perception, 156

Gag reflex, 32
  cerebral palsy, 130, 134
Gait
  biomechanical pattern development, 28
  cerebral palsy, 61, 62–63
    energy cost, 63
  Duchenne muscular dystrophy, 282–283
  motor development, 28–30
    independent ambulation, 29–30
    locomotor inactivity period, 28, 29
    mature walking pattern, 29
    neonatal stepping, 28
    supported walking, 29
  see also Walking
Galant reflex, 387–388, 395
  cerebral palsy, 130

torticollis, 295
Genu valgum (knock knees), 93, 275, 277
  associated flat feet, 277
  clinical measurements, 277
  management, 277
  splinting, 277
Genu varum (bow legs), 275, 277–278
  clinical measurements, 278
  flat feet, 278
  management, 278
  rickets, 278
Glasgow Coma Scale (GCS), 146–147, 148
Goal identification, 44, 47–48
Goal-directed activity, 5, 6
Goniometry
  cerebral palsy, 131
  Duchenne muscular dystrophy, 284, 286
  inflammatory joint/soft tissue disorders, 315
  talipes equinovarus, 212
  torticollis, 295
Grasp, 15
  anticipatory hand opening/orientation, 31
  aperture, 70–71
  bimanual actions, preparatory adjustments, 76–77
  cerebellar maturation, 92
  cerebral palsy, 120
  description of activity, 71
  Down's syndrome, 169
  dynamic tripod, 23
  essential components of movement, 72
  fetal, 13
  inflammatory joint/soft tissue disorders, 18
  minimal brain dysfunction, 158
  motor development, 21–22
  motor dysfunction, 73
  neonates, 22, 30
  pincer, 23
  reaching approach, 70–71
    environmental context, 71
    thumb stabilization, 71
  release, 23
  tactile feedback control, 71
  see also Manipulation
Grasp reflex
  brachial plexus lesions, 198
  torticollis, 295
Guided reaching behaviour, 15
Guillain-Barré syndrome, 91, 185, 193–194
  clinical features, 193
  management, 194
  pathology, 193

Haemophilia, 319–320
  haemarthrosis, 319
  treatment, 319–320
Hand
  anticipatory opening/orientation for grasp, 31
  closure timing, 31–32
  inflammatory joint/soft tissue disorders, 318

movement in visual field, 31
support in balance, 18
Handedness establishment, 25
Harrington rods, 307
Head control, 16
  athetoid cerebral palsy, 119
  brain lesions, 73
  development, 11, 12
    prone lying, 13
  environmental modification, 49–50
  mental retardation, 168
  myelomeningocele, 252, 253
    with hydrocephalus, 243, 252
  neonate/young infant, 79
  optimal position, 12, 16
Head injury, 380
  cerebellar lesions, 100
  mental retardation, 165
  upper motorneuron lesions, 95
  see also Brain injury, acute
Head lag, 16–17
  hypotonus, 115
Head position training, 46
Heart disease, congenital, 344
Heat treatment, arthritic pain relief, 315, 316
Heel raising, 67
Herpes virus, congenital infection, 165
Hip disarticulation prosthesis, 266
Hip dislocation, congenital, 228–233
  aetiology, 229
  associated congenital abnormalities, 207, 212,
    224, 229, 264
  description, 228
  diagnosis, 229
    Barlow's test, 229, 230
    Ortolani's manoeuvre, 229, 230
  hip instability screening, 229
  management, 229, 231–233
  myelomeningocele, 242, 247, 250, 251
    treatment, 250
  physical treatment, 233
  splinting, 228, 229, 231–233
    Denis Browne hip harness, 231, 232, 233
    Frejka pillow, 231
    Pavlik hip harness, 231, 232
    plaster hip spica, 232–233
    von Rosen splint, 229, 231
  surgery, 228, 229
Hitching, 11
Home-based treatment, 4, 5
Hopping, 21
Hospitalization
  myelomeningocele, 244, 252
  parent visiting, 4
  separation effects, 4
Hyaline membrane disease, *see* Respiratory
  distress syndrome
Hydraulic hoist, 289
Hydrocephalus, 91

mental retardation, 165
myelomeningocele, 241, 242, 255
  carrying position, 244
  treatment, 242–243
  ventriculoperitoneal shunt surgery, 243
Hydrotherapy
  burns, 325
  inflammatory joint/soft tissue disorders, 317
Hyperactivity
  attention deficit disorder, 159–160
  with cognitive impairment, 165
  treatment, 161
Hypermobility
  athetoid cerebral palsy, 119
  congenital hip dislocation, 228
Hyperreflexia/hypertonus, 96, 97
  acute brain injury, 147
  clumsiness (motor control deficit), 157
  drug treatment, 139
  muscle changes, 99
  myelomeningocele, 241
  righting reactions, 80
  spastic cerebral palsy, 114, 115–116
  therapeutic interventions, 99–100
    control of force generation, 100
    soft tissue shortening prevention, 99–100
  upper motor neurone syndrome, 96–98
Hypothyroidism, congenital, 165
Hypotonia, 96
  acute brain injury, 147
  cerebellar lesions, 101
  cerebral palsy, 114, 115
    oral musculature training, 134
  cognitive impairment, 166–167
  differential diagnosis, 115
  Down's syndrome, 166–167
  secondary flat feet, 278
  upper motorneuron lesions, 95
Hypoxic-ischaemic brain damage, 344–345
  cerebral palsy, 113, 114
  minimal brain dysfunction, 155

Ileal loop diversion, 246
Ileocutaneous ureterostomy, 246
Incentive spirometry, 378
  Duchenne muscular dystrophy, 285
Incontinence with myelomeningocele, 242, 245–247
  bowel training, 246–247
  conservative management methods, 246
  urinary diversion surgery, 246
  urinary tract infection, 246
Incubator nursed-infants, 376–377
Infections, 185–194
Inflammatory joint/soft tissue disorders, 275,
  311–320
  anti-inflammatory drug treatment, 314
  assessment, 315
  breathing exercises, 318
  hand function, 318

Inflammatory joint/soft tissue disorders (*continued*)
  home therapy programme, 319
  immobility avoidance, 314
  joint range improvement, 317
  management 314–319
  mobility improvement, 316–318
  muscle strengthening exercises, 317
  pain relief, 314–316
    cold, 315, 316
    heat, 315, 316, 317
    rest, 315, 316
    TENS, 315
    ultrasound, 315
  postural development, 318
  protective spasm relief, 316, 317
  respiratory function, 318–319
  splinting, 314, 316, 318
  swimming/hydrotherapy, 317–318
  walking aids, 318
Inhaled foreign body, 344, 350–351
Instruction, 44, 48
Intelligence tests, 165, 166
Intensive care, 374–375
  cardiac surgery, 376
  handling, 375
  prone position, 375
Intention tremor, 101
Intermittent negative pressure ventilation, 378
Intermittent positive pressure breathing (IPPB),
    377–378
  asthma management, 354
  bronchodilator drug delivery, 354
    status asthmaticus, 358
  cardiac surgery post-operative care, 376
  contraindications, 377
  cystic fibrosis, 360
  Duchenne muscular dystrophy, 285
Intracranial haemorrhage
  cerebral palsy, 113–114
  head injury, 145–146
  pre-term infant, 345
  respiratory distress syndrome, 347
Involuntary movements
  athetoid cerebral palsy, 114, 118
  basal ganglia lesions, 102
  drug treatment, 139
IQ score, 165
Isoprenaline, 354

Jaundice, neonatal, 92
Jobst elastic pressure supports, 326–327
Joint position sense
  biofeedback in training, 46, 47
  cerebral palsy, 133
  minimal brain dysfunction, 158
Jumping, 21
Juvenile ankylosing spondylitis, 311, 314
  physiotherapy, 314

Juvenile chronic arthritis (Still's disease), 311–313,
    314
  aetiological factors, 312
  clinical features, 312
  fitness, 318–319
  pathology, 312–313
  prognosis, 312
  reparative process promotion, 312–313
  respiratory function, 318
  see also Inflammatory joint/soft tissue disorders

Kartagener's syndrome, 351
Kicking movements
  cerebral palsy, 119–120
  patterns in infants, 15–16, 64
Klinefelter's syndrome, 165
Knee-ankle foot orthoses, 254
Knock knees, *see* Genu valgum
Kugelberg-Welander disease, 280
Kyphosis with myelomeningocele, 242, 247

Labyrinthine-righting reaction, 388–389
Landau reaction, 25, 79, 389, 395
  cerebral palsy, 389
  mental retardation, 389
Language development, 32–34
Language difficulty, 5
Laryngeal development, 33, 338–339
Laryngeal intubation, 339
Laughter, 33
Laurence-Moon syndrome, 165
Lead poisoning-associated neuropathy, 91, 185
  minimal brain dysfunction, 154
Learning capacity improvement programmes, 172
Learning disability, 154, 155
  attention deficit disorder, 159
  cerebral palsy, 123
  clinical features, 156–157
  diagnosis, 155–156
  minimal brain dysfunction, 154–162
Leg length discrepancy, 275
Legg-Calvé-Perthes disease, 275, 276
  casting/orthoses, 276
  orthopaedic treatment, 276
Limb deficiencies, congenital , 261–270
  amelia, 261
  balance problems, 262–263
  causes, 261–262
  classification, 261
  clinical features, 263–264
    associated deformities, 263–264
    loss of surface area, 264
    motor deficits, 263
  cognitive/perceptual development, 263
  environmental exploration, 262, 266
  longitudinal, 261
  management, 264–266
  mobility aids, 265, 268
  parental support/adjustment, 262, 264, 265

phocomelia, 261
physiotherapy, 266–270
  assessment, 266
  functional independence training, 267
  mobility of limbs/trunk, 267–269
  prehension, 266–267
  rolling, 267–268
prostheses, 264–265
  changes with age, 263
  cosmetic, 264–265
  functional, 264, 265
  lower-limb, 265–266
  prehension, 266–267
  training, 265
  upper-limb, 265
sensory/motor exploration, 263
soft tissue contractures, 264
substitute use of foot/mouth, 263, 266–267
surgery, 264
transverse, 261
upper limb remnant use, 263, 265, 266, 267
wheelchair ambulation, 265, 266
see also Lower limb deficiencies, congenital
Limb load monitors, 46
Lower limb activity
  extension from crouch, 51
  motor development, 17–21
  neonatal standing/stepping, 17
  prone lying, 16
  pulling to standing, 17
  sit-to-stand, 51
Lower limb deficiencies, congenital
  balance training, 270
  deformities correction, 269–270
  limb remnant potential, 269, 270
  physiotherapy, 269
  postural adjustments, 270
  prostheses, 268
  talipes equinovarus, 269
Lung development
  at birth, 340–341
  embryonic/fetal period, 338–340
Luque rods, 307

Magnetic resonance imaging (MRI)
  acute brain injury, 148
  cerebral palsy/perinatal asphyxia, 114
  mental retardation, 166
  occult spinal dysraphism, 240
Malnutrition
  cerebral palsy, 113
  mental retardation, 166
  minimal brain dysfunction, 154
Manipulation
  associated movements, 14
  bimanual activity development, 32
  blind infant, 398
  cerebral palsy, 120, 133
  description of activity, 71
  development, 21–22
    associated movements, 23, 25
    child-rearing practices influencing, 36
    corticomotorneuronal synapse, 23
    handedness establishment, 25
  essential components, 72
  hand closure timing, 31–32
  inflammatory joint/soft tissue disorders, 318
  kinaesthetic control, 32
  mental retardation, 169, 170, 173
  motor dysfunction, 72–73
  motor training, 68–78, 133
    bimanual actions, 76
    environmental modification, 77–78
    hand orientation options, 76
    restraint of unaffected arm, 73, 75
  moving objects, 32
  myelomeningocele, 252, 256–257
  visual control, 30, 31, 32
Manual dexterity loss, 95
Manual guidance, 44, 48–49
  passive movement, 48
  sit-to-stand training, 56–57
  spatial constraint, 48
Manual hyperinflation, 376
Measles, 351
  cerebral palsy, 113
  neurological syndromes, 185
Median nerve lesion, 91
Memory deficit, 156
Meningitis, 91, 185, 380
  cerebral palsy, 113
  mental retardation, 165
Meningocele, 240
Mental retardation, 165–181
  adaptive motor behaviours, 169
  aetiology, 165–166
  arrest of development, 168
  associated ophthalmological problems, 166
  balance dysfunction
    adaptive motor behaviours, 81
    postural adjustments, 168, 169
    righting reactions, 80
  cerebral palsy, 123
  classification (IQ score), 165
  developmental assessment, 166
  Duchenne muscular dystrophy, 281
  feeding problems, 167
  food aspiration, 181
  head injury, 146, 147
  head rolling prevention, 173
  home-based care, 181
  hydrocephalus with myelomeningocele, 243
  hypotonia/muscle strength deficit, 167–167, 168
  interventions, 170–181
    behaviour modification, 172–173, 181
    eating/drinking training, 179–181
    environmental modification, 173

Mental retardation (*continued*)
  learning capacity improvement programmes,
    172
  measures of effectiveness, 171–172
  motor learning approach, 170–171
  movement control training, 173–178
  physical fitness promotion, 173
  postural adjustments training, 178–179
  swimming instruction, 177–178
  Landau reaction, 389
  manipulation, 169
  motor development/performance, 166–170
  motor milestones, 167–168
  mouthing, 167
  myelomeningocele, 252
    with hydrocephalus, 242
  orofacial dysfunction, 169
  parental attitudes, 181
  persistent hand regard, 167
  social unresponsiveness, 167
  vocalization, 167
Microcephaly, 91
  mental retardation, 165
  righting reactions, 80
Mikity-Wilson syndrome, 347
Milwaukee brace, 306–307
Minimal brain dysfunction, 119, 154–162
  aetiology, 154
  assessment, 160
  attention deficit disorder, 154, 155, 159–160
  clumsiness (motor control deficit), 154, 157–158
  diagnosis, 155–156
    IQ tests, 156
    neurological examination, 155
    psychometric testing, 156
  dyslexia, 154
  hyperactivity treatment, 161
  intervention, 160–161
    behavioural management, 161
    group activity, 161
    motor training, 161
  learned adaptive behaviours, 155
  learning disability, 154, 155, 156–157
  pathogenesis, 154–155
  specific problems, 158-159
    balance, 158
    dominance, 159
    hand function, 158
    inadequate sensory discrimination, 158
    oculomotor deficit, 158
    sensory integrative function, 158–159
    vestibular dysfunction, 159
    visuospatial orientation, 158
Minnesota Child Development Inventory, 166
Mirror movements, *see* Associated movements
Mobility aids
  limb deficiencies, congenital, 265, 268
  myelomeningocele, 245
Möbius syndrome, 165

Moro reflex, 30, 388, 393, 394
  brachial plexus lesions, 198, 388
  cerebral palsy, 130
  preterm infant, 34
  torticollis, 295
Motor cortex lesions, 73
Motor development, 9–37
  active body movement, 15
  associated movements, 14–15
  cross-cultural comparisons, 36–37
  ecological approach/dynamic systems perspective,
    10, 12–13
  environmental effects, 35–37
  gait, 28–30
  lower limb activity, 17–21
  maturation, 10–13
    cephalocaudal direction, 11
    child-rearing/parental handing influence, 11–12
    hierarchical model, 12
    as invariant neurodevelopmental sequence, 11
  neonatal reflexive behaviours, 10, 13–14
  oral function, 32–34
  parental expectations, effects of, 37
  postural control, 25–28
  prehension, 30–32
  preterm infant, 34–35
  righting/equilibrium reactions, 10
  speech, 32–34
  upper limb activity, 21–25
  visual monitoring, 15
Motor learning, 45–50
  inhibition of unwanted muscular activity, 46
  optimization, 43–84
  techniques, 46–50
    demonstration, 48
    environmental modification, 49–50
    feedback, 46–47
    goal identification, 47–48
    instruction, 48
    manual guidance, 48–49
    practice, 49
    visual monitoring of performance, 50
Motor milestones, 10, 11, 36
  mental retardation, 167
  parental expectations, 37
Motor training, 50–84
  biomechanical models of actions, 44, 50
  cerebral palsy, 100, 133–137
  child-rearing practices, 35, 36
    cross-cultural comparisons, 36
  crouch-to-stand, 58
  erect body positions, 44
  inhibition of unwanted muscular activity, 46
  methods, 44
  motor control, 43–84
    mental retardation, 173–178
  reaching/manipulation, 68–78
  sit-to-stand, 51–58
  walking, 58–68